Mayo Clinic Infectious Diseases Board Review

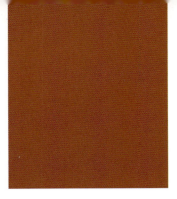

Mayo Clinic Scientific Press

Mayo Clinic Atlas of Regional Anesthesia and Ultrasound-Guided Nerve Blockade
Edited by James R. Hebl, MD, and Robert L. Lennon, DO

Mayo Clinic Preventive Medicine and Public Health Board Review
Edited by Prathibha Varkey, MBBS, MPH, MHPE

Mayo Clinic Internal Medicine Board Review, 9th edition
Edited by Amit K. Ghosh, MD

Mayo Clinic Challenging Images for Pulmonary Board Review
Edward C. Rosenow III, MD

Mayo Clinic Gastroenterology and Hepatology Board Review, 4th edition
Edited by Stephen C. Hauser, MD

Mayo Clinic Infectious Diseases Board Review

EDITOR-IN-CHIEF

Zelalem Temesgen, MD

Consultant, Division of Infectious Diseases
Mayo Clinic, Rochester, Minnesota
Professor of Medicine
College of Medicine, Mayo Clinic

ASSOCIATE EDITORS

Larry M. Baddour, MD

James M. Steckelberg, MD

MAYO CLINIC SCIENTIFIC PRESS

OXFORD UNIVERSITY PRESS

The triple-shield Mayo logo and the words MAYO, MAYO CLINIC, and MAYO CLINIC SCIENTIFIC PRESS are marks of Mayo Foundation for Medical Education and Research.

OXFORD
UNIVERSITY PRESS

Oxford University Press, Inc., publishes works that further
Oxford University's objective of excellence
in research, scholarship, and education.

Oxford New York
Auckland Cape Town Dar es Salaam Hong Kong Karachi
Kuala Lumpur Madrid Melbourne Mexico City Nairobi
New Delhi Shanghai Taipei Toronto

With offices in
Argentina Austria Brazil Chile Czech Republic France Greece
Guatemala Hungary Italy Japan Poland Portugal Singapore
South Korea Switzerland Thailand Turkey Ukraine Vietnam

Copyright ©2011 by Mayo Foundation for Medical Education and Research.

Published by Oxford University Press, Inc.
198 Madison Avenue, New York, New York 10016
www.oup.com

Oxford is a registered trademark of Oxford University Press

All rights reserved. No part of this publication may be reproduced, stored in a retrieval system, or transmitted, in any form or by any means, electronic, mechanical, photocopying, recording, or otherwise, without the prior permission of Mayo Foundation for Medical Education and Research. Inquiries should be addressed to Scientific Publications, Plummer 10, Mayo Clinic, 200 First St SW, Rochester, MN 55905

Library of Congress Cataloging-in-Publication Data

Mayo Clinic infectious diseases board review / editor-in-chief, Zelalem Temesgen; associate editors, Larry M. Baddour, James M. Steckelberg.
   p. ; cm.
 Mayo Clinic infectious diseases board review
 Includes bibliographical references and index.
 ISBN 978-0-19-982762-6 (alk. paper)
  1. Communicable diseases—Outlines, syllabi, etc. 2. Communicable diseases—Examinations, questions, etc. I. Temesgen, Zelalem. II. Baddour, Larry M. III. Steckelberg, James M. IV. Mayo Clinic. V. Title: Mayo Clinic infectious diseases board review.
 [DNLM: 1. Communicable Diseases—Examination Questions. 2. Communicable Diseases—Outlines. WC 18.2]
 RC112.M39 2012
 616.90076—dc22   2011007326

Mayo Foundation does not endorse any particular products or services, and the reference to any products or services in this book is for informational purposes only and should not be taken as an endorsement by the authors or Mayo Foundation. Care has been taken to confirm the accuracy of the information presented and to describe generally accepted practices. However, the authors, editors, and publisher are not responsible for errors or omissions or for any consequences from application of the information in this book and make no warranty, express or implied, with respect to the contents of the publication. This book should not be relied on apart from the advice of a qualified health care provider.

The authors, editors, and publisher have exerted efforts to ensure that drug selection and dosage set forth in this text are in accordance with current recommendations and practice at the time of publication. However, in view of ongoing research, changes in government regulations, and the constant flow of information relating to drug therapy and drug reactions, readers are urged to check the package insert for each drug for any change in indications and dosage and for added wordings and precautions. This is particularly important when the recommended agent is a new or infrequently employed drug.

Some drugs and medical devices presented in this publication have US Food and Drug Administration (FDA) clearance for limited use in restricted research settings. It is the responsibility of the health care providers to ascertain the FDA status of each drug or device planned for use in their clinical practice.

9 8 7 6 5 4 3 2 1

Printed in China
on acid-free paper

We dedicate this book to our infectious diseases fellows, who inspire and teach us with their compassion, intellect, diligence, and accomplishments.

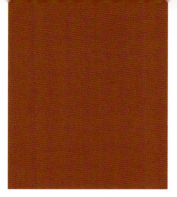

Foreword

"There are two objects of medical education: To heal the sick, and to advance the science." These words written by Dr Charles H. Mayo in 1926 underscore the long-standing commitment of Mayo Clinic to education. At the turn of the 20th century, medicine had a guild mentality, and many practitioners jealously guarded their skills and knowledge. Dr William Worrall Mayo, father of the brothers who founded Mayo Clinic, firmly believed in collaboration and sharing of medical knowledge at a time when medicine was the province of solo practitioners. His sons, William and Charles Mayo, joined their father and developed a shared vision and practice: One of the brothers would stay home to care for patients while the other sought best practices in the United States and abroad; the brothers organized, sponsored, and developed programs to share these best practices; and they worked to develop a framework to provide structure and standardization for medical education.

As the brothers traveled widely to learn and to teach, they invited physicians from around the world to Rochester, Minnesota, to share knowledge. Doctors flocked to the observation gallery at Saint Marys Hospital to observe surgical procedures performed by the Mayo brothers and other surgeons. In 1906, physicians visiting Rochester formed the Surgeons Club, an informal group that discussed what they had seen in the operating room. The visiting physicians described these educational sessions as the "Mayos' clinic," a nickname that later led to the official name of Mayo Clinic in 1914. In 1915, collaborating with the University of Minnesota, the Mayo brothers established the country's first graduate education program in clinical medicine. In 1919, the Mayo brothers transformed the private practice into a nonprofit institution. Commitment to medical education became an integral part of the mission of Mayo Clinic that is symbolized in the institutional logo: 3 shields represent practice, education, and research.

The Mayo brothers' deep commitment to education helped to usher in a new era of transparency and openness among medical institutions throughout the United States. Together with leading medical centers in the Midwest and along the eastern seaboard, Mayo Clinic contributed substantial financial and other resources to support collaborative, multidisciplinary medical and surgical meetings. For the first time, Mayo Clinic physicians and other physicians presented results of their experience with thyroid, abdominal, urologic, obstetrical, and other surgical procedures. Presentations at their meetings also included results of the medical management of many conditions, including postoperative infection, prevention of nosocomial infection, epidemiology of infectious diseases, and trials of vaccine use.

The Division of Infectious Diseases was founded in 1940 by Dr Wallace Herrell, who was one of the pioneers of anti-infective therapy in the United States. Dr Herrell organized some of the first annual meetings devoted exclusively to infectious diseases and invited experts from around the country as speakers. The published proceedings of these meetings began a long tradition at Mayo Clinic to provide source documents in infectious diseases for residents in training at Mayo Clinic and for infectious diseases practitioners. *Mayo Clinic Infectious Diseases Board Review*, edited by Dr Temesgen and associate editors Drs Baddour and Steckelberg, extends and expands upon this tradition established by Dr Herrell. While this book is intended primarily to help infectious diseases fellows and practitioners prepare for the subspecialty board examination, I believe this book will be a useful, concise, practical, and up-to-date guide for the diagnosis, treatment, and prevention of infectious diseases.

Walter R. Wilson, MD
Consultant, Division of Infectious Diseases
Mayo Clinic, Rochester, Minnesota
Assistant Professor of Microbiology and
Professor of Medicine
College of Medicine, Mayo Clinic

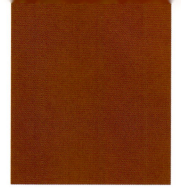

Preface

While infections have always played an important role in the history of mankind, advances in science and technology as well as rapid globalization have resulted in an unprecedented wave of new and old infections thrust into the limelight. The recent pandemic of H1N1 influenza virus infection demonstrates the recurrent theme of emerging and reemerging pathogens that continue to impact public health and patient care areas. Drug resistance among various organisms (not limited to bacteria) has unfortunately become the expectation and, not infrequently, we have been left with few or no efficacious treatment options, an experience not witnessed in more than 7 decades. Human immunodeficiency virus infection continues to challenge our abilities to provide the desired level of care in most areas of the world. Novel syndromes of infection continue to be defined as newer forms of immunosuppression and the development of unique medical devices become standard practice in all areas of medicine and surgery. For trainees and practitioners in the field of infectious diseases today, these factors mandate intense study to establish an expertise in the field that is required to provide best practices now and beyond. This board review will be pivotal in that education. This book is designed and intended primarily for infectious diseases trainees and practitioners preparing for the infectious disease subspecialty examination of the American Board of Internal Medicine. We believe that this book will also be useful to infectious diseases practitioners as well as general internists and other clinicians who desire a comprehensive but practical overview of contemporary infectious diseases topics.

Larry M. Baddour, MD
James M. Steckelberg, MD
Zelalem Temesgen, MD

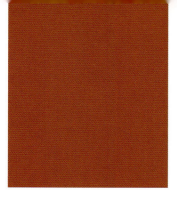

Contents

Contributors *xv*

I General

1. Pharmacokinetics and Pharmacodynamics of Antimicrobials *3*
   Lynn L. Estes, PharmD, RPh

2. Antimicrobials *14*
   Lynn L. Estes, PharmD, RPh, and John W. Wilson, MD

3. Health Care–Associated Infection Prevention and Control Programs *31*
   W. Charles Huskins, MD, MSc

4. Mycobacterial and Fungal Diagnostics *41*
   Matthew J. Binnicker, PhD, Glenn D. Roberts, PhD, and Nancy L. Wengenack, PhD

   Questions and Answers *53*

II Etiologic Agents

5. Select Viruses in Adults *61*
   Randall C. Walker, MD

6. Select Gram-positive Aerobic Bacteria *80*
   Robin Patel, MD

7. Select Gram-negative Aerobic Bacteria *90*
   David R. McNamara, MD, and Franklin R. Cockerill III, MD

8. Select Anaerobic Bacteria: *Clostridium tetani* and *Clostridium botulinum* *102*
   M. Rizwan Sohail, MD

9 *Borrelia* and *Leptospira* Species *110*
Julio C. Mendez, MD

10 Tick-Borne Infections *116*
Alan J. Wright, MD

11 Mycobacteria *126*
Irene G. Sia, MD

12 *Nocardia* and *Actinomyces* *138*
Christine L. Terrell, MD

13 *Candida* Species *147*
Shimon Kusne, MD, and Ann E. McCullough, MD

14 *Aspergillus* Species *153*
Shimon Kusne, MD, and Ann E. McCullough, MD

15 *Histoplasma capsulatum* *157*
Janis E. Blair, MD

16 *Blastomyces dermatitidis* *164*
Janis E. Blair, MD

17 *Coccidioides* Species *168*
Janis E. Blair, MD

18 *Paracoccidioides brasiliensis* *171*
Janis E. Blair, MD

19 *Sporothrix schenckii* *174*
Janis E. Blair, MD

20 *Cryptococcus neoformans* *177*
Shimon Kusne, MD, and Ann E. McCullough, MD

21 Emerging Fungal Infections *182*
Holenarasipur R. Vikram, MD, FACP, FIDSA

22 Parasitic Infections *190*
Jon E. Rosenblatt, MD, and Bobbi S. Pritt, MD

Questions and Answers *218*

III Select Major Clinical Syndromes

23 Fever of Unknown Origin *237*
Mary J. Kasten, MD

24 Infections of the Oral Cavity, Neck, and Head *244*
Lisa M. Brumble, MD

25 Pneumonia *256*
Priya Sampathkumar, MD

26 Urinary Tract Infections *267*
Walter C. Hellinger, MD

27 Sepsis Syndrome *274*
Andrew D. Badley, MD

28 Infectious Diarrhea *280*
Robert Orenstein, DO

29 Intra-abdominal Infections *285*
    Robert Orenstein, DO

30 Viral Hepatitis *295*
    Stacey A. Rizza, MD

31 Infective Endocarditis *301*
    Larry M. Baddour, MD, and Daniel Z. Uslan, MD

32 Infections of the Central Nervous System *319*
    Michael R. Keating, MD

33 Skin and Soft Tissue Infections *341*
    Imad M. Tleyjeh, MD, MSc, and Larry M. Baddour, MD

34 Osteomyelitis, Infectious Arthritis, and Orthopedic Device Infection *351*
    Elie F. Berbari, MD, and Douglas R. Osmon, MD

35 Sexually Transmitted Diseases *360*
    Randall S. Edson, MD

Questions and Answers *375*

IV Special Hosts and Situations

36 Human Immunodeficiency Virus Infection *391*
    Zelalem Temesgen, MD

37 HIV-Associated Opportunistic Infections and Conditions *417*
    Anne M. Meehan, MB, BCh, PhD, and Eric M. Poeschla, MD

38 Infections in Patients With Hematologic Malignancies *428*
    John W. Wilson, MD, and Michelle A. Elliott, MD

39 Infections in Transplant Recipients *443*
    Raymund R. Razonable, MD

40 Health Care–Associated Infections *458*
    Rodney L. Thompson, MD, and Priya Sampathkumar, MD

41 Obstetric and Gynecologic Issues Related to Infectious Diseases *464*
    Kristi L. Boldt, MD

42 Pediatric Infectious Diseases *485*
    Thomas G. Boyce, MD

43 Travel Medicine *495*
    Abinash Virk, MD

44 Adult Immunizations *516*
    Priya Sampathkumar, MD

45 Agents of Bioterrorism *525*
    Mark P. Wilhelm, MD, FACP

Questions and Answers *537*

Index *551*

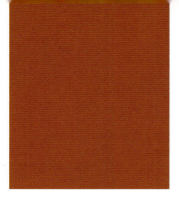

Contributors

Larry M. Baddour, MD
Chair, Division of Infectious Diseases, Mayo Clinic, Rochester, Minnesota; Professor of Medicine, College of Medicine, Mayo Clinic

Andrew D. Badley, MD
Consultant, Division of Infectious Diseases, Mayo Clinic, Rochester, Minnesota; Professor of Medicine, College of Medicine, Mayo Clinic

Elie F. Berbari, MD
Consultant, Division of Infectious Diseases, Mayo Clinic, Rochester, Minnesota; Associate Professor of Medicine, College of Medicine, Mayo Clinic

Matthew J. Binnicker, PhD
Consultant, Division of Clinical Microbiology, Mayo Clinic, Rochester, Minnesota; Assistant Professor of Laboratory Medicine and Pathology, College of Medicine, Mayo Clinic

Janis E. Blair, MD
Consultant, Division of Infectious Diseases, Mayo Clinic, Scottsdale, Arizona; Professor of Medicine, College of Medicine, Mayo Clinic

Kristi L. Boldt, MD
Consultant, Department of Obstetrics and Gynecology, Mayo Clinic, Rochester, Minnesota; Assistant Professor of Obstetrics and Gynecology, College of Medicine, Mayo Clinic

Thomas G. Boyce, MD
Consultant, Division of Pediatric Infectious Diseases, Mayo Clinic, Rochester, Minnesota; Associate Professor of Pediatrics, College of Medicine, Mayo Clinic

Lisa M. Brumble, MD
Consultant, Division of Infectious Diseases, Mayo Clinic, Jacksonville, Florida; Assistant Professor of Medicine, College of Medicine, Mayo Clinic

Franklin R. Cockerill III, MD
Chair, Department of Laboratory Medicine and Pathology and Consultant, Division of Pediatric Infectious Diseases, Mayo Clinic, Rochester, Minnesota; Professor of Medicine and of Microbiology, College of Medicine, Mayo Clinic

Randall S. Edson, MD
Consultant, Division of Infectious Diseases, Mayo Clinic, Rochester, Minnesota; Professor of Medicine, College of Medicine, Mayo Clinic

Michelle A. Elliott, MD
Consultant, Division of Hematology, Mayo Clinic, Rochester, Minnesota; Associate Professor of Medicine, College of Medicine, Mayo Clinic

Lynn L. Estes, PharmD, RPh
Infectious Diseases Pharmacy Specialist, Mayo Clinic, Rochester, Minnesota; Assistant Professor of Pharmacy, College of Medicine, Mayo Clinic

Walter C. Hellinger, MD
Consultant, Division of Infectious Diseases, Mayo Clinic, Jacksonville, Florida; Associate Professor of Medicine, College of Medicine, Mayo Clinic

W. Charles Huskins, MD
Consultant, Division of Pediatric Infectious Diseases, Mayo Clinic, Rochester, Minnesota; Assistant Professor of Pediatrics, College of Medicine, Mayo Clinic

Mary J. Kasten, MD
Consultant, Division of General Internal Medicine, Mayo Clinic, Rochester, Minnesota; Assistant Professor of Medicine, College of Medicine, Mayo Clinic

Michael R. Keating, MD
Chair, Division of Infectious Diseases, Mayo Clinic, Jacksonville, Florida; Associate Professor of Medicine, College of Medicine, Mayo Clinic

Shimon Kusne, MD
Chair, Division of Infectious Diseases, Mayo Clinic, Scottsdale, Arizona; Professor of Medicine, College of Medicine, Mayo Clinic

Ann E. McCullough, MD
Consultant, Department of Laboratory Medicine and Pathology, Mayo Clinic, Scottsdale, Arizona; Assistant Professor of Laboratory Medicine and Pathology, College of Medicine, Mayo Clinic

David R. McNamara, MD
Fellow in Infectious Diseases, Mayo School of Graduate Medical Education, College of Medicine, Mayo Clinic, Rochester, Minnesota; presently, on staff at Gundersen Lutheran Health System, La Crosse, Wisconsin

Anne M. Meehan, MB, BCh, PhD
Fellow in Molecular Medicine, Mayo School of Graduate Medical Education, College of Medicine, Mayo Clinic, Rochester, Minnesota

Julio C. Mendez, MD
Consultant, Division of Infectious Diseases, Mayo Clinic, Jacksonville, Florida; Assistant Professor of Medicine, College of Medicine, Mayo Clinic

Robert Orenstein, DO
Consultant, Division of Infectious Diseases, Mayo Clinic, Scottsdale, Arizona; Associate Professor of Medicine, College of Medicine, Mayo Clinic

Douglas R. Osmon, MD
Consultant, Division of Infectious Diseases, Mayo Clinic, Rochester, Minnesota; Associate Professor of Medicine, College of Medicine, Mayo Clinic

Robin Patel, MD
Chair, Division of Clinical Microbiology and Consultant, Division of Infectious Diseases, Mayo Clinic, Rochester, Minnesota; Professor of Medicine and of Microbiology, College of Medicine, Mayo Clinic

Eric M. Poeschla, MD
Consultant, Division of Infectious Diseases, Mayo Clinic, Rochester, Minnesota; Professor of Medicine, College of Medicine, Mayo Clinic

Bobbi S. Pritt, MD
Senior Associate Consultant, Division of Clinical Microbiology, Mayo Clinic, Rochester, Minnesota; Assistant Professor of Laboratory Medicine and Pathology, College of Medicine, Mayo Clinic

Raymund R. Razonable, MD
Head, Section of Transplantation Infectious Diseases and Consultant, Division of Infectious Diseases, Mayo Clinic, Rochester, Minnesota; Associate Professor of Medicine, College of Medicine, Mayo Clinic

Stacey A. Rizza, MD
Consultant, Division of Infectious Diseases, Mayo Clinic, Rochester, Minnesota; Assistant Professor of Medicine, College of Medicine, Mayo Clinic

Glenn D. Roberts, PhD
Consultant, Division of Clinical Microbiology, Mayo Clinic, Rochester, Minnesota; Professor of Laboratory Medicine and Pathology and of Microbiology, College of Medicine, Mayo Clinic

Jon E. Rosenblatt, MD
Consultant, Division of Infectious Diseases, Mayo Clinic, Rochester, Minnesota; Professor of Medicine and of Microbiology, College of Medicine, Mayo Clinic

Priya Sampathkumar, MD
Consultant, Division of Infectious Diseases, Mayo Clinic, Rochester, Minnesota; Assistant Professor of Medicine, College of Medicine, Mayo Clinic

Irene G. Sia, MD
Consultant, Division of Infectious Diseases, Mayo Clinic, Rochester, Minnesota; Assistant Professor of Medicine, College of Medicine, Mayo Clinic

M. Rizwan Sohail, MD
Senior Associate Consultant, Division of Infectious Diseases, Mayo Clinic, Rochester, Minnesota; Assistant Professor of Medicine, College of Medicine, Mayo Clinic

James M. Steckelberg, MD
Consultant, Division of Infectious Diseases, Mayo Clinic, Rochester, Minnesota; Professor of Medicine, College of Medicine, Mayo Clinic

Zelalem Temesgen, MD
Consultant, Division of Infectious Diseases, Mayo Clinic, Rochester, Minnesota; Professor of Medicine, College of Medicine, Mayo Clinic

Christine L. Terrell, MD
Consultant, Division of Infectious Diseases, Mayo Clinic, Rochester, Minnesota; Assistant Professor of Medicine, College of Medicine, Mayo Clinic

Rodney L. Thompson, MD
Consultant, Division of Infectious Diseases, Mayo Clinic, Rochester, Minnesota; Assistant Professor of Medicine, College of Medicine, Mayo Clinic

Imad M. Tleyjeh, MD, MSc
Fellow in Infectious Diseases, Mayo School of Graduate Medical Education, College of Medicine, Mayo Clinic, Rochester, Minnesota; presently, Chair, Division of Infectious Diseases, King Fahd Medical City, Riyadh, Saudi Arabia

Daniel Z. Uslan, MD
Fellow in Infectious Diseases, Mayo School of Graduate Medical Education, College of Medicine, Mayo Clinic, Rochester, Minnesota; presently, Division of Infectious Diseases, David Geffen School of Medicine at UCLA, Los Angeles, California

Holenarasipur R. Vikram, MD, FACP, FIDSA
Consultant, Division of Infectious Diseases, Mayo Clinic, Scottsdale, Arizona; Assistant Professor of Medicine, College of Medicine, Mayo Clinic

Abinash Virk, MD
Consultant, Division of Infectious Diseases, Mayo Clinic, Rochester, Minnesota; Associate Professor of Medicine, College of Medicine, Mayo Clinic

Randall C. Walker, MD
Consultant, Division of Infectious Diseases, Mayo Clinic, Rochester, Minnesota; Assistant Professor of Medicine, College of Medicine, Mayo Clinic

Nancy L. Wengenack, PhD
Consultant, Division of Clinical Microbiology, Mayo Clinic, Rochester, Minnesota; Associate Professor of Laboratory Medicine and Pathology and Assistant Professor of Microbiology, College of Medicine, Mayo Clinic

Mark P. Wilhelm, MD, FACP
Consultant, Division of Infectious Diseases, Mayo Clinic, Rochester, Minnesota; Assistant Professor of Medicine, College of Medicine, Mayo Clinic

John W. Wilson, MD
Consultant, Division of Infectious Diseases, Mayo Clinic, Rochester, Minnesota; Assistant Professor of Medicine, College of Medicine, Mayo Clinic

Alan J. Wright, MD
Consultant, Division of Infectious Diseases, Mayo Clinic, Rochester, Minnesota; Assistant Professor of Medicine, College of Medicine, Mayo Clinic

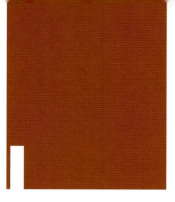

General

Lynn L. Estes, PharmD, RPh

Pharmacokinetics and Pharmacodynamics of Antimicrobials

I. Introduction
   A. Definitions
      1. *Pharmacokinetics:* the disposition of drugs in the body (how the body acts on the drug); it incorporates terms such as *absorption, bioavailability, distribution, protein binding, metabolism,* and *elimination*
      2. *Pharmacodynamics:* the interaction between the drug concentration at the site of action over time (drug exposure) and the pharmacologic effect, which, in the case of antimicrobials, is eradication of microorganisms
   B. Interrelationships
      1. Pharmacokinetics and pharmacodynamics are interrelated
      2. Both need to be taken into account to optimize antimicrobial therapy (Figure 1.1)
II. Pharmacokinetic Concepts
   A. Dosing
      1. Patient variability in pharmacokinetics needs to be considered in choosing the most effective dose
      2. Individualizing the dose to the patient and to the site of infection is very important
   B. Absorption
      1. Route of administration
         a. Intravenous bolus administration: absorption is assumed to be rapid and complete
         b. Extravascular administration with oral or intramuscular preparations: absorption is generally slower; thus, there is a delay in the time to peak serum concentrations (usually 1-2 hours, but varies by drug) as well as lower peak serum levels
      2. Oral route
         a. Some oral drugs are incompletely or erratically absorbed
            1) *First-pass effects* relate to metabolism of a drug in the intestine or liver before reaching the systemic circulation
            2) First-pass effects can decrease the serum levels obtained with some oral drugs; thus, the *bioavailability* (the amount of active drug that reaches the systemic circulation) of oral preparations is often lower than that with intravenous administration
         b. In contrast, some oral drugs have excellent oral bioavailability and serum levels are similar to those with intravenous administration (Box 1.1)
            1) For highly bioavailable drugs, oral therapy should be used whenever feasible (Box 1.2)
            2) However, oral therapy may not be appropriate for patients with

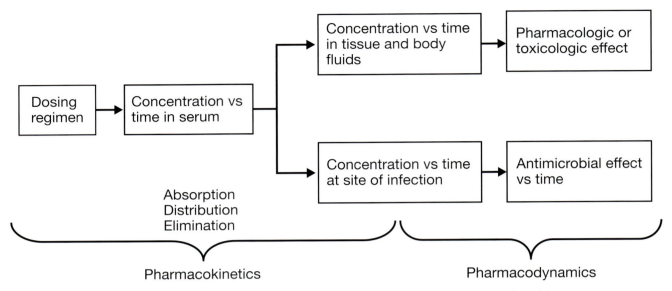

Figure 1.1. Interrelationship Between Pharmacokinetics and Pharmacodynamics. (Adapted from Craig WA. Pharmacokinetic/pharmacodynamic parameters: rationale for antibacterial dosing of mice and men. Clin Infect Dis. 1998 Jan;26[1]:1–10.)

conditions such as ileus, short bowel syndrome, bowel ischemia, vomiting, or diarrhea since they may hinder oral absorption

c. Some oral drugs are given as a *prodrug* (inactive form of the drug that is converted in the body to the active compound)
   1) Prodrugs are given to enhance absorption though chemical modification of the drug
   2) For example, bioavailability of ganciclovir with oral capsules is only 5% to 10%; however, bioavailability of ganciclovir after administration of the prodrug, valganciclovir, is about 60%
   3) Prodrugs include cefuroxime axetil, cefpodoxime proxetil, valacyclovir, valganciclovir, famciclovir, and fosamprevanir

d. Drug interactions in the gastrointestinal tract may impair absorption of some agents after oral administration
   1) Administration of divalent or trivalent cations (present in antacids, iron preparations, some multivitamin and mineral preparations, sucralfate, etc) can markedly impair absorption of the quinolones or tetracyclines through chelation, leading to failure of antibiotic therapy unless there is adequate spacing of administration (refer to prescribing information for spacing recommendations)
   2) Elevated gastric pH can decrease absorption of itraconazole capsules,

---

Box 1.1

Highly Bioavailable Antimicrobials

Fluoroquinolones
Fluconazole
Voriconazole
Metronidazole
Linezolid
Minocycline
Doxycycline
Cotrimoxazole (trimethoprim-sulfamethoxazole)
Rifampin

Box 1.2

Potential Benefits of Oral Therapy With Highly Bioavailable Drugs Compared With Intravenous Therapy

Decreased hospital-associated adverse events related to intravenous lines (eg, phlebitis, extravasation, line infections, and bacteremia)
Early discharge (in several studies of patients with respiratory tract infections, a switch to oral drugs has decreased time to discharge by 2-4 days)
Increased patient mobility and decreased risk of deep venous thrombosis and pulmonary embolism
Patient preference for oral therapy over intravenous therapy
Decreased drug cost
Avoids compatibility issues with other intravenous medications

ketoconazole, cefuroxime axetil, cefpodoxime proxetil, and atazanivir since they require gastric acidity for maximal absorption; thus, the administration of drugs that affect gastric pH (eg, H_2 receptor antagonists, proton pump inhibitors, and antacids) can decrease absorption of these drugs

3) The presence or absence of food, and even the type of food (eg, fat or caloric content), can affect oral absorption of many antimicrobials (eg, absorption of posaconazole is increased about 4-fold when taken with a full meal, but absorption of azithromycin capsules is decreased about 2-fold when given with food); the manufacturer's information should be consulted before prescribing oral antimicrobials to determine the proper timing in relation to food

C. Distribution
1. Drug distribution and tissue penetration characteristics are important to review to ensure that the drug reaches the site of infection
   a. Examples of sites of infection and drug considerations
      1) Cerebrospinal fluid: if the infecting organism is methicillin-susceptible *Staphylococcus* species, cefazolin would not be effective because it does not penetrate the blood-brain barrier; nafcillin would be effective because it penetrates the blood-brain barrier in the presence of meningeal inflammation
      2) Lower urinary tract: drugs must be at least partially renally excreted
      3) Blood: macrolides, which do not achieve good blood levels, should not be used
      4) Lungs: daptomycin would not be a good choice since it is inactivated by surfactant and thus does not reach the site of infection
   b. Similarly, doses may need to be adjusted on the basis of how well the drug distributes to the site of infection (eg, larger doses of appropriate β-lactams are used for meningitis, in which penetration is impaired; lower doses of renally excreted drugs are used for a lower urinary tract infection because they concentrate in the urine)

2. Apparent *volume of distribution* (V_d): the size of a hypothetical compartment necessary to account for the total amount of drug in the body if it were present throughout the body at the same concentration as found in the plasma
   a. The V_d is not a true physiologic space; it is a mathematical proportionality constant represented by the following equation:

   $$V_d = \frac{\text{Amount of Drug in Body (the Dose)}}{\text{Measured Peak Plasma Concentration}}$$

   b. The V_d gives an estimate of the extent of distribution but does not indicate to which body sites the drug distributes
   c. A drug that distributes primarily to extracellular fluid or plasma (ie, more hydrophilic drugs, including the aminoglycosides and many β-lactams) will have a small V_d that approximates that of the extracellular fluid compartment
      1) For these drugs, changes in extracellular fluid volume (such as may occur with fluid overload or dehydration, congestive heart failure, sepsis, extensive burns, pregnancy, etc) can affect the V_d and thus the subsequent serum concentrations
         a) If doses are not modified accordingly, drug serum levels may be unexpectedly low (in the case of a V_d higher than normal) or high (in the case of a V_d lower than normal)
   d. In contrast, the V_d is high for drugs that distribute widely into tissues or intracellular compartments and have relatively low plasma concentrations; these are typically more lipophilic drugs, such as azithromycin
   e. Morbid obesity can alter the V_d of many drugs, so that an increased dose may be needed (eg, surgical prophylaxis guidelines suggest a cefazolin dose of 2 g, rather than 1 g, in patients heavier than 80 kg); package inserts or other references can be consulted for information about dosing in obesity (eg, whether ideal body weight, adjusted body weight, or actual body weight should be used for dosing calculations)
   f. An important application of the V_d is determination of the loading dose

3. A loading dose can be used to achieve therapeutic antibiotic concentrations immediately rather than waiting for steady state to occur
   a. Loading doses are often used in patients with serious infections, in patients with renal failure (which increases half-lives and time to reach steady state), and for agents with long half-lives
   b. The intravenous loading dose is higher than the maintenance dose and can be estimated from the following equation:

   $$\text{Loading Dose} = V_d \times \text{Desired Peak Plasma Concentration}$$

   (if the dose is given orally and bioavailability is <100%, a correction is made by dividing this equation by the oral bioavailability)
   c. From the loading dose equation, it is apparent that alterations in elimination characteristics (renal or liver dysfunction) do not affect the loading dose; thus, the loading dose need not be modified for renal or liver function, but alterations in elimination characteristics must be taken into account for subsequent maintenance dosing

D. Clearance
   1. *Clearance*: the volume of blood or serum completely cleared of drug per unit of time
   2. Clearance is often expressed as the number of liters per hour or milliliters per minute

E. Metabolism and Elimination
   1. Renal elimination
      a. Elimination of many antimicrobials (including most β-lactams, vancomycin, and aminoglycosides) occurs primarily through the kidneys—either by glomerular filtration or tubular secretion (or both)
      b. For these antimicrobials, maintenance doses need to be adjusted for renal dysfunction by prolonging the dosing interval or by decreasing the dose and using the usual dosing interval or by a combination of both
         1) Increasing the dosing interval, while keeping the dose constant, typically results in a larger difference between the peak and trough concentrations and may be preferred for drugs whose efficacy is correlated with high peak concentrations (eg, aminoglycosides)
         2) Decreasing the dose and maintaining the regular dosing interval results in less fluctuation between the peak and trough concentrations (compared with a longer dosing interval and constant dose) and may, at least in theory, be better for drugs whose efficacy is related to keeping the drug concentration above the minimum inhibitory concentration for the organism for the majority of the dosing interval (eg, β-lactams)
      c. The calculated creatinine clearance is an estimate of renal function and can be determined from several equations, but the Cockcroft-Gault equation is the most widely used in practice and in dosing studies:

      Creatinine Clearance for Adult Males

      $$= \frac{(140 - \text{Age})(\text{Weight in kg})}{72 \times \text{Serum Creatinine}}$$

      (for adult females, multiply the creatinine clearance for adult males by 0.85)
         1) A common error in designing a dosing regimen with a renally excreted drug is to assume that if the serum creatinine level is normal, the dosage does not need to be adjusted
            a) This is an issue for elderly patients who may have a relatively normal serum creatinine level but a somewhat diminished renal clearance due to age-related factors
         2) Calculating the creatinine clearance, rather than relying on the serum creatinine level, is considerably more accurate, since the creatinine clearance equation also takes into account the patient's age, weight, and sex
         3) This creatinine clearance equation does not work well for patients with rapidly changing renal function, patients with low muscle mass, and patients who are very obese; for these patients, consider measuring the clearance or the glomerular filtration rate (iothalmate clearance, measured creatinine clearance, etc)
   2. Hepatic metabolism
      a. Drugs eliminated primarily hepatically include the macrolides, clindamycin, chloramphenicol, voriconazole, itraconazole, posaconazole, rifampin,

rifabutin, caspofungin, and the protease inhibitors
b. Most drugs have *linear pharmacokinetics* (ie, the drug concentration increases proportionally as the dose is increased)
c. Some drugs have *nonlinear* (also known as Michaelis-Menten) *pharmacokinetics* (ie, beyond a certain point, the concentration increase is more than expected after a dose increase), most commonly when there is saturation of metabolizing enzymes
   1) For these drugs, an increase in dose produces a nonproportional increase in serum concentrations and can lead to toxicity
   2) Examples of this type of drug are voriconazole and phenytoin
   3) Serum levels may be useful to guide dosing
d. *Phase 1 metabolism* occurs by reduction, hydrolysis, or oxidation (most common)
e. *Phase 2 metabolism* occurs by conjugation—that is, attachment of an ionized group to the drug, making it more water soluble (eg, glucoronidation, methylation, or acylation)
f. The type and severity of liver disease, as well as the type of metabolic process, may influence drug clearance, but it is often difficult to determine the extent of liver disease and the effects of specific drugs on liver metabolism
g. Additional factors that affect metabolism are race, sex, age, and genetic variability in hepatic enzymes
   1) Some whites (5%-10%) do not have an active form of the cytochrome P450 2D6 (CYP2D6) isoenzyme, and in 20% to 30% of Asians the CYP2C19 enzyme is absent; these patients may have supratherapeutic levels of drugs metabolized by these isoenzymes when usual doses are used (eg, voriconazole and many selective serotonin reuptake inhibitor antidepressants)
   2) There are large variations of the slow acetylator phenotype among ethnic groups (40%-70% of whites and African Americans, 10%-20% of Japanese and Eskimos, >80% of Egyptians, and certain Jewish populations are slow acetylators); these patients do not metabolize certain drugs well (eg, isoniazid, procainamide, and dapsone) and may be more prone to side effects
h. There are no sensitive and specific criteria for determining the extent of liver function impairment
   1) Liver enzyme elevations are a clue, but the effects on metabolism cannot be directly calculated and liver enzymes may actually be low in severe liver dysfunction; in that case, elevations in the international normalized ratio may be an important clue to more severe liver dysfunction
   2) The Child-Pugh score (sometimes called the Child-Turcotte-Pugh score) is used to assess the prognosis of patients with chronic liver disease (mainly cirrhosis)
      a) It includes scoring based on bilirubin, albumin, international normalized ratio prolongation, ascites, and encephalopathy
      b) Dosing adjustment recommendations in package inserts often refer to this classification
      c) Assessing how acute liver dysfunction and liver dysfunction by other mechanisms might affect drug metabolism is more challenging
   3) When possible, therapeutic and clinical drug monitoring are advised for liver-metabolized drugs in patients with liver disease
i. Drug interactions for hepatically metabolized drugs
   1) Numerous important drug interactions can occur with drugs that are eliminated hepatically, particularly if they are metabolized by the cytochrome P450 system (Box 1.3)
      a) Erythromycin, clarithromycin, azole antifungals, and the protease inhibitors are cytochrome P450 enzyme inhibitors
         i) They can inhibit metabolism and thus increase serum levels of other drugs that are metabolized through the same isoenzymes
         ii) Doses of concomitant medications often need to be decreased

Box 1.3
Common Drug Substrates, Inhibitors, and Inducers of CYP3A, According to Drug Class[a]

CYP3A Substrates	CYP3A Inhibitors	CYP3A Inducers
Calcium channel blockers	Calcium channel blockers	Rifamycins
Diltiazem	Diltiazem	Rifabutin
Felodipine	Verapamil	Rifampin
Nifedipine	Azole antifungal agents	Rifapentine
Verapamil	Itraconazole	Anticonvulsant agents
Immunosuppressant agents	Ketoconazole	Carbamazepine
Cyclosporine	Macrolide antibiotics	Phenobarbital
Tacrolimus	Clarithromycin	Phenytoin
Benzodiazepines	Erythromycin	Anti-HIV agents
Alprazolam	Troleandomycin	Efavirenz
Midazolam	(Not azithromycin)	Nevirapine
Triazolam	Anti-HIV agents	Others
Statins	Delavirdine	St John's wort
Atorvastatin	Indinavir	
Lovastatin	Ritonavir	
(Not pravastatin)	Saquinavir	
Macrolide antibiotics	Others	
Clarithromycin	Grapefruit juice	
Erythromycin	Mifepristone	
Anti-HIV agents	Nefazodone	
Idinavir		
Nelfinavir		
Ritonavir		
Saquinavir		
Others		
Losartan		
Sildenafil		

Abbreviations: CYP3A, cytochrome P450 3A isoenzyme; HIV, human immunodeficiency virus.

[a] These inhibitors and inducers can interact with any CYP3A substrate and may have important clinical consequences.

Adapted from Wilkinson GR. Drug metabolism and variability among patients in drug response. N Engl J Med. 2005 May 26;352(21):2211-21. Used with permission.

  b) In contrast, antimicrobials such as rifampin, rifabutin, nevirapine, and efavirenz induce liver metabolism of other drugs that are substrates for the same enzymes, potentially leading to subtherapeutic concentrations
    i) Higher doses of concomitant medications metabolized through the same pathway are often needed
    ii) Some combinations are contraindicated
  c) Antimicrobials that are metabolized through the P450 isoenzymes (ie, they are substrates) can be affected by other drugs that induce or inhibit the same isoenzymes; even some herbal medicines (eg, St John's wort) and foods (eg, grapefruit juice) can inhibit drug metabolism
2) Thus, drug interactions should be closely evaluated when starting or stopping the use of medications that are inducers, inhibitors, or substrates of the P450 system

3) A good reference on substrates, inducers, and inhibitors can be found at http://www.medicine.iupui.edu/Flockhart/table.htm
F. Elimination Half-life
1. The rate of elimination of a drug from the body is often described by the half-life of the drug
   a. *Half-life*: the amount of time necessary to decrease the serum levels by one-half
   b. The half-life applies to drugs that are eliminated according to *first-order pharmacokinetics* (ie, the rate of elimination is proportional to the drug concentration)
   c. Most drugs have first-order elimination
2. Applications of half-life
   a. Knowledge of the half-life of a drug can be used to determine when steady state will occur
   b. *Steady state*: with successive doses, drugs accumulate in the body until equilibrium is achieved and the amount of drug administered during a dosing interval equals the amount of drug eliminated during the dosing interval
   c. The time to reach steady state depends entirely on the half-life of the drug
      1) In most clinical situations, steady state is assumed to occur after 3 to 5 half-lives of the drug (Figure 1.2)
      2) Measuring drug levels at steady state is often desirable since drug levels with subsequent doses can be assumed to remain the same at corresponding time points in the dosing interval, unless there is a change in the dosing regimen or pharmacokinetic parameters (eg, renal function)
   d. In addition, if peak and trough levels are measured at steady state, patient-specific pharmacokinetic variables such as the half-life and V_d can be calculated from only 2 serum levels
      1) This information can be used to predict, through a series of equations, the serum levels that will result from a particular dosing change
      2) This type of calculation is most commonly done with aminoglycosides to tailor the dose; pharmacists can assist with this calculation
   e. In contrast, if drug levels are measured before steady state, the result indicates

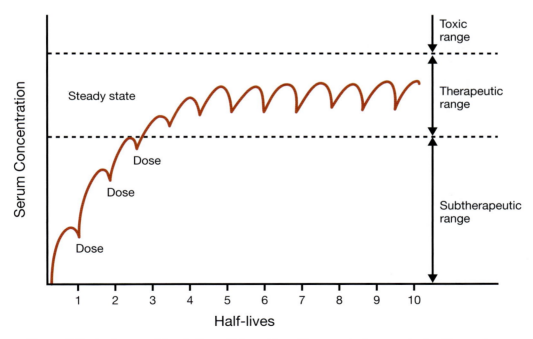

Figure 1.2. Attainment of Steady State. (Adapted from Therapeutic drug monitoring [Internet]. Burlington [NC]: Laboratory Corporation of America and Lexi-Comp, Inc.; c2007 [cited 2008 Dec 17]. Available from: http://www.labcorp.com/datasets/labcorp/html/appendix_group/appendix/section/tdm.htm.)

only the serum levels with that particular dose, since the levels will change with subsequent doses until steady state is achieved
G. Interpretation of Serum Levels
1. The therapeutic range (both the toxic range and the effective range) of the drug must be known; however, for many drugs there are no good studies relating particular serum levels to efficacy or toxicity (eg, peak and trough levels of vancomycin are often measured, but there are no good studies correlating peak levels with efficacy or toxicity)
    a. Whether the levels are measured at steady state is important (as described above)
    b. Serum levels are only a measure of the concentration of drug in the serum
        1) Serum levels do not necessarily represent the concentration at the site of infection
        2) One must know where and how the drug distributes in the body, the relationship of serum levels to levels of the drug at the site of infection, and whether the drug has activity at the site of infection to determine whether the serum concentration is appropriate
    c. Serum levels of the total drug are usually measured, but only the free drug has antimicrobial activity; this distinction is important for highly protein-bound drugs
    d. If peak levels are measured, they should be measured after the absorption and α distribution phases; manufacturers' information can be consulted to determine when this occurs
2. If serum levels are unexpectedly high or low, several potential reasons should be considered
    a. Clearance of the drug in the patient may be higher or lower than expected because of changes in the V_d or elimination half-life (or both)
    b. The drug may not be at steady state; even though it is often assumed that steady state always occurs on the third or fourth dose, this is not the case for many drugs (eg, itraconazole is dosed once or twice daily but has a long half-life of 35-64 hours, so steady state does not occur until 7-10 days)
    c. Missed or late doses need to be considered when serum levels are unusually low
    d. Drug interactions affect serum levels and should be reviewed closely
    e. If the level of an intravenous drug is unexpectedly high after a dose was given, determine whether the sample was drawn through the intravenous line in which the drug was infused (drug remaining in the line can artificially elevate serum levels)
    f. The timing of the samples in relation to when the dose was given should be considered (for various reasons, the samples may have been drawn earlier or later than the times they were ordered to be drawn)
    g. Samples drawn before complete absorption of oral drugs and samples drawn during the α distribution phase of the drug may lead to erroneous conclusions
    h. Preparation errors in the pharmacy, improper processing or storage of the drug sample, and assay errors in the laboratory are less common reasons for an unusually high or low serum level
    i. If the cause of an unexpected level cannot be determined, the wisest action may be to repeat the measurement before making a dosing decision
III. Pharmacodynamic Concepts
A. Minimum Inhibitory Concentration
1. *Minimum inhibitory concentration* (MIC): the lowest concentration that inhibits visible growth in vitro
2. Various methods are used to measure the MIC: broth (or microbroth) dilution, agar diffusion, agar dilution, and E-test; the results are typically compared against standards for the organism-drug combination set forth by the Clinical and Laboratory Standards Institute (CLSI) and reported as *sensitive*, *intermediate*, or *resistant*
3. Limitations of MIC testing
    a. Uses static drug concentrations and does not account for the time course of antimicrobial activity
    b. MIC breakpoints may not correlate well with the free drug concentration at the site of infection (eg, meningitis); it is necessary to know whether the drug reaches the site of infection
    c. May be affected by test conditions (pH, oxygen concentration, cation concentrations, growth phase of the bacteria, etc) and may not represent the local conditions at the infection site
    d. Does not account for host factors that may affect antimicrobial efficacy (immune function, disease states, etc)

e. May not characterize well the activity of antimicrobial agents when used in combination (ie, synergy and antagonism) and does not reflect the likelihood of resistance development
f. The standardized organism inoculum used in determining the MIC may not be indicative of the inoculum and antimicrobial activity of a drug at the site of action
4. Pharmacodynamic parameters used in combination with MIC and pharmacokinetic information may assist with determining goals for optimal effect

B. Postantibiotic Effect
1. *Postantibiotic effect* (PAE): persistent suppression of bacterial regrowth after the antibiotic is removed or levels decrease to below the MIC for the organism
2. The duration of the PAE varies with the particular organism-drug combination and may be influenced by the concentration of the antimicrobial used, the duration of exposure to the antimicrobial, the inoculum of organisms, the particular combination of antimicrobials used, the growth rate of the organisms, and host defenses
3. Antibiotics that inhibit protein and nucleic acid synthesis (eg, aminoglycosides, quinolones, macrolides, and ketolides) generally have a relatively large PAE that can help to support the use of a longer dosing interval since bacterial growth is inhibited even after the drug concentrations have decreased to less than the MIC
4. In contrast, β-lactam antibiotics, which act on the cell wall, generally have a PAE against gram-positive organisms but not against gram-negative organisms (an exception is that carbapenems may have a PAE against some gram-negative organisms)

C. Pharmacodynamic Time Course Factors
1. Three factors are generally recognized as being predictive of antimicrobial efficacy (Figure 1.3), but their importance varies among drug classes
   a. *Peak concentration to MIC ratio*: ratio of the peak concentration of the drug to the MIC of the drug
   b. *AUC/MIC*: ratio of the area under the drug concentration–time curve (AUC) to the

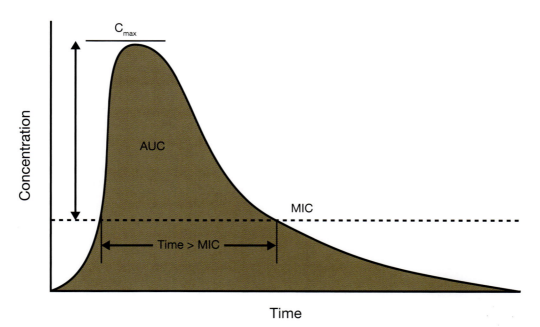

Figure 1.3. Pharmacokinetic and pharmacodynamic predictors of efficacy: 1) ratio of the peak concentration of the drug (C_{max}) to the minimum inhibitory concentration (MIC) of the drug; 2) ratio of the area under the drug concentration–time curve (AUC) to the MIC of the drug; and 3) time during which the drug concentration is greater than the MIC. (Adapted from A PK/PD approach to antibiotic therapy [Internet]. Plattsburg [MO]: RxKinetics; c2008 [cited 2008 Dec 17]. Available from: http://www.rxkinetics.com/antibiotic_pk_pd.html.)

MIC of the drug; the area under the inhibitory curve (AUIC) can be normalized over 24 hours (AUIC24), which allows for comparison of agents with different dosing intervals
c. *T>MIC*: time (T) that the drug concentration is greater than the MIC for the organism during the dosing interval; typically expressed as the percentage of the dosing interval in which the drug concentration is greater than the MIC
D. Patterns of Antimicrobial Activity (Box 1.4)
1. Concentration-dependent killing
   a. Drugs that exhibit this pattern of killing include aminoglycosides, fluoroquinolones, metronidazole, amphotericin, echinocandins, telithromycin, and daptomycin
   b. Parameters that have been associated with efficacy with these agents include the peak concentration to MIC ratio and the AUC/MIC ratio or the similar term, AUIC
   c. The specific goal targets differ slightly according to various studies, but in general a high peak concentration to MIC ratio appears to minimize development of resistance and enhance killing
      1) Thus, giving larger doses less often may be more beneficial than giving smaller doses more frequently
      2) This is the rationale for giving 1 large daily dose (single daily dosing or pulse dosing) of aminoglycosides for gram-negative infections (rather than giving smaller doses several times a day); this approach also takes advantage of the concentration-dependent PAE of aminoglycosides, and in some studies this approach has been associated with less toxicity
      3) With quinolones, it may be difficult to reach an optimal peak concentration to MIC ratio owing to toxicity concerns at high doses
         a) In this case, the AUC/MIC ratio (or AUIC) may be the most important parameter in predicting efficacy
         b) For gram-negative organisms, the target AUC/MIC ratio over 24 hours is greater than 125 (>250 may be optimal for killing)
         c) For gram-positive organisms, the target AUC/MIC ratio over 24 hours is greater than 30 to 50 (some studies support higher AUC/MIC ratios, similar to those for gram-negative organisms, but this is somewhat controversial)
2. Time-dependent killing without a substantial PAE
   a. Drugs that exhibit this pattern include penicillins, cephalosporins, clindamycin, and erythromycin

---

Box 1.4
Patterns of Microbial Killing, With Parameters and Representative Drugs

Concentration-Dependent Killing	*Time-Dependent Killing Without a Substantial PAE*	*Time-Dependent Killing With a Moderate to Prolonged PAE*
Parameters	Parameter	Parameters
Peak/MIC ratio	T>MIC	AUC/MIC
AUC/MIC ratio		T>MIC
Drugs	Drugs	Drugs
Aminoglycosides	Penicillins	Azithromycin
Fluoroquinolones	Cephalosporins	Tigecycline
Metronidazole	Carbapenems	Vancomycin
Amphotericin	Vancomycin	Linezolid
Echinocandins	Clindamycin	Tetracyclines
Telithromycin	Macrolides	Clindamycin
Daptomycin	Flucytosine	Streptogrammins (eg, Synercid)
Colistin		Azole antifungals
		Fluoroquinolones

Abbreviations: AUC, area under the drug concentration–time curve; MIC, minimum inhibitory concentration; PAE, postantibiotic effect; Peak, peak concentration of the drug; T>MIC, time that the drug concentration is greater than the MIC.

b. With these agents, killing of microorganisms is primarily time dependent, and efficacy is enhanced by maximizing the duration that the drug concentration is greater than the MIC
   1) Peak levels greater than 4 to 6 times the MIC do not usually provide additional benefit
   2) It is thought that higher peak levels of cephalosporins and penicillins do not enhance killing because of their mechanism of action: a maximal proportion of the penicillin-binding proteins can be acylated (which typically occurs at 4-6 times the MIC) and after this maximal acylation occurs, the killing rate does not increase further with higher concentrations
   3) For penicillins and cephalosporins, a reasonable goal is to have serum levels greater than the MIC of the organism for at least 40% to 50% of the dosing interval
   4) For carbapenems, the goal is to have serum levels greater than the MIC for 20% to 30% of the dosing interval
   5) Continuous-infusion β-lactams maximize this pharmacodynamic pattern, since drug levels can be maintained greater than the MIC continuously; this has been most widely studied with penicillin G, but it has also been used with drugs such as nafcillin and ceftazidime
   6) Vancomycin is often included in this group (as well as in the time-dependent killing group with a moderate to prolonged PAE): trough levels of 10 to 15 mcg/mL are suggested for endocarditis infections and 15 to 20 mcg/mL for nosocomial pneumonia and meningitis; lower levels (7-15 mcg/mL) may be adequate for less serious infections
   7) Less information is available for macrolides: it appears that keeping the T>MIC for 50% of the dosing interval may be appropriate for patients with normal host defenses and that keeping T>MIC for the entire dosing interval may be appropriate for neutropenic patients
3. Time-dependent killing with a moderate to prolonged PAE
   a. This pattern of killing is less well described, and some do not distinguish it from the other time-dependent pattern
   b. Drugs that exhibit this pattern include newer macrolides, tetracyclines, tigecycline, linezolid, and vancomycin
   c. These agents typically have a moderate to prolonged PAE, so drug concentrations decrease to less than the MIC at the end of the dosing interval and maintain efficacy
   d. Some of these agents have a degree of concentration dependence (eg, azithromycin and clarithromycin)
   e. For these drugs, the AUC/MIC ratio appears to be the parameter most closely associated with efficacy, although the exact targets have not been as well established

IV. Conclusion
   A. Antimicrobial Regimen
      1. Choose a regimen with appropriate spectra and distribution characteristics for the particular infection
      2. Dose the antimicrobial appropriately to achieve maximal results and avoid toxicity
   B. Optimal Dosing Regimen
      1. Understand and apply patient-specific pharmacokinetic principles, including absorption, distribution, metabolism, drug interactions, and elimination
      2. Consider pharmacodynamic principles such as the peak concentration to MIC ratio, the duration that drug levels exceed the MIC, and the AUC/MIC ratio

Suggested Reading

Andes D, Anon J, Jacobs MR, Craig WA. Application of pharmacokinetics and pharmacodynamics to antimicrobial therapy of respiratory tract infections. Clin Lab Med. 2004 Jun;24(2):477–507.

Craig WA. Pharmacokinetic/pharmacodynamic parameters: rationale for antibacterial dosing of mice and men. Clin Infect Dis. 1998 Jan;26(1):1–10.

McKinnon PS, Davis SL. Pharmacokinetic and pharmacodynamic issues in the treatment of bacterial infectious diseases. Eur J Clin Microbiol Infect Dis. 2004 Apr;23(4):271–88. Epub 2004 Mar 10.

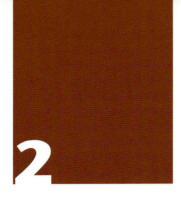

Lynn L. Estes, PharmD, RPh
John W. Wilson, MD

Antimicrobials[a]

I. Antibacterial Agents
  A. Penicillins
    1. Prototypic agents
       a. Natural penicillins: penicillin G, penicillin V, penicillin G benzathine, and penicillin G procaine
       b. Aminopenicillins: ampicillin, amoxicillin, ampicillin sodium-sulbactam sodium (Unasyn), and amoxicillin-clavulanate potassium (Augmentin)
       c. Penicillinase-resistant penicillins: nafcillin, oxacillin, and dicloxacillin
       d. Carboxypenicillins and ureidopenicillins: ticarcillin, piperacillin, ticarcillin disodium-clavulanate potassium (Timentin), and piperacillin sodium-tazobactam sodium (Zosyn)
    2. Mechanism of action: bind to penicillin-binding proteins in the cell wall and inhibit cross-linking, thus inhibiting cell wall synthesis
    3. Spectrum of activity
       a. Natural penicillins
          1) Most streptococci and enterococci
          2) Most *Neisseria gonorrhoeae*, susceptible anaerobes (*Clostridium* species, most oral bacteroides, *Fusobacterium*, and *Peptostreptococcus*), *Listeria*, *Pasteurella*, *Treponema pallidum* (syphilis), and *Borrelia* (Lyme disease)
          3) Most staphylococci and gram-negative organisms produce β–lactamase, which renders these agents inactive
       b. Aminopenicillins
          1) Similar to penicillin but somewhat expanded gram-negative spectrum (although many organisms originally susceptible have developed resistance)
          2) Active against most streptococci, enterococci, *Listeria*, *Proteus mirabilis*, *Borrelia*, *Pasteurella*, and β-lactamase–negative *Haemophilus influenzae*
          3) May be active against some strains of *Escherichia coli*, *Salmonella*, and *Shigella*, but resistance is increasing and thus they should not be used as empirical therapy without susceptibility results

---

[a] Portions of the text have been adapted from Oliveira GHM, Nesbitt GC, Murphy JG. Mayo Clinic medical manual. Boca Raton (FL): Mayo Clinic Scientific Press, Taylor & Francis Group; c2006. Used with permission of Mayo Foundation for Medical Education and Research.

4) Addition of a β-lactamase inhibitor (amoxicillin-clavulanate and ampicillin-sulbactam) extends the spectrum to include methicillin-sensitive staphylococci, *Bacteroides fragilis*, many *Klebsiella*, *Haemophilus influenzae*, *Moraxella catarrhalis*, and other select gram-negative bacteria
   c. Penicillinase-resistant penicillins
      1) Narrow spectrum: includes methicillin-susceptible staphylococcus and group A streptococci
      2) Useful for serious staphylococcal infections and skin or soft tissue infections
      3) No gram-negative, enterococcal, or anaerobic activity
   d. Carboxypenicillins and ureidopenicillins
      1) Expanded gram-negative spectrum beyond penicillin and ampicillin, with some loss of gram-positive activity
      2) Active against many gram-negative bacteria, including most Enterobacteriaceae
      3) Ticarcillin does not reliably cover enterococci; piperacillin does have activity against them
      4) Addition of a β-lactamase inhibitor (piperacillin-tazobactam or ticarcillin-clavulanate) extends the spectrum to methicillin-sensitive staphylococci, *Bacteroides fragilis*, and some other gram-negative bacteria (ticarcillin-clavulanate has activity against many *Stenotrophomonas* species)
      5) Used when broad-spectrum empirical therapy is needed and for gram-negative or mixed nosocomial infections
      6) Piperacillin and piperacillin-tazobactam have activity against many *Pseudomonas* isolates and should generally be used in higher doses for these organisms
4. Toxicities
   a. All: hypersensitivity reactions (if allergic to 1 penicillin, allergic to all penicillins), gastrointestinal tract (GI) side effects (nausea, vomiting, diarrhea, and *Clostridium difficile*), and phlebitis with intravenous (IV) therapy
   b. High-dose IV penicillin: can cause central nervous system (CNS) side effects, including seizures (especially without a dose adjustment for kidney disease); hyperkalemia (potassium salt form) or hypernatremia (sodium salt form)
   c. Penicillinase-resistant penicillins: can cause interstitial nephritis, phlebitis, hepatitis, and neutropenia with prolonged use
   d. Ticarcillin and ticarcillin-clavulanate: can cause sodium overload, hypokalemia, and platelet dysfunction
   e. Nafcillin, ticarcillin, and piperacillin: can cause neutropenia with long-term therapy
   f. Piperacillin-tazobactam: has been associated with false-positive galactomannan antigen assays (for *Aspergillus*)
5. Major route of elimination
   a. Natural penicillins: renal
   b. Aminopenicillins: renal
   c. Penicillinase-resistant penicillins: hepatobiliary for nafcillin; primary renal for oxacillin and dicloxacillin
   d. Carboxypenicillins and ureidopenicillins: renal
B. Cephalosporins
   1. Prototypic agents
      a. First-generation cephalosporins: cefazolin sodium (Ancef), cephalexin (Keflex), and cefadroxil (Duricef)
      b. Second-generation cephalosporins: cefuroxime (Zinacef), cefoxitin (Mefoxin), cefotetan (Cefotan), cefaclor (Celor), cefprozil (Cefzil), and loracarbef (Lorabid)
      c. Third-generation cephalosporins
         1) IV: cefotaxime (Claforan), ceftriaxone (Rocephin), and ceftazidime (Fortaz)
         2) Oral: cefpodoxime-proxetil (Vantin), cefixime (Suprax), cefdinir (Omnicef), ceftibuten (Cedax), and cefditoren pivoxil (Spectracef)
      d. Fourth-generation cephalosporins: cefepime (Maxipime)
      e. Advanced-generation cephalosporin: ceftaroline
   2. Mechanism of action: bind to penicillin-binding proteins in the cell wall and inhibit cross-linking, thus inhibiting cell wall synthesis
   3. Spectrum of activity
      a. None of the agents currently approved by the US Food and Drug Administration (FDA) are active against enterococcus; however, ceftobiprole does have enterococcal activity
      b. First-generation cephalosporins

1) Highly active against methicillin-susceptible staphylococci, β–hemolytic streptococci, and many strains of *P mirabilis*, *E coli*, and *Klebsiella* species
2) Used commonly for methicillin-sensitive staphylococcal or streptococcal infections, skin or other soft tissue infections, and surgical prophylaxis for clean surgery

c. Second-generation cephalosporins
1) Improved gram-negative activity but slightly less gram-positive activity than first-generation agents
2) Cefuroxime and oral agents: activity against community-acquired respiratory pathogens (*Streptococcus pneumoniae*, *H influenzae*, and *M catarrhalis*)
3) Cefotetan and cefoxitin: their expanded gram-negative and anaerobic activities make them potentially useful for obstetric-gynecologic and colorectal surgical prophylaxis, for treatment of community-acquired abdominal infections, and for pelvic inflammatory disease; they have some resistance with *B fragilis*, so they are not drugs of choice

d. Third-generation cephalosporins
1) Improved gram-negative activity compared with first- and second-generation agents
2) Cefotaxime and ceftriaxone: enhanced gram-negative activity compared with second-generation agents but not active against *Pseudomonas*
   a) Good streptococcal activity (eg, against viridans streptococci and *S pneumoniae*) and moderate activity against methicillin-susceptible staphylococci
   b) Good activity against community-acquired respiratory, urinary, and meningeal pathogens
3) Ceftazidime: less active against staphylococci and streptococci, but good activity against many gram-negative organisms, including *Pseudomonas aeruginosa*
4) Cefixime and ceftibuten: best gram-negative activity of oral cephalosporins; neither is very active against staphylococci, and ceftibuten has poor streptococcal activity
5) Cefpodoxime and cefdinir: better gram-positive activity than other oral third-generation cephalosporins, particularly against staphylococci and streptococci

e. Fourth-generation cephalosporins
1) Cefepime: highly active and durable gram-negative activity (including *P aeruginosa* and *Enterobacter* species)
2) Cefepime: similar gram-positive activity as cefotaxime and ceftriaxone (methicillin-susceptible *Staphylococcus aureus* and *Streptococcus* species)

f. Advanced-generation cephalosporin: ceftaroline
1) The only currently available cephalosporin with activity against methicillin-resistant staphylococci
2) Good activity against community-acquired respiratory pathogens (*S pneumoniae*, *H influenzae*, and *M catarrhalis*)

4. Toxicities
a. Most common: GI effects (nausea, vomiting, and diarrhea)
b. Hypersensitivity reactions (cross-reactivity with penicillins is about 5%), drug fever, and *C difficile* colitis
c. Cefotetan, cefamandole, cefoperazone, moxalactam, and cefmetazole have a methyltetrazolethiol side chain that is associated with hypoprothrombinemia (increased international normalized ratio), and a disulfiram-like reaction when ethanol is consumed
d. Ceftriaxone: associated with pseudocholelithiasis, cholelithiasis, and biliary colic, especially in young children; avoid concomitant use of ceftriaxone and calcium products in neonates (deaths related to precipitation in organs have been reported)

5. Major route of elimination: renal (except ceftriaxone, which has dual renal and hepatic elimination)

C. Monobactam
1. Agent: aztreonam
2. Mechanism of action: binds to penicillin-binding proteins in the cell wall and inhibits cross-linking, thus inhibiting cell wall synthesis

3. Spectrum of activity: active against gram-negative aerobic organisms, including most strains of *Pseudomonas aeruginosa*; not active against gram-positive organisms or anaerobes
4. Toxicities
   a. Similar to other β-lactams
   b. Low risk of cross-allergenicity, so it can often be used in patients who have allergic reactions to penicillin or cephalosporin (but cross-reactivity with ceftazidime may occur since aztreonam has the same side chain)
5. Major route of elimination: renal

D. Carbapenems
1. Agents: imipenem, meropenem, doripenem, and ertapenem
2. Mechanism of action: bind to penicillin-binding proteins in the cell wall and inhibit cross-linking, thus inhibiting cell wall synthesis
3. Spectrum of activity: very broad antibacterial activity against gram-positive, gram-negative, and anaerobic organisms
   a. Gram-positive spectrum
      1) Includes β-hemolytic streptococci, *S pneumoniae*, and methicillin-susceptible *S aureus*
      2) Imipenem, doripenem, and meropenem cover susceptible *Enterococcus* species, but ertapenem does not
   b. Gram-negative spectrum
      1) Includes the Enterobacteriaceae (including organisms with extended-spectrum β-lactamase production), *H influenzae*, and *M catarrhalis*
      2) Meropenem, doripenem, and imipenem cover most *P aeruginosa* and *Acinetobacter* species; however, ertapenem is not clinically active against either
   c. Anaerobic activity
      1) Excellent
      2) Includes *Bacteroides*, *Clostridium*, *Fusobacterium*, *Peptostreptococcus*, and *Prevotella*
4. Toxicities
   a. Can cause GI side effects, hypersensitivity reactions (may have cross-reactivity with penicillins), drug fever, and overgrowth of resistant organisms (yeast, *Stenotrophomonas*, and *C difficile*)
   b. Seizures occur rarely with these agents; especially if patients have a history of seizure disorder, renal insufficiency without proper dosage adjustment, or structural CNS defects
5. Major route of elimination: renal

E. Aminoglycosides
1. Agents: prototypic agents are gentamicin, tobramycin, amikacin, and streptomycin
2. Mechanism of action: inhibit protein synthesis (bind to 30S subunit of the bacterial ribosome)
3. Spectrum of activity
   a. Includes most aerobic gram-negative bacilli, mycobacteria (varies by agent), *Brucella* (streptomycin), *Nocardia* (amikacin), *Francisella tularensis* (streptomycin), and *Yersinia pestis* (streptomycin)
   b. Synergistic with certain β-lactams and vancomycin against susceptible enterococci (gentamicin and streptomycin), staphylococci, and several aerobic gram-negative organisms; they should not be used as monotherapy for gram-positive organisms
4. Toxicities
   a. Can cause nephrotoxicity, auditory or vestibular toxicity, and rarely neuromuscular blockade
   b. Nephrotoxicity
      1) Usually reversible
      2) Risk is increased in the presence of other nephrotoxins, so drug levels and renal function should be monitored to minimize risk
   c. Ototoxicity
      1) May be irreversible
      2) Auditory toxicity is more frequent with amikacin and gentamicin; vestibular toxicity is more common with streptomycin
   d. Individualized dosing and monitoring of serum levels is important to minimize toxic reactions
5. Major route of elimination: renal
   a. Traditional dosing and serum levels are shown in Table 2.1
      1) Adjust dosing interval for renal dysfunction
   b. Single daily (pulse) dosing
      1) Theoretically maximizes pharmacodynamics by providing high serum levels compared with the minimum inhibitory

Table 2.1
Aminoglycoside Dosing and Serum Level Targets for Normal Renal Function

Condition	Gentamicin and Tobramycin			Amikacin and Streptomycin		
	Traditional dosing, mg/kg every 8 h[a]	Target Peak	Target Trough	Traditional dosing, mg/kg every 8-12 h	Target Peak	Target Trough
Pneumonia, sepsis	2-2.5	7-10	<1.2	7-8	25-40	2.5-8
Bacteremia, skin and soft tissue infections, pyelonephritis	1.5-1.7	6-8	<1.2	6	20-30	2.5-4
Lower urinary tract infection	1-1.3	4-5	<1.2	5-6	15-20	2.5-4
Gram-positive synergy	1	3-4	<1.2	…	…	…

[a] Must adjust doses and intervals for renal dysfunction.

concentration and produces similar or slightly reduced nephrotoxicity by allowing a drug-free interval between doses
2) Gentamicin and tobramycin: 5 to 7 mg/kg daily
3) Amikacin and streptomycin: 15 to 20 mg/kg daily
4) Adjust dosing interval for renal dysfunction

F. Vancomycin
 1. Mechanism of action: inhibits cell wall synthesis (at an earlier step than β-lactams)
 2. Spectrum of activity
    a. Includes most aerobic and anaerobic gram-positive organisms
    b. Active against methicillin-resistant staphylococci, susceptible enterococci, and highly penicillin-resistant S pneumoniae
    c. An alternative agent for infections caused by methicillin-sensitive staphylococci (less active than cefazolin, nafcillin, and oxacillin), ampicillin-sensitive enterococci, or streptococci in patients intolerant of β-lactam antimicrobials
    d. Not active against certain strains of Lactobacillus, Leuconostoc, Actinomyces, and vancomycin-resistant enterococci
    e. Use should be minimized when feasible owing to emergence of vancomycin-resistant enterococci and, more recently, vancomycin-intermediate/resistant staphylococci
    f. Do not use simply for more convenient dosing (eg, in patients with renal dysfunction)
    g. Oral vancomycin is not systemically absorbed and can be used for treatment of C difficile colitis
 3. Toxicities
    a. Rare ototoxicity and nephrotoxicity (especially in combination with other nephrotoxins)
    b. Infusion-related pruritus and rash or flushing reaction involving the face, neck, and upper body (called red man syndrome or red neck syndrome) due to nonimmunologic release of histamine (not an allergic reaction); minimize by slowing the rate of infusion or administering an antihistamine
 4. Dosing
    a. Usual dosing with normal renal function: 15 to 20 mg/kg every 12 hours (loading dose of 25-30 mg/kg can be considered for seriously ill patients)
    b. With renal dysfunction: decrease the dose or prolong the interval
    c. Target trough levels for most infections: 10 to 20 mcg/mL
 5. Major route of elimination: renal

G. Telavancin
 1. Mechanism of action: inhibits cell wall synthesis (similar to vancomycin)
 2. Spectrum of activity
    a. Semisynthetic derivative of vancomycin with activity against methicillin-resistant staphylococci, streptococci, and vancomycin-susceptible enterococci
 3. Toxicities
    a. Nephrotoxicity: somewhat higher incidence than with vancomycin
    b. Infusion-related effects: similar to those with vancomycin
    c. Interference with anticoagulation tests (international normalized ratio, activated partial thromboplastin time, activated clotting time, and factor Xa tests should be performed ≥18 hours after a dose of telavancin)
 4. Major route of elimination: renal

H. Fluoroquinolones
1. Prototypic agents: ciprofloxacin, levofloxacin, moxifloxacin, and gemifloxacin
2. Mechanism of action: inhibit nucleic acid synthesis by binding to DNA topoisomerases II and IV, which are enzymes involved in DNA supercoiling and chromosome partitioning
3. Spectrum of activity
   a. Active against most aerobic gram-negative bacilli, including the Enterobacteriaceae, *H influenzae*, and some staphylococci
   b. Against gram-positive and anaerobic organisms, activity varies
   c. Ciprofloxacin and levofloxacin have the best activity against *P aeruginosa*
   d. Ciprofloxacin has poor activity against *S pneumoniae*, and clinical failures have been reported
   e. Levofloxacin, moxifloxacin, and gemifloxacin
      1) Relatively good activity against *S pneumoniae* and other gram-positive organisms
      2) Good activity against atypical pneumonia pathogens such as *Chlamydia pneumoniae*, *Mycoplasma pneumoniae*, and *Legionella* and thus are useful for community-acquired respiratory infections
      3) They are not optimal for serious staphylococcal infections since resistance can develop during therapy
   f. Moxifloxacin and gemifloxacin have appreciable anaerobic activity but are not drugs of choice for serious anaerobic infections
4. Toxicities
   a. GI effects, including *C difficile* colitis
   b. Rash is most frequent with gemifloxacin
   c. CNS effects
      1) Uncommon
      2) Seizures in predisposed patients, especially without dose adjustment for renal function
      3) Occasionally, hallucinations and other CNS effects
   d. Musculoskeletal effects
      1) Cartilage erosions in animals; thus, quinolones are generally not recommended for pregnant women or for patients younger than 18 years
      2) Tendinitis and tendon rupture are rare complications even in adults
   e. QT prolongation and rare cases of torsades de pointes have been reported; fluoroquinolones should generally not be given with other QT-prolonging agents or to patients who have prolonged QT syndrome
   f. Gatifloxacin: hyperglycemia or hypoglycemia has been reported; drug was removed from the market
   g. Space dosing apart from oral chelating agents that can inhibit absorption (aluminum, calcium, magnesium, iron, zinc, etc)
5. Major route of elimination
   a. Ciprofloxacin: renal (hepatic)
   b. Levofloxacin: renal
   c. Moxifloxacin: hepatic
I. Tetracyclines and Glycylcycline (Tigecycline)
1. Prototypic agents: tetracycline, doxycycline, minocycline, and tigecycline
2. Mechanism of action: inhibit protein synthesis (bind to 30S ribosomal subunit)
3. Spectrum of activity
   a. Includes *Rickettsia*, *Chlamydia*, *M pneumoniae*, *Vibrio*, *Brucella*, *Borrelia burgdorferi* (early stages), *Helicobacter pylori*, *S pneumoniae*, *Treponema pallidum*, and some mycobacteria
   b. Minocycline is also active against methicillin-resistant staphylococci (for mild disease in patients who cannot tolerate vancomycin), *Stenotrophomonas*, and *Mycobacterium marinum*
   c. Tigecycline: compared with tetracyclines, tigecycline has an expanded spectrum of activity
      1) Gram-positive activity includes methicillin-sensitive and methicillin-resistant staphylococci and vancomycin-resistant enterococci
      2) Gram-negative activity is broad
         a) Includes *E coli*, *Klebsiella*, *Enterobacter*, *Citrobacter*, *Acinetobacter*, *Stenotrophomonas*, *Haemophilus*, and *Moraxella*
         b) No appreciable activity against *Proteus* or *Pseudomonas*
      3) Good anaerobic and nontuberculous mycobacterial activity, although not studied extensively
      4) Not studied extensively for serious infections such as bacteremia (and blood levels remain low, so not the drug of choice)

4. Toxicities
   a. GI effects (especially prominent with tigecycline), rash, and photosensitivity
   b. Avoid in pregnant females and children because the drugs impair fetal bone growth and stain children's teeth
   c. Coadministration of antacids, iron, calcium, magnesium, or aluminum substantially decreases the enteric absorption of oral agents
   d. Tigecycline: FDA issued warning about increased mortality among patients treated for hospital-acquired pneumonia (which is not an FDA-approved use)
5. Major route of elimination
   a. Doxycyline and minocycline: hepatic
   b. Tetracycline: renal
   c. Tigecycline: biliary and fecal

J. Macrolides and Ketolides (Telithromycin)
   1. Prototypic agents: erythromycin, clarithromycin, azithromycin, and telithromycin
   2. Mechanism of action: inhibit protein synthesis (bind to 50S ribosomal subunit)
   3. Spectrum of activity
      a. Most β-hemolytic streptococci, *S pneumoniae* (resistance is increasing with macrolides), some methicillin-sensitive staphylococci, *Bordetella pertussis*, *Campylobacter jejuni*, *T pallidum*, *Ureaplasma*, *M pneumoniae*, *Legionella pneumophila*, *Chlamydia* species, and some mycobacteria
      b. Azithromycin and clarithromycin have enhanced activity over erythromycin against *H influenzae* and several nontuberculous mycobacterial species
      c. Telithromycin has enhanced activity against *S pneumoniae* (including strains resistant to macrolides) and activity against *H influenzae*, *M catarrhalis*, Mycoplasma, *Legionella*, and *C pneumoniae*
      d. Azithromycin and clarithromycin can be used for prophylaxis or treatment (in combination with other drugs) of *Mycobacterium avium* and other select nontuberculous mycobacterial infections
   4. Toxicities
      a. GI side effects (more common with erythromycin and telithromycin), diplopia (telithromycin), and rare reversible hearing loss with high doses
      b. Can prolong the QT interval, with rare reports of torsades de pointes (possibly less significant with azithromycin)
      c. Agents except azithromycin inhibit metabolism of other drugs through the cytochrome P450 3A4 isozyme (CYP3A4) system; the potential for drug interactions should be reviewed closely
      d. Telithromycin: recent case reports of serious hepatotoxicity including death
         1) Do not use in patients with underlying hepatic dysfunction
         2) Stop use with symptoms or laboratory evidence of hepatotoxicity
   5. Major route of elimination
      a. Hepatic metabolism
      b. Clarithromycin: also renal excretion

K. Trimethoprim-Sulfamethoxazole
   1. Mechanism of action: interferes with folic acid synthesis at sequential steps
   2. Spectrum of activity
      a. Includes various aerobic gram-positive cocci and gram-negative bacilli, including staphylococci (moderate activity), most *S pneumoniae*, *H influenzae*, *M catarrhalis*, *Listeria monocytogenes*, and many of the Enterobacteriaceae
      b. Active against *Pneumocystis*, *Stenotrophomonas*, *Nocardia*, *Shigella*, and *Isospora*
      c. Inactive against *Pseudomonas*, *Enterococcus*, and group A streptococcus
   3. Toxicities
      a. Most common: hypersensitivity reactions and GI side effects
      b. Less frequent: nephrotoxicity, myelosuppression, and hyperkalemia may occur, especially with high-dose therapy
      c. Use with caution or avoid during the last trimester of pregnancy (to minimize risk of fetal kernicterus) and in patients with known glucose-6-phosphate dehydrogenase deficiency
   4. Major route of elimination: renal

L. Clindamycin
   1. Mechanism of action: inhibits protein synthesis (binds to 50S ribosomal subunit)
   2. Spectrum of activity
      a. Includes aerobic and anaerobic gram-positive organisms
      b. Anaerobic activity includes *Actinomyces* species, *Clostridium* (except *C difficile*), *Peptostreptococcus*, and many *Bacteroides* species (but 10%-20% of *B fragilis* organisms are resistant)
      c. Clindamycin is active against gram-positive aerobes, such as many

staphylococci and group A streptococci (resistance is increasing)
   d. Emergence of resistance by staphylococci can occur during treatment
   e. The double-disk diffusion test should be performed to look for inducible resistance in staphylococci or streptococci that are erythromycin resistant
  3. Toxicities
   a. Most common: rash and GI side effects
   b. Antibiotic-associated diarrhea in up to 20% of patients
   c. *C difficile* colitis in 1% to 10%
  4. Major route of elimination: hepatic metabolism
M. Metronidazole
  1. Mechanism of action: disrupts bacterial DNA
  2. Spectrum of activity
   a. Includes most anaerobic microorganisms, including *Bacteroides* species (drug of choice)
   b. Exceptions include some anaerobic gram-positive organisms, including *Peptostreptococcus*, *Actinomyces*, and *Propionibacterium acnes*
   c. A drug of choice for *C difficile*, *Entamoeba histolytica*, *Giardia*, and *Gardnerella*
  3. Toxicities
   a. Include nausea, vomiting, reversible neutropenia, metallic taste, and a disulfiram reaction when coadministered with alcohol
   b. Neuropathies and seizures with high doses
  4. Major route of elimination: hepatic metabolism
N. Quinupristin-Dalfopristin (Synercid)
  1. Mechanism of action: block protein synthesis (the 2 components are synergistic) by binding to the 50S ribosomal subunit
  2. Spectrum of activity
   a. Good activity against gram-positive cocci, including vancomycin-resistant *Enterococcus faecium* and staphylococcus and methicillin-resistant strains
   b. Substantially decreased activity against *Enterococcus faecalis*
  3. Toxicities
   a. Include a relatively high rate of inflammation and irritation at the infusion site, arthralgias, myalgias, and hyperbilirubinemia
   b. Inhibits the metabolism of other drugs metabolized through the CYP3A4 enzyme; guard against possible drug interactions
  4. Major route of elimination: hepatic
O. Linezolid
  1. Mechanism of action: inhibits bacterial ribosome assembly (thus inhibits protein synthesis)
  2. Spectrum of activity
   a. Active against gram-positive bacteria, including methicillin-resistant staphylococci, most vancomycin-resistant enterococci, and penicillin-resistant *S pneumoniae*
   b. Active against *Nocardia* and some mycobacterial species
  3. Toxicities
   a. Most prominent: myelosuppression, especially with prolonged use
   b. Headache, diarrhea, and peripheral or optic neuropathy can occur
   c. Rare: lactic acidosis
   d. Linezolid is a weak monoamine oxidase inhibitor that interacts with some medications, such as selective serotonin reuptake inhibitors and monoamine oxidase inhibitors (there are reports of serotonin syndrome)
  4. Major route of elimination: hepatic metabolism
P. Daptomycin
  1. Mechanism of action: acts on cell membrane, causing rapid membrane depolarization and a potassium ion efflux, which is followed by arrest of DNA, RNA, and protein synthesis, resulting in bacterial cell death
  2. Spectrum of activity: gram-positive organisms, including *Staphylococcus* (including methicillin-resistant strains), group A streptococcus, and *Enterococcus* (including many vancomycin-resistant strains, but not well studied for serious infections)
  3. Toxicities
   a. Include GI effects, hypersensitivity reactions, headache, insomnia, myalgias, and creatine phosphokinase elevations
   b. The manufacturer suggests stopping use of statins during daptomycin therapy and monitoring creatine kinase values weekly
  4. Major route of elimination: renal
Q. Colistimethate or Colistin
  1. Given IV (or by inhalation for local effect in the lungs)
  2. Mechanism of action: colistimethate is converted to colistin, which disrupts the permeability of the bacterial membrane, leading to leakage of the cell contents and cell death
  3. Spectrum of activity
   a. Broad activity against gram-negative aerobes, including many multidrug resistant *Acinetobacter baumannii*, *P aeruginosa*, and *Klebsiella pneumoniae*

b. Its activity against resistant organisms has led to a resurgence in its use
4. Toxicities
   a. Administered IV
      1) Nephrotoxicity is the predominant adverse effect (usually reversible) but is less common than previously thought
      2) Neurotoxicity (rare) includes paresthesias, vertigo, and possible neuromuscular blockade
   b. Administered by inhalation (not FDA approved)
      1) FDA reported a possible connection between use of premixed colistimethate and death of a cystic fibrosis patient
      2) Colistimethate should be reconstituted as close to the administration time as possible
5. Major route of elimination: renal
   a. Requires dose adjustment of IV formulation with renal dysfunction

II. Antiviral Agents
   A. Anti–Herpes Simplex Agents
      1. Agents: acyclovir, valacyclovir, and famciclovir
      2. Mechanism of action: activated by viral thymidine kinase and blocks viral DNA synthesis
      3. Spectrum of activity
         a. Clinical activity against herpes simplex virus (HSV)-1, HSV-2, and varicella-zoster virus (VZV)
         b. Not effective for treatment of cytomegalovirus (CMV)
      4. Toxicities
         a. Acyclovir has been associated with neurotoxicity and nephrotoxicity (IV, especially if dose not adjusted for renal dysfunction)
         b. GI effects
         c. Patients receiving high doses of acyclovir IV should be well hydrated to minimize renal tubule drug precipitation
         d. Famciclovir is associated uncommonly with headache, nausea, diarrhea, and rare CNS effects, specifically confusion or hallucinations; neutropenia and liver function test elevations may occur rarely
      5. Major route of elimination: renal
   B. Anti-CMV Agents
      1. Agents: ganciclovir, valganciclovir, cidofovir, and foscarnet
      2. Mechanism of action
         a. Cidofovir: metabolized intracellularly (by thymidine kinase for herpesvirus and by a viral protein for CMV) to the active diphosphate form; inhibits viral DNA synthesis
         b. Ganciclovir and valganciclovir: intracellularly phosphorylated; inhibit viral DNA synthesis
         c. Foscarnet: directly inhibits viral DNA synthesis; does not require phosphorylation
      3. Spectrum of activity
         a. Ganciclovir (and its prodrug, valganciclovir): clinically active against CMV, HSV-1, HSV-2, human herpesvirus (HHV)-6, and VZV
         b. Cidofovir and foscarnet: clinically active against CMV (including many ganciclovir-resistant strains), HSV-1, HSV-2 (including many acyclovir-resistant strains), HHV-6, and VZV
      4. Toxicities
         a. Ganciclovir and valganciclovir
            1) Myelosuppression (generally neutropenia or thrombocytopenia)
            2) Less common: nephrotoxicity, liver function test elevations, and fever
            3) Rare: CNS effects, including headache, confusion, seizures, and coma
         b. Cidofovir
            1) Dose-related nephrotoxicity, neutropenia, iritis, uveitis, and GI effects
            2) Saline hydration and probenecid should be used to decrease the risk of nephrotoxicity
            3) Avoid use if possible in patients with renal dysfunction
         c. Foscarnet
            1) Nephrotoxicity (minimize with saline hydration), electrolyte disturbances, and CNS effects
            2) Fever, nausea, vomiting, and diarrhea are common
      5. Major route of elimination: renal
   C. Anti–Influenza Virus Agents
      1. Agents: rimantadine, amantadine, oseltamivir, and zanamivir
      2. Mechanism of action
         a. Amantadine and rimantadine inhibit entry and uncoating of influenza A
         b. Zanamivir and oseltamivir are selective inhibitors of influenza A and B neuraminidase
            1) Neuraminidase is required for infectivity of influenza virus
            2) Neuraminidase is thought to be essential for the release of newly assembled virions from infected cells

3. Spectrum of activity
   a. Rimantadine and amantadine are active against only influenza A; resistance is variable (see annual recommendations from the Centers for Disease Control for use and resistance patterns)
   b. Oseltamivir and zanamivir are active against influenza A (including most novel H1N1 strains) and B and have some activity against avian influenza (optimal dose and duration are unclear)
4. Toxicities
   a. Rimantadine and amantadine
      1) Commonly associated with GI complaints and CNS effects, including insomnia, anxiety, and difficulty concentrating
      2) Neurotoxicity, including tremor, seizures, and coma, has been seen at high doses and at doses unadjusted for renal dysfunction
      3) CNS effects are less pronounced with rimantadine
      4) Dose-related cardiac arrhythmias have rarely been reported
   b. Zanamivir and oseltamivir
      1) Generally well tolerated
      2) Oseltamivir: GI complaints most frequently reported
      3) Zanamivir: given by inhalation, rarely causes cough and bronchospasm, and not recommended in patients with underlying chronic pulmonary disease
5. Major route of elimination
   a. Amantadine: renal
   b. Rimantadine: hepatic metabolism
   c. Oseltamivir: renal
   d. Zanamavir: given by inhalation; little oral absorption
D. Anti–Hepatitis Virus Agents
   1. See Chapter 32, "Viral Hepatitis"
E. Antiretroviral Agents
   1. See Chapter 38, "HIV/AIDS"
III. Antifungal Agents
   A. Triazoles
      1. Agents: fluconazole, itraconazole, voriconazole, and posaconazole
      2. Mechanism of action: inhibit ergosterol synthesis and cell membrane formation
      3. Spectrum of activity
         a. Fluconazole
            1) Active against many *Candida* species (less activity against *Candida glabrata*; inactive against *Candida krusei*), *Cryptococcus*, and *Coccidioides immitis*
            2) An alternative agent for *Histoplasma capsulatum*, *Blastomyces dermatitidis*, and *Paracoccidioides* species
         b. Itraconazole
            1) Active against some filamentous fungi, including *Aspergillus* species, *Pseudallescheria*, *Alternaria*, and *Sporothrix*
            2) Has similar activity as fluconazole against most yeasts
            3) Has greater activity than fluconazole against *Histoplasma* and *Blastomyces* and is a drug of choice
         c. Voriconazole
            1) Active against many filamentous fungi, including *Aspergillus* species, *Pseudallescheria*, *Scedosporium*, and *Fusarium*
            2) Active against most strains of *Candida*, *Coccidioides*, *Cryptococcus*, *Histoplasma*, and *Blastomyces*
         d. Posaconazole
            1) Similar activity as voriconazole against yeasts, endemic fungi, and filamentous fungi
            2) Adds activity against the Zygomycetes
         e. Itraconazole, voriconazole, and posaconazole
            1) May be active against some fluconazole-resistant *Candida* strains
            2) Cross-resistance occurs (especially with *C glabrata*)
      4. Toxicities
         a. All azoles can elevate liver function test results and, less commonly, cause overt hepatotoxicity
         b. Triazoles inhibit hepatic metabolism (and secondarily increase serum drug concentrations) of many drugs, including cyclosporine, tacrolimus, sirolimus, midazolam, triazolam, and statins, so that potential drug interactions should be reviewed closely
         c. In about 10% of patients receiving voriconazole, transient visual disturbances develop (acuity, field, or color)
         d. Rash is more common with voriconazole
         e. Itraconazole is a negative inotrope (congestive heart failure has been reported rarely); it should not be used in patients who have congestive heart failure
         f. IV voriconazole
            1) Contains a cyclodextrin vehicle that can accumulate with renal dysfunction, but clinical significance is unclear
            2) Use with caution in patients with renal dysfunction (assess risks and benefits)

g. All triazoles may have cardiac effects
   1) Prolonged QT interval
   2) Torsades de pointes, particularly when triazoles are used in combination with other drugs that prolong the QT interval or in patients with QT syndrome
5. Major route of elimination
   a. Fluconazole: renal
   b. Itraconazole and voriconazole: hepatic metabolism through cytochrome P450 isoenzymes
   c. Posaconazole: metabolized primarily by glucoronidation

B. Polyenes: Amphotericin B Products
1. Agents: amphotericin B deoxycholate, amphotericin B liposomal complex (AmBisome), and amphotericin B lipid complex (Abelcet)
2. Mechanism of action: bind to ergosterol in the fungal cell membrane and cause cell damage by increasing permeability and allowing efflux
3. Spectrum of activity
   a. Broadest antifungal activity against yeasts (*Candida*, *Cryptococcus*, etc), dimorphic fungi (including *Histoplasma*, *Coccidioides*, and *Blastomyces*), and filamentous fungi (including *Aspergillus*)
   b. Less active against *Aspergillus terreus*
   c. Variable activity against *Aspergillus flavus*, the Zygomycetes, and dematiaceous molds
4. Toxicities
   a. Infusion-related: fever, chills, rigors, nausea, and vomiting
      1) Pretreatment with diphenhydramine, acetaminophen, and meperidine may lessen such reactions
      2) Reactions are less frequent with AmBisome
   b. Nephrotoxicity (usually reversible)
      1) Can be lessened with sodium crystalloid loading
      2) Lipid formulations are associated with a significantly smaller incidence of nephrotoxicity
   c. Other: hypokalemia, hypomagnesemia, anemia, phlebitis, changes in blood pressure, and neurologic effects
5. Major route of elimination: nonrenal, nonhepatic, slow release from peripheral compartments

C. Echinocandins
1. Agents: caspofungin, micafungin, and anidulafungin
2. Mechanism of action: inhibition of 1,3-β-D-glucan synthesis (cell wall inhibitor)
3. Spectrum of activity
   a. Active against *Candida* species (including most azole-resistant strains) and *Aspergillus* species
   b. Not active against *Cryptococcus* or Zygomycetes
4. Toxicities
   a. Not common
   b. Possible histamine-related effects: rash and facial swelling
   c. Abnormal results on liver function tests (not common)
   d. Caspofungin
      1) Can slightly increase levels of cyclosporine
      2) Enzyme inducers (rifampin, efavirenz, nevirapine, phenytoin, etc) can decrease levels, so use higher daily dosage (70 mg)
5. Major route of elimination
   a. Caspofungin and micafungin: hepatic metabolism
   b. Anidulafungin: nonhepatic chemical degradation

IV. Antimycobacterial Agents
A. Antitubercular Agents
1. First-line agents
   a. Isoniazid, rifamycins (rifampin, rifabutin, and rifapentine), pyrazinamide, and ethambutol
   b. Toxicities
      1) Isoniazid: hepatitis, peripheral neuropathy, rash and other skin eruptions, and seizures (rarely)
      2) Rifampin
         a) Hepatitis (may show cholestatic pattern), orange discoloration of urine and tears (not a toxicity), rash and other skin eruptions, thrombocytopenia, anemia, flulike symptoms, nephritis, and proteinuria
         b) Rifampin induces the hepatic cytochrome P450 metabolic pathway, resulting in decreased serum concentrations of concomitantly administered drugs metabolized by this same pathway, including azathioprine, digoxin, propranolol, azole antifungals, haloperidol, protease inhibitors, calcium channel blockers, imidazoles, quinidine,

        corticosteroids, opioids, methadone, theophylline, cyclosporine, oral contraceptives, tolbutamide, dapsone, oral hypoglycemic agents, warfarin, diazepam, and phenytoin
    3) Rifabutin
        a) Similar profile as rifampin
        b) Also uveitis, arthritis and arthralgias, neutropenia and leukopenia, and bronze skin pigmentation
        c) Less hepatic cytochrome P450 induction than rifampin
    4) Pyrazinamide: hepatitis, arthralgias, hyperuricemia (not a toxicity), and rash
    5) Ethambutol: optic neuritis (decreased visual acuity or red-green color discrimination)
    2. Second-line agents: fluoroquinolones (moxifloxacin and levofloxacin), aminoglycosides (streptomycin, amikacin, and kanamycin), capreomycin, ethionamide, cycloserine, p-aminosalicylic acid (PAS), linezolid, and clofazimine
  B. Nontubercular Antimycobacterial Agents
    1. Selection of drugs depends on the species of Mycobacterium
    2. Macrolides (clarithromycin, and azithromycin), fluoroquinolones (moxifloxacin, levofloxacin, and ciprofloxacin), doxycycline, tigecycline, trimethoprim-sulfamethoxazole, amikacin, tobramycin, imipenem, linezolid, cefoxitin, and clofazimine
V. Quick Reference Tables
  A. Laboratory and Clinical Toxicity Monitoring for Antimicrobials (Table 2.2)
  B. Select Bacterial Resistance Issues (Table 2.3)

Table 2.2
Laboratory and Clinical Toxicity Monitoring for Antimicrobials[a]

Medication	Select Toxicities	Minimum Laboratory Monitoring[b]	Clinical Monitoring
Antibacterials			
Aminoglycoside class (eg, gentamicin, tobramycin, amikacin, streptomycin)	Nephrotoxicity, auditory toxicity, vestibular toxicity, neuromuscular blockade	SCr at least twice weekly (for dose-adjustment and nephrotoxicity assessments), serum levels if therapy to continue >72 h	Baseline and periodic hearing and vestibular function questioning (audiologic testing with prolonged therapy)
Aztreonam	GI effects, hypersensitivity	SCr weekly (for dose-adjustment assessment)	Hypersensitivity, diarrhea
Carbapenem class (eg, ertapenem, doripenem, imipenem, meropenem)	Hypersensitivity, GI effects, Clostridium difficile, seizures (especially with high dose or doses not adjusted for renal function)	SCr weekly (for dose-adjustment assessment)	Hypersensitivity, GI effects, seizures (rare but often seen with renal dysfunction without dose adjustment or with underlying seizure disorder)
Cephalosporin class	GI effects, hypersensitivity reactions, C difficile	For IV cephalosporins: SCr weekly (for dose-adjustment assessment) except for ceftriaxone, which does not require dose adjustment for renal function	Hypersensitivity, diarrhea, other GI effects
With MTT side chain (eg, cefotetan, cefmetazole, moxalactam, cefoperazone, cefamandole)	As for cephalosporin class plus hypoprothrombinemia and disulfiram-like reactions with alcohol	As for IV cephalosporins plus INR for prolonged use	As for cephalosporin class plus avoid alcohol; bleeding with long-term use; diarrhea
Ceftriaxone	As for cephalosporin class plus biliary sludging (especially in young children), gallstones	As for IV cephalosporins plus consider LFTs in pediatric patients with prolonged use	As for cephalosporin class plus signs of biliary sludge or gallstones
Clindamycin	Diarrhea, C difficile colitis, nausea, vomiting	Not routinely indicated	Hypersensitivity, GI effects, photosensitivity

(continued)

Table 2.2
(continued)

Medication	Select Toxicities	Minimum Laboratory Monitoring[b]	Clinical Monitoring
Dalfopristin-quinupristin	Pain or inflammation at infusion site, arthralgia or myalgia, hyperbilirubinemia	LFTs weekly	Phlebitis, arthralgias, myalgias
Daptomycin	GI effects, hypersensitivity, headache, elevated CK, myalgias; rarely rhabdomyolysis	CK weekly; SCr weekly (dose-adjustment assessment)	Hypersensitivity, GI effects, myalgias, rhabdomyolysis
Fluoroquinolone class (eg, ciprofloxacin, ofloxacin, levofloxacin, moxifloxacin, gemifloxacin)	GI effects, arthropathy (especially in pediatric patients), tendon rupture, prolongation of QT interval, hypersensitivity (especially gemifloxacin), CNS effects (especially with ciprofloxacin)	Consider periodic SCr and LFTs with prolonged use	Hypersensitivity, GI effects, drug-drug interactions, prolongation of QT interval with risk factors (avoid use with other QT-prolonging agents), CNS effects, photosensitivity
Ketolides (eg, telithromycin)	Nausea, diarrhea, dizziness, headache, prolongation of QT interval, visual effects, rash, hepatotoxicity	LFTs at baseline (do not use with significant hepatic impairment) and weekly for prolonged use	Symptoms associated with liver dysfunction, hypersensitivity, diarrhea, other GI effects, visual disturbances, QT prolongation with risk factors (avoid use with other QT-prolonging agents), photosensitivity, drug-drug interactions
Linezolid	Myelosuppression, diarrhea, nausea, rash, optic neuritis, peripheral neuropathy	CBC baseline and weekly; consider periodic LFTs with prolonged use	Hypersensitivity, GI effects, optic or peripheral neuropathy (with prolonged use), drug-drug interactions (eg, with serotonergic or adrenergic drugs)
Macrolide class (eg, erythromycin, clarithromycin, azithromycin)	GI effects (less with clarithromycin and azithromycin), cholestatic jaundice, transient hearing loss (at high doses), prolongation of QT interval or torsades de pointes (primarily with erythromycin and clarithromycin), allergic reaction	Consider periodic LFTs with prolonged use; baseline SCr for clarithromycin (dose-adjustment assessment)	Hypersensitivity, GI effects, drug-drug interactions, QT prolongation with risk factors (avoid use with other QT-prolonging agents), hearing deficits (especially with high-dose IV erythromycin)
Metronidazole	Nausea, diarrhea, disulfiram-like reactions with alcohol, metallic taste, reversible neutropenia	Consider baseline LFTs (dose-adjustment assessment)	GI effects (avoid alcohol)
Penicillin class	Hypersensitivity reactions, GI effects (nausea, vomiting, diarrhea, *C difficile*)	For IV penicillins: SCr weekly (dose-adjustment assessment except penicillinase-resistant penicillins)	Hypersensitivity, diarrhea, other GI effects
Natural penicillins	IV form: as for penicillin class plus seizures (with high dose), phlebitis, pain during infusion, sodium or potassium excess (depending on salt form)	As for IV penicillins plus sodium or potassium (depending on salt form)	As for penicillin class plus phlebitis
Aminopenicillins (eg, ampicillin, amoxicillin, amoxicillin-clavulanate, ampicillin-sulbactam)	As for penicillin class: amoxicillin-clavulanate results in greater incidence of diarrhea and hepatitis	As for IV penicillins plus periodic LFTs with prolonged use	As for penicillin class plus higher incidence of diarrhea

Table 2.2
(continued)

Medication	Select Toxicities	Minimum Laboratory Monitoring[b]	Clinical Monitoring
Penicillinase-resistant penicillins (eg, nafcillin, oxacillin)	As for penicillin class plus thrombophlebitis, hepatitis, neutropenia (with prolonged use), interstitial nephritis	As for IV penicillins plus weekly WBC and weekly LFTs	As for penicillin class plus phlebitis
Carboxypenicillins (eg, ticarcillin, ticarcillin-clavulanate)	As for penicillin class plus hypokalemia, hypernatremia, platelet dysfunction, neutropenia	As for IV penicillins plus weekly CBC, weekly potassium, weekly sodium	As for penicillin class plus bleeding
Ureidopenicillins (eg, piperacillin, piperacillin-tazobactam)	As for penicillin class plus neutropenia or thrombocytopenia (with prolonged use)	As for IV penicillins plus weekly CBC with prolonged use	As for penicillin class
Tetracycline class (eg, tetracycline, doxycycline, minocycline)	Photosensitivity, permanent staining of developing teeth (avoid in pregnant women and children <8 y), GI effects, rash, vestibular toxicity (minocycline)	Consider periodic LFTs with prolonged use	Hypersensitivity, diarrhea, other GI effects, drug-drug interactions (chelators with oral tetracyclines), vestibular toxicity (minocycline), photosensitivity
Tigecycline	Nausea and vomiting (higher incidence than comparable agents), permanent staining of developing teeth (avoid in pregnancy and in children <8 y)	LFTs weekly	GI effects
Trimethoprim-sulfamethoxazole	Nausea, vomiting, hypersensitivity reactions, bone marrow suppression, hyperkalemia	With high dose: consider baseline and periodic measurement of SCr (dose-adjustment and nephrotoxicity assessments), CBC, potassium, and LFTs	Hypersensitivity, GI effects
Vancomycin	Ototoxicity, red man syndrome, nephrotoxicity (usually in combination with other nephrotoxins), phlebitis, reversible neutropenia	SCr baseline and weekly (for potential dose-adjustment and nephrotoxicity assessments); CBC weekly; serum levels as appropriate	Phlebitis, consider audiologic testing for long-term use, hypersensitivity, GI effects
Antitubercular Agents (Also See Fluoroquinolones and Linezolid)			
Isoniazid	Hepatitis, hypersensitivity reactions, lupus-like reactions, peripheral neuropathy	LFTs monthly in patients with underlying liver dysfunction	Hypersensitivity, neuropathy, drug-drug interactions
Rifamycins (eg, rifampin, rifabutin, rifapentine)	Orange discoloration of body fluids, thrombocytopenia, hepatitis, uveitis (with rifabutin)	LFTs monthly in patients with underlying liver dysfunction	Uveitis (especially with rifabutin), numerous drug-drug interactions, hypersensitivity
Pyrazinamide	Hepatitis, hyperuricemia, nausea, anorexia, polyarthralgia	LFTs monthly in patients with underlying liver dysfunction; uric acid as indicated	GI effects, hypersensitivity
Ethambutol	Retrobulbar neuritis, optic neuritis, hyperuricemia	Not routinely indicated	Baseline vision or color discrimination testing and monthly questioning (repeat testing with prolonged use or with doses >25 mg/kg daily); consider monthly vision or color discrimination testing; GI effects

(continued)

Table 2.2
(continued)

Medication	Select Toxicities	Minimum Laboratory Monitoring[b]	Clinical Monitoring
Ethionamide	High incidence of GI effects, drowsiness, asthenia, psychiatric effects, hepatitis, hypothyroidism	LFTs in patients with underlying liver dysfunction; TSH baseline and monthly	GI effects, CNS effects
p-Aminosalicylic acid	Rash, GI effects, hypersensitivity, hypothyroidism	LFTs and TSH at baseline; TSH every 3 mo for prolonged use	Hypersensitivity, GI effects
Cycloserine	CNS toxic effects (somnolence, headache, tremor, psychosis, seizures)	Serum levels may help establish optimum dose	Monthly assessment of neuropsychiatric effects
Streptomycin, amikacin, kanamycin, capreomycin	Nephrotoxicity, auditory toxicity, vestibular toxicity, neuromuscular blockade	SCr baseline and weekly; serum levels when available	Baseline hearing, vestibular, or Romberg testing; monthly questioning of symptoms; repeat testing as indicated
Antifungal Agents			
Amphotericin B deoxycholate	Infusion-related reactions (fever, chills, rigors, nausea, hypertension, hypotension), nephrotoxicity, hypokalemia, hypomagnesemia, reversible anemia	Twice-weekly SCr, twice-weekly potassium, and twice-weekly magnesium; weekly LFTs and weekly CBC	Infusion-related effects, blood pressure monitoring as indicated
Lipid amphotericin B product	Lower incidence of nephrotoxicity than amphotericin B deoxycholate; lower incidence of infusion-related effects with amphotericin B liposomal complex	Twice-weekly SCr, twice-weekly potassium, and twice-weekly magnesium; weekly LFTs and weekly CBC	Infusion-related effects
Flucytosine	Bone marrow suppression, GI effects, hepatitis	Twice-weekly SCr (dose-adjustment assessment) and twice-weekly CBC; weekly LFTs; periodic serum levels as indicated	Nausea and vomiting (often associated with elevated serum levels)
Triazole antifungal class (eg, fluconazole, itraconazole, voriconazole, posaconazole)	GI effects, hepatitis, prolongation of QT interval, hypersensitivity	Baseline and periodic LFTs and SCr (dose-adjustment assessment with fluconazole; cyclodextrin vehicle accumulation with IV voriconazole or itraconazole)	GI effects, prolongation of QT interval with risk factors (avoid if possible with other QT-prolonging agents), hypersensitivity, photosensitivity, many drug-drug interactions
Itraconazole	As for triazole class plus CHF, cyclodextrin vehicle accumulation with IV formulation in patients with renal dysfunction (clinical significance of risk and benefit unknown), high doses may produce endocrine effects similar to those of ketoconazole	As for triazole class plus periodic SCr with IV or oral solution (cyclodextrin vehicle accumulation with renal dysfunction, so avoid or consider risk and benefit); consider periodic potassium and sodium; consider serum levels as indicated	As for triazole class plus edema, signs of CHF (uncommon)
Voriconazole	Transient visual disturbances, cyclodextrin vehicle accumulation with IV formulation in patients with renal dysfunction (clinical significance of risk and benefit unknown)	As for triazole class plus periodic SCr with IV (cyclodextrin vehicle accumulation with renal dysfunction, so avoid or consider risk and benefit); consider serum levels as indicated	As for triazole class plus visual side effects, hallucinations

Table 2.2
(continued)

Medication	Select Toxicities	Minimum Laboratory Monitoring[b]	Clinical Monitoring
Echinocandin class (eg, caspofungin, micafungin, anidulafungin)	Facial flushing or swelling (histamine mediated but rare), hypersensitivity, hepatitis	LFTs weekly	Hypersensitivity, a few drug-drug interactions with caspofungin
Anti-Cytomegalovirus Agents			
Cidofovir	Renal impairment, neutropenia, ocular hypotonia, headache, asthenia, alopecia, rash, GI effects	SCr (also give saline load and probenecid), WBC, and UA, all twice weekly and before each dose	GI effects, hypersensitivity (especially with probenecid)
Foscarnet	Renal impairment, electrolyte disturbances, seizures, GI effects	SCr twice weekly (dose-adjustment and nephrotoxicity assessments); electrolytes weekly	GI effects, hypersensitivity
Ganciclovir or valganciclovir	Myelosuppression, GI effects	CBC once or twice weekly; SCr weekly (dose-adjustment assessment)	GI effects
Anti–Influenza Virus Agents			
Oseltamivir	GI effects (usually well tolerated)	SCr at baseline (dose-adjustment assessment)	GI effects
Zanamivir	Bronchospasm in patients with underlying lung disease	None	Bronchospasm (avoid in patients with lung injury or asthma)
Anti-Herpesvirus Agents			
Acyclovir or valacyclovir	Malaise, nausea, vomiting, diarrhea; phlebitis (with IV acyclovir); nephrotoxicity and CNS effects more common with high-dose IV therapy	SCr weekly with IV acyclovir (dose-adjustment and nephrotoxicity assessments)	Phlebitis, CNS effects (IV), GI effects
Famciclovir	Headache, dizziness, nausea, diarrhea, fatigue	SCr at baseline (dose-adjustment assessment)	GI effects

Abbreviations: CBC, complete blood cell count; CHF, congestive heart failure; CK, creatine kinase; CNS, central nervous system; GI, gastrointestinal tract; INR, international normalized ratio; IV, intravenous; LFT, liver function test; MTT, methyltetrazolethiol; SCr, serum creatinine; TSH, thyrotropin; UA, urinalysis; WBC, white blood cell count.

[a] Also monitor for signs or symptoms of infection improvement or worsening.

[b] Monitor more frequently if tests are abnormal or changing and in critically ill patients.

Adapted from Wilson JW, Estes LL. Mayo Clinic antimicrobial therapy: quick guide. Rochester (MN): Mayo Clinic Scientific Press; c2008. Used with permission of Mayo Foundation for Medical Education and Research.

Table 2.3
Select Bacterial Resistance Issues

Pertinent Organisms	Resistance Issues	Treatment
Extended-Spectrum β-Lactamase–Producing (ESBL) Gram-negative Bacilli		
Escherichia coli, Klebsiella species Less common: Proteus mirabilis, Enterobacter species	Generally resistant to penicillins and cephalosporins[a]; may appear susceptible to piperacillin-tazobactam but with a potentially higher failure rate than with carbapenem	First-line: carbapenem (carbapenem resistance may occur by a different mechanism in Klebsiella species) Alternates: fluoroquinolone or tigecycline, but there is less clinical experience with these

(continued)

Table 2.3
(continued)

Pertinent Organisms	Resistance Issues	Treatment
ampC-Mediated Resistance in Gram-negative Bacilli		
Enterobacter and *Citrobacter* species (also may be seen in *Morganella morganii*, *Providencia*, *Serratia*, and indole-positive *Proteus* species)	Generally avoid second- and third-generation cephalosporins even if organism is reported to be susceptible, because of potential for induction or selection of AmpC-type β-lactamase (derepressed β-lactamase production), which can lead to development of resistance during treatment	First-line: carbapenem
Alternates (depending on susceptibility testing): fluoroquinolone, trimethoprim-sulfamethoxazole, tigecycline, piperacillin-tazobactam, aminoglycoside, cefepime (better activity than third-generation cephalosporin[b])
If *ampC*-mediated resistance occurs, a carbapenem is typically the only active β-lactam
Klebsiella pneumoniae Carbapenemases (KPC)		
Klebsiella pneumoniae
Less common: other Enterobacteriaceae, *Pseudomonas aeruginosa*	Resistance to carbapenems and other β-lactams; often have coresistance to other classes of drugs	Based on susceptibility testing
Colistin, polymyxin, tigecycline, and aminoglycosides often have in vitro activity
Methicillin-Resistant *Staphylococcus aureus* (MRSA)		
S aureus	Oxacillin-resistant (methicillin-resistant) staphylococci are resistant to all currently available β-lactams; both nosocomial and community-acquired strains are seen
Community-acquired MRSA isolates tend to be more susceptible to non–β-lactams (eg, trimethoprim-sulfamethoxazole, clindamycin, tetracycline, fluoroquinolone) than nosocomial isolates	First-line: vancomycin, linezolid, daptomycin[c]
Alternates (depending on susceptibility testing): doxycycline, minocycline, trimethoprim-sulfamethoxazole, clindamycin (test for inducible resistance), dalfopristin-quinupristin, tigecycline, newer fluoroquinolone[d]
Vancomycin-Intermediate *S aureus* (VISA) or Vancomycin-Resistant *S aureus* (VRSA)		
S aureus with vancomycin minimum inhibitory concentration ≥4 mcg/mL	Organisms with reduced susceptibility or complete resistance to vancomycin have been reported	Contact infection control immediately and obtain infectious diseases consultation
Vancomycin-Resistant Enterococci (VRE)		
Enterococcus species	Enterococci with resistance to vancomycin	First-line: linezolid
Alternates: daptomycin[c], dalfopristin-quinupristin (only for *Enterococcus faecium*), tigecycline; may be susceptible to penicillin and ampicillin
Strenotrophomonas		
Stenotrophamonos maltophilia	May cause invasive disease but frequently is a colonizer (and treatment is not required); treatment should be guided by susceptibility testing (resistance to multiple drugs is typical)	First-line: trimethoprim-sulfamethoxazole, ticarcillin-clavulanate, tigecycline
Alternates (depending on susceptibility testing): fluoroquinolones, minocycline

[a] May show in vivo susceptibility to cephamycin (eg, cefotetan, cefoxitin), but failures have been reported and other mechanisms can confer resistance.

[b] Cefepime is less likely than third-generation agents to induce resistance, but resistance has been reported. If inducible β-lactamase production occurs, organisms should be considered resistant to penicillins and cephalosporins.

[c] Daptomycin should not be used for pneumonia because it is inactivated by surfactant. It has in vitro activity against enterococci, but studies are limited for serious enterococcal infections.

[d] Newer fluoroquinolone (eg, moxifloxacin, levofloxacin, gemifloxacin). Staphylococcal resistance to fluoroquinolone has been reported to develop while patients are receiving therapy.

Adapted from Wilson JW, Estes LL. Mayo Clinic antimicrobial therapy: quick guide. Rochester (MN): Mayo Clinic Scientific Press; c2008. Used with permission of Mayo Foundation for Medical Education and Research.

Suggested Reading

Gorbach SL, Bartlett JG, Blacklow NR. Infectious diseases. 3rd Edition. Philadelphia (PA): Lippincott Williams & Wilkins; c2004.

Mandell GL, Bennett JE, Dolin R. Mandell, Douglas, and Bennett's principles and practice of infectious diseases. 7th Edition. Philadelphia (PA): Churchill Livingstone Elsevier; c2010.

Wilson JW, Estes LL. Mayo Clinic antimicrobial therapy: quick guide. Rochester (MN): Mayo Clinic Scientific Press; c2008.

W. Charles Huskins, MD, MSc

Health Care–Associated Infection Prevention and Control Programs

I. Introduction
   A. Rationale
      1. Infectious diseases subspecialists should have basic knowledge of interventions necessary to prevent and control health care–associated infections (HAIs)
   B. Scope of Chapter
      1. Reviews key components and activities of HAI prevention and control programs
      2. Addressed in other chapters: interventions to prevent specific HAIs, such as intravascular catheter–associated bloodstream infections, ventilator-associated pneumonia, urinary catheter–associated urinary tract infections, and surgical site infections
II. Organizations in the United States That Influence HAI Prevention and Control Programs
   A. State Health Departments
      1. Generally have requirements for programs and for reporting of communicable diseases
      2. Some states require public reporting of HAI rates
   B. The Joint Commission (TJC)
      1. Private, not-for-profit organization
      2. Has accreditation requirements for the structure and activity of HAI programs
      3. Has performance indicators, including several that are HAI rates
   C. United States Department of Labor's Occupational Safety and Health Administration (OSHA)
      1. Promulgates regulations regarding workplace exposure to bloodborne pathogens and tuberculosis
      2. Bloodborne pathogen regulations
         a. Specific exposure prevention strategies
         b. Health care worker education
         c. Evaluation and management of exposures
         d. Voluntary hepatitis B vaccination at no cost to employees
         e. Detailed record-keeping (see "Employee and Occupational Health" section below)
   D. Centers for Disease Control and Prevention (CDC)
      1. Division of Healthcare Quality Promotion (DHQP)
         a. Has major role in providing information and guidance to HAI prevention and control programs
         b. Has extensive experience in nosocomial infection outbreak investigation
      2. Healthcare Infection Control Practices Advisory Committee (HICPAC)
         a. Provides advice and guidance to DHQP
         b. Develops evidence-based guidelines for infection control and prevention

3. Advisory Committee on Immunization Practices (ACIP) provides recommendations on immunization practices relevant to health care workers
    E. Other Organizations That Develop Recommendations and Guidelines
        1. Society of Healthcare Epidemiology of America (SHEA)
        2. Association for Professionals in Infection Control and Epidemiology (APIC)
        3. Infectious Diseases Society of America (IDSA)
        4. In 2008, SHEA and IDSA collaborated on compendium of guidelines to prevent HAIs
        5. Institute for Healthcare Improvement (IHI)
            a. Conducts voluntary campaigns to improve patient safety in US health care facilities
            b. Includes efforts to reduce HAIs
III. Program Organization, Responsibilities, Staffing, and Activities
    A. Consensus Panel Report
        1. Published in 1998 in *Infection Control and Hospital Epidemiology*
        2. Requirements for infrastructure and essential activities of HAI prevention and control programs
        3. Endorsed by SHEA, APIC, DHQP, and TJC
        4. Principal goals of programs
            a. Protect the patient
            b. Protect the health care worker, visitors, and others in the health care environment
            c. Accomplish goals in a cost-effective manner whenever possible
        5. Recommendation of report: all hospitals should have the continuing services of 1 or more trained hospital epidemiologists and infection control professionals and provide them with appropriate support
    B. Key Activities of Program
        1. Comply with relevant regulatory and accreditation requirements
        2. Perform surveillance of HAI
        3. Identify infection outbreaks, conduct comprehensive and timely investigations, and implement appropriate prevention and control measures
        4. Establish, implement, update, and monitor written infection prevention and control policies and procedures
        5. Provide ongoing educational programs to employees
        6. Collaborate with local and state health departments as required
IV. Surveillance of HAIs
    A. Reporting HAI Data
        1. More than 300 US hospitals voluntarily collect and confidentially report data on the incidence of HAIs to the DHQP's National Healthcare Safety Network (NHSN)
            a. Formerly called the National Nosocomial Infections Surveillance (NNIS) System
            b. NHSN collects data on HAIs to serve as national benchmarks
                1) Adult and pediatric intensive care units (ICUs)
                2) High-risk nurseries
                3) Surgical site infections in surgical patients
                4) Antimicrobial use and resistance in ICUs and non-ICU areas
        2. NHSN regularly reports various rates
            a. Device-associated infection rates in ICUs (eg, central line–associated infections per 1,000 central line–days, ventilator-associated pneumonias per 1,000 ventilator-days, urinary catheter–associated infections per 1,000 urinary catheter–days)
            b. Risk-adjusted surgical site infection rates for specific operative procedures
            c. Device utilization ratios in ICUs (ie, ratios of central line–days, mechanical ventilation–days, and urinary catheter–days to patient-days)
            d. Prevalence of antimicrobial resistance among pathogens causing HAIs in ICU patients
            e. Antimicrobial use rates in ICUs and non-ICU areas
        3. Facility-based surveillance of HAI has many purposes
            a. Establish baseline endemic HAI rates and monitor trends in these rates over time
            b. Benchmark HAI rates with local, regional, and national networks
            c. Detect outbreaks of HAIs
            d. Demonstrate the seriousness of HAIs and the importance of improvement efforts to institutional leaders and health care providers
            e. Guide and evaluate HAI prevention and control efforts
            f. Satisfy regulatory and reporting requirements
        4. Health care facilities should have a written surveillance plan
            a. Guided by the needs and resources of the facility
            b. Outlines the surveillance methodology
            c. Updated regularly

5. Hospital-wide surveillance of HAI (surveillance of all HAI in all patients)
   a. Was frequently performed in the 1970s and 1980s
   b. Rarely performed now because of the substantial time commitment required for data collection
   c. Most facilities use focused (or targeted) surveillance of a specific feature
      1) Specific high-risk groups (eg, ICU patients, surgical patients)
      2) Specific types of HAI (eg, bloodstream infections, surgical site infections)
      3) Specific pathogens (eg, respiratory virus infections, toxin-producing *Clostridium difficile*, multidrug-resistant microorganisms)
B. Other Strategic Surveillance Considerations
   1. Sensitivity and specificity of the case finding
   2. Adjustment for the risk of infection whenever possible
   3. Calculation of appropriate rates
   4. Audience and timing of feedback of the HAI rates to staff and administrators
V. Investigation of Clusters of Infection
   A. Clusters of HAIs Are Encountered Commonly
      1. Investigate to determine whether there is an outbreak
         a. Epidemiologic links
         b. Microbiologic factors
      2. Also investigate a single, highly unusual infection, such as a postoperative group A streptococcal infection
      3. Features of infections in a cluster of HAIs that suggest an outbreak
         a. Tightly clustered in space and time
         b. Caused by an uncommon microorganism
         c. Caused by a common microorganism with a distinctive antimicrobial susceptibility pattern
   B. Systematic Approach to Investigation of HAI Clusters
      1. Confirm each infection in the cluster
      2. Make a case definition
      3. Search for additional infections and record basic information on each case
      4. Prepare a preliminary line listing of relevant information
      5. Plot an epidemic curve
      6. Compare the infection rate during the cluster with the rate during a period before the cluster; if the rate during the cluster is significantly higher, an outbreak is likely occurring
      7. Communicate with leaders of relevant departments, the microbiology laboratory, and the hospital administration
      8. Record details of events in the investigation
      9. Review the medical literature to identify reports of similar outbreaks
      10. Review all cases in more detail and refine the line listing of relevant information
      11. Develop hypothesis about a likely reservoir and mode of transmission
      12. Institute temporary control measures as needed
      13. Perform an epidemiologic study (eg, case control or cohort study) to collect data to test the hypotheses
      14. Update control measures
      15. Document microbiologically the reservoir and mode of transmission, and confirm the relatedness of isolates with molecular genotyping techniques if necessary
      16. Determine the effectiveness of the control measures
      17. Write a report and distribute it to appropriate individuals
      18. Change policies and procedures if necessary
VI. Hand Hygiene, Standard Precautions, and Transmission-Based Precautions
   A. Modes of Transmission
      1. Mechanisms by which microorganisms are transferred from the reservoirs where they live and replicate to susceptible hosts (Table 3.1)

Table 3.1

Principal Modes of Transmission in Health Care Settings

Mode of Transmission	Examples	
	Infection	Source
Airborne	Pulmonary tuberculosis, measles, varicella[a]	Airborne droplet nuclei
Direct or indirect contact	*Clostridium difficile*–associated diarrhea MRSA skin or soft tissue infection	Infectious material, hands of caregivers, fomites
Droplet contact	Pertussis, adenovirus infection, invasive meningococcal disease	Large respiratory droplets

Abbreviation: MRSA, methicillin-resistant *Staphylococcus aureus*.

[a] Varicella may be spread by airborne transmission and by direct or indirect contact transmission.

2. Principal modes of transmission in health care settings
   a. Airborne
      1) Transfer of microorganisms on droplet nuclei
      2) *Droplet nuclei*: very small particles (<5 μm), light enough to be carried substantial distances on air currents
   b. Direct contact and indirect contact
      1) Direct contact transmission and indirect contact transmission are usually considered together
      2) Often difficult to distinguish between direct and indirect
   c. Droplet contact
      1) Transfer of microorganisms on large respiratory droplets, such as those generated by sneezing or coughing
      2) Travel only short distances
3. Other modes of transmission
   a. Endogenous transmission or *autoinfection*
      1) Transfer of a microorganism from a contaminated body site (ie, skin or gastrointestinal tract) to a sterile body site
      2) Usually a consequence of the use of an invasive device or procedure
   b. Common vehicle transmission
      1) Examples: contaminated blood products or intravenous fluids
      2) Rare but can lead to widespread infection
   c. Vector-borne transmission (rare in most health care settings)
4. Reservoirs of microorganisms often cannot be eliminated; therefore, use strategies to interrupt the principal modes of transmission in health care settings

B. Hand Hygiene
1. Hand hygiene is an essential practice to prevent transmission of infectious agents in any setting
   a. *Hand rubbing*: use of a waterless, alcohol-based (antiseptic) hand rub, gel, or foam
   b. *Hand washing*: scrubbing with soap (which may or may not contain antiseptic agents) and water
   c. *Surgical hand antisepsis* (ie, surgical scrub): preoperative hand rubbing or hand washing by surgical personnel with antiseptic agents that have persistent activity
2. Antiseptic agents in soaps: chlorhexidine, hexachlorophene, iodine, triclosan, chloroxylenol, and quaternary ammonium compounds
3. Hand hygiene is primarily intended to remove *transient flora*
   a. Microorganisms that colonize the superficial layers of skin
   b. Typical causes of HAIs (eg, *Staphylococcus aureus*, gram-negative bacilli)
4. Use of antiseptic agents decreases *resident flora*
   a. Microorganisms that colonize deeper skin structures
   b. Examples: coagulase-negative staphylococci, diphtheroids
5. Alcohol-based hand rubs
   a. Very effective in decreasing colony counts quickly (15-30 seconds)
   b. Magnitude of reduction depends on the type of alcohol, concentration, and formulation
   c. In combination with an appropriate moisturizer, they reduce skin dryness and irritation compared with hand washing
   d. Convenient and easy
6. Antiseptic agents with residual activity
   a. Examples: chlorhexidine, hexachlorophene
   b. Suppress growth of skin flora for hours after application
7. HICPAC guideline discusses indications and procedures for hand hygiene
   a. Before performing an invasive procedure
   b. Before and after other patient contact
   c. After contact with body fluids and substances, mucous membranes, nonintact skin, and objects and surfaces that are likely to be contaminated, including the immediate patient care environment
   d. After removing gloves
   e. Hand washing: to remove organic material and associated microorganisms when hands are visibly soiled
      1) Hand rubbing: when hands are not visibly soiled

C. Standard Precautions
1. Standard Precautions: a set of precautions, including hand hygiene, to be used for all patients at all times regardless of their diagnosis or presumed infection status
2. Synthesizes elements of 2 previous precautions systems
   a. Universal Precautions: developed in the mid 1980s in response to the human immunodeficiency virus (HIV) epidemic

b. Body Substance Isolation: developed in the late 1980s as a simpler alternative to the isolation precautions systems in use at that time
3. Purpose of Standard Precautions
   a. To protect health care workers from bloodborne pathogens
   b. To protect health care workers and patients from transmission of microorganisms from moist body substances and surfaces
      1) Blood and all body fluids
      2) Secretions and excretions (except sweat), regardless of whether they contain visible blood
      3) Mucous membranes
      4) Nonintact skin
4. Scope of Standard Precautions recommendations
   a. Practicing hand hygiene
   b. Using gloves, mask and eye protection (or face shield), and gowns, as needed, to prevent contact with body substances or surfaces
   c. Reducing environmental contamination
   d. Appropriately handling sharps, patient care equipment, and linen
D. Transmission-Based Precautions
   1. Transmission-Based Precautions: used with Standard Precautions
      a. To prevent transmission of contagious diseases (eg, tuberculosis, measles, varicella, pertussis)
      b. To prevent transmission of other epidemiologically important microorganisms (eg, toxin-producing *C difficile*, multidrug-resistant microorganisms) from infected or colonized patients
   2. HICPAC guideline describes precautions
   3. Three types of Transmission-Based Precautions to use alone or in combination, as indicated (Table 3.2)
      a. Airborne Precautions
      b. Droplet Precautions
      c. Contact Precautions
VII. Reprocessing of Reusable Patient Care Items
   A. Collaboration Between Departments and HAI Prevention and Control Programs
      1. To ensure appropriate reprocessing of reusable patient care items
      2. Highly technical process: standardized procedures, careful monitoring, and close supervision by skilled personnel
   B. Wide Range of Susceptibility (or Resistance) to Reprocessing Methods
      1. Prions
         a. Most resistant microorganisms (Figure 3.1)
         b. Inactivation requires special conditions of steam sterilization (higher temperature, longer exposure)
      2. *Mycobacteria*: more resistant than vegetative bacteria
      3. Small viruses: more resistant than medium to large viruses
      4. Viruses with nonlipid envelopes: more resistant than viruses with lipid envelopes
   C. Spaulding Approach to Disinfection and Sterilization
      1. Foundation for reprocessing methods for decades, although it has been expanded and refined extensively
      2. Three categories of items
         a. *Critical items*

Table 3.2
General Requirements of Transmission-Based Precautions[a]

		Need for Protective Covering		
Type of Precaution	Type of Room	Face Protection	Gown	Gloves
Airborne	Private with negative pressure	Fit-tested N95 mask or powered air-purifying respirator	None	None
Contact	Private	None	Yes, for contact with patient or environment	Yes, when clothing will have direct contact with patient or potentially contaminated environmental surfaces or equipment
Droplet	Private	Mask with eye protection	None	None

[a] Detailed recommendations are provided at http://www.cdc.gov/ncidod/dhqp/gl_isolation.html. Some infections, such as avian or pandemic influenza, may require additional precautions.

Resistant

Prions (Creutzfeldt-Jakob disease) — Prion reprocessing

Bacterial spores (*Bacillus atrophaeus*) — Sterilization

Coccidia (*Cryptosporidium*)

Mycobacteria (*Mycobacterium tuberculosis, Mycobacterium terrae*) — High

Viruses with nonlipid envelopes or small viruses (poliovirus, coxsackievirus) — Intermediate

Fungi (*Aspergillus, Candida*)

Vegetative bacteria (*Staphylococcus aureus, Pseudomonas aeruginosa*) — Low

Viruses with lipid envelopes or medium-sized viruses (human immunodeficiency virus, herpesvirus, hepatitis B virus)

Susceptible

Figure 3.1. Resistance of Microorganisms to Disinfection and Sterilization. Microorganisms are listed in decreasing order of resistance. (Adapted from Guideline for disinfection and sterilization in healthcare facilities, 2008 [Internet]. [cited 2009 Jun 10]. Available from: http://www.cdc.gov/ncidod/dhqp/pdf/guidelines/Disinfection_Nov_2008.pdf.)

1) Items that can cause infection if they are contaminated with microorganisms, even in very small amounts
2) These items have contact with sterile body fluids and sites
3) Sterilization is required for inactivation of all microorganisms, including any bacterial spores
  b. *Semicritical items*
   1) Items that can cause infection unless they are nearly free of microorganisms, except small numbers of bacterial spores
   2) These items have contact with mucous membranes or nonintact skin
   3) High-level disinfection (which will inactivate *Mycobacteria* and less-resistant microorganisms) is sufficient
  c. *Noncritical items*
   1) Items that are unlikely to cause infection even if contaminated by small numbers of microorganisms
   2) These items have contact with intact skin
   3) Low-level disinfection is sufficient (it will inactivate vegetative bacteria and large and medium-sized viruses or those with lipid envelopes)
 D. Other Factors Affecting Reprocessing Methods
  1. Degree of cleaning before reprocessing
   a. To decrease the number of contaminating microorganisms
   b. To remove organic matter, which may make reprocessing methods less effective
  2. Other variables that affect the efficacy of reprocessing methods: time, concentration, temperature, humidity, etc
  3. Probability that the reprocessed items will be damaged from reprocessing methods
  4. Turnaround time requirements for the items
 E. HICPAC Guideline on Disinfection and Sterilization
VIII. Environmental Sources of Infection
 A. Transmission of Microorganisms Causing HAIs
  1. Air, water, and environmental surfaces are rarely involved

2. Exception: airborne fungal spores and aerosols from plumbing systems heavily contaminated with *Legionella*
    a. Hazard for immunocompromised patients
    b. Particularly patients with severe neutropenia after cancer chemotherapy or stem cell transplant
  B. HICPAC Guideline on Environmental Infection Control
    1. Key approaches to minimizing environmental sources of infection
      a. System for evaluating environmental risks and monitoring for environmentally related HAIs (eg, fungal and *Legionella* pneumonia in immunocompromised hosts)
      b. Air-handling systems to provide appropriate air exchanges and circulation
      c. Dust-control procedures and barriers during construction, repair, renovation, or demolition, with air sampling to ensure effectiveness
      d. Prompt remediation of water system disruptions, water leaks, and natural disasters (eg, flooding)
      e. Proper design and maintenance of equipment that uses water from main lines (eg, water systems for hemodialysis, ice machines, hydrotherapy equipment, dental unit water lines, and automated endoscope reprocessors)
      f. Environmental surface cleaning and disinfection strategies for contamination by antibiotic-resistant microorganisms and *C difficile*
IX. Medical Waste Management
  A. Medical Waste
    1. Various types of waste have various risks
      a. Contaminated sharps (eg, needles, scalpel blades)
        1) Significant risk of injury and infection
        2) All sharps must be disposed of in designated, puncture-resistant containers
      b. Body-fluid specimens
        1) Microbiology waste (eg, cultures of microorganisms), pathology and anatomy waste, blood and blood products
        2) Require special processing
        3) Handling and disposal requirements may vary by jurisdiction
      c. Other contaminated, nonsharp waste items carry an extremely low risk of infection
  B. Proper Waste Management
    1. Appropriate procedures for separation and segregation of different types of waste
    2. Proper containment, handling, transport, storage, and disposal of waste
X. Employee and Occupational Health
  A. Health Care Workers
    1. Require protection from infectious risks inherent in patient care
    2. Patients and health care workers require protection from exposure to health care workers with communicable diseases
    3. Management and prevention strategies must be integrated
    4. Requires close collaboration
    5. Hospital infection prevention and control program
    6. Employee and occupational health department
  B. HICPAC Guideline on Infection Control in Health Care Workers
  C. Evaluation of Illnesses in Health Care Workers
    1. Symptoms that should prompt evaluation for contagious disease
      a. Persistent fever
      b. Conjunctivitis
      c. Skin lesions or rashes
      d. Diarrhea
      e. Persistent cough
    2. Conditions that should be investigated promptly and confirmed with laboratory tests if necessary
      a. Varicella
      b. Herpes zoster on an exposed area of the body
      c. Herpetic whitlow
      d. Adenoviral conjunctivitis
      e. Measles, mumps, rubella
      f. Pertussis
      g. Staphylococcal skin infection
      h. Enteric infection in a food service worker
      i. Active pulmonary tuberculosis
  D. Postexposure Evaluation and Management of Health Care Workers
    1. Evaluate promptly and systematically all exposures of health care workers to patients with infectious diseases
      a. Provide postexposure prophylaxis, if indicated
      b. Allay anxiety
      c. Avoid unnecessary interventions and loss of workdays
    2. Steps in process
      a. Confirm the infection involved in the exposure

b. Confirm that an exposure occurred, according to accepted criteria
c. Review the susceptibility of the exposed health care worker to infection and the risks of infection
d. Prescribe postexposure prophylaxis, as indicated
e. Restrict the health care worker from work, as indicated
f. Assess the risk of secondary exposure of other health care workers and patients
g. Perform follow-up evaluations, as indicated: determine whether infection occurred and, if so, whether it has resolved
h. Provide counseling, as needed
3. Specific postexposure prophylaxis regimens are discussed in several HICPAC and CDC publications
4. Significant exposure to bloodborne pathogen
   a. OSHA standard
      1) Hospitals must test the source patient for evidence of a bloodborne infection, when consent can be obtained
      2) Hospitals must provide postexposure prophylaxis in accordance with current recommendations
5. *Significant exposures*: percutaneous, mucous membrane, or nonintact skin exposure to tissue or various fluids
   a. Blood or other potentially infectious body fluids
      1) Cerebrospinal, pericardial, pleural, peritoneal, synovial, or amniotic fluid
      2) Semen or cervical or vaginal secretions
   b. Visibly bloody fluids, excretions, or secretions
6. Summary risk estimates
   a. Helpful in counseling persons after an exposure
   b. Several factors may affect the risk of infection in an individual case
      1) Level of viremia in the source patient
      2) Amount of blood involved in the exposure
      3) Nature of the exposure
7. Summary risk estimates for specific infections
   a. Hepatitis B virus
      1) After percutaneous exposure to blood
         a) For hepatitis B e antigen–negative blood: 23% to 37%
         b) For hepatitis B e antigen–positive blood: 37% to 62%
      2) After mucous membrane or nonintact skin exposure to blood: not well quantified, but infection can occur
   b. Hepatitis C virus
      1) After percutaneous exposure to blood: 1.8%
      2) After mucous membrane exposure to blood: not well quantified but rare
      3) After nonintact skin exposure to blood: no infection has been documented
   c. Human immunodeficiency virus
      1) After percutaneous exposure to blood: 0.3%
      2) After mucous membrane exposure to blood: 0.09%
8. Postexposure prophylaxis for hepatitis B virus infection: highly effective
   a. Hepatitis B immune globulin or hepatitis B vaccine (or both)
   b. As indicated by the source information and the vaccination and serologic status of the exposed health care worker
9. Postexposure prophylaxis for hepatitis C virus infection: none is effective
10. Postexposure prophylaxis for HIV: efficacy has not been established definitively
    a. Use of antiretroviral agents as postexposure prophylaxis
       1) Supported by several lines of evidence, including a case-control study conducted among exposed health care workers
       2) Is standard practice in the United States
    b. Evaluation, counseling, and treatment should be provided by experts using current guidelines
11. Persons exposed to active pulmonary tuberculosis
    a. Evaluate with purified protein derivative (PPD) skin testing if they do not have a history of PPD reactivity
       1) Administer skin test after the exposure and, if negative, 12 weeks later
       2) Skin test converters and persons with signs of active tuberculosis: treat according to published recommendations
       3) All skin tests should be administered and interpreted by trained personnel
    b. Exposure to tuberculosis may be unrecognized
       1) Hospitals should require health care workers to undergo periodic PPD skin testing

2) Baseline PPD skin test
   a) Use 2-step method to detect booster phenomenon (could be misinterpreted as skin test conversion)
   b) Test persons without a history of prior PPD reactivity and without a documented negative PPD within the preceding 12 months
3) Subsequent testing
   a) Use a single PPD skin test
   b) Frequency of testing dictated by risk of exposure
   c) Persons with a history of prior PPD reactivity: assess periodically for evidence of active disease
4) To ensure compliance, many hospitals require periodic skin tests as prerequisite for reappointment of physicians or continuing employment of other hospital staff

E. Prevention of Occupationally Acquired Infections in Health Care Workers
   1. Vaccination against infectious diseases is a highly cost-effective prevention strategy
   2. Hospitals should offer indicated vaccinations to health care workers
      a. Hepatitis B vaccine
      b. Measles, mumps, rubella vaccine
      c. Annual influenza vaccine
      d. Tetanus-diphtheria-acellular pertussis booster vaccine
      e. Varicella vaccine
   3. OSHA bloodborne pathogens standard mandates specific prevention measures
      a. Hepatitis B vaccination
      b. Development of exposure control plan that identifies employees with occupational risk of exposure to bloodborne pathogens
      c. Annual training for these persons on the risk of bloodborne infection and prevention measures
      d. Provision of personal protective clothing and equipment
      e. Work practice controls, including equipment and procedures for safe handling and disposal of sharps
      f. Procedures for identification, transportation, storage, and disposal of contaminated items and waste
   4. CDC guideline emphasizes hierarchy of prevention and control measures
      a. First level: implementation of administrative controls
         1) Effective written policies and protocols to ensure rapid identification, isolation, diagnostic evaluation, and treatment of persons likely to have tuberculosis
         2) Effective work practices among health care workers (eg, using and correctly wearing respiratory protection, keeping doors to isolation rooms closed)
         3) Educating, training, and counseling health care workers about tuberculosis
         4) Screening for *M tuberculosis* infection and disease among health care workers
      b. Second level: use of environmental controls
         1) Eliminate or decrease the concentration of droplet nuclei
         2) Control the amount, direction, and exhaust of ventilation systems
         3) Use high-efficiency particulate air (HEPA) filtration or ultraviolet irradiation
      c. Third level: respiratory protection controls
         1) Prevent the inhalation of droplet nuclei
         2) Impossible to eliminate infectious droplet nuclei in some areas of the hospital (eg, patient isolation rooms, treatment rooms where cough-inducing procedures are performed)
         3) Satisfactory particulate respirators
            a) National Institute for Occupational Safety and Health (NIOSH) certification of N95 or better
            b) Personal respirators with HEPA filtration
            c) Must be fit tested on the persons using them, according to OHSA standards

XI. Antimicrobial Resistance
   A. Health Care–Associated Infections Are Increasingly Caused by Antimicrobial-Resistant Organisms
      1. Methicillin-resistant *S aureus*
      2. Vancomycin-resistant *Enterococcus*
      3. Multidrug-resistant gram-negative bacilli
      4. HICPAC guideline provides recommendations for programs to control multidrug-resistant organisms
   B. Interventions
      1. Use of Contact Precautions
         a. During care of patients who are colonized or infected with these types of organisms
         b. Appropriate to reduce transmission to other patients

2. Active surveillance may be used to prospectively identify patients who are colonized with these organisms
3. Appropriate use of antimicrobial agents to control spread of antimicrobial resistance
4. Monitor trends in antimicrobial resistance
5. Apply interventions as indicated to control emergence and spread of these important pathogens

XII. Antimicrobial Stewardship
   A. Antimicrobial Use Contributes to Antimicrobial Resistance
      1. Extent to which the use of specific agents facilitates emergence and spread of particular organisms varies
      2. All facilities should encourage appropriate antimicrobial use
         a. Benefits: effective antimicrobial prophylaxis and treatment of individuals
         b. Risks: increasing the prevalence of antimicrobial resistance at the population level
   B. Facility Programs for Antimicrobial Stewardship
      1. Through HAI prevention and control program
      2. Through other departments
   C. Infectious Diseases Society of America Guideline
      1. Published in 2007 in *Clinical Infectious Diseases*
      2. Reviews the evidence for specific interventions
      3. Provides recommendations for key elements of program

Suggested Reading

Dellit TH, Owens RC, McGowan JE Jr, Gerding DN, Weinstein RA, Burke JP, et al; Infectious Diseases Society of America; Society for Healthcare Epidemiology of America. Infectious Diseases Society of America and the Society for Healthcare Epidemiology of America guidelines for developing an institutional program to enhance antimicrobial stewardship. Clin Infect Dis. 2007 Jan 15;44(2):159–77.

Guidelines for environmental infection control in health-care facilities: recommendations from CDC and the Healthcare Infection Control Practices Advisory Committee (HICPAC) [Internet]. [cited 2009 Jun 10]. Available from: http://www.cdc.gov/ncidod/dhqp/gl_environinfection.html.

Guideline for hand hygiene in healthcare settings: recommendations of the Healthcare Infection Control Practices Advisory Committee and the HICPAC/SHEA/APIC/IDSA Hand Hygiene Task Force [Internet]. [cited 2009 Jun 10]. Available from: http://www.cdc.gov/ncidod/dhqp/gl_handhygiene.html.

Guideline for isolation precautions: preventing transmission of infectious agents in healthcare settings 2007 [Internet]. [cited 2009 Jun 10]. Available from: http://www.cdc.gov/ncidod/dhqp/gl_isolation.html.

Guidelines for infection control in health care personnel, 1998 [Internet]. [cited 2009 Jun 10]. Available from: http://www.cdc.gov/ncidod/dhqp/gl_hcpersonnel.html.

Guidelines for preventing the transmission of *Mycobacterium tuberculosis* in health-care settings, 2005 [Internet]. [cited 2009 Jun 10]. Available from: http://www.cdc.gov/mmwr/preview/mmwrhtml/rr5417a1.htm.

Management of multidrug-resistant organisms in healthcare settings, 2006 [Internet]. [cited 2009 Jun 10]. Available from: http://www.cdc.gov/ncidod/dhqp/pdf/ar/mdroGuideline2006.pdf.

National Healthcare Safety Network [Internet]. [cited 2009 Jun 10]. Available from: http://www.cdc.gov/nhsn.

Scheckler WE, Brimhall D, Buck AS, Farr BM, Friedman C, Garibaldi RA, et al. Requirements for infrastructure and essential activities of infection control and epidemiology in hospitals: a consensus panel report. Society for Healthcare Epidemiology of America. Infect Control Hosp Epidemiol. 1998 Feb;19(2):114–24.

SHEA/IDSA HAI prevention compendium [Internet]. [cited 2009 Jun 10]. Available from: http://www.cdc.gov/ncidod/dhqp/HAI_shea_idsa.html.

Updated U.S. Public Health Service guidelines for the management of occupational exposures to HBV, HCV, and HIV and recommendations for postexposure prophylaxis [Internet]. [cited 2009 Jun 10]. Available from: http://www.cdc.gov/mmwr/preview/mmwrhtml/rr5011a1.htm.

Updated U.S. Public Health Service guidelines for the management of occupational exposures to HIV and recommendations for postexposure prophylaxis [Internet]. [cited 2009 Jun 10]. Available from: http://www.cdc.gov/mmwr/preview/mmwrhtml/rr5409a1.htm.

Matthew J. Binnicker, PhD
Glenn D. Roberts, PhD
Nancy L. Wengenack, PhD

Mycobacterial and Fungal Diagnostics

I. Classification of Mycobacteria
   A. *Mycobacterium tuberculosis* Complex (MTBC)
   B. Nontuberculous Mycobacteria (NTM)
      1. Slowly growing NTM
         a. Require more than 7 days to appear on solid media
         b. Examples: *Mycobacterium avium* complex, and *Mycobacterium kansasii*
      2. Rapidly growing NTM
         a. Require less than 7 days to appear on solid media
         b. Examples: *Mycobacterium fortuitum* complex, *Mycobacterium chelonae*, and *Mycobacterium abscessus*
      3. Noncultivatable NTM: *Mycobacterium leprae*
II. Laboratory Diagnosis of Tuberculosis
   A. Key Features of MTBC
      1. At the DNA level, MTBC members share more than 95% homology
      2. Identification of MTBC members to the species level requires spoligotyping or molecular method such as polymerase chain reaction (PCR)
      3. Members of MTBC
         a. *Mycobacterium tuberculosis*
            1) Most common member of MTBC causing tuberculosis (TB)
            2) Highest prevalence among homeless persons, prison inmates, the elderly, alcoholics, intravenous drug users, and persons born in countries other than the United States
            3) Human immunodeficiency virus (HIV) infection is greatest risk factor for progression to active TB
         b. *Mycobacterium bovis*
            1) Causes TB in warm-blooded animals
            2) Clinical presentation similar to that of *M tuberculosis*
            3) Inherent resistance to pyrazinamide
         c. *Mycobacterium bovis* bacille Calmette-Guérin (BCG)
            1) Attenuated in virulence through serial passage
            2) Used in some areas of the world for vaccination
         d. *Mycobacterium africanum*
            1) Causes TB in humans in tropical Africa
         e. *Mycobacterium microti*
            1) "Croissant-like" morphology in stained smears
            2) Often does not grow in culture
            3) TB in voles
         f. *Mycobacterium canettii*
            1) May be more prevalent in Africa
            2) Phenotypically different from other members of MTBC

B. Specimen Collection in the Diagnosis of TB
1. Appropriate specimens for the diagnosis of TB
   a. Sputum
      1) Most common specimen used in the diagnosis of pulmonary TB
      2) Collect early-morning, expectorated or induced sputum specimen on 3 consecutive days
   b. Other respiratory specimens
      1) Bronchoalveolar lavage
      2) Bronchial aspirate
      3) Lung biopsy
   c. Gastric aspirate
      1) Gastric aspirate is often the specimen of choice from children or from those unable to produce sputum
      2) Collect fasting, early-morning specimens on 3 consecutive days
      3) Specimen should be adjusted to neutral pH with sodium carbonate to prevent mycobacterial degradation from exposure to stomach acid
   d. Urine
      1) Collect midstream voided sample in a sterile container on 3 consecutive days
2. Additional specimens that may be submitted
   a. Tissue
   b. Aseptically collected body fluid (eg, cerebrospinal fluid, peritoneal, pleural)
   c. Stool
3. Inappropriate specimens for smear and culture
   a. Pooled sputum
   b. Pooled urine
   c. Fixed tissue

C. Laboratory Identification of *M tuberculosis*
1. Direct examination of specimens using acid-fast staining procedures and microscopy
   a. Rapid method of identifying patients who are highly contagious
   b. Termed *acid-fast bacilli* (AFB) because mycolic acid residues in the cell wall of mycobacteria retain the primary stain even after exposure to acid-alcohol or mineral acids
   c. A smear that is positive for AFB has at least 10^4 AFB per milliliter of sputum
   d. Staining methods
      1) Ziehl-Neelsen staining method: phenol and high temperature are used to promote penetration of the stain
      2) Carbolfuchsin stain (Figure 4.1)

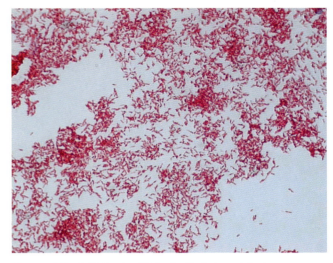

Figure 4.1. Acid-fast bacilli (carbolfuchsin, original magnification ×1,000).

      3) Auramine-rhodamine stain (Figure 4.2): fluorescent stain that enhances the sensitivity of direct smear examination
   e. Serpentine cording in direct examination of liquid media is characteristic of *M tuberculosis* but is not sufficient for identification
   f. Interpretation of smear microscopy
      1) Positive AFB results also occur with NTM
      2) Various nonmycobacterial organisms may exhibit acid-fast staining characteristics: *Nocardia* species, *Legionella micdadei*, *Rhodococcus*

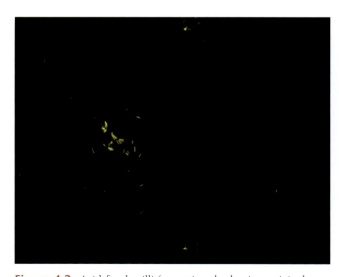

Figure 4.2. Acid-fast bacilli (auramine-rhodamine, original magnification ×1,000).

species, *Cryptosporidium*, *Cyclospora*, and *Isospora*
      3) Negative smear does not rule out TB
  2. Culture of *M tuberculosis* on solid media
     a. Growth in culture represents the gold standard for the diagnosis of TB
     b. May take 4 to 8 weeks for growth on standard solid culture media (eg, Löwenstein-Jensen culture medium)
     c. Identification in laboratory requires biosafety level 3 facility
     d. Colonies of *M tuberculosis* often exhibit a "rough and buff" phenotype
     e. Members of the MTBC are nonchromogens (nonpigmented in light and in darkness)
     f. Key phenotypic tests used in the identification of *M tuberculosis*
        1) Positive niacin accumulation
        2) Positive nitrate reduction
        3) Positive pyrazinamidase test: useful in distinguishing most *M tuberculosis* (positive result) from *M bovis* (negative result)
        4) Resistance to thiophene-2-carboxylic acid hydrazide test
        5) Negative 68°C catalase test
  3. Culture of *M tuberculosis* in liquid media
     a. Cultivation in broth media allows for more rapid growth and identification
     b. Several automated, continuously monitoring systems have been developed
        1) In broth media, mean time to detection for smear-positive specimens is generally 12 to 14 days
        2) Growth on solid media may require 4 to 8 weeks
  4. Molecular identification of *M tuberculosis* in culture
     a. Commercially available chemiluminescent DNA probes (eg, Gen-Probe AccuProbe) allow for rapid identification of culture isolates
        1) Target 16S ribosomal RNA
        2) Identifies to level of MTBC
  5. DNA sequencing
     a. Can be performed on extracts from liquid cultures or from colonies on solid media
        1) Target 16S ribosomal DNA or *hsp65* (heat shock protein)
        2) Identifies to level of MTBC
  6. Direct detection of MTBC in clinical specimens
     a. Several nucleic acid amplification tests (NAATs) are commercially available
        1) Amplified *M tuberculosis* direct (MTD) test
           a) Approved by US Food and Drug Administration (FDA) for both smear-positive and smear-negative respiratory specimens
        2) AMPLICOR MTB PCR assay for *M tuberculosis*
           a) FDA-approved for smear-positive respiratory specimens
     b. Limitations of NAATs
        1) May detect nonviable organisms after appropriate therapy
        2) Sensitivity results may be affected by inhibitors in the specimen
        3) Need culture for most susceptibilities to be performed
D. Immunodiagnostics for TB
  1. Mantoux tuberculin skin test (TST)
     a. Screening test to identify persons who are latently infected with TB
     b. Tuberculin purified protein derivative (0.1 mL) is injected intradermally
     c. Reaction is measured in millimeters of induration (not erythema) at 48 to 72 hours after the injection (Box 4.1)
     d. Limitations of TST
        1) False-positive reactions
           a) Infection with NTM
           b) BCG vaccination
           c) Improper TST administration or interpretation
        2) False-negative reactions
           a) Anergy in immunocompromised host
           b) Recent infection

Box 4.1

Interpretive Criteria for a Positive Tuberculin Skin Test Result: Cutoffs Among Groups of People

Induration ≥5 mm
  HIV-infected persons
  Persons with recent TB contact
  Immunosuppressed persons
  Persons with chest radiograph consistent with TB
Induration ≥10 mm
  Intravenous drug users
  Recent immigrants
  Laboratory personnel working with TB
  Infants and children
Induration ≥15 mm
  Any person

Abbreviations: HIV, human immunodeficiency virus; TB, tuberculosis.

c) Improper TST administration or interpretation
3) Boosted reactions possible from prior TST
2. QuantiFERON-TB Gold test
   a. In vitro whole blood test for use as an aid in diagnosing latent TB infection and tuberculous disease
   b. FDA approved in 2005
   c. Indirect test for MTBC
      1) Measures interferon-γ release from lymphocytes in response to a peptide cocktail simulating early secreted antigenic target 6 (ESAT-6) and culture filtrate protein 10 (CFP-10)
      2) ESAT-6 and CFP-10 are antigens that are present in *M tuberculosis* but absent in all BCG strains and most NTM
   d. Advantages of QuantiFERON-TB Gold test
      1) Requires only 1 patient visit
      2) Does not show "boost response"
      3) Is not subject to placement error or reader bias
      4) Is not affected by prior BCG vaccination
   e. Limitations of QuantiFERON-TB Gold test
      1) Can yield false-positive results with some NTM infections (eg, *M kansasii*, *Mycobacterium szulgai*, and *M marinum*)
      2) Limited data on use in children 17 years or younger, pregnant women, and immunocompromised hosts
E. Susceptibility Testing
   1. Recommendations
      a. Test the first isolate of *M tuberculosis* obtained from each individual
      b. Repeat susceptibility tests if cultures are still positive after 3 months of therapy or if the patient does not respond clinically
   2. Methods
      a. Agar proportion method
      b. Several automated, continuously monitoring systems that allow for growth and susceptibility testing in parallel
   3. Drugs to test
      a. First-line drugs recommended by the Clinical Laboratory Standards Institute (CLSI): isoniazid, rifampin, ethambutol, and pyrazinamide
      b. Streptomycin is considered a second-line drug for TB
III. Laboratory Diagnosis of NTM
   A. Key Features of NTM
      1. Ubiquitous environmental organisms
      2. More than 100 valid species, most of which have been reported to cause disease in humans (some in single case reports only)
      3. Infection occurs through inhalation, ingestion, or direct contact
      4. No person-to-person spread
      5. Common colonizers or contaminants (American Thoracic Society requires >1 positive culture for diagnosis)
      6. Runyon classification
         a. Slowly growing NTM
            1) Photochromogens: nonpigmented in the absence of light; pigment develops when exposed to light
               a) *Mycobacterium kansasii*: pulmonary disease similar in presentation to TB
               b) *Mycobacterium marinum*: exposure to fresh and saltwater, fish tank granulomas; "sporotrichoid-like" lesions
            2) Scotochromogens: always pigmented
               a) *Mycobacterium scrofulaceum*: cervical lymphadenopathy in children
               b) *Mycobacterium xenopi*: required elevated temperature for growth (42°C); associated with hot water tanks
               c) *Mycobacterium gordonae*: most commonly encountered species and common contaminant; occasionally pathogenic in immunocompromised hosts
            3) Nonchromogens: never pigmented
               a) *Mycobacterium avium* complex
                  i) *Mycobacterium avium*
                  ii) *Mycobacterium intracellulare*
                  iii) Other subspecies (eg, MAC-X)
                  iv) Pulmonary disease strongly associated with decreased cellular immunity (AIDS)
                  v) Most common mycobacterial disease in the United States
                  vi) Can be a colonizer or a contaminant
               b) *Mycobacterium genavense*: difficult to grow; requires mycobactin J supplement
               c) *Mycobacterium haemophilum*: associated with cervical lymphadenopathy, especially in children; grows at lower temperatures (30°C) and requires X factor (hemin) in cultures

d) *Mycobacterium ulcerans*: causes Buruli ulcer (mainly in Africa), grows at lower temperatures (30°C), and is highly drug resistant
   b. Rapidly growing NTM
      1) From traumatic implantation, surgical infections, or line infections
      2) *Mycobacterium fortuitum*
      3) *Mycobacterium chelonae*: often nodular skin disease
      4) *Mycobacterium abscessus*: often pulmonary infection
      5) *Mycobacterium smegmatis*: often nonpathogenic
   7. Noncultivatable NTM: leprosy
      a. Called also Hansen disease
      b. Caused by *M leprae*, noncultivatable; diagnosis by visualization of AFB in pathology sections, growth in mouse footpad (extremely slow, >6 months), or PCR at specialized centers
      c. Hypopigmented skin patches, gradual destruction of tissue with loss of sensation
      d. *Tuberculoid leprosy* is synonymous with *paucibacillary leprosy*; localized form
      e. *Lepromatous leprosy* is synonymous with *multibacillary leprosy*; disseminated form
B. Diagnostic Tools for NTM
   1. Direct examination of specimens using acid-fast staining procedures and microscopy
      a. Positive smear: at least 10^4 AFB per milliliter of sputum
      b. Staining methods
         1) Ziehl-Neelsen
         2) Carbolfuchsin
         3) Auramine-rhodamine: preferred for direct examinations; most sensitive since fluorescence allows for detection of AFB in the presence of large amounts of background material found in sputa
      c. Interpretation of smear microscopy
         1) Smear is nonspecific; cannot distinguish between MTBC and NTM
         2) Acid-fast staining characteristics may be seen with various nonmycobacterial organisms, including *Nocardia* species, *Legionella micdadei*, *Rhodococcus* species, *Cryptosporidium*, *Cyclospora*, and *Isospora*
         3) Negative smear does not rule out mycobacterial disease
   2. Culture of NTM
      a. Repeated isolation from clinical material represents the gold standard for the diagnosis of NTM infection
      b. May take 4 to 8 weeks for growth on standard solid culture media (eg, Löwenstein-Jensen or Middlebrook media)
      c. Cultivation in broth media allows for more rapid growth and identification
      d. Several automated, continuously monitoring systems have been developed
      e. Several difficult-to-cultivate species require incubation at alternative temperatures (*M xenopi*, *M ulcerans*, and *M haemophilum*) or additives (*M haemophilum*, *M genavense*, and *Mycobacterium paratuberculosis*)
   3. Molecular identification of NTM from culture
      a. Commercially available chemiluminescent DNA probes (eg, AccuProbe) allow for rapid identification of culture isolates
         1) Target 16S rRNA
         2) Identifies *M gordonae*, *M avium* complex, *M avium*, *M intracellulare*, and *M kansasii*
   4. DNA sequencing: performed directly or on extracts from either liquid cultures or colonies on solid media
      a. Common targets are 16S rDNA or *hsp65* (heat shock protein)
      b. Identifies most NTM to the species level in about 24 hours after growth in culture
   5. Other methods of NTM identification
      a. High-performance liquid chromatography (HPLC)
         1) Analyzes mycolic acid content of cell wall
         2) Limitation: mycolic acid content of all NTM species has not been characterized
      b. PCR restriction endonuclease analysis (PRA)
         1) PCR followed by fragmentation of DNA with restriction enzymes
         2) Visualize fragment size on gel; patterns are used to identify species
         3) Complex procedure; patterns are not defined for all species
      c. Reverse hybridization probe (line probe) assays
         1) Use PCR on target DNA (16S region or intergenic spacer region of 16S-23S region)
         2) Hybridize target DNA to nitrocellulose strip containing individual probes for 16 NTM species
      d. PCR: individual methods are available for a limited number of NTM species

6. Susceptibility testing of NTMs
    a. Slowly growing NTM
        1) Not routinely recommended
        2) Perform when therapy is failing or to obtain baseline pattern from clinically significant specimen sources
        3) Broth dilution or E test methods available
        4) Minimum inhibitory concentrations (MICs) available for only selected species: *M avium* complex, *M kansasii*, and *M marinum*
    b. Rapidly growing NTM
        1) Recommended panel of drugs and MIC break points are available from CLSI
        2) Broth dilution method

IV. Diagnosis of Fungi
    A. Common Diagnostic Tools for Identification of Fungi
        1. Of the thousands of species of fungi, only about 200 are recognized as causing disease in humans
        2. Stains for fungi
            a. Potassium hydroxide (KOH) and calcofluor white
                1) KOH: digests proteinaceious material present in specimen
                2) Calcofluor white: binds chitin of fungal cell wall
            b. Gomori methenamine silver (GMS); also called methenamine silver stain
            c. Periodic acid-Schiff (PAS)
            d. Lactophenol-aniline blue
        3. Culture media
            a. Inhibitory mold agar: contains chloramphenicol; inhibits wide range of gram-positive and gram-negative organisms
            b. Sabouraud dextrose (SAB) agar
                1) SAB agar with gentamicin: used primarily for respiratory sources that can be heavily contaminated with bacteria
                2) SAB agar with cycloheximide: inhibits rapidly growing saphrophytic fungi that can overgrow slower-growing pathogens (eg, *Histoplasma capsulatum*, *Blastomyces dermatitidis*); inhibits some important pathogens (Zygomycetes, *Pseudallescheria boydii*, some *Aspergillus*, and *Candida* species)
        4. Macroscopic characterization
            a. Colony morphology (color on front and reverse, texture, pigment production in media)
        5. Microscopic morphology
            a. Visualization of hyphae, macroconidia, and microconidia
            b. Cornmeal morphology
        6. Phenotypic methods for fungi identification
            a. Substrate use (API strips and Vitek Yeast Biochemical Card)
        7. Molecular identification of fungi from culture
            a. Commercially available, FDA-approved chemiluminescent DNA probes (Gen-Probe AccuProbe) allow for rapid identification of culture isolates
            b. Identify *H capsulatum*, *B dermatitidis*, *Coccidioides immitis*
        8. Antigen detection
            a. *Aspergillus*: commercially available, FDA-approved assay (Platelia *Aspergillus* galactomannan antigen test) allows for rapid identification of possible invasive aspergillosis with serum or bronchoalveolar lavage fluid
                1) Patients with possible invasive aspergillosis should be monitored twice weekly with this assay
                2) May be used to monitor response to therapy: antigen levels typically decrease after treatment
                3) Causes of false-positive results
                    a) Infection with *Histoplasma*, *Penicillium*, *Paecilomyces*, or *Alternaria* species
                    b) Treatment with semisynthetic antibiotics (eg, piperacillin, amoxicillin, augmentin)
                    c) Use of Plasma-Lyte for intravenous hydration
            b. *Histoplasma*: antigen detection in urine, serum, or bronchoalveolar lavage fluid for the diagnosis of disseminated histoplasmosis
                1) May be used to monitor response to therapy: antigen levels typically decrease after treatment
                2) Cross reactivity occurs in patients who have other dimorphic fungal infections (eg, blastomycosis, coccidioidomycosis)
            c. Detection of (1,3)-β-D-glucan in serum samples: commercially available, FDA-approved assay (Fungitell) for diagnosis of invasive fungal infection
                1) Assay detects (1,3)-β-D-glucan produced by several organisms
                    a) *Candida* species
                    b) *Aspergillus* species
                    c) *Fusarium* species

            d) *Trichosporon* species
            e) *Saccharomyces cerevisiae*
            f) *Acremonium*
            g) *Coccidioides immitis*
            h) *Histoplasma capsulatum*
            i) *Sporothrix schenckii*
            j) *Blastomyces dermatitidis*
            k) *Pneumocystis jiroveci*
        2) Assay does *not* detect infections caused by *Cryptococcus* species or Zygomycetes, which are not known to produce (1,3)-β-D-glucan
    9. DNA sequencing
        a. Can be performed directly or on extracts from liquid cultures or from colonies on solid media
        b. Common target is D2 region of the large ribosomal subunit or the internal transcribed spacer region
B. Superficial and Cutaneous Mycoses
    1. Tinea nigra
        a. Pigmented lesions of hands and feet (darkly pigmented hyphae)
        b. Tropical areas
        c. Etiologic agent: *Hortaea werneckii*
    2. Black piedra
        a. Infection of scalp hair shaft
        b. Dark brown to black nodules on hair shaft
        c. Hard nodule contains ascospores
        d. Etiologic agent: *Piedraia hortae*
    3. White piedra
        a. Etiologic agent: *Trichosporon asahii*
        b. White nodules on hair shaft of facial, axillary, and genital regions
        c. Visualization of nodules; microscopic examination of arthroconidia
    4. Tinea versicolor
        a. Etiologic agent: *Malessezia furfur*
        b. Smooth, hyperpigmented or hypopigmented lesion of the trunk
        c. Microscopic hyphal fragments and yeast cells seen ("spaghetti and meatballs" appearance) (Figure 4.3)
        d. Culture requires lipid overlay for *M furfur* growth
        e. Common skin flora; infections in patients receiving intralipid therapy and in patients with AIDS
    5. Dermatophytes
        a. Tinea (popularly called ringworm)
            1) Tinea capitis: scalp, eyebrows, and eyelashes; *Trichophyton tonsurans* is the most common cause in the United States

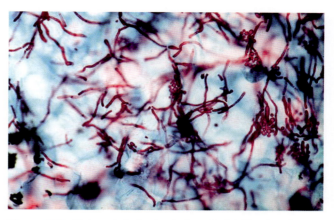

Figure 4.3. *Malessezia furfur* (periodic acid-Schiff, original magnification ×400). (Adapted from Koneman EW. Practical laboratory mycology. 3rd ed. Baltimore [MD]: Williams & Wilkins; c1985. p. 33. Used with permission.)

            2) Tinea barbae: beard; *Trichophyton mentagrophytes* or *Trichophyton verrucosum*
            3) Tinea corporis: smooth or glabrous skin; *Microsporum canis* or *Trichophyton rubrum*
            4) Tinea cruris: groin; *T rubrum* or *Epidermophyton floccosum* most commonly
            5) Tinea pedis: foot; *T mentagrophytes* or *T rubrum*
            6) Tinea unguium: nails (also known as onychomycosis); *T rubrum* or *T mentagrophytes*
        b. Trichophyton
            1) Most common genus causing dermatophyte infections
            2) *Trichophyton rubrum*, *T mentagrophytes*, and *T tonsurans*
            3) Numerous microconidia or smooth-walled, pencil-shaped macroconidia (or both)
        c. Microsporum
            1) Large rough-walled macroconidia and few microconidia
        d. Epidermophyton
            1) Club-shaped macroconidia with 1 to 3 cells and no microconidia
        e. Diagnostics
            1) KOH wet preparation
            2) Culture confirmation necessary
C. Subcutaneous Fungal Infections
    1. Sporotrichosis
        a. Chronic nodular and ulcerative lesions along the lymphatics; suppurative and granulomatous tissue response; dissemination is rare

b. Rose gardener's disease
   c. Etiologic agent: *Sporothrix schenckii*
   d. Dimorphic (mold at 25°C, yeast at 37°C and in tissue)
   e. Mold form has cluster of conidia like a floret
   f. Yeast form: spherical, oval, or cigar-shaped cells (Figure 4.4)
 2. Chromoblastomycosis
   a. Chronic infection of skin and subcutaneous tissue characterized by formation of slow-growing cauliflower-like, warty nodules or plaques
   b. Common in tropics (warm, moist environment; barefoot people); may be acquired by traumatic implantation
   c. Pigmented (dematiaceous) fungi
      1) *Fonsecaea* species: principal cause in the Americas
      2) *Cladosporium* species
      3) *Exophiala* species
      4) *Cladophialophora bantiana*
      5) *Phialophora* species
   d. Brown sclerotic bodies (copper pennies) divided by horizontal and vertical septations
 3. Eumycotic mycetoma
   a. Tropics
   b. Mycetoma: localized, chronic, granulomatous, infectious process involving cutaneous or subcutaneous tissue
   c. *Acremonium*, *Fusarium*, *Madurella*, *Exophiala*, and *Scedosporium*
   d. Most common cause in North America is *P boydii*

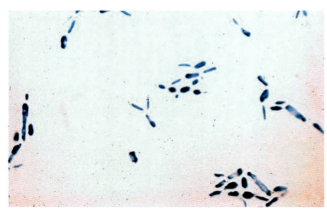

Figure 4.4. *Sporothrix schenckii* (lactophenol aniline blue, original magnification ×400.) (Adapted from Koneman EW. Practical laboratory mycology. 3rd ed. Baltimore [MD]: Williams & Wilkins; c1985. p. 141. Used with permission.)

   e. Dematiaceous (black grain) hyphae or hyaline (white grain); large thick-walled chlamydoconidia are often present; hyphae are often embedded in cement-like material; Splendore-Hoeppli material is often interdigitated
   f. Infected through percutaneous implantation of the etiologic agent
   g. Foot and hand are most common; also back, shoulders, and chest
   h. Diagnosis: demonstration of grains or granules in draining sinus tracts or expressed from mycetoma; tumor-like appearance (Madura foot)
 4. Phaeohyphomycosis
   a. Black molds appear as dark-walled irregular hyphal and yeastlike forms in tissue
   b. Pleomorphic hyphae and chlamydoconidia: *Exophiala jeanselmei*, *Exophiala dermatitidis*, *Bipolaris* species, *Exserohilum*, *Curvularia*, and *Alternaria*
   c. Commonly a single inflammatory cyst; usually painless
   d. Traumatic implantation
D. Systemic Fungal Infections
 1. Blastomycosis
   a. *Blastomyces dermatitidis*
   b. Endemic in Mississippi, Missouri, and Ohio river valleys
   c. Associated with aerosolization of the organism from soil and wood near water
   d. Dimorphic
      1) Yeast: broad-based, budding cells; 8 to 15 μm; double refractile cell wall (Figure 4.5)
      2) Mold: pear-shaped conidia on single stalks (lollipop appearance) (Figure 4.6); in vitro conversion to yeast form or nucleic acid probes useful for identification
      3) Easily seen on KOH preparation from skin
      4) Serology: immunodiffusion and complement fixation detect less than 50% of cases
 2. Coccidioidomycosis
   a. *Coccidioides immitis* and *Coccidioides posadasii*
   b. Endemic in San Joaquin Valley of California (valley fever), southwestern states (Arizona and New Mexico), South America, and Central America
   c. Associated with semi-arid desert regions; acquired by inhalation of arthroconidia

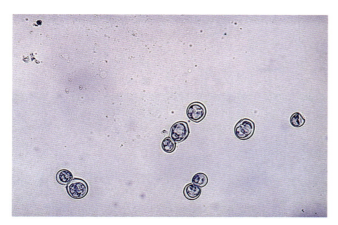

Figure 4.5. *Blastomyces dermatitidis*, yeast form (lactophenol aniline blue, original magnification ×500). (Adapted from Forbes BA, Sahm DF, Weissfeld AS. Bailey & Scott's diagnostic microbiology. 11th ed. St. Louis [MO]: Mosby; c2002. p. 761. Used with permission.)

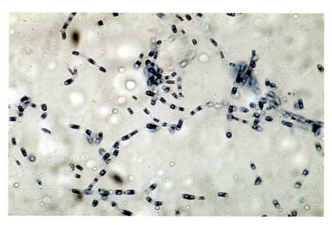

Figure 4.7. *Coccidioides* species, arthroconidia (lactophenol aniline blue, original magnification ×400).

    d. Associated activities: construction, dust storms, archeologic digs, and any other activities that aerosolize soil
    e. Dimorphic
       1) Mold: alternate arthroconidia (infectious form) (Figure 4.7)
       2) Spherule form: found in tissue (40-100 μm); spherule contains endospores; granulomatous; suppurative when endospores are released (Figure 4.8)
    f. Detection
       1) Direct visualization of spherule in KOH or histopathology
       2) Hyphae in cavitary lesions
       3) Culture: rapid growth (3-5 days); nucleic acid hybridization probe
       4) Serology: complement fixation (titer ≥1:2) and immunodiffusion detect 90% of primary symptomatic cases
  3. Histoplasmosis
    a. *Histoplasma capsulatum* var *capsulatum*; *H capsulatum* var *duboisii* in Africa
    b. Endemic in Mississippi, Missouri, and Ohio river valleys; Central America; and South America
    c. Associated with caves, construction sites, bird roosting sites
    d. Acquired by inhalation of microconidia and hyphal fragments
    e. Dimorphic

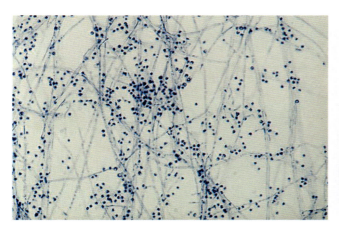

Figure 4.6. *Blastomyces dermatitidis*, mold form (lactophenol aniline blue, original magnification ×400). (Adapted from Forbes BA, Sahm DF, Weissfeld AS. Bailey & Scott's diagnostic microbiology. 11th ed. St. Louis [MO]: Mosby; c2002. p. 764. Used with permission.)

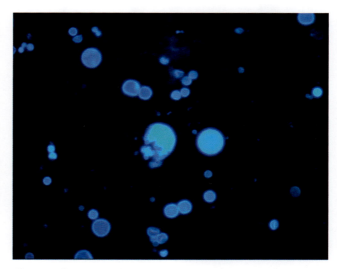

Figure 4.8. *Coccidioides* species, spherule form (calcofluor white, original magnification ×400).

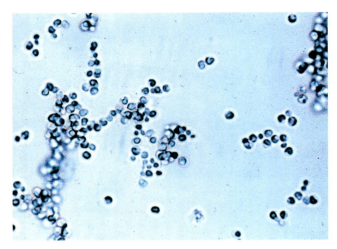

Figure 4.9. *Histoplasma capsulatum,* yeast form (lactophenol aniline blue, original magnification ×400). (Adapted from Dolan CT, Funkhouser JW, Koneman EW, Miller NG, Roberts GD. Atlas of clinical mycology. Chicago [IL]: American Society of Clinical Pathologists, Commission on Continuing Education; c1975. Slide 24. Used with permission.)

        1) Small (2-5 μm), intracellular, narrow-necked budding yeast (Figure 4.9)
        2) Mold: tuberculate macroconidia and microconidia (Figure 4.10)
   f. Optimal sources for culture: bone marrow and blood
   g. Granulomatous response
   h. May take days to weeks for growth in culture

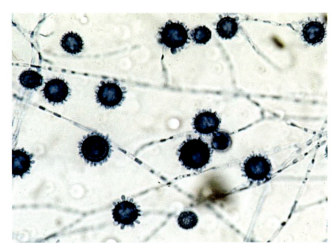

Figure 4.10. *Histoplasma capsulatum,* tuberculate macroconidia (lactophenol aniline blue, original magnification ×400). (Adapted from Forbes BA, Sahm DF, Weissfeld AS. Bailey & Scott's diagnostic microbiology. 11th ed. St. Louis [MO]: Mosby; c2002. p. 765. Used with permission.)

   i. Diagnosis by nucleic acid hybridization probe from culture
   j. Direct visualization is not diagnostic owing to potential for confusion with other yeast (eg, *Candida glabrata*)
   k. PCR is promising for diagnosis
   l. Serology
        1) Complement fixation: titer of 1:32 or more is associated with active infection
        2) Immunodiffusion: present together, H and M bands indicate active infection; M band alone indicates active infection or past infection
        3) Urine antigen test: more than 1 enzyme immunoassay unit is highly sensitive for disseminated disease; cross-reactions occur frequently with other fungi (eg, *Blastomyces*)
4. Paracoccidioidomycosis
   a. *Paracoccidioides brasiliensis*
   b. Endemic to Central America and South America
   c. Acquired by contact with vegetation and wood
   d. Inhalation or traumatic implantation
   e. Dimorphic
        1) Yeast: central bud with numerous peripheral buds resembling a ship's wheel; 5 to 60 μm
        2) Tissue response: granulomatous and suppurative
        3) Mold: slowly growing colonies; resembles *Blastomyces* mold form
        4) In vitro conversion from mold to yeast is readily accomplished
   f. Serology: *Blastomyces* nucleic acid probe cross-reacts with *Paracoccidioides* as indirect method of detection
5. Penicilliosis
   a. *Penicillium marneffei*
   b. Endemic in southeastern Asia (in rice paddies and the bamboo rat)
   c. Found exclusively in immunocompromised patients (eg, patients with HIV)
   d. Blood and bone marrow
   e. Dimorphic
        1) Yeast: reproduces by binary fission (2 cells with single septation) (Figure 4.11)
        2) Mold: reverse of colony produces red diffusible pigment
E. Opportunistic Fungal Infections
   1. Aspergillosis

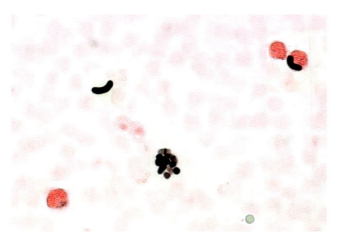

Figure 4.11. *Penicillium marneffei* (Gomori methenamine silver, original magnification ×500).

   a. *Aspergillus fumigatus*: blue-green to gray-green; some isolates may be white; fruiting heads are uniserate; phialides cover surface of the upper half to two-thirds of the vesicle
   b. *Aspergillus niger*: colonies are black, reverse is often yellow; fruiting heads are biserate; phialides cover entire surface of spherical vesicle; conidia are black and often rough
   c. *Aspergillus flavus*: colonies are yellow to green and rapidly growing; fruiting heads may be uniserate or biserate or both; phialides cover entire surface of the vesicle
   d. *Aspergillus terreus*: colonies are cinnamon to brown; fruiting heads are biserate; phialides cover entire surface of hemispherical vesicle; aleuriospores may be found on submerged hyphae
   e. KOH preparation or histopathology shows dichotomous branching (45° branches) and septate hyphae with parallel walls
   f. Serology: galactomannan antigen found in *Aspergillus* cell wall; serial positive specimens necessary owing to high false-positive rate (Zosyn, food, and Plasma-Lyte)
2. Other hyaline molds
   a. *Fusarium*: highly resistant to amphotericin B
   b. *Acremonium*
   c. *Scopulariopsis*
   d. *Paecilomyces lilacinus*
3. Dematiacious molds
   a. *Bipolaris*
   b. *Drechslera*
   c. *Curvularia*
   d. *Alternaria*: sinusitis; can cause disseminated disease
4. Zygomycosis
   a. Most common: *Rhizopus*, *Mucor*, and *Absidia*
   b. Pauciseptate, ribbon-like hyphae; often fragmented; nonparallel walls, irregular branching (often 90°) (Figure 4.12)
   c. Distinguished by identification of characteristic sporangia or sporangiospores and the presence or absence of rhizoids on submerged hyphae
   d. Rapidly growing (may push up lid of Petri dish); highly angioinvasive
   e. It is the only fungal infection considered to be a medical emergency
5. Yeasts
   a. Candida
      1) Oval to round budding yeast; pseudohyphae and true hyphae
      2) Suppurative infection
      3) Identification: biochemical profiles and microscopic features
      4) *Candida albicans*: most common species; positive results on germ tube test; produces pseudohyphae
      5) *Candida tropicalis*
      6) *Candida glabrata*: often fluconazole resistant
      7) *Candida parapsilosis*
      8) *Candida lusitaniae*
      9) *Candida guilliermondii*
      10) Endogenous organism; normal flora of skin and gastrointestinal, genitourinary, and respiratory tracts
      11) Serology is generally not useful

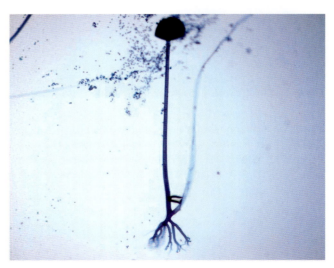

Figure 4.12. Zygomycetes (lactophenol aniline blue, original magnification ×100).

b. Cryptococcus
1) Species
    a) *Cryptococcus neoformans* (var *neoformans* or var *grubii*) is primary species responsible for disease in patients with AIDS or other immune dysfunction
    b) *Cryptococcus neoformans* var *gatti* causes meningoencephalitis and pulmonary cryptococcosis in healthy hosts
    c) Other species (*Cryptococcus albidus*, *Cryptococcus laurentii*, etc) are not usually associated with disease
2) Round and small with variation in size (2-5 μm); budding; can have polysaccharide capsule (Figure 4.13); produces urease; pigment production on Niger (birdseed) agar
3) India ink capsule stain: insensitive
    a) Detects less than 50% in nonimmunocompromised patients
    b) Detects more than 50% in immunocompromised patients
4) Associated with pigeons and bats
5) Marked predilection for central nervous system
6) Identification based on morphology and biochemical profile
7) Serology: latex agglutination test for antigen is highly sensitive and specific for disseminated disease and meningitis
8) Tissue response: generally inert; granulomatous in some instances

6. Pneumocystis
   a. *Pneumocystis jiroveci* (formerly *Pneumocystis carinii*)
   b. *Pneumocystis jiroveci* pneumonia (PCP)
   c. Cannot be routinely cultured
   d. Seen in immunocompromised patients; can be a colonizer
   e. Detection
      1) Cyst form with extracystic bodies seen in clinical specimen
      2) Stain with Gomori methenamine silver stain, calcofluor white
      3) May be difficult to distinguish from *Histoplasma* by stain
      4) Molecular methods available: PCR

Suggested Reading

Mazurek GH, Jereb J, Lobue P, Iademarco MF, Metchock B, Vernon A; Division of Tuberculosis Elimination, National Center for HIV, STD, and TB Prevention, Centers for Disease Control and Prevention (CDC). Guidelines for using the QuantiFERON-TB Gold test for detecting *Mycobacterium tuberculosis* infection, United States. MMWR Recomm Rep. 2005 Dec 16;54(RR-15):49–55. Erratum in: MMWR Morb Mortal Wkly Rep. 2005 Dec 23;54(50):1288.

Pfyffer GE. *Mycobacterium*: general characteristics, laboratory detection, and staining procedures. In: Murray PR, Baron EJ, Jorgensen JH, Landry ML, Pfaller MA, editors. Manual of clinical microbiology. 9th ed. Washington (DC): ASM Press; c2007. p. 543–72.

Vincent V, Gutierrez MC. *Mycobacterium*: laboratory characteristics of slowly growing Mycobacteria. In: Murray PR, Baron EJ, Jorgensen JH, Landry ML, Pfaller MA, editors. Manual of clinical microbiology. 9th ed. Washington (DC): ASM Press; c2007. p. 573–88.

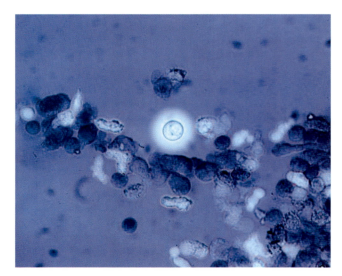

Figure 4.13. *Cryptococcus neoformans*, with polysaccharide capsule (India ink, original magnification ×400). (Adapted from Balows A, Hausler WJ Jr, Herrmann KL, Isenberg HD, Shadomy HJ, editors. Manual of clinical microbiology. 5th ed. Washington [DC]: ASM Press; c1991. p. 595. Used with permission.)

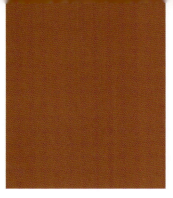

General
Questions and Answers

Questions

Multiple Choice (choose the best answer)

1. A 24-year-old woman who has tested positive for human immunodeficiency virus (HIV) presents to your office with mild fever and symptoms of an upper respiratory tract infection. She is currently in her 26th week of pregnancy and has a recent positive tuberculin skin test (TST) conversion with a 22-mm induration. Additionally, she has genital ulcerative lesions that test positive for herpes simplex virus. Which antimicrobial agent should you avoid prescribing for this patient?
   a. Acyclovir
   b. Amoxicillin
   c. Tetracycline
   d. Azithromycin
   e. Isoniazid

2. A 41-year-old man complains of a productive cough for the past 2 days with general malaise and fever up to 37.8°C. Chest radiography shows a right mid-lung infiltrate. A sputum sample is collected and the Gram stain shows many white blood cells, no epithelial cells, and many gram-positive diplococci. The culture results are pending. The patient states that 4 years ago he had a penicillin reaction that consisted of laryngeal edema, wheezing, and breathing problems that required emergent medical treatment. Which of the following is the most appropriate outpatient antimicrobial agent to use in this patient?
   a. Cefuroxime axetil
   b. Amoxicillin-clavulanate
   c. Meropenem
   d. Ciprofloxacin
   e. Moxifloxacin

3. A 57-year-old woman reports 3 days of dysuria and right-sided flank pain. In your office, her temperature is 38.4°C. On further questioning, she describes previous urinary tract infections with similar symptoms and a history of calcium oxalate renal stones in the right kidney and ureteral tract. Her most recent urinary infection was approximately 2 weeks ago for which she received a 3-day supply of an antibiotic. Her previous urine culture grew more than 10^5 colony-forming units/mL *Enterococcus faecalis*. You are concerned that enterococcus is again the most likely urinary pathogen. Which of the following drugs is *not* active against *E faecalis*?
   a. Vancomycin
   b. Cefazolin
   c. Ampicillin
   d. Piperacillin-tazobactam
   e. Linezolid

4. A 51-year-old woman who had been receiving chemotherapy through a surgically placed central catheter for acute myelogenous leukemia was admitted to the hospital

for management of a presumed line-related infection. Blood cultures begun at admission are now growing a coagulase-negative, oxacillin-resistant staphylococcus. Intravenous vancomycin is administered, but approximately 20 minutes into the infusion of the first dose, a diffuse "flushing-like" red rash develops over the patient's face, neck, and torso. The infusion is stopped and within an hour the rash has disappeared. What should you do next?
   a. Discontinue use of vancomycin, and give chloramphenicol.
   b. Discontinue use of vancomycin, and give nafcillin and rifampin.
   c. Continue use of vancomycin, but first give antihistamine and corticosteroids.
   d. Continue use of vancomycin, but use a slower infusion rate.
   e. Discontinue use of vancomycin, and observe the patient without giving any antibiotics.

5. What is the preferred method for hand hygiene during routine patient care?
   a. Hand washing with plain soap and water
   b. Hand washing with antimicrobial soap and water
   c. Hand rubbing with an alcohol-based, waterless product
   d. Either hand washing or hand rubbing
   e. Surgical scrub

6. What is the first step in conducting an investigation of a possible cluster of health care–associated infections?
   a. Perform molecular typing of the isolates.
   b. Confirm each infection in the cluster.
   c. Develop a hypothesis about a likely reservoir and mode of transmission.
   d. Institute control measures.
   e. Write a report and distribute it to appropriate individuals.

7. Which statement about Standard Precautions is correct?
   a. It is designed to protect health care workers from transmission of bloodborne pathogens only.
   b. It applies to patients with specific infections only.
   c. It does not include use of gloves, mask and eye protection (or a face shield), or gowns.
   d. It applies to potential contact with moist body surfaces and substances (except sweat).
   e. It does not include recommendations for reducing environmental contamination.

8. How does the risk of infection for a health care worker after a needlestick injury compare (from greatest to least risk) for hepatitis B virus (HBV), hepatitis C virus (HCV), and human immunodeficiency virus (HIV)?
   a. HIV > HCV > HBV
   b. HCV > HBV > HIV
   c. HBV > HIV > HCV
   d. HIV > HBV > HCV
   e. HBV > HCV > HIV

9. Which of the following conditions in a health care worker does *not* require prompt evaluation and confirmation with laboratory tests, if necessary?
   a. Vesicular rash suggestive of varicella
   b. Fever and rash suggestive of measles
   c. Cough for more than 2 weeks suggestive of pertussis
   d. Nasal congestion suggestive of an uncomplicated viral upper respiratory tract infection
   e. Diarrhea suggestive of bacterial enteritis in a food service worker

10. Which is *false* about the absorption of oral antimicrobials?
    a. Chelation interactions in the gastrointestinal tract with divalent or trivalent cations can decrease the absorption of fluoroquinolones.
    b. Antibiotics with low oral bioavailability (eg, most cephalosporins and penicillins) should be given orally rather than intravenously (IV) to patients with serious infections.
    c. Some antimicrobials (eg, valacyclovir) are given as prodrugs to enhance oral absorption of the active compound.
    d. The presence or absence of food in the stomach can affect the absorption of several antimicrobials.
    e. The time to reach peak concentration is longer for a drug administered orally than for a drug given IV.

11. Which is *true* about drug distribution?
    a. The volume of distribution is used in calculating an appropriate loading dose of an antimicrobial.
    b. Drug levels in the cerebrospinal fluid are similar to drug levels in the blood for most drugs.
    c. The apparent volume of distribution of a drug is a true physiologic body space.
    d. Larger than usual doses of renally excreted antimicrobials are required when treating lower urinary tract infections.
    e. Patients who are morbidly obese typically have a lower volume of distribution than patients with normal weight, and thus lower antimicrobial doses can be used.

12. Which of the following is *true*?
    a. Drug interactions should be closely reviewed when adding drugs that are cytochrome P450 inducers, inhibitors, or substrates.
    b. Rifampin is an inducer of cytochrome P450 enzymes and often results in supratherapeutic (potentially toxic) levels of other drugs metabolized by the P450 enzymes.
    c. Determining the serum creatinine concentration is as useful as calculating the creatinine clearance for

deciding whether to modify the dosage of renally eliminated drugs.
d. Since steady state always occurs with the third dose of a drug, drug levels should always be drawn with the third dose of an antimicrobial.
e. Both answer *a* and answer *c* are true.

13. Which is *true* for antimicrobials with concentration-dependent killing?
    a. The parameter most associated with efficacy is the duration of time the drug level is above the minimum inhibitory concentration (MIC) for the organism.
    b. Giving antimicrobials as a continuous infusion maximizes the pharmacodynamics of concentration-dependent antimicrobials.
    c. Concentration-dependent killing is the rationale for the use of single daily (or pulse) dosing of aminoglycosides.
    d. A high peak concentration to minimum inhibitory concentration (MIC) ratio enhances killing.
    e. Both answer *c* and answer *d* are true.

14. For *Mycobacterium tuberculosis*, first-line drug susceptibility testing should include which of the following antimicrobial agents?
    a. Isoniazid, rifampin, amikacin, pyrazinamide
    b. Isoniazid, rifampin, clarithromycin, streptomycin
    c. Isoniazid, rifampin, streptomycin, pyrazinamide
    d. Isoniazid, rifampin, ethambutol, pyrazinamide
    e. Streptomycin, pyrazinamide, clarithromycin, minocycline

15. Which component of the mycobacterial cell wall is responsible for retention of the primary stain after exposure to acid-alcohol or mineral acids?
    a. Lipopolysaccharide
    b. Ergosterol
    c. Mycolic acid
    d. Peptidoglycan
    e. Porin

16. Which of the following is a limitation of interferon-γ release assays (eg, QuantiFERON-TB Gold) for the immunodiagnosis of latent tuberculosis?
    a. False-positive results due to prior vaccination with bacilli Calmette-Guérin (BCG)
    b. False-positive results due to infection with *Mycobacterium avium*
    c. "Boost" response due to prior testing
    d. Placement error and reader bias
    e. False-positive results due to infection with *Mycobacterium kansasii*

17. Which of the following characteristics of *Mycobacterium tuberculosis* can be used to distinguish it from *Mycobacterium bovis*?
    a. Nonchromogenic pigmentation
    b. Positive pyrazinamidase test
    c. Negative 68°C catalase test
    d. Positive nucleic acid probe for *M tuberculosis* complex
    e. Negative arylsulfatase test

Answers

1. Answer c.
Acyclovir, amoxicillin, azithromycin, and isoniazid are all safe to use during pregnancy. No adverse or teratogenic effects have been reported to occur when these drugs are administered to pregnant women. Tetracyclines have an affinity for developing teeth and bone. They can inhibit fetal bone development and produce tooth discoloration in infants and children. Additionally, acute hepatotoxicity with fatty necrosis has been reported in pregnant women taking tetracyclines. For these reasons, tetracyclines should be avoided in pregnant women, nursing mothers, and children younger than 8 years.

2. Answer d.
This patient has had a severe reaction to penicillin. Therefore, he should not receive another agent in the penicillin class. Because the reaction was anaphylactoid and potentially life threatening, the prudent action is to avoid all β-lactam antimicrobials since cross-reactions occur. The β-lactams include the penicillins, cephalosporins, and carbapenems. The quinolones, macrolides, and tetracyclines are acceptable alternatives. Ciprofloxacin is not an optimal choice for outpatient treatment of community-acquired pneumonia because it is not overly active against *Streptococcus pneumoniae*. Moxifloxacin is the most suitable antimicrobial choice among the agents listed.

3. Answer b.
Ampicillin, piperacillin-tazobactam, linezolid, and vancomycin all provide excellent anti-enterococcal activity (for susceptible strains). The cephalosporins are not active against enterococci. Additionally, the quinolones do not generally produce reliable activity against *Enterococcus* species.

4. Answer d.
Red man syndrome or red neck syndrome is an infusion-associated reaction that is frequently associated with vancomycin. Typical manifestations include an erythematous rash that involves the face, neck, and upper torso. Itching is common and hypotension occasionally develops. The reaction can occur within a few minutes after initiation of vancomycin infusion, or it may develop soon after the infusion is complete. This peculiar syndrome is due to a nonimmunologic release of histamine and is related to the rate of vancomycin infusion. The complication is not a classic drug allergy, and it can be avoided by slowing the infusion rate of vancomycin or by administering vancomycin over at least 1 hour. Larger doses of vancomycin (eg, 1,500 mg) are typically infused over more than 1 hour. If slowing the rate of infusion does not prevent this reaction, the addition of an antihistamine (eg, diphenhydramine) may be useful if it is given before the infusion of vancomycin.

5. Answer c.
Hand rubbing with an alcohol-based, waterless product is the preferred method for hand hygiene in routine patient care. Hand washing with soap and water (with or without antimicrobial soap) is indicated if hands are visibly soiled with organic material. A surgical scrub is not necessary during routine patient care.

6. Answer b.
Molecular typing of the isolates is an important tool to examine the genetic relatedness of isolates, but it is not the first step in an outbreak investigation. Steps that should be performed first include the following: confirm each infection in the cluster; make a case definition; search for additional infections and record basic information on each case; and prepare a preliminary line listing of relevant information.

7. Answer d.
Standard Precautions applies to all patients and is designed to prevent transmission of bloodborne pathogens and other microorganisms from moist body surfaces and substances, including blood, all body fluids, secretions and excretions (except sweat) regardless of whether they contain visible blood, mucous membranes, and nonintact skin.

8. Answer e.
The risk of infection after a needlestick injury is greatest with HBV, particularly if the patient is hepatitis e antigen–positive, and least with HIV.

9. Answer d.
In a health care worker, nasal congestion (without fever and cough) that is suggestive of an uncomplicated viral upper respiratory tract infection does not require prompt evaluation or confirmation with laboratory tests. The worker may be excluded from direct patient contact depending on the nature of the work and the patient population. All the other conditions require prompt evaluation and confirmation with laboratory tests, if necessary.

10. Answer b.
Antibiotics with low oral bioavailability (such as β-lactams) have much lower serum levels when given orally rather than IV. For serious infections, these drugs should be given IV at least initially. In contrast, drugs with good oral bioavailability (eg, fluoroquinolones, linezolid, fluconazole) reach similar levels when given orally or IV. Thus, they can often be given orally as long as the patient is expected to have normal absorption (eg, no ileus, vomiting, or short bowel syndrome).

11. Answer a.
With serious infections, a loading dose is often used to reach near steady-state levels very quickly rather than waiting 3 to 5 half-lives. The equation for calculating a loading dose for an intravenous drug is the following: Loading Dose = Volume of Distribution × Desired Peak Plasma Concentration.

12. Answer a.
Numerous drug interactions can occur with drugs that are eliminated hepatically, particularly if they are metabolized by the cytochrome P450 system. Drug levels of cytochrome

P450 substrates are decreased by concomitant administration of an enzyme inducer (therapeutic failure can result); they are increased by concomitant administration of an enzyme inhibitor (toxicity can result).

13. Answer e.

Parameters that have been associated with efficacy for concentration-dependent killing drugs include the peak concentration to MIC ratio and the ratio of the area under the drug concentration–time curve (AUC) to the MIC (AUC/MIC ratio). Additionally, higher peak levels can enhance the duration of the postantibiotic effect. This is the rationale for single daily (pulse) dosing of aminoglycosides.

14. Answer d.

First-line drugs for *M tuberculosis* include isoniazid, rifampin, ethambutol, and pyrazinamide. The Clinical and Laboratory Standards Institute (CLSI) states that the first isolate of *M tuberculosis* from each patient should be tested to obtain antimicrobial susceptibility results for the first-line drugs. In addition, if culture results are not negative or if there is clinical evidence of treatment failure after 3 months of therapy, susceptibility testing should be repeated.

15. Answer c.

Mycolic acids and free lipids present in the mycobacterial cell wall create a hydrophobic permeability barrier that prevents access of common aniline dyes. However, mycobacteria can form complexes with arylmethane dyes (eg, fuchsin or auramine O) and special staining procedures. The mycolic acid residues in the cell wall retain the primary stain even after exposure to acid-alcohol; therefore, mycobacteria are termed *acid-fast*.

16. Answer e.

Interferon-γ release assays (eg, QuantiFERON-TB Gold) do not demonstrate cross-reactivity in patients who have received the BCG vaccination or are infected with most nontuberculous mycobacteria. However, known cross-reactions have been observed in patients infected with *M kansasii, Mycobacterium szulgai,* or *Mycobacterium marinum*.

17. Answer b.

Mycobacterium tuberculosis and *M bovis* are members of the *M tuberculosis* complex and share several phenotypic properties, including nonchromogenic pigmentation and negative reactions with both the 68°C catalase test and the arylsulfatase test. In the pyrazinamidase test, however, *M tuberculosis* shows a positive reaction, and *M bovis* has a negative reaction. In addition, results on the niacin and nitrate reduction tests are positive for *M tuberculosis* and negative for *M bovis*.

Etiologic Agents

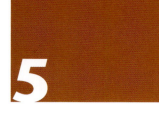

Randall C. Walker, MD

5

Select Viruses in Adults

I. Introduction
   A. Viral Infections Discussed in Other Chapters
      1. Infections specific to organ systems (eg, central nervous system [CNS], respiratory system)
      2. Infections specific to special populations (eg, transplant patients, patients with human immunodeficiency virus [HIV], international travel patients, pediatric patients)
   B. Viral Infections Discussed in This Chapter
      1. Viral infections that have the capacity for multiorgan or systemic disease
      2. Viral infections that affect adults who may be otherwise healthy or at least not in the above special populations
      3. Specifically, herpes simplex virus (HSV) type 1, varicella-zoster virus (VZV), Epstein-Barr virus, adenovirus, mumps virus, human parvovirus B19, and coxsackievirus
      4. Topics: reviews of these viruses, focusing on differentiating clinical features, diagnostic tools and treatment, and salient microbiologic and epidemiologic factors
II. Herpes Simplex Virus Type 1
   A. Characteristics
      1. HSV type 1 (HSV-1) attains latency in sensory neurons
      2. Virus reactivation results in shedding from mucosal and cutaneous tissues supplied by these latently infected nerves, which, in turn, is the basis for transmission to other human hosts
      3. Latency-associated transcript (LAT)
         a. A viral gene expressed during latent infection in neurons
         b. Inhibits apoptosis through modulation of transforming growth factor β signaling
         c. Maintains latency by promoting the survival of infected neurons
            1) LAT is not a protein gene product (which would be recognized by the host immune system)
            2) Instead, LAT is microRNA (a molecule that the host immune system cannot recognize), illustrating another aspect of latency
      4. Reactivation of HSV-1 is precipitated by physical, thermal, or ultraviolet light trauma to the mucosa
      5. Reactivation can also occur with transient reductions in immune function, including other illnesses (thus, the term *cold sore*), chemotherapy, immunotherapy, and sleep deprivation

6. Latency in the trigeminal nerve produces a characteristic distribution for reactivation lesions
B. Clinical Manifestations
 1. Primary HSV-1 infections in adults
    a. Occur at mucocutaneous sites that contact the mucosa of another person shedding HSV-1, including oral lesions, genital lesions from sexual contact, finger lesions (herpetic whitlow), and generalized skin lesions (eg, skin contact between athletes causing herpes gladiatorum)
    b. Can be severe, presenting as a gingival stomatitis (Figure 5.1), and spread through other oropharygeal and esophageal structures
    c. Fever, dysphagia, myalgia, and cervical adenopathy are common and can last for several days to 2 weeks
 2. Generally, HSV-1 is tropic for oral mucosa and HSV type 2 (HSV-2) for anogenital mucosa, but they can cause lesions at any location
 3. Manifestations of HSV-1 in immunosuppression (eg, transplant, AIDS, and malignancy) are worse at local sites but also include disseminated cutaneous infection and involvement of visceral organs, such as the lungs and the liver (Figure 5.2)
 4. Bell palsy: both HSV and VZV can cause paralysis of the mandibular portion of the facial nerve

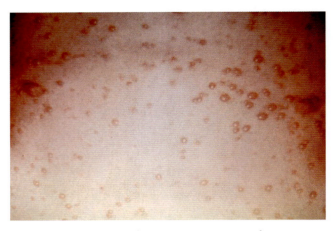

Figure 5.2. Disseminated Cutaneous Herpes Simplex Virus. (Adapted from Centers for Disease Control and Prevention. Public Health Image Library (PHIL): photographs, illustrations, multimedia files. [cited 2009 May 15] Available from: http://phil.cdc.gov/phil/home.asp.)

 5. Ophthalmologic conditions
    a. Necrotizing retinitis: can be caused by HSV and VZV, even in nonimmunocompromised hosts
    b. HSV keratitis: may be falsely diagnosed as a noninfectious inflammatory condition needing topical corticosteroids, which would make the condition worse
 6. When primary HSV-1 affects the anogenital mucosa, complications resulting from spinal cord involvement (eg, bladder dysfunction, aspectic meningitis, rarely transverse myelitis) are more severe
 7. Community-acquired encephalitis: HSV-1 is the main cause (Figure 5.3)
C. Diagnosis
 1. Usually based on appearance: painful vesicular lesion with a surrounding erythematous base on oral mucosal or skin surfaces
 2. If diagnosis of primary HSV-1 infection is not readily made on clinical appearance alone, perform polymerase chain reaction (PCR) testing
    a. Begin empirical antiviral therapy while awaiting confirmation
    b. Direct swab of ulcerative lesion tested for viral DNA by PCR can confirm the diagnosis within 1 day and can be used to distinguish HSV-1 from HSV-2
    c. PCR testing is several times more sensitive for HSV in oral lesions than in genital lesions

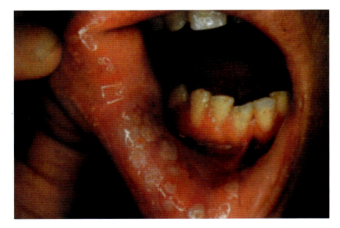

Figure 5.1. Primary Herpes Simplex Virus Stomatitis. (Adapted from Schrier RW. Atlas of diseases of the kidney. Vol 5. Philadelphia: Current Medicine. c1999. [cited 2009 May 15]. Available from: http://cnserver0.nkf.med.ualberta.ca/cn/Schrier/Default5.htm. Used with permission.)

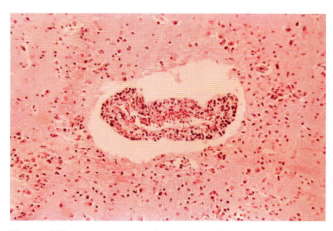

Figure 5.3. Herpes Encephalitis. Histopathologic changes are apparent in brain tissue (hematoxylin-eosin, original magnification ×125). (Adapted from Centers for Disease Control and Prevention. Public Health Image Library (PHIL): photographs, illustrations, multimedia files. [cited 2009 May 15]. Available from: http://phil.cdc.gov/phil/home.asp.)

Table 5.1

Use of Acyclovir for HSV and VZV Infections

Location	Host	Route	Dosage[a]	Duration, d
HSV				
Mucocutaneous junction	Healthy	Oral	200 mg 5 times daily[b]	5 (recurrence) or 10 (primary infection)
Mucocutaneous junction	ICH	IV	5 mg/kg every 8 h	7
Brain	Healthy or ICH	IV	10 mg/kg every 8 h	10
Varicella				
Skin	Healthy	Oral	800 mg 4 or 5 times daily	5
Lungs	Healthy	IV	10 mg/kg every 8 h	7
Any	ICH	IV	10 mg/kg every 8 h	7-10
Zoster				
Dermatome	Healthy, older than 50 y	Oral	800 mg 4 or 5 times daily[c]	7-10
Dermatome	ICH	IV	10 mg/kg every 8 h	7
Disseminated or CNS	ICH	IV	10 mg/kg every 8 h	10-14

Abbreviations: CNS, central nervous system; HSV, herpes simplex virus; ICH, immunocompromised host; IV, intravenous; VZV, varicella-zoster virus.

[a] All dosages are for patients with normal renal function; adjustments are required if renal function is abnormal.

[b] Valacyclovir is also available for healthy hosts with cutaneous HSV infection. Dosages differ from those for acyclovir, reflecting valacyclovir's higher bioavailability.

[c] Instead of oral acyclovir for varicella or zoster in healthy hosts, oral valacyclovir can be used at a dosage of 1 g orally 3 times daily for 7 days.

  d. PCR testing is several times more sensitive than viral culture
 D. Treatment
  1. Considerations
   a. Intravenous, oral, and topical antiviral treatments are variably indicated
   b. Doses and durations depend on various factors: whether disease is primary or reactivation; whether disease affects deeper structures, viscera, or CNS; and the immune status of the patient (Table 5.1)
   c. Earlier treatment improves outcome, shortens duration of symptoms and viral shedding, and decreases the frequency of reactivation symptoms
  2. Antiviral agents
   a. Acyclovir, valacyclovir, and famciclovir are all active against HSV
   b. Acyclovir resistance develops rarely but increasingly (and usually only in compromised hosts who have already taken much acyclovir)
    1) Resistant strains lack thymidine kinase, the enzyme needed to phosphorylate acyclovir into an active form
    2) Resistant strains are also usually resistant to famciclovir and ganciclovir but susceptible to foscarnet or cidofovir
III. Varicella-Zoster Virus
 A. Varicella
  1. Introduction
   a. Primary infection with VZV causes chickenpox (varicella) in susceptible hosts
    1) The disease in adults is generally more severe than in children
   b. Latent VZV: in sensory nerve root ganglia
   c. Reactivation of latent VZV: typically a localized eruption in a single dermatome
  2. Transmission
   a. Chickenpox is highly contagious: high secondary household attack rates (>90%) among susceptible persons

b. Transmission by aerosolized droplets from nasopharyngeal secretions or by direct cutaneous contact with vesicle fluid
c. Airborne transmission to susceptible nursing staff
d. Average incubation period: 2 weeks (range, 10-21 days); longer incubation after administration of varicella zoster immune globulin (VZIG) if given immediately after exposure
e. Infectivity begins 48 hours before onset of rash and ends when skin lesions have fully crusted

3. Epidemiology
   a. Before the varicella vaccine was licensed in 1995, there were about 4 million cases of varicella in the United States each year, with nearly 11,000 hospital admissions and 100 deaths
      1) Persons older than 20 years had a 10-fold higher mortality rate than those younger than 20
   b. Since 1995, the incidence of chickenpox appears to have declined by 3-fold to 10-fold, with greater decreases in states with higher vaccination rates

4. Clinical manifestations
   a. Skin lesions
      1) Varicella lesions are present in different stages of development on the face, trunk, and extremities
      2) New lesions generally stop forming within 4 days, and most lesions have fully crusted by day 6 in healthy hosts
   b. Visceral disease
      1) Varicella pneumonia: most frequent complication of varicella infection in healthy adults
         a) Incidence: about 1 in 400 cases
         b) Overall mortality: 10% to 30%
         c) Mortality rate nearly 50% among patients who require mechanical ventilation even if they receive intensive therapy and appropriate supportive measures
         d) Risk factors: cigarette smoking, pregnancy, and immunosuppression
            i) Pregnant women with chickenpox: risk of pneumonia does not appear to be higher than for other adults
            ii) Pregnant women with varicella pneumonia: pneumonia is more severe than in other adults
         e) Varicella pneumonia usually develops 1 to 6 days after the rash has appeared: patients present with progressive hypoxemia, impaired gas exchange, and diffuse bilateral infiltrates
            i) Early stage: nodular
            ii) Subsequently calcified
         f) Prompt administration of intravenous acyclovir can decrease mortality
         g) Use of adjunctive corticosteroids for life-threatening varicella pneumonia is controversial
      2) Varicella encephalitis
         a) More diffuse in adults than in children
         b) Associated with vasculopathy, hemorrhage, and demyelination
         c) More severe in immunosuppressed hosts, such as patients with AIDS and transplant recipients
         d) Relatively unresponsive to antiviral therapy
      3) Varicella hepatitis
         a) Generally affects immunosuppressed hosts, including transplant recipients and AIDS patients
         b) Frequently fatal
         c) Patients usually present with cutaneous vesicular lesions, fever, and acute abdominal or back pain
            i) Rash may appear after the onset of hepatitis, which can delay the diagnosis
            ii) In bone marrow transplant patients, rash may not appear at all
         d) Early high-dose intravenous acyclovir (10 mg/kg every 8 hours, with dose adjustment for renal dysfunction) has proved effective in varicella hepatitis
      4) Disseminated varicella
         a) Patients with impaired cellular immunity are particularly susceptible to fatal disseminated varicella, affecting multiple visceral organs, skin, and CNS

5. Treatment
   a. The use of antiviral therapy for varicella depends on the host, the time of presentation, and comorbidities

b. Acyclovir is effective therapy for primary varicella in both healthy hosts and immunosuppressed hosts
  1) VZV is less susceptible to acyclovir than HSV
  2) To inhibit VZV replication in vitro, acyclovir levels must be about 10-fold higher than those required for HSV
c. Use of acyclovir in children
  1) In general, acyclovir is not recommended for otherwise healthy children
  2) Indications for use of acyclovir in children who are at increased risk of moderate to severe varicella
    a) Older children
    b) Secondary household cases
    c) Children who have chronic cutaneous or cardiopulmonary disorders and who are at risk of secondary bacterial infections
    d) Children receiving intermittent oral or inhaled corticosteroid therapy
d. Varicella is uncomplicated in most healthy adults who become infected
  1) Nonetheless, adults are at increased risk of pneumonia, CNS disease, hospitalization, and death
  2) Oral acyclovir
    a) Recommended if therapy can be initiated within 24 hours of symptom onset
    b) Usual oral dose for adults: 800 mg 4 times daily
  3) Intravenous acyclovir
    a) Use to treat any immunosuppressed host (adult or child)
    b) Treat even if more than 24 hours has passed since the onset of symptoms
    c) Intravenous dose: 10 mg/kg every 8 hours
    d) Use same dose in immunocompromised patients and in immunocompetent patients who have serious complications, such as varicella pneumonia or encephalitis (Table 5.1)
e. Famciclovir and valacyclovir have activity against VZV in vitro, but most data relate to their effectiveness in herpes zoster infections and not varicella
6. Varicella vaccine
  a. A live, attenuated strain of VZV
  b. All susceptible children should be vaccinated by their 13th birthday
  c. Indications for vaccinating adults
    1) Ongoing risk of exposure (eg, day care employees)
    2) Household contacts of immunosuppressed hosts
    3) Women of childbearing age
    4) Outbreaks characterized by intense exposure
    5) Postexposure prophylaxis in unvaccinated or nonimmune family members of children presenting with chickenpox
  d. Contraindications for vaccinating adults: pregnancy or immunocompromised status
  e. Vaccine-induced immunity appears to wane over time
    1) Patients with "breakthrough varicella" have mild symptoms
    2) Associated rash may be atypical for varicella
      a) Papular or papulovesicular characteristics rather than the usual vesicular lesions
      b) Patients can still be infectious
  f. Effect of the VZV vaccine
    1) Rate of varicella-related hospitalizations has decreased about 4-fold
    2) Rate of death has decreased sharply in all age groups younger than 50 years, with the greatest reduction (92%) among children 1 to 4 years old
  g. Health care and child-care workers who do not have a history of varicella
    1) Test serologically
    2) If seronegative and without a contraindication, immunize
7. Postexposure prophylaxis
  a. Use of postexposure prophylaxis depends on several conditions
    1) Patient susceptibility (ie, negative history of varicella and no prior vaccination)
    2) High-level exposure (eg, household or close indoor contact lasting >1 hour, or other prolonged face-to-face contact)
    3) Underlying diseases or conditions that put the patient at higher risk of varicella-related complications
    4) Adults should undergo antibody testing for varicella before receiving VZIG (VariZIG)

- a) Among adults with a negative or uncertain history of varicella, 70% to 90% are seropositive
- b) Seropositive adults do not require postexposure prophylaxis
  - 5) Bone marrow transplant recipients: considered at risk of varicella infection regardless of prior history of infection or vaccination in either the recipient or the donor
- b. Agents
  - 1) Acyclovir, VZIG (VariZIG), or vaccine can be administered
  - 2) The manufacture of US Food and Drug Administration–approved VZIG has been discontinued
  - 3) A new VZIG product from Canada, VariZIG, is now available
    - a) Similar to VZIG, VariZIG is a purified human immune globulin made from plasma containing high levels of anti-varicella IgG antibodies
    - b) Any patient who receives VariZIG should also receive varicella vaccine 5 or more months later (provided that live vaccine is not contraindicated)
    - c) If VZIG (VariZIG) cannot be administered within 96 hours of exposure, consider use of intravenous immunoglobulin (IVIG)
      - i) Anti-varicella antibody titers vary from lot to lot of IVIG
- c. Options for pregnant women who cannot receive VariZIG
  - 1) Administer IVIG
  - 2) Alternatively, closely monitor for signs and symptoms of varicella and preemptively treat with acyclovir at the first sign of illness
- d. Options for healthy adults
  - 1) Administer postexposure VariZIG
  - 2) Alternatively, treat acute varicella with acyclovir only if infection develops
    - a) If the exposed adult is given acyclovir with the first development of skin lesions, clinical illness is milder and acyclovir does not interfere with an antibody response to natural infection
    - b) Recommended dosage of oral acyclovir for adults with uncomplicated varicella: 20 mg/kg orally 4 times daily for 5 days
- e. The Advisory Committee on Immunization Practices (ACIP) recommends vaccination with live virus vaccine for the postexposure management of adults
  - 1) Rationale: to improve protection against subsequent contact with the virus
  - 2) Ideally, the vaccine should be administered within 3 days of exposure to chickenpox
- f. If varicella develops despite prophylaxis, acyclovir therapy can decrease the risk of severe disease in adult contacts and in health care workers who have contact with immunosuppressed patients
- g. Patients hospitalized with varicella should be kept in strict isolation in a negative pressure room to prevent spread of aerosolized virus particles to other patients and staff in the hospital who are at risk of primary infection

B. Zoster
  1. Latency
     a. After primary infection with VZV, latent infection is established in the sensory dorsal root ganglia
     b. Special viral mechanisms enable VZV to remain latent in both neurons and satellite cells surrounding the sensory neuron; cellular immunity of the host keeps the virus in a latent state
  2. Reactivation
     a. Reactivation results in herpes zoster (also called shingles): a painful, unilateral vesicular eruption in a restricted dermatomal distribution
     b. With reactivation, the virus spreads to other cells within the ganglion, involving multiple sensory neurons and thereby the skin
     c. The dermatomal distribution of the vesicular rash of herpes zoster corresponds to the sensory fields of many infected neurons within a specific ganglion
  3. Epidemiology
     a. Older age groups have the highest incidence of zoster, presumably related to decreased VZV-specific cell-mediated immunity
     b. Emerging data suggest that the vaccine-induced decrease in varicella disease since the 1990s has not led to an increase in herpes zoster in the general population

c. The incidence of shingles in blacks: one-fourth the rate in whites, but fewer elderly black persons have had primary varicella and thus are not at risk of zoster
4. Clinical manifestations
   a. In immunocompetent hosts, a prodrome of fever, malaise, dysesthesias, and headache often precedes the vesicular dermatomal eruption by several days
   b. Groups of vesicles or bullae initially appear along the dermatome and then become pustular or hemorrhagic lesions within 3 to 4 days
   c. In 7 to 10 days, the lesions crust and are no longer infectious
   d. Complete resolution requires 3 to 4 weeks
   e. Deep burning pain is the most common symptom, usually preceding the rash by days to weeks
   f. Zoster is generally limited to 1 dermatome in healthy hosts but occasionally affects 2 or 3 neighboring dermatomes
   g. Some otherwise healthy patients have a few scattered vesicles located away from the involved dermatome
      1) These vesicles are thought to be the result of small quantities of VZV being released from the infected ganglion into the bloodstream
   h. Thoracic and lumbar dermatomes are the most common sites of zoster
   i. Zoster keratitis and herpes zoster ophthalmicus can result from involvement of the ophthalmic branch of the trigeminal cranial nerve and can be sight-threatening infections
5. Complications
   a. Complications occur in up to 20% of immunocompetent patients
   b. Advanced age is associated with postherpetic neuralgia, bacterial superinfection of the skin, ocular complications, and motor neuropathy
   c. Patients with comorbidities (eg, patients with diabetes mellitus, cancer, HIV, or transplant) also have complications more frequently
   d. Postherpetic neuralgia
      1) Most common complication (10%-15% of patients)
      2) The pain results from injury of the peripheral nerves and altered CNS processing of pain signals
      3) Patients older than 60 years
         a) Account for 50% of cases
         b) Are 25 times more likely to have postherpetic neuralgia (PHN) that lasts for at least 2 months
      4) Immunosuppression
         a) An additional risk factor
         b) Tenfold increase in the risk of prolonged (>2 months) PHN
      5) Gabapentin
         a) Anticonvulsant drug that is a structural analogue of γ-aminobutyric acid
         b) Moderately effective in the management of PHN that is refractory to analgesia
   e. Ocular infection
      1) Herpes zoster ophthalmicus
         a) A sight-threatening VZV reactivation within the trigeminal ganglion
         b) Prodromal headache, malaise, and fever
         c) Patients may present with unilateral pain or hypesthesia in the affected eye, forehead, and top of the head
         d) When vesicles erupt along the trigeminal dermatome, hyperemic conjunctivitis, episcleritis, and lid droop can occur
         e) Many have corneal involvement (keratitis) or iritis (or both)
         f) Early diagnosis is critical to prevent progressive corneal involvement and potential loss of vision
         g) Treatment of herpes zoster ophthalmicus
            i) Prompt antiviral therapy to limit VZV replication
            ii) Adjunctive topical corticosteroid drops to decrease the inflammatory response and to control immune keratitis and iritis
      2) Acute retinal necrosis
         a) Occurs in immunocompetent and immunocompromised hosts
         b) Blurred vision and eye pain
         c) Complications: acute iridocyclitis, vitritis, necrotizing retinitis, and occlusive retinal vasculitis, with rapid loss of vision and eventual retinal detachment
         d) The other eye becomes involved in 33% to 50% of patients

e) Treatment: intravenous acyclovir
    i) Clinical improvement in 48 to 72 hours
    ii) Decreases the risk of contralateral eye involvement
f. Ramsay Hunt syndrome (herpes zoster oticus)
    1) Reactivation of VZV from the geniculate ganglion
    2) Often involves cranial nerves V, IX, and X
    3) Typical presentation: triad of ipsilateral facial paralysis, ear pain, and vesicles in the auditory canal and auricle
    4) Alterations in taste perception, hearing (tinnitus and hyperacusis), and lacrimation are common
    5) Facial paralysis in Ramsay Hunt syndrome
        a) More severe than in Bell palsy attributed to HSV
        b) Lower rate of complete recovery
    6) Vestibular disturbances are common
    7) Ramsay Hunt syndrome has also been reported with HSV
g. Neurologic complications
    1) Aseptic meningitis
        a) Reactive cerebrospinal fluid (CSF) pleocytosis
            i) Occurs in 40% to 50% of patients with herpes zoster
            ii) Some patients have symptoms of headache and neck stiffness
        b) Peripheral motor neuropathy
            i) Segmental motor weakness occurs rarely
            ii) Time of appearance and dermatomal distribution are the same as for the pain and cutaneous eruption
            iii) Most patients gradually recover full motor strength
    2) Myelitis
        a) Noted more frequently in immunocompromised patients
        b) Caused by direct spread of VZV from dorsal root ganglia centrally into spinal cord
        c) Associated with zoster in thoracic dermatomes
        d) Occurs within days to weeks after the rash (or sometimes occurs without rash)
    3) Encephalitis
        a) Occurrence
            i) Usually within days after vesicular eruption
            ii) Also occurs before the eruption, several months after resolution of the eruption, or without any cutaneous eruption (especially in immunosuppressed patients)
        b) Major risk factors
            i) Cranial or cervical dermatomal involvement
            ii) Two or more prior episodes of zoster
            iii) Disseminated herpes zoster
            iv) Impaired cell-mediated immunity
        c) CSF PCR assays for VZV DNA, in conjunction with magnetic resonance brain imaging, now permit more rapid diagnosis of VZV-induced encephalitis (Figure 5.4)
    4) Stroke syndrome
        a) VZV eye infections can be complicated, rarely, by contralateral thrombotic stroke due to zoster-associated cerebral angiitis

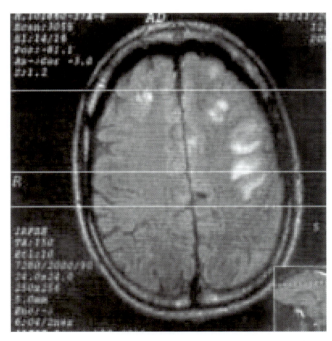

Figure 5.4. Zoster Encephalitis. [cited 2009 May 15]. (Available from: http://www.scielo.br/img/revistas/bjid/v8n3/21624f2.jpg. Used with permission.)

b) Occurs within several weeks to a few months after the zoster eruption
c) Abrupt onset of severe headache
d) Rapid evolution to contralateral weakness
e) Angiography shows multifocal occlusion of the proximal branches of the anterior and middle cerebral arteries
f) Granulomatous vasculitis of the large and small arteries, with VZV antigens detectable in the smooth muscle cells of the intima media, suggesting direct VZV invasion of the arterial surface by spreading along the intracranial branches of the trigeminal nerve
h. Zoster complications in immunosuppressed hosts
1) Immunosuppressed hosts are at substantial risk of severe VZV-related complications
a) Zoster pneumonitis in transplant recipients has been associated with high mortality even with prompt diagnosis and empirical institution of antiviral therapy
b) Zoster dissemination is 1 of the most frequent late infections of allogeneic bone marrow transplant recipients
c) Treatment of disseminated or CNS zoster requires high-dose intravenous acyclovir (10 mg/kg every 8 hours)

6. Treatment
a. Uncomplicated herpes zoster
1) Antiviral therapy should be initiated within 72 hours of clinical presentation
2) Oral acyclovir (800 mg 5 times daily) has been the mainstay of herpes zoster treatment
3) Newer antiviral agents (valacyclovir and famciclovir) have better pharmacokinetics
4) Treatment within 48 to 72 hours of the onset of rash can accelerate resolution of the pain associated with acute neuritis, especially in patients older than 50 years
5) Prompt treatment can also decrease the incidence of prolonged PHN
b. Valacyclovir
1) Provides a 3- to 5-fold increase in acyclovir bioavailability
2) May be more efficacious than acyclovir
a) Clears pain symptoms more rapidly (20% faster)
b) Reduces the frequency and duration of PHN by about 20%
c. Famciclovir
1) Well absorbed from the gastrointestinal tract
2) Rapidly converted in the intestinal wall and liver to penciclovir, the active compound that has broad activity against VZV
3) Is at least as effective as oral acyclovir for uncomplicated zoster in immunocompetent hosts
4) Requires less frequent dosing than acyclovir
5) Adjunctive corticosteroid therapy
a) Does not appear to improve the incidence or duration of PHN
b) Results may be no better than when antiviral therapy is used alone
c) May increase risk of secondary bacterial skin infections
d) Optimal duration of corticosteroid use is unknown: extended administration after antiviral therapy could potentiate viremia and complications such as visceral and cutaneous dissemination
d. HIV-infected and other immunosuppressed patients, regardless of age, should receive antiviral therapy for episodes of uncomplicated herpes zoster
e. Adjunctive corticosteroids are not recommended in immunosuppressed patients
f. Treatment of disseminated or CNS zoster requires high-dose intravenous acyclovir (10 mg/kg every 8 hours)
g. Acyclovir-resistant zoster
1) Foscarnet, an inhibitor of viral DNA polymerase, has in vitro activity against acyclovir-resistant VZV strains
2) Efficacy of foscarnet has varied in treating complicated herpes zoster that has been refractory to prolonged acyclovir therapy in severely immunosuppressed hosts
h. Herpes zoster ophthalmicus
1) Current treatment is usually administered orally

2) Intravenous acyclovir (10 mg/kg 3 times daily for 7 days) should be considered in immunocompromised patients and in any patient with zoster eye infection who is extremely ill and requires hospitalization
7. Issues of infectivity
   a. Localized herpes zoster in an immunocompetent host
      1) Contagious only through direct contact with open lesions
      2) Contact precautions are instituted for hospitalized patients who can keep lesions covered with clothing or dressings
   b. Immunocompromised patients with disseminated zoster or localized zoster (who are nonetheless at risk of dissemination)
      1) Isolated in the same way as patients with varicella infection, in which airborne spread is possible
      2) These patients are usually hospitalized and placed in strict isolation
   c. Individuals who have not had varicella and are exposed to a patient with herpes zoster are at risk of primary varicella
8. Prevention
   a. Herpes zoster reactivation disease
      1) Occurs in 30% of allogeneic hematopoietic cell transplant recipients with a past history of varicella
      2) Clinical trials are being conducted to determine the optimal regimen and required duration of prophylaxis to decrease VZV reactivation among these patients
   b. For adults 60 years or older, a live attenuated VZV vaccine (Zostavax zoster vaccine)
      1) Decreases the incidence of herpes zoster by 50%
      2) Among those who do get zoster, the incidence of prolonged PHN is decreased by two-thirds
      3) These results are clinically meaningful given that the vaccine is administered after primary infection

IV. Epstein-Barr Virus
   A. Introduction
      1. Epstein-Barr virus (EBV) is spread by intimate contact between asymptomatic EBV shedders and susceptible persons
      2. Worldwide, 90% to 95% of adults are EBV-seropositive
      3. EBV is associated with the B-cell lymphomas, T-cell lymphomas, Hodgkin disease, nasopharyngeal carcinomas, and posttransplant lymphoproliferative disorders
   B. Primary Infection
      1. Majority occur in childhood and are subclinical
      2. Older patients usually present with infectious mononucleosis
      3. Majority of primary EBV infections originate in the oropharynx
         a. Oropharyngeal epithelial cells are permissive for viral replication
         b. From these cells, transmission to B cells occurs
   C. Latency
      1. After primary infection, EBV is latent in B lymphocytes, T lymphocytes, epithelial cells, and myocytes
      2. Latency in B lymphocytes
         a. Persistence is the result of a dynamic interaction between viral evasion strategies and host immune responses
         b. Two genes, *LMP-1* and *LMP-2*, allow an EBV-infected B blast cell to become a resting memory cell, where EBV can persist in a transcriptionally quiescent state, thereby minimizing immune recognition
      3. Intracellular persistence of the entire viral genome is achieved through circularization of the linear EBV genome and maintenance of multiple copies of this covalently closed episomal DNA
      4. During convalescence, there is sporadic replication in epithelial cells lining the oropharynx and 1 in every 100,000 to 1 million small resting B lymphocytes
      5. Latently infected B cells typically contain between 1 and 10 complete EBV episomes per cell
      6. Although most EBV DNA persists in latently infected cells in an episomal form, the EBV genome also integrates into chromosomal DNA
      7. The integrated form of EBV DNA is limited in its ability to infect new cells, since episomal DNA is probably necessary for lytic cycle EBV replication
   D. Infectivity
      1. The EBV receptor on human cells is the B-cell surface molecule CD21, the receptor for the C3d component of complement
      2. EBV can enter and replicate within monocytes

a. Infected monocytes have decreased phagocytic activity
b. They serve as another potential early site for viral replication and for a blunted immune response to the virus
3. EBV can infect resting naive B cells that go to germinal centers within lymphoid follicles; these cells escape immune surveillance by turning off production of viral proteins such as EBV-determined nuclear antigen (EBNA)-2
4. The EBNA-1 protein is required for episome maintenance and probably for episome amplification

E. Differences With Other Herpesviruses
1. Unlike other herpesviruses, such as herpes simplex or cytomegalovirus, EBV is capable of transforming its host cells (ie, B cells) and does not routinely have a cytopathic effect in cell culture
2. Reactivation disease with EBV in normal hosts is not seen

F. Clinical Manifestations
1. Acute infectious mononucleosis: main form of primary EBV infection
   a. Young adults have typical symptom constellations; presentation in older adults can be less typical
      1) Initially, malaise, headache, and low-grade fever; then signs of tonsillitis or pharyngitis (or both), cervical lymph node enlargement and tenderness, and moderate to high fever
      2) Lymphadenopathy is usually bilateral, involving the posterior more than the anterior cervical chain
      3) May have tonsillar exudate with a white, gray-green, or necrotic appearance
      4) Less common findings: palatal petechiae, periorbital or palpebral edema, subconjunctival hemorrhages, and maculopapular and morbilliform rashes (Figure 5.5)
      5) Splenomegaly: in as many as 50% of patients
      6) Jaundice and hepatomegaly: uncommon
      7) Mild hepatitis: in about 90% of patients
         a) Often produces nausea, vomiting, and anorexia
         b) Some patients have hepatitis without other typical features of infectious mononucleosis

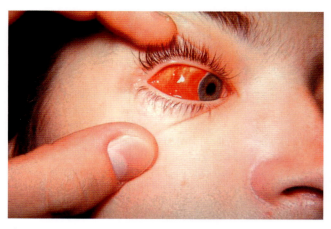

Figure 5.5. Conjunctival Hemorrhage in Infectious Mononucleosis. (Adapted from Centers for Disease Control and Prevention. Public Health Image Library (PHIL): photographs, illustrations, multimedia files. [cited 2009 May 15]. Available from: http://phil.cdc.gov/phil/home.asp.)

      8) Peripheral blood smears: lymphocytosis, mostly atypical lymphocytes
      9) Frequently, a morbilliform rash develops after the administration of ampicillin (and, to a lesser extent, penicillin)
         a) Mechanism may involve circulating antibodies to ampicillin
         b) Even though a rash develops with ampicillin, patients can subsequently tolerate ampicillin without an adverse reaction
      10) Acute symptoms resolve in 1 to 2 weeks, but fatigue often persists for months
      11) Splenic rupture: estimated to occur in about 2 patients per thousand
         a) Not correlated with the clinical severity of infectious mononucleosis or with laboratory findings
         b) Almost all cases have been in males
         c) In most cases, splenic rupture is spontaneous, without specific injury
         d) Management is similar to that for other splenic injuries
         e) Despite its life-threatening potential, EBV-based splenic rupture rarely results in death
      12) Airway obstruction (from massive lymphoid hyperplasia and mucosal

edema) is an uncommon and potentially fatal complication
- a) Severe obstruction may require tracheotomy or endotracheal intubation
- b) Corticosteroids can decrease pharyngeal edema and lymphoid hypertrophy in patients with incipient obstruction
b. Most patients recover completely, with a high degree of durable immunity
2. Various syndromes have been associated with primary EBV infection
   a. Neurologic syndromes
      1) Guillain-Barré syndrome
      2) Facial nerve palsy
      3) Meningoencephalitis
      4) Aseptic meningitis
      5) Transverse myelitis
      6) Peripheral neuritis
      7) Optic neuritis
   b. Hematologic abnormalities
      1) Hemolytic anemia
      2) Thrombocytopenia
      3) Aplastic anemia
      4) Thrombotic thrombocytopenic purpura or hemolytic uremic syndrome
      5) Disseminated intravascular coagulation
3. EBV can affect any organ system and cause various conditions
   a. Pneumonia
   b. Myocarditis
   c. Pancreatitis
   d. Mesenteric adenitis
   e. Myositis
   f. Glomerulonephritis
   g. Genital ulceration
4. Oral hairy leukoplakia
   a. Involves lingual squamous epithelium
      1) Generally affects lateral portions of tongue
      2) Also may involve floor of mouth, palate, or buccal mucosa
   b. Lesions are white, corrugated, painless plaques that, unlike candidal lesions, cannot be scraped from the mucosal surface with a tongue depressor
5. Lymphoproliferative disorders
   a. Hemophagocytic lymphohistiocytosis
      1) Rare but potentially fatal EBV complication
      2) Generalized histiocytic proliferation and hemophagocytosis
      3) T-cell proliferation is a primary feature
      4) Patients usually present with fever, generalized lymphadenopathy, hepatosplenomegaly, hepatitis, pancytopenia, and coagulopathy
   b. Lymphomatoid granulomatosis
      1) An angiodestructive disorder of the lymphoid system involving clonal B-cell proliferation
      2) Lung, kidney, liver, skin and subcutaneous tissue, and CNS may be involved
      3) Patients often have evidence of immunodeficiency and may respond to interferon-alfa
   c. X-linked lymphoproliferative disease (Duncan syndrome)
      1) Selective immunodeficiency to EBV
      2) Severe or fatal infectious mononucleosis and acquired immunodeficiency
      3) Usually occurs in childhood
      4) Fatal EBV infections in males: usually result from extensive liver necrosis
      5) Survivors of acute EBV infection have global cellular immune defects with deficient T-cell, B-cell, and natural killer cell responses
   d. Burkitt lymphoma
      1) Most common childhood malignancy in equatorial Africa
      2) Typically localized in the jaw of young patients
      3) Malaria and EBV may be cofactors in Burkitt lymphoma
         a) Malaria may provide a long-term stimulus for proliferation of B lymphocytes, some of which carry latent EBV
         b) Alternatively, malaria infection may impair EBV-specific T-cell immunity and lead to loss of viral control
   e. Nasopharyngeal carcinoma
      1) One of the most common cancers in southern China but relatively rare in other populations
      2) Although malignancy does not develop in most EBV-infected patients in China, EBV nonetheless appears to be the primary etiologic agent in the pathogenesis of nasopharyngeal carcinoma
         a) EBV is present in every anaplastic nasopharyngeal carcinoma cell
         b) The presence of a single clonal form of EBV in preinvasive lesions,

such as nasopharyngeal dysplasia or carcinoma in situ, indicates that EBV-induced cellular proliferation precedes invasion of these tumors
- f. Hodgkin disease
  1) In up to 50% of cases in western countries, the malignant cells (including the characteristic Reed-Sternberg cells) contain the EBV genome; this finding supports a pathogenic role for EBV in this malignancy
  2) Healthy persons in western populations are infected with predominantly type 1 EBV; not surprisingly, the majority of EBV detected in persons with Hodgkin disease in western countries is also type 1
  3) In contrast, the frequencies of type 1 and type 2 EBV in HIV-associated non-Hodgkin lymphoma and endemic Burkitt lymphoma are nearly equal, reflecting the equal rates of EBV-1 and EBV-2 infections in countries where these malignancies are endemic
- g. T-cell lymphoma
  1) Develops in immunosuppressed persons with chronic EBV infection
  2) A fulminant form may occur after acute EBV infection
- h. Nasal or nasal-type angiocentric lymphoma
  1) Rare malignancy endemic in Asia, Central America, and South America
  2) Affected sites: nasal septum, palate, gastrointestinal tract, and, less commonly, skin, testes, and peripheral nerves
  3) EBV is found in virtually all cases in the neoplastic cells; these tumors are probably of natural killer cell origin

G. Diagnosis
 1. EBV infection is suspected from the clinical presentation
 2. Supportive evidence of infection is derived from the peripheral blood smear and serology studies
 3. PCR for viral DNA
   a. Not used in healthy hosts
   b. May be useful with immunocompromised hosts and in CSF of persons with suspected EBV-associated CNS disease

H. Treatment and Prevention
 1. Primary EBV infections rarely require more than supportive therapy
 2. Even in clinical situations in which an antiviral or immunomodulatory treatment would be desirable, it is not clear that EBV responds
 3. Corticosteroids
   a. Use of corticosteroids in the treatment of EBV-induced infectious mononucleosis is controversial
   b. A trial of corticosteroids is warranted for persons with impending airway obstruction
 4. Antiviral treatment
   a. Acyclovir inhibits permissive EBV infection through inhibition of EBV DNA polymerase but has no effect on latent infection
   b. Short-term suppression of viral shedding can be shown, but there is no clinically significant benefit
 5. In most EBV-associated malignancies, there is little evidence of permissive (lytic) infection
 6. Acyclovir may be useful in EBV-induced hemophagocytic lymphohistiocytosis, in which evidence of replicating EBV has been demonstrated
 7. Other therapies
   a. Anecdotal reports of interleukin-2, interferon-alfa, and intravenous immunoglobulins in EBV-associated diseases
   b. These agents have not shown any clear benefit, except for possible effects in lymphomatoid granulomatosis and posttransplant lymphoproliferative disease
   c. Clinical trials of a recombinant vaccinia virus vaccine containing the EBV glycoprotein 350/220 are now in progress in China, where EBV-associated nasopharyngeal carcinoma is common

V. Adenovirus
 A. Introduction
  1. Adenoviruses: an important cause of febrile illnesses in young children
  2. Most adenoviral diseases are self-limiting, although fatal infections can occur in immunocompromised hosts and, occasionally, in healthy children and adults
 B. Epidemiology
  1. Most persons have serologic evidence of prior adenoviral infection by the age of 10, most commonly to serotypes that are associated

primarily with upper respiratory tract diseases
2. Adenoviruses are nonenveloped
   a. They can survive for long periods (>30 days) on environmental surfaces
   b. They are resistant to lipid disinfectants
   c. They can be inactivated by heat, formaldehyde, or bleach (sodium hypochlorite)
3. Transmission: by aerosol droplets, fecal-oral route, or contact with contaminated fomites
4. Adenovirus infections are prevalent in day care centers and in households with young children
5. Nosocomial transmission has been documented
6. Epidemics of adenoviral disease: pharyngoconjunctival fever among persons at summer camps and public swimming pools, keratoconjunctivitis at medical facilities, and serious acute respiratory disease in military recruits
7. Adenoviruses can be shed in feces for months to years after acute infection
8. Adenoviruses can be transmitted from kidney and liver transplants; therefore, these organs may harbor adenoviruses in a latent form
9. Reactivation of endogenous virus is involved in adenoviral diseases in immunocompromised patients

C. Clinical Manifestations
1. Acute respiratory disease
   a. In young adults, a syndrome of acute respiratory disease may occur under the special conditions of fatigue and crowding in military training camps
   b. Symptoms: fever, pharyngitis, cough, hoarseness, and conjunctivitis
   c. Pneumonia can develop, occasionally resulting in death
2. Eyes
   a. Pharyngoconjunctival fever
      1) Benign follicular conjunctivitis, often with febrile pharyngitis and cervical adenitis
      2) Outbreaks can occur at summer camps with swimming pools or lakes
   b. Epidemic keratoconjunctivitis
      1) A more serious disease, characterized by bilateral conjunctivitis and preauricular adenopathy, with subsequent development of painful corneal opacities
      2) Self-limited and virtually never results in permanent corneal damage; however, it causes severe pain and blurred vision
      3) Up to 50% of patients with epidemic keratoconjunctivitis carry virus on their hands
3. Gastrointestinal tract
   a. Symptomatic gastroenteritis occurs with range of adenovirus serotypes in immunocompromised hosts
   b. Hepatitis
      1) Occurs in immunocompromised hosts, especially with subgroup C type 5
      2) Adenovirus hepatitis is a particular problem in pediatric liver transplant recipients and may be fatal
4. Genitourinary tract
   a. Nonimmunocompromised adults: adenovirus subgroup D types 19 and 37 have been occasionally associated with urethritis
   b. Immunocompromised patients: adenovirus subgroup B types 11, 34, and 35 can cause hemorrhagic cystitis and tubulointerstitial nephritis
5. Nervous system
   a. Meningitis and encephalitis have been reported occasionally in association with adenovirus infection
   b. Neurologic involvement may be a primary manifestation or may occur with severe pneumonia, especially when infection is due to type 7
6. Other
   a. With PCR, adenoviruses have been detected in myocardial biopsies in some cases of acute myocarditis
   b. Adenovirus has also been found in viral myositis accompanied by rhabdomyolysis
7. Immunocompromised hosts
   a. Allogeneic stem cell transplant recipients and, in particular, recipients of unrelated or mismatched related grafts have an increased risk of infection; cidofovir treatment can lead to clinical improvement in these patients
   b. In solid organ transplant recipients, adenoviral disease typically involves the donor organ
      1) For example, renal transplant is sometimes complicated by interstitial nephritis and acute hemorrhagic cystitis
      2) Similarly, adenoviral pneumonia is described as an early complication after lung transplant

- c. Despite the frequency with which they are found in stool or urine specimens, adenoviruses are an uncommon cause of morbidity or death in HIV-infected patients
- D. Diagnosis
  1. Adenovirus infection cannot be diagnosed with clinical criteria alone
  2. Viral culture
     - a. Most sensitive and specific method for detecting most adenoviruses
     - b. In cell culture, a cytopathic effect generally occurs within 2 to 7 days with the common serotypes, although some can require up to 28 days
     - c. Appropriate samples: nasopharyngeal swabs or aspirates, throat swabs or washes, conjunctival swabs or scrapings, urine, CSF, stool or rectal swabs, and tissue samples
     - d. Immunocompromised hosts
       1) Adenoviruses may be continuously shed from stool or urine for months without symptoms
       2) Positive culture result must be interpreted in the context of current clinical manifestations
  3. PCR testing
     - a. Highly sensitive and specific
     - b. Detection of adenovirus DNA from various clinical specimens, including fixed tissues
     - c. Blood samples: quantitative PCR is promising for evaluation of adenovirus infections in immunocompromised patients
  4. Histopathology
     - a. Adenoviruses can cause characteristic intranuclear inclusions
       1) Early stages of infection: eosinophilic
       2) Later stages of infection: basophilic inclusions, which initially may be surrounded by a clear halo within the nucleus
     - b. Occasionally, adenovirus inclusions may resemble cytomegalovirus (CMV) inclusions, but unlike CMV, adenoviruses cause neither intracytoplasmic inclusions nor multinucleated cells
- E. Treatment
  1. Most adenovirus infections are self-limited, but they can be fatal in neonates and immunocompromised hosts
  2. Cidofovir (HPMPC)
     - a. The most promising antiviral agent for adenoviral infection
     - b. Currently approved for the treatment of CMV infections
     - c. Compared with ganciclovir, cidofovir is much more active against adenovirus in vitro
     - d. Variants resistant to cidofovir can be isolated after exposure of adenoviruses to cidofovir in vitro
- F. Infection Control
  1. Decontamination of environmental surfaces and instruments
     - a. May be difficult
     - b. Requires specific agents, such as chlorine, formaldehyde, or heat
  2. Handwashing does not reliably remove adenoviruses from contaminated fingers
     - a. Use gloves to examine patients with epidemic keratoconjunctivitis
     - b. Decontaminate instruments with 10% bleach
  3. Adenoviruses can cause serious nosocomial infections
     - a. In 1 report, an epidemic of adenovirus 7a in a neonatal unit resulted in the death of 2 patients and symptomatic infection in 9 patients, 10 staff, and 3 parents
     - b. Outbreak was controlled by grouping patients into cohorts; using gloves, gowns, and goggles; and excluding symptomatic staff from the unit
  4. Outbreaks of pharyngoconjunctival fever in swimming pools are usually associated with inadequate chlorination

VI. Mumps Virus
- A. Epidemiology
  1. The incidence of mumps in the United States decreased dramatically (100-fold) after the approval and introduction in 1967 of a live, attenuated mumps vaccine, which was initially intended for adolescents and adults (but is now given to infants)
  2. Sporadic mumps outbreaks still occur, though, usually in cohorts of susceptible persons from military posts, high schools, colleges, and summer camps
  3. Hospital-based and workplace outbreaks have frequently involved older persons who are at risk of more serious morbidity and complications requiring hospital admission
  4. In 2006, an outbreak of mumps in Iowa tripled the annual rate of cases in the United States since 2001
     - a. Most of the affected persons were young (18-25 years), and two-thirds had received 2 doses of vaccine

b. The source of the Iowa outbreak is unknown, but the mumps strain was genotype G, the same genotype that had caused an outbreak involving more than 70,000 people in the United Kingdom between 2004 and 2006
c. To control the outbreak, the Iowa Department of Public Health recommended isolation of patients for 5 days, and full vaccination of susceptible students and staff at colleges and health care professionals

B. Clinical Manifestations
1. Parotitis
   a. Nonspecific prodrome: anorexia, headache, malaise, low-grade fever
   b. Earache and tenderness of ipsilateral parotid
   c. Progressive increase in size of the involved parotid gland
2. Epididymo-orchitis
   a. The second most common manifestation of mumps infection in men (38%)
   b. Abrupt onset of fever (39°C-41°C)
   c. Severe testicular pain, accompanied by swelling and erythema of the scrotum
   d. Bilateral involvement in up to 30% of cases
3. Aseptic meningitis
   a. Asymptomatic CSF pleocytosis occurs in more than 50% of patients with clinical mumps
   b. Clinical aseptic meningitis due to mumps occurs in 4% to 6% in larger clinical series of mumps outbreaks
   c. Over half the patients who present with clinical mumps meningitis do not have parotitis
   d. CSF profile in mumps meningitis
      1) Typically less than 500 white blood cells per microliter, usually with a lymphocytic predominance
      2) Early polymorphonuclear predominance, with more than 1,000 white blood cells per microliter are occasionally seen
      3) CSF total protein is generally normal but can be slightly elevated
      4) CSF glucose levels are usually slightly decreased, but values less than 30 to 40 mg/dL (1.7-2.2 mmol/L) have been reported
      5) Occasionally mimics bacterial meningitis
   e. Patients generally have full neurologic recovery and no permanent deficits
4. Other, less frequent, neurologic complications of mumps: encephalitis, deafness, Guillain-Barré syndrome, transverse myelitis, and facial palsy
5. Mumps-associated arthropathy
   a. Infrequent
   b. Affects males more often than females
   c. Affects monoarticular large joints (knee and hip)
   d. Polyarticular syndromes have been reported
6. Acute pancreatitis
   a. Infrequent
   b. Typically benign
   c. Serum lipase can be used instead of amylase (which could be of salivary origin)
7. Myocardial involvement
   a. Transient electrocardiographic changes (depressed ST segments) in up to 15% of patients with mumps
   b. Rarely: myocarditis with dilated cardiomyopathy

C. Diagnosis
1. For acute parotitis
   a. The diagnosis of mumps does not warrant specific laboratory confirmation
   b. Standard blood testing: leukopenia, with a relative lymphocytosis, and an elevated serum amylase may be noted
2. For extrasalivary disease or during a mumps outbreak
   a. Serology
   b. Culture
   c. PCR testing

D. Treatment
1. Therapy for parotitis is symptomatic and includes analgesics or antipyretics

E. Prevention
1. Stay home from school or work for 9 days after onset of clinical symptoms
2. Active immunization with attenuated mumps virus vaccine
   a. Patients who have not been vaccinated in the past
   b. Patients who received only 1 dose of vaccine
3. Immunization after exposure has not been demonstrated to be protective, although it is recommended by the Centers for Disease Control and Prevention
   a. Rationale for vaccination: decrease the risk of disease with possible future exposures
4. Persons born before 1957 are considered immune

5. Vaccine should not be administered to pregnant women, immunosuppressed patients, or persons with advanced malignancies

VII. Human Parvovirus B19
  A. Pathology
   1. The B19 virus replicates in erythroid progenitor cells of the bone marrow and blood, leading to inhibition of erythropoiesis
   2. The parvovirus cellular receptor, P blood group antigen (globoside), is found in high concentrations on red blood cells and their precursors and accounts for this special tropism
   3. The B19 virus causes cell lysis
   4. The cytopathic effect induced during B19 virus infection is seen as giant pronormoblasts in the bone marrow
  B. Clinical Manifestations
   1. Most immunocompetent people with detectable IgG specific for B19 virus do not recall ever having any specific symptoms
   2. In children, human parvovirus B19 causes erythema infectiosum
      a. A mild febrile illness with rash (Figure 5.6)
      b. Often occurs in outbreaks among school-aged children, although it can occur in adults as well
      c. Recrudescence of rash after various nonspecific stimuli, such as change in temperature, exposure to sunlight, exercise, or emotional stress

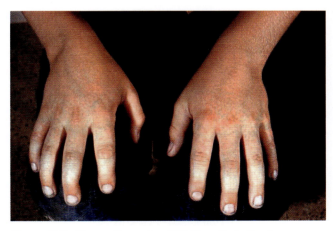

Figure 5.6. Human Parvovirus B19 Virus Rash. Erythema infectiosum is also called fifth disease. (Adapted from Centers for Disease Control and Prevention. Public Health Image Library (PHIL): photographs, illustrations, multimedia files. [cited 2009 May 15]. Available from: http://phil.cdc.gov/phil/home.asp.)

   d. In most patients, symptoms resolve within a few weeks, but symptoms can last for months or, rarely, years
   3. Transient aplastic crisis can develop in patients with underlying hemolytic disorders
   4. Infection during pregnancy can lead to fetal death
   5. Most B19 virus infections are acquired through the respiratory system, usually from contact with children
      a. Approximately 25% are asymptomatic during infection
      b. Nonspecific flulike symptoms in 50%
      c. Other symptoms of B19 virus infection are present in the remaining 25%
         1) In symptomatic hosts, intense viremia in the first week
            a) Fever, malaise, myalgia, coryza, headache, and pruritus
            b) Reticulocytopenia, decreased hemoglobin concentration, and leukopenia or thrombocytopenia (or both)
         2) In the second week, symptoms of rash or arthralgia (or both)
      d. Patients with human parvovirus B19 infection can present with acute arthritis
         1) May be mistaken for acute rheumatoid arthritis in the absence of rash
         2) Arthralgia or arthritis is more common in women
            a) Usually symmetric, involving the small joints of the hands, wrists, knees, and feet
            b) Usually resolving in about 3 weeks
      e. Patients with history of hematologic abnormalities, including increased red blood cell destruction (eg, sickle cell disease, hereditary spherocytosis) or decreased red blood cell production (eg, iron deficiency anemia), are at increased risk of transient aplastic crisis
         1) Rapid decrease in or lack of reticulocytes is a key laboratory finding in B19 virus infection (associated with high viral titers of parvovirus DNA)
         2) Red blood cell production returns to baseline level after resolution of infection
      f. Immunosuppressed patients are at risk of acute or chronic anemia after B19 virus infection owing to lack of protective antibodies

1) Life-threatening anemia can develop from inability to mount an immune response to clear viremia
2) Usually not accompanied by rash or arthropathy
3) These patients respond well to intravenous immune globulin
4) Some patients require recurrent treatment for relapses
g. Pregnant women: 30% to 40% lack measurable levels of IgG to B19 virus and are therefore presumed to be susceptible
1) A pregnant woman who has young children at home or who works in a day care is at highest risk of acquiring B19 virus infection
2) B19 virus infection during pregnancy can result in fetal complications, including miscarriage, intrauterine fetal death, or nonimmune hydrops fetalis
3) Determine the serologic status of a pregnant woman who has a history of known meaningful exposure to the virus or who has any of the classic symptoms of B19 virus infection
4) Seronegative health care workers may also be at increased risk of transmission, depending on their degree of contact with infected patients
C. Laboratory Diagnosis
1. Recommendation for immunocompetent patient: serologic testing for B19 virus–specific IgM and IgG
2. Recommendation for immunosuppressed patient, fetus, or neonate: nucleic acid amplification testing for detecting B19 virus–specific DNA
3. PCR analysis can be performed on serum, plasma, bone marrow, synovial fluid, amniotic fluid, and placental and fetal tissues
4. B19 virus DNA can often be detected in synovial fluid or bone marrow even in patients with no recent history of infection or disease
D. Prevention
1. Patients with transient aplastic crisis: implement droplet isolation precautions for 7 days
2. Immunodeficient patients with chronic human parvovirus B19 infection: implement droplet precautions for the duration of hospitalization
3. Patients with normal immune systems: probably not infectious after the onset of rash, arthralgias, or arthritis
4. Good infection control practices in the home, workplace, and hospital should be emphasized to decrease the risk of transmission to persons with compromised immune systems, those with red blood cell disorders such as homozygous sickle cell disease, and pregnant women

VIII. Coxsackievirus and Other Nonpolio Enteroviruses
A. Introduction
1. Nonpolio enteroviruses (groups A and B coxsackieviruses, echoviruses, and enteroviruses) cause infection in adults and children
B. Clinical Manifestations
1. Most infected persons (>90%) are asymptomatic or have undifferentiated febrile illness
2. Disease features reflect the age, sex, and immune status of the host
3. Various enterovirus serotypes can cause the same clinical syndromes (eg, viral meningitis, some exanthems)
4. Specific enterovirus subgroups cause other specific clinical syndromes (eg, coxsackieviruses cause pleurodynia and myocarditis)
5. Exanthems and enanthems
a. Some exanthems, which may be accompanied by enanthems, are caused by coxsackieviruses and echoviruses
b. Appearances of the eruptions are too similar for a visual diagnosis (except for hand-foot-and-mouth disease)
6. CNS infections
a. Acute CNS infection occurs at all ages
b. Meningitis is the most common CNS infection and is usually caused by group B coxsackieviruses and echoviruses
c. Encephalitis is less frequent
d. Certain nonpolio enteroviruses (eg, enterovirus 71) preferentially target, as polio does, the motor nuclei and anterior horn cells of the brain and spinal cord, affecting cranial and spinal nerves and causing acute paresis
7. Ocular infections
a. Worldwide pandemics, mostly in tropical coastal areas, of enterovirus 70 and coxsackievirus A24 have produced a highly contagious ocular infection
1) Pain, lid edema, and subconjunctival hemorrhage
2) Self-limited and rarely leads to permanent visual impairment

8. Pleurodynia
    a. Patients present with acute fever and paroxysmal spasms of the chest and abdominal muscles
    b. Most cases occur in summer outbreaks among adolescents and adults
    c. The group B coxsackieviruses are the most important cause of epidemic pleurodynia
    d. Pleurodynia sometimes mimics bacterial pneumonia, pulmonary embolus, myocardial infarction, and acute surgical abdomen
    e. Symptoms usually resolve in 4 to 6 days
9. Myopericarditis
    a. The group B coxsackieviruses are the most frequent viral cause of myocarditis in the United States
    b. In older children and adults, the severity ranges from asymptomatic cardiac involvement to fulminate disease with intractable heart failure and death
10. Infections in immunocompromised patients
    a. The enteroviruses cause persistent, sometimes fatal, infections in patients with hereditary or acquired defects in B lymphocyte function
        1) Children with X-linked agammaglobulinemia
        2) Adults with common variable immunodeficiency
        3) Allogeneic stem cell transplant patients
    b. Nonpolio enteroviruses
        1) Persistent CNS infections
        2) Dermatomyositis-like syndrome
        3) Chronic hepatitis
    c. In severe cases, large doses of intravenous immune globulin have been reported to improve outcome

Suggested Reading

Ahmad NM, Boruchoff SE. Multiple cerebral infarcts due to varicella-zoster virus large-vessel vasculopathy in an immunocompetent adult without skin involvement. Clin Infect Dis. 2003 Jul 1;37(1):e16-8. Epub 2003 Jun 24.

Crawford DH, Macsween KF, Higgins CD, Thomas R, McAulay K, Williams H, et al. A cohort study among university students: identification of risk factors for Epstein-Barr virus seroconversion and infectious mononucleosis. Clin Infect Dis. 2006 Aug 1;43(3):276–82. Epub 2006 Jun 20. Erratum in: Clin Infect Dis. 2006 Sep 15;43(6):805.

Graff JM, Beaver HA. Adenoviral conjunctivitis: 38 y.o. WF with watery, red irritated eyes; left more than right. EyeRounds.org. The University of Iowa Department of Ophthalmology & Visual Sciences; c2008. Updated 2005 Jun 14 [cited 2009 May 15]. Available from: http://webeye.ophth.uiowa.edu/eyeforum/cases/case28.htm.

Lin JC, Wang WY, Chen KY, Wei YH, Liang WM, Jan JS, et al. Quantification of plasma Epstein-Barr virus DNA in patients with advanced nasopharyngeal carcinoma. N Engl J Med. 2004 Jun 10;350(24):2461–70.

Oxman MN, Levin MJ, Johnson GR, Schmader KE, Straus SE, Gelb LD, et al; Shingles Prevention Study Group. A vaccine to prevent herpes zoster and postherpetic neuralgia in older adults. N Engl J Med. 2005 Jun 2;352(22):2271–84.

Ryan MA, Gray GC, Smith B, McKeehan JA, Hawksworth AW, Malasig MD. Large epidemic of respiratory illness due to adenovirus types 7 and 3 in healthy young adults. Clin Infect Dis. 2002 Mar 1;34(5):577–82. Epub 2002 Jan 16.

Select Gram-positive Aerobic Bacteria

Robin Patel, MD

I. Gram-positive Cocci
  A. Staphylococci
    1. Features
       a. Gram-positive cocci in clusters
       b. Catalase-positive
       c. Multiple species (Table 6.1)
    2. *Staphylococcus aureus*
       a. Cell wall: peptidoglycan and ribitol teichoic acid
       b. Protein A: binds Fc region of IgG, competes with phagocytic cells for IgG Fc sites, prevents opsonization
       c. Yellow colonies, β-hemolytic, ferments mannitol
       d. Free coagulase: if incubated with rabbit or human plasma, *S aureus* causes clotting (coagulase activates prothrombin) (tube coagulase test)
       e. Bound coagulase: dense emulsion of *S aureus* mixed with plasma; fibrin deposits on cell cause clumping (slide coagulase test)
       f. α-Toxin: inserts in lipid bilayer and forms transmembrane pores
       g. Panton-Valentine leukocidin
          1) Potent cytotoxin that causes leukocyte destruction, tissue necrosis, severe skin infections, and necrotizing pneumonia
          2) Associated with methicillin-resistant *S aureus*
       h. Superantigens (Figure 6.1)
          1) Toxic shock syndrome toxin-1
          2) Enterotoxins (eg, enterotoxin A, B, C) cause gastroenteritis by acting on neural receptors in the upper gastrointestinal tract, resulting in vomiting
          3) Bacteriophage
          4) Stable to boiling and digestive enzymes
       i. Can produce hyaluronidase, nuclease, lipase, and protease
       j. Surface proteins bind fibronectin, fibrinogen, and collagen
       k. Capsule blocks complement deposition and prevents opsonization
       l. Antimicrobial resistance

Table 6.1
Common Species of Staphylococci

Species	Coagulase	Novobiocin
Staphylococcus aureus	Positive	Susceptible
Staphylococcus epidermidis	Negative	Susceptible
Staphylococcus saprophyticus	Negative	Resistant
Staphylococcus lugdunensis	Negative	Susceptible

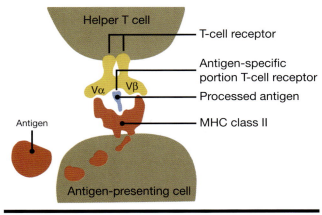
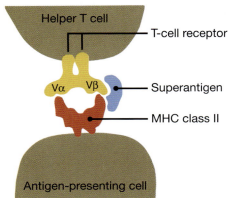

Figure 6.1. Mechanism of Action of Bacterial Superantigens. Bacterial superantigens are microbial polypeptide exotoxins that are very potent T-cell activators at low concentrations. In contrast to conventional antigens (upper), which are processed before binding to the peptide-binding groove of major histocompatibility complex (MHC) class II molecules, superantigens (lower) are not processed before they bind outside the peptide-binding groove.

        1) Penicillin resistance: plasmid penicillinase (β-lactamase)
        2) Methicillin-resistant *S aureus* (MRSA): penicillin-binding proteins 2′ (PBP2′) and 2a (PBP2a) are produced with decreased affinity for methicillin (also nafcillin, oxacillin) and all available β-lactam antimicrobial agents (except ceftobiprole)
        3) Vancomycin-intermediate and vancomycin-resistant *S aureus*
    3. Coagulase-negative *Staphylococcus* species
      a. Skin: frequent contaminants in clinical specimens
      b. *Staphylococcus saprophyticus*: 10% to 20% of urinary tract infections in young women; resistance to novobiocin

      c. *Staphylococcus lugdunensis*: endocarditis (including native valve endocarditis); bone and joint infection
      d. Emerging pathogens: barrier disruption, prosthetic materials, immunocompromised hosts, premature infants, and adherence to foreign material (biofilm formation)
  B. Streptococci
    1. Features
      a. Ovoid
      b. Chains: divide in 1 plane and remain attached
      c. Some produce hyaluronic acid or polysaccharide capsules
      d. Blood agar hemolytic reactions: α, β, and γ
      e. Catalase-negative
      f. Multiple species (Table 6.2)
    2. *Streptococcus pyogenes* (group A streptococcus)
      a. β-Hemolysis
        1) Streptolysin S: oxygen stable, occasionally absent, nonantigenic
        2) Streptolysin O (pore forming): lyses leukocytes, tissue cells, and platelets, antigenic
        3) Antistreptolysin O (ASO): used in quantitation; oxygen labile within agar
      b. Bacitracin test
        1) Detection of group A antigen in throat swab specimens with polymerase chain reaction (PCR) or enzyme immunoassay
      c. ASO, anti-DNAse B, antistreptokinase, and antihyaluronidase (for sequelae)
      d. Pyrogenic exotoxins
        1) Nine streptococcal pyrogenic exotoxins (A, B, C, F, G, H, J, streptococcal superantigen, streptococcal mitogenic exotoxin Z)
        2) Fever, rash (scarlet fever), T-cell proliferation, B-cell suppression, sensitivity to endotoxin, superantigens (streptococcal toxic shock syndrome)
        3) Streptococcal pyrogenic exotoxin B has enzymatic activity: cleaves elements of extracellular matrix (eg, fibronectin, vitronectin)
      e. M protein: shed into circulation, forms a complex with fibrinogen that binds to integrins on the surface of polymorphonuclear leukocytes
        1) Degranulation, release of hydrolytic enzymes, and respiratory burst

Table 6.2

Features of Select Streptococci and Enterococci

Species	Appearance of Gram-positive Cocci	Common Term	Hemolysis	Lancefield Group	Capsule	Virulence Factors	Disease
Pyogenic Streptococci							
Streptococcus pyogenes	Chains	Group A streptococcus (GAS)	β	A	Hyaluronic acid	M protein, lipoteichoic acid, streptococcal pyrogenic exotoxins, streptolysin O, streptokinase	Strep throat, impetigo, pyogenic infections, toxic shock, rheumatic fever, glomerulonephritis
Streptococcus agalactiae	Chains	Group B streptococcus (GBS)	β, γ	B	Sialic acid (9 types of antigens)	Capsule	Neonatal sepsis, meningitis, pyogenic infections
Streptococcus equi	Chains		β	C	—	—	Pyogenic infections
Streptococcus bovis species group	Chains		α, γ	D	—	—	Pyogenic infections
Other species	Chains		α, β, γ	E-W	—	—	Pyogenic infections
Pneumococcus							
Streptococcus pneumoniae	Diplococci	Pneumococcus	α	—	Polysaccharide (>90 serotypes)	Capsule, pneumolysin, neuraminidase	Pneumonia, meningitis, otitis media, pyogenic infections
Viridans Group and Nonhemolytic Streptococci							
Streptococcus sanguinis	Chains		α	—	—	—	Low virulence, endocarditis
Streptococcus salivarius	Chains		α	—	—	—	Low virulence, endocarditis
Streptococcus mutans	Chains		α	—	—	—	Dental caries
Other species	Chains		α, γ	—	—	—	Low virulence, endocarditis
Enterococci							
Enterococcus faecalis	Chains	Enterococcus	α, γ	D	—	—	Urinary tract, pyogenic infections, endocarditis
Enterococcus faecium	Chains	Enterococcus	α, γ	D	—	—	Urinary tract, pyogenic infections, endocarditis
Other species	Chains		α, γ	D or none	—	—	Urinary tract, pyogenic infections, endocarditis

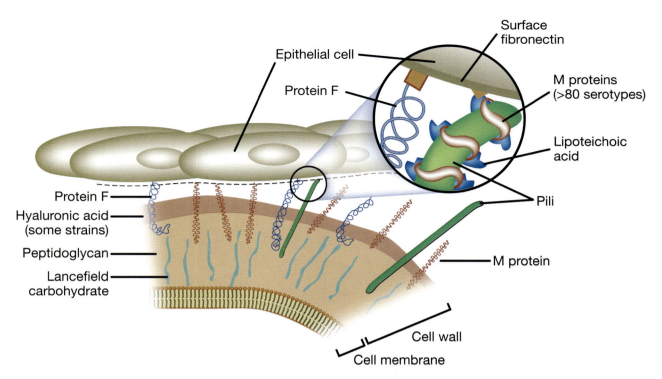

Figure 6.2. Antigenic Structure of *Streptococcus pyogenes* Showing Adhesion to an Epithelial Cell. (Adapted from Ryan KJ, Ray CG. Sherris medical microbiology: an introduction to infectious diseases. 4th ed. New York [NY]: McGraw-Hill; c2004. Used with permission.)

2) Vascular damage, hypercoagulability, hypotension, disseminated intravascular coagulation, and organ damage
f. Adherence (Figure 6.2)
  1) Mucosal surface: lipoteichoic acid (LTA), protein F, M protein (scaffold LTA)
  2) Epidermis: keratinocyte (CD46) and M protein
  3) Langerhans cells: protein F
g. Invasion phagocytes: M protein, fibronectin-binding proteins (eg, protein F), integrin receptors, cytoskeletal rearrangements
h. Resistance to opsonophagocytosis (Figure 6.3)
  1) M protein binds fibrinogen and serum factor H, diminishing the availability of C3b for deposition on streptococcal surface
  2) Opsonization with type-specific antibody binds complement C3b by classical mechanism, facilitating phagocyte recognition
  3) C5a peptidase degrades C5a, the main factor attracting phagocytes to sites of complement deposition
  4) Hyaluronic acid capsule
i. Streptokinase: converts plasminogen to plasmin (lysis of fibrin clots); antigenic, tissue injury, toxic to phagocytic cells
j. Hyaluronidase: may help bacteria spread through tissues
k. Nucleases (DNAses) protect
l. Repeated infections and rheumatic fever result from multiple antigenic types of M proteins
m. Acute rheumatic fever
  1) Autoimmune state induced by pharyngeal streptococcal infection
  2) Anti-M protein antibody cross-reacts with heart sarcolemma
  3) Anti–group A carbohydrate reacts with heart valves

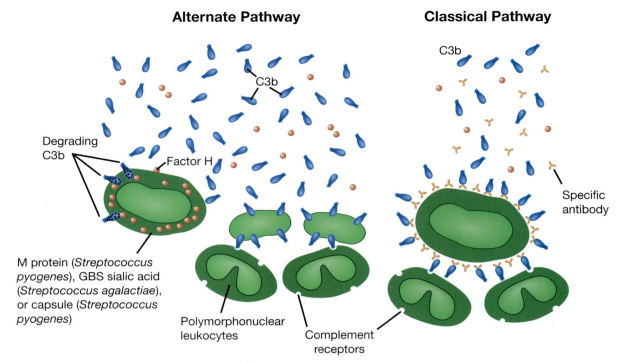

Figure 6.3. Streptococcal Resistance to Opsonophagocytosis. Left, In the alternate pathway, C3b binds to the surface of bacteria, providing a recognition site for professional phagocytes. Organisms with capsules or M protein bind serum factor H to their surface, interfering with complement deposition by accelerating the breakdown of C3b. Right, In the classical pathway, specific antibody binding to an antigen on the surface provides another binding site for C3b, enabling phagocyte recognition independently of serum factor H. GBS indicates group B streptococci. (Adapted from Ryan KJ, Ray CG. Sherris medical microbiology: an introduction to infectious diseases. 4th ed. New York [NY]: McGraw-Hill; c2004. Used with permission.)

4) Genetic factors: host and increased cell-mediated immune response
5) Aschoff bodies: lymphocytes and macrophages aggregated around fibrinoid deposits in the heart
6) Diagnostic criteria
   a) Major criteria: carditis, polyarthritis, chorea, erythema marginatum, and subcutaneous nodules
   b) Minor criteria: clinical (arthralgia or fever) and laboratory (increased leukocyte count, increased erythrocyte sedimentation rate, increased concentration of C-reactive protein, and prolonged PR interval)
   c) Two major criteria *or* 1 major plus 2 minor criteria are highly suggestive if supported by positive throat culture, antigen test or PCR results, increased levels of antistreptococcal antibodies (ASO and DNAse), or scarlet fever
   n. Acute glomerulonephritis
      1) Antigen-antibody complexes, complement activation, inflammation, diffuse proliferative (mesangial and endothelial) exudate (neutrophils and monocytes), deposits of IgG and C3
      2) M proteins of some nephritogenic strains share antigenic determinants with glomeruli
3. *Streptococcus agalactiae* (group B streptococcus)
   a. Large colonies, less β-hemolytic than group A streptococci, CAMP (Christie, Atkins, Munch-Peterson) test positive
   b. Polysaccharide capsular antigens: 9 types (Ia, Ib, and II-VIII) with sialic acid terminal side chain residues
   c. Gastrointestinal tract, vagina (10%-30% of women), amniotic fluid, newborn passing through birth canal

d. Capsular sialic acid moiety binds serum factor H, accelerating degradation of C3b
   1) Renders alternative pathway–mediated opsonophagocytosis ineffective (Figure 6.3)
   2) Complement-mediated phagocyte recognition through classical pathway requires specific antibody
   3) Transplacental type-specific anticapsular IgG is protective
e. C5a peptidase is a polymorphonuclear neutrophil chemoattractant
4. *Streptococcus pneumoniae*
   a. α-Hemolytic; dimpled on blood agar (autolysis); susceptible to optochin; bile soluble
   b. Autolysis from peroxidases and autolysins produced by organism (accentuated by bile; "bile soluble")
   c. More than 90 serotypes of polysaccharide polymer capsules (Pneumovax 23 vaccine contains 23 serotypes): inhibit phagocytosis by interfering with C3b binding to cell (Figure 6.3)
   d. Choline-binding protein on pneumococcal cell wall binds choline and carbohydrates on nasopharyngeal cells
   e. Pneumolysin: forms pores in pulmonary endothelial cells; stimulates cytokines, suppresses host inflammatory and immune function, and disrupts respiratory epithelial cell cilia
   f. Neuraminidase cleaves sialic acid in host mucin, glycoproteins, and glycolipids
   g. Pneumococcal surface protein A interferes with complement deposition
   h. Peptidoglycan and teichoic acid stimulate inflammation and cerebral edema
   i. Most common in persons younger than 2 years or older than 60 years
   j. Predisposing conditions: alcoholism, diabetes mellitus, chronic renal or lung disease, asplenia, some malignancies, smoking, and viral respiratory infections
   k. Nasopharyngeal colonization: 5% to 40% (highest in children, in winter, and in patients with aspiration pneumonia)
   l. Transmitted person to person through direct contact or microaerosols (cough or sneeze in close quarters)
5. Viridans group streptococci
   a. α-Hemolytic streptococci
   b. Normal oral and nasopharyngeal flora
   c. Low virulence: bacterial endocarditis (Table 6.2)
   d. Glucans: complex polysaccharide polymers enhance attachment to cardiac valves
   e. *Streptococcus mutans*: dental caries
C. Enterococci
   1. Growth in 6.5% sodium chloride; nonhemolytic or α-hemolytic
   2. Group D antigen: teichoic acid (Table 6.2)
   3. Colonize gut (resistant to bile salts)
   4. Inhibited only by high concentrations of penicillin; combination of penicillin and aminoglycoside is synergistic
   5. Glycopeptide-resistant enterococci: phenotypically and genotypically heterogeneous (Table 6.3)
   6. Genes *vanA*, *vanB*, and *vanD* encode ligase responsible for synthesis of the depsipeptide D-alanyl-D-lactate, which is incorporated into a pentapeptide peptidoglycan cell wall precursor to which vancomycin binds poorly (Figure 6.4)
   7. VanA-type glycopeptide resistance is mediated by Tn*1546* or closely related elements; Tn*1546* consists of 10,851 base pairs and encodes 9 polypeptides assigned to different functional groups
      a. Transposition functions and regulation of glycopeptide resistance genes (*vanR* and *vanS*)
      b. Synthesis of depsipeptide D-alanyl-D-lactate, which, when incorporated into pentapeptide peptidoglycan precursor, forms pentapeptide precursor to which neither vancomycin nor teicoplanin binds (*vanH* and *vanA*)
      c. Hydrolysis of precursors of normal peptidoglycan (*vanX* and *vanY*); function of *vanZ* is unknown (Figure 6.5)
      d. Genes *vanR*, *vanS*, *vanH*, *vanA*, and *vanX* are necessary and sufficient for inducible expression of resistance to vancomycin (Figure 6.5)
   8. VanB-type glycopeptide resistance is homologous to VanA glycopeptide resistance
   9. VanC-type glycopeptide resistance
      a. Low-level vancomycin resistance but teicoplanin susceptibility
      b. Intrinsic property: *Enterococcus gallinarum* and *Enterococcus casseliflavus* (*Enterococcus flavescens*)
      c. Chromosomally encoded
      d. Pentapeptide peptidoglycan precursors in strains with VanC vancomycin resistance terminate in D-alanyl-D-serine (rather than D-alanyl-D-alanine)

Table 6.3
Resistance to Glycopeptides Among Enterococci

Phenotype	Genotype	MIC, mcg/mL		Expression	Transfer[a]	Species
		Vancomycin	Teicoplanin			
VanA	vanA	64-1,000	16-512	Inducible	+	E faecium E faecalis E avium E gallinarum E durans E mundtii E casseliflavus E raffinosus E hirae
VanB	vanB	4-1,000	0.25-2	Inducible	+	E faecium E faecalis E gallinarum E durans
VanC	vanC-1	2-32	0.12-2	Constitutive, inducible	−	E gallinarum
VanC	vanC-2	2-32	0.12-2	Constitutive	−	E casseliflavus
VanC	vanC-3	2-32	0.12-2	Constitutive	−	E flavescens
VanD	vanD	16-256	2-64	Constitutive	−	E faecium E faecalis
VanE	vanE	16	0.5		−	E faecalis
VanF	vanF	800	<1		−	P popilliae
VanG	vanG	16	0.5		−	E faecalis

Abbreviations: E, Enterococcus; MIC, minimum inhibitory concentration; P, Paenibacillus.

[a] Plus sign indicates transferability; minus sign, lack of transferability.

Adapted from Patel R. Vancomycin-resistant enterococci in solid organ transplantation. Curr Opin Organ Transplant. 1999;4(3):271–80. Used with permission.

II. Gram-positive Bacilli
  A. Corynebacterium Species
    1. Small, pleomorphic, catalase-positive non–spore-forming, club-shaped Gram-positive rods in "Chinese letter" or palisade arrangements
    2. Corynebacterium diphtheriae
      a. Diphtheria toxin (Figure 6.6)
        1) Lysogenic phage carries tox gene
        2) Repressor protein DtxR increases toxin biosynthesis in iron-limiting conditions
        3) Immunity: antibodies neutralize toxin
        4) Toxoid is produced from formalin treatment of toxin
      b. Culture requires special medium
        1) Tellurite medium (eg, Tindale agar) inhibits growth of normal flora; C diphtheriae reduces tellurite to tellurium, turning colonies black
        2) Loeffler medium inhibits growth of normal flora; promotes metachromatic granules, which are visualized with methylene blue stain
      c. Toxin production: Elek test
    3. Corynebacterium jeikeium: antimicrobial resistance
  B. Listeria monocytogenes
    1. Identification
      a. Gram-positive, non–spore-forming bacillus
      b. Catalase-positive
      c. Motility agar: motile at 25°C, not at 37°C
      d. Cold enrichment for isolation
      e. Wet mount: tumbling motility
      f. Narrow zone of β-hemolysis
      g. Fluorescent antibody with anti-Listeria antibody
    2. Thirteen serotypes
      a. Based on teichoic acid composition
      b. Human disease from 3 food-borne strains: 1/2a, 1/2b, and 4b
    3. Reservoir: intestines of animals and humans
    4. At risk: persons who are elderly, pregnant, neonatal, or immunocompromised
    5. Food-borne disease from animal products: soft cheeses (eg, feta, Brie, Camembert,

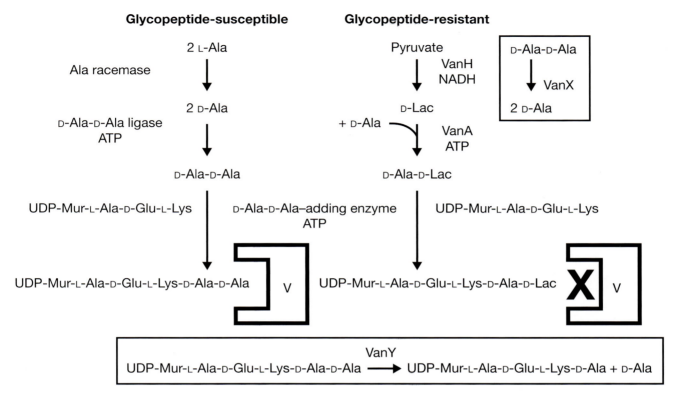

Figure 6.4. Vancomycin Resistance. Mechanism of action of vancomycin and mechanism of vancomycin resistance are shown for enterococci with *vanA*-associated vancomycin resistance. ATP indicates adenosine triphosphate; Mur, muramic acid; NADH, reduced form of nicotinamide adenine dinucleotide; UDP, uridine diphosphate; V, vancomycin. (Adapted from Patel R. Vancomycin-resistant enterococci in solid organ transplantation. Curr Opin Organ Transplant. 1999;4[3]:271–80. Used with permission.)

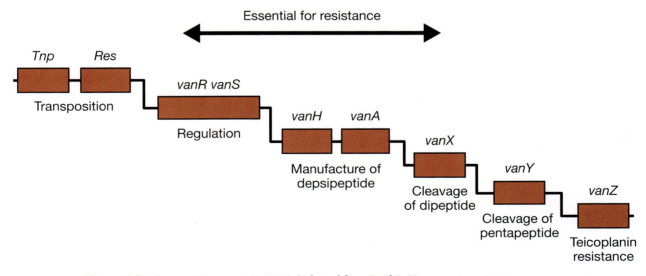

Figure 6.5. The *vanA* Operon in Tn*1546*. (Adapted from Patel R. Vancomycin-resistant enterococci in solid organ transplantation. Curr Opin Organ Transplant. 1999;4[3]:271–80. Used with permission.)

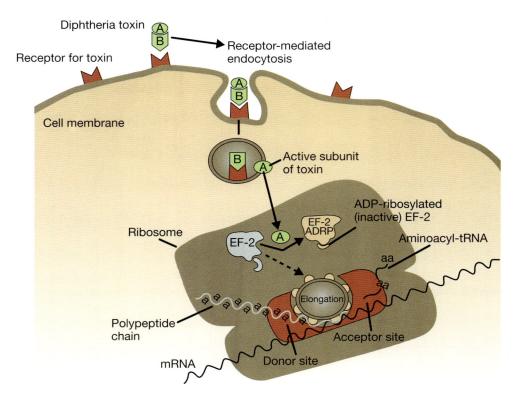

Figure 6.6. Mechanism of Action of Diphtheria Toxin. The B (toxin-binding) subunit attaches to the cell membrane, and the whole molecule enters the cell. Thereafter, the 2 subunits dissociate, and the A subunit catalyzes a reaction that results in adenosine diphosphate (ADP)-ribosylated elongation factor-2 (EF-2), which inhibits protein synthesis. ADRP indicates ADP-ribosylated; mRNA, messenger RNA; tRNA, transfer RNA. (Adapted from Ryan KJ, Ray CG. Sherris medical microbiology: an introduction to infectious diseases. 4th ed. New York [NY]: McGraw-Hill; c2004. Used with permission.)

blue-veined, Mexican-style), unpasteurized milk, ready-to-eat sausages, and delicatessen products
6. Mechanisms
   a. Grows in nonimmune macrophages
   b. Attaches to and internalizes into enterocytes, fibroblasts, dendritic cells, hepatocytes, endothelial cells, M cells, and macrophages
   c. Internalin (surface protein): induces local reorganization of cytoskeleton and stimulates entry into membrane-bound vacuole
   d. Listeriolysin O (pore-forming cytotoxin) aids escape to cytosol
   e. *Listeria monocytogenes* moves through cell by controlling cell's actin filaments, stimulated by surface proteins (ActA and gelsolin), which control actin polymerization so that monomers are sequentially concentrated behind the bacterium
   f. Distinctive comet tail structure (highly cross-linked F-actin) develops and pushes the bacterium through the cytoplasm; "rockets" push bacteria to neighboring cells, propagating infection
C. *Bacillus* Species
   1. Identification
      a. Gram-positive, spore-forming rods
      b. Catalase-positive
      c. Spores: location (central, subterminal, or terminal) and structure (oval or spherical) are used for species identification
   2. Ubiquitous: survive in diverse environments
   3. Many species are part of normal human flora; most often, skin or environmental contaminants

4. *Bacillus anthracis*
   a. Identification
      1) Centrally located elliptical spores
      2) Sheep blood agar: off-white colonies, comma-shaped outgrowth ("Medusa head"), nonhemolytic, nonmotile
   b. Primarily a disease of herbivores: 80% mortality
   c. Humans
      1) Inoculated through skin
      2) Ingestion
      3) Inhalation: infectious dose is 8,000-10,000 spores
   d. Capsule
      1) Encapsulated in vivo
      2) Enhanced capsule production in elevated carbon dioxide concentrations in vitro
      3) Capsule is associated with virulence, D-glutamic acid polypeptide, and antiphagocytic properties
   e. Toxins
      1) Plasmid mediated
      2) Protective antigen elicits protective immune response
      3) Lethal factor (zinc metalloproteinase) stimulates release of tumor necrosis factor and interleukin 1β and impairs dendritic cell maturation
      4) Edema factor (calmodulin-dependent adenyl cyclase) increases levels of cyclic adenosine monophosphate, impairs neutrophil function, disrupts water balance, resulting in massive tissue edema
5. *Bacillus cereus*
   a. Food poisoning
      1) Enterotoxin stimulates adenyl cyclase production
      2) Not usually diagnosed unless large outbreak
      3) Found in healthy persons
      4) Isolation not an indication of infection
      5) Same serotype from suspected food
      6) Clinically significant concentration: >10^5 colony-forming units per gram of food
   b. Infections: eye, soft tissues, lung in association with trauma, foreign body infection, etc
6. *Bacillus subtilis*
   a. Infections: eye, soft tissues, lung in association with trauma, foreign body infection, etc
D. *Erysipelothrix rhusiopathiae*
   1. Catalase-negative
   2. Hydrogen sulfide–positive
E. *Tropheryma whipplei*
   1. Actinomycete (gram-positive bacillus) phylogenetically
   2. Periodic acid-Schiff stain of tissue
   3. Polymerase chain reaction

Suggested Reading

Frank KL, Del Pozo JL, Patel R. From clinical microbiology to infection pathogenesis: how daring to be different works for *Staphylococcus lugdunensis*. Clin Microbiol Rev. 2008 Jan;21(1):111–33.

Gorwitz RJ. Community-associated methicillin-resistant *Staphylococcus aureus*: epidemiology and update. Pediatr Infect Dis J. 2008 Oct;27(10):925–6.

Jacobs MR. Antimicrobial-resistant *Streptococcus pneumoniae*: trends and management. Expert Rev Anti Infect Ther. 2008 Oct;6(5):619–35.

Nordmann P, Naas T, Fortineau N, Poirel L. Superbugs in the coming new decade; multidrug resistance and prospects for treatment of *Staphylococcus aureus*, *Enterococcus* spp. and *Pseudomonas aeruginosa* in 2010. Curr Opin Microbiol. 2007 Oct;10(5):436–40. Epub 2007 Aug 30.

David R. McNamara, MD
Franklin R. Cockerill III, MD

Select Gram-negative Aerobic Bacteria

I. Introduction
   A. Diversity of Gram-negative Bacteria
      1. May be rod-shaped (bacilli), spherical (cocci), oval, helical, or filamentous
         a. Cytoplasmic membrane is surrounded by a cell wall consisting of a peptidoglycan layer and an outer cell membrane
         b. Flagellae that are present on some species confer motility
      2. Widely distributed in the natural environment
         a. Commensals with many animals
         b. Vital role in normal human physiology as intestinal commensals
   B. Cause of Various Human Illnesses
      1. The gram-negative bacterial cell wall contains various lipopolysaccharide endotoxins
      2. Endotoxins trigger intense inflammation and the sepsis syndrome during infection
II. Specific Organisms
   A. Gram-negative Cocci
      1. *Neisseria meningitidis*
         a. A gram-negative diplococcus (Figure 7.1)
         b. Can cause fulminant meningitis and bacteremia, typically in children and young adults
         c. Infection is acquired through the nasopharyngeal route, and the frequency of asymptomatic colonization increases during disease outbreaks
         d. Persons with terminal complement component (C5-C9) and properdin deficiencies are predisposed to meningococcal infection

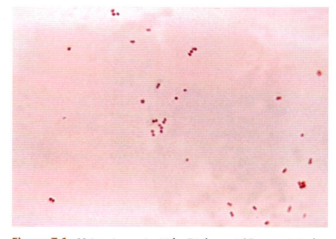

Figure 7.1. *Neisseria meningitides* Diplococci (Gram, original magnification ×1,150). (Adapted from Centers for Disease Control and Prevention. Public Health Image Library [PHIL]: photographs, illustrations, multimedia files. [cited 2006 Aug 23]. Available from: http://phil.cdc.gov/phil/home.asp.)

e. Antimicrobial therapy of choice: penicillin, ampicillin, or ceftriaxone
f. Close contacts of persons with meningococcal disease should receive prophylaxis with rifampin, ciprofloxacin, or ceftriaxone
g. Vaccination against serogroups A, C, Y, and W-135 is available and should be considered for students living in dormitories

2. *Moraxella catarrhalis*
    a. A common respiratory tract pathogen and commensal organism
    b. On Gram stain, it appears as a gram-negative diplococcus, resembling *N meningitidis*
    c. Nasopharyngeal colonization of children and adults is common
    d. In children: associated with acute otitis media
    e. In adults: associated with exacerbation of chronic obstructive pulmonary disease, sinusitis, and pneumonia
    f. Commonly produces an inducible β-lactamase
    g. Antibacterials with reliable activity against *M catarrhalis*: amoxicillin-clavulanate, trimethoprim-sulfamethoxazole, macrolides, quinolones, and second- and third-generation cephalosporins

3. *Acinetobacter calcoaceticus-baumannii* complex
    a. Coccobacillary to rod-shaped gram-negative bacteria
    b. Occasionally appears gram-positive, especially if isolated from blood culture media
    c. Can be part of commensal flora on skin and in pharynx
    d. Typically with low intrinsic virulence
    e. Common infections associated with *Acinetobacter*
        1) Ventilator-associated pneumonia
        2) Bacteremia
        3) Infected traumatic wounds, particularly in soldiers
    f. Multidrug-resistant *Acinetobacter* are increasingly common
        1) Nosocomial pathogens, especially with broad-spectrum antimicrobial use: intensive care units, surgical wounds, and burn units
        2) Many strains are resistant to multiple drug classes
        3) Carbapenems (except ertapenem), quinolones, aminoglycosides, colistin, and tigecycline may possess activity

B. Gram-negative Bacilli
    1. *Vibrio*
        a. *Vibrio cholerae*
            1) Causes profuse, watery diarrhea that can lead to fatal volume depletion
            2) Endemic to South America (Peru)
            3) Fecal-oral transmission, usually in areas with poor wastewater treatment facilities and poverty
            4) Direct examination of stool during an outbreak
            5) Supports clinical diagnosis if gram-negative bacilli with a polar flagellum are present
            6) May see characteristic darting motility in wet mount preparations
            7) Primary therapy: fluid and electrolyte replacement
            8) Secondary therapy: antibacterials active against *V cholerae*, including tetracyclines, ampicillin, trimethoprim-sulfamethoxazole, and quinolones
        b. *Vibrio vulnificus* and *Vibrio parahaemolyticus*
            1) In the United States, *Vibrio* infections usually involve *V vulnificus* or *V parahaemolyticus*
            2) *Vibrio* bacteria live in marine waters and can cause enteritis and soft tissue infection with sepsis
                a) Ingestion of raw or undercooked seafood
                b) Exposure to saltwater
            3) Persons with liver cirrhosis are particularly at risk of fulminant soft tissue infections
                a) Septic shock
                b) Hemorrhagic, bullous skin lesions
    2. Enterobacteriaceae
        a. Enterobacteriaceae is a family of gram-negative bacilli
            1) Widely distributed in nature
            2) Normal intestinal commensals of humans and other animals
            3) Can cause disease in hospital environments
        b. Oxidase-negative, in contrast to *Pseudomonas* species
        c. Includes the genera *Citrobacter*, *Enterobacter*, *Escherichia*, *Klebsiella*, *Proteus*, and *Serratia*
            1) Commonly associated with extraintestinal, nosocomial infection
            2) Can cause bacteremia, nosocomial pneumonia, urinary tract infections, and wound infections

3) *Citrobacter* and *Enterobacter* species can possess inducible *ampC* β-lactamase resistance
d. Some Enterobacteriaceae, especially *Escherichia coli* and *Klebsiella pneumoniae*, produce extended-spectrum β-lactamase (ESBL)
   1) Occasionally appear gram-positive, especially if isolated from blood culture media
   2) Confers inducible resistance to third-generation cephalosporins, which have been mainstays in the treatment of infections caused by these bacteria
   3) ESBL-producing organisms can also be resistant to quinolones and aminoglycosides
   4) Empirical therapy for gram-negative infections suspected to be from ESBL-producing strains: carbapenems (meropenem and imipenem), which generally have the most reliable activity against these organisms
e. Various Enterobacteriaceae carry a transmissible plasmid that encodes *Klebsiella pneumoniae* carbapenemase (KPC)
   1) Confers resistance to β-lactam antibacterials, including carbapenems
   2) Positive modified Hodge test in the microbiology laboratory
   3) Treatment options include aminoglycosides, tigecycline, and colistin; most are resistant to quinolones
f. In addition to causing extraintestinal disease, *E coli* can cause enterocolitis: diarrhea (watery, mucoid, or bloody), abdominal pain, and fever
   1) Transmitted through fecally contaminated food or water
   2) Enterohemorrhagic *E coli* (EHEC) produce verotoxin, a Shiga toxin
      a) Maintained in the intestinal tracts of domestic livestock, EHEC are spread to humans through consumption of fecally contaminated food (eg, ground beef, contaminated produce) or water
      b) EHEC, including the *E coli* O157:H7 strain, can also cause hemolytic uremic syndrome
         i) Characterized by microvascular hemolytic anemia, renal failure, and thrombocytopenia
         ii) Serious, multisystem illness that can cause irreversible renal failure and is a leading cause of renal failure in children
         iii) Other *E coli* strains besides O157:H7 cause 30% to 50% of enterohemorrhagic *E coli* infections (the rate appears to be similar for hemolytic uremic syndrome) but have a lower propensity to cause bloody diarrhea
      c) EHEC-related diarrhea should not be treated with antibiotics
         i) Outcomes may be worse
         ii) Perturbation of verotoxin production by antibiotics
g. Some *Klebsiella pneumoniae* strains have a mucoid phenotype characterized by production of a hyperviscous mucoid polysaccharide capsule
   1) These strains are less susceptible to complement-mediated clearance
   2) They are associated with invasive clinical illness, including liver abscess and meningitis
h. Treatment of infection caused by Enterobacteriaceae is typically guided by results of susceptibility testing
   1) Common empirical therapy choices in hospitalized patients with extraintestinal infection: third- and fourth-generation cephalosporins, piperacillin, and quinolones
   2) Other antibacterials active against many strains: ampicillin, aztreonam, trimethoprim-sulfamethoxazole, tigecycline, colistin, and aminoglycosides
   3) Because antibacterial therapy for EHEC strains (including *E coli* O157:H7) may increase the risk of renal failure and worsen the clinical outcome, empirical antibacterial therapy is not recommended for diarrhea possibly due to *E coli* O157:H7
   4) Antimotility agents may worsen the clinical course by increasing intestinal contact with bacterial toxins
i. *Salmonella typhi*, *Salmonella paratyphi*, and nontyphi *Salmonella* species
   1) *Salmonella* species are members of the family Enterobacteriaceae and are

an important cause of gastroenteritis worldwide
2) Taxonomy of *Salmonella* species has been revised
   a) Older classification based on serotypes (referred to as separate species) is still in clinical use
   b) *Salmonella* species were classically differentiated into *S typhi* or *S paratyphi* and numerous (>2,000) nontyphi serotypes
3) *Salmonella* species are nonfastidious Enterobacteriaceae that do not ferment lactose, unlike other Enterobacteriaceae
4) Infection with *Salmonella* species causes 2 major clinical syndromes: enteric fever and enteritis
   a) Enteric fever
      i) Febrile systemic disease with abdominal pain and headache that may be preceded by gastrointestinal tract symptoms such as diarrhea or constipation
      ii) Commonly due to ingestion of food or water that is fecally contaminated with *S typhi* or *S paratyphi* from their human reservoirs
      iii) Clues to diagnosis on physical examination: evanescent maculopapular rash on abdomen and thorax (rose spots) (Figure 7.2) and hepatosplenomegaly
      iv) Enteric fever due to *S typhi* was classically referred to as typhoid fever owing to its similarity to typhus, the systemic febrile rickettsiosis
      v) Recovery of *S typhi* (or *S paratyphi*) in cultures of blood or bone marrow is common in enteric fever
      vi) Small proportion of persons with enteric fever become chronic, asymptomatic carriers of *Salmonella*
         (a) Colonization of gallbladder
         (b) Chronic fecal shedding and fecal-oral contact allow perpetuation of infection in the human population

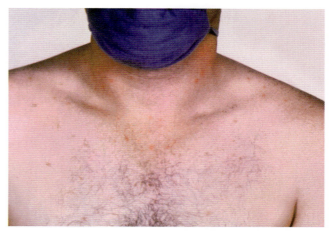

Figure 7.2. Rose Spots on Chest of Patient With Typhoid Fever Due to *Salmonella typhi*. (Adapted from Centers for Disease Control and Prevention. Public Health Image Library [PHIL]: photographs, illustrations, multimedia files. [cited 2006 Aug 23]. Available from: http://phil.cdc.gov/phil/home.asp.)

   b) Enteritis
      i) Localized gastrointestinal tract infection with watery diarrhea that may progress to bloody stools
      ii) Usually associated with ingestion of *Salmonella* species (nontyphi *Salmonella* or *S paratyphi*) from undercooked eggs or other foods
      iii) Nontyphi *Salmonella* serotypes are widely distributed in animal reservoirs, particularly in reptiles and birds
      iv) Complications of infection: bacteremia, metastatic foci of infection (such as osteomyelitis), dehydration due to severe diarrhea, and a postinfectious arthritis in patients with HLA-B27 antigen
5) Treatment of *Salmonella* infection: complicated by increased resistance to antibiotics
   a) Currently, ceftriaxone or ciprofloxacin are first-line therapies
   b) Ampicillin and trimethoprim-sulfamethoxazole are alternative agents for susceptible isolates

j. *Shigella sonnei*, *Shigella boydii*, *Shigella dysenteriae*, and *Shigella flexneri*
   1) *Shigella* species are oxidase-negative, nonmotile, gram-negative bacilli that are members of the family Enterobacteriaceae
   2) Infection with *Shigella*
      a) Important cause of enteritis or intestinal inflammation with resulting diarrhea
      b) Often accompanied by abdominal pain and fever
      c) The severe diarrhea can lead to fatal dehydration
      d) Transmitted through contact with hands of infected persons or ingestion of fecally contaminated food or water
      e) Notable for the small gastrointestinal inoculum (<200 organisms) required to produce disease
   3) Treatment of *Shigella* enteritis
      a) Rehydration (with oral rehydration solutions or intravenous fluids) and antibacterial therapy
      b) In contrast to *E coli* enteritis, antibiotic therapy is beneficial in *Shigella* enteritis in limiting the clinical course of disease
      c) Antibiotics of choice: quinolones in adults and trimethoprim-sulfamethoxazole in children
k. *Yersinia pestis*, *Yersinia pseudotuberculosis*, and *Yersinia enterocolitica*
   1) Short gram-negative rods with characteristic bipolar "safety pin" appearance on Gram stain (Figure 7.3)
   2) Plague
      a) Caused by *Y pestis*
      b) Transmission from natural reservoir of rodents (including rats and prairie dogs) through the bite of an infected flea
      c) Rapid onset of fever and prostration 2 to 8 days after the bite of an infected flea
      d) Three forms of plague
         i) Bubonic plague: most common; characteristically tender regional lymphadenopathy (buboes) (Figure 7.4)
         ii) Pneumonic plague: lower respiratory tract infection with *Y pestis*; transmissible from person-to-person through droplet nuclei
         iii) Septicemic plague: bacteremia without regional lymphadenopathy; has a high mortality rate
      e) Antimicrobials of choice for *Y pestis* infection: streptomycin, gentamicin, or tetracycline

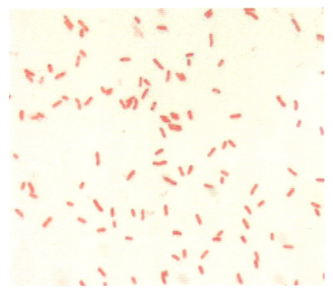

Figure 7.3. Blood From Person With Plague. Stained bipolar ends of *Yersinia pestis* are apparent (Wright stain, original magnification ×1,000). (Adapted from Centers for Disease Control and Prevention. Public Health Image Library [PHIL]: photographs, illustrations, multimedia files. [cited 2006 Aug 23]. Available from: http://phil.cdc.gov/phil/home.asp.)

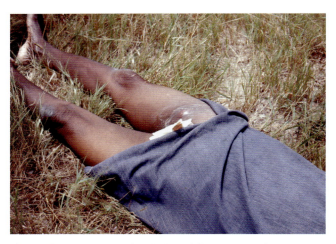

Figure 7.4. Inguinal Bubo. (Adapted from Centers for Disease Control and Prevention. Public Health Image Library [PHIL]: photographs, illustrations, multimedia files. [cited 2006 Aug 23]. Available from: http://phil.cdc.gov/phil/home.asp.)

- f) Like *Francisella tularensis*, *Y pestis* is a potential agent of bioterrorism
3) *Yersinia pseudotuberculosis* and *Y enterocolitica* cause yersiniosis
    - a) Gastrointestinal tract infection is characterized by fever, abdominal pain, and diarrhea (which is often bloody)
    - b) Pathologically, terminal ileitis and adenitis are common
    - c) Patients with iron overload (transfusion-dependent patients or those with hemochromatosis) may be at increased risk of yersiniosis
    - d) Patients with HLA-B27 antigen are at risk of a postinfectious arthritis (Reiter syndrome) and erythema nodosum
3. *Pseudomonas aeruginosa*
    a. Oxidase-positive, motile, gram-negative bacillus that is widely distributed in nature
    b. Occurs commonly in water, soil, and hospital environments, where it can colonize ventilator circuits and water sources and contaminate pharmaceutical preparations
    c. *Pseudomonas* is a common cause of infection in patients with defects in host defense mechanisms and immunosuppression (eg, hospitalized patients, patients with burns, patients undergoing chemotherapy, and patients with cystic fibrosis)
        1) Nosocomial pneumonia
        2) Line-associated bacteremia
        3) Sepsis
        4) Wound infections
    d. Contact lens–associated keratitis: associated with pseudomonal contamination of contact lens cleaning solution
    e. Antibiotics: antipseudomonal penicillins such as piperacillin, carbapenems (except ertapenem), ceftazidime and cefepime, aztreonam, quinolones, colistin, and aminoglycosides
        1) Resistance is common
            a) May develop during therapy
            b) Multidrug-resistant isolates are increasingly common
        2) Mechanisms of resistance: efflux mechanisms, production of β-lactamases, altered outer membrane permeability, and aminoglycoside inactivating enzymes
4. *Stenotrophomonas maltophilia*
    a. Gram-negative bacillus that was formerly classified as *Pseudomonas maltophilia*
    b. Like *Pseudomonas*, it can colonize hospital water sources and respiratory equipment from environmental sources
    c. An increasingly recognized cause of nosocomial infection, including ventilator-associated pneumonia, wound infection, and pulmonary infection in patients with cystic fibrosis
    d. Produces β-lactamases and carbapenemases, conferring resistance to many commonly used antibiotics, including most cephalosporins and carbapenems
        1) Often susceptible to ticarcillin-clavulanate and trimethoprim-sulfamethoxazole
        2) Rifampin and minocycline may possess activity against many *S maltophilia* strains
        3) Resistance to quinolones and aminoglycosides is common
5. *Burkholderia*
    a. *Burkholderia cepacia*
        1) Formerly classified as *Pseudomonas cepacia*
        2) Occurs naturally in environmental water sources
            a) Minimal nutritional needs
            b) Can survive for extended periods
            c) Like *Pseudomonas* and *Stenotrophomonas*, it can colonize hospital water sources
        3) The most common human disease associated with *B cepacia* is chronic colonization and progressive lung infection in patients with cystic fibrosis
        4) Commonly resistant to many antibacterials, including many β-lactams and aminoglycosides
            a) Therapy should be guided by results of susceptibility testing
            b) Third-generation cephalosporins, quinolones, trimethoprim-sulfathoxazole, and carbapenems are variably active against *B cepacia* strains
    b. *Burkholderia pseudomallei*
        1) Formerly classified as *Pseudomonas pseudomallei*
        2) Gram-negative bacillus
        3) Environmental saprophyte

a) Endemic to Thailand, Southeast Asia, and Northern Australia
b) Sporadic cases are also seen in South America and Africa
4) Causes melioidosis: spectrum of human disease
   a) Skin abscesses, subacute pulmonary cavitary disease, and fulminant sepsis
   b) High case fatality rate
   c) Therapy for acute illness: ceftazidime or a carbapenem for 2 to 4 weeks
   d) Subsequent therapy: 3 to 12 months of oral therapy with trimethoprim-sulfamethoxazole, amoxicillin-clavulanate, or doxycycline
   e) Often resistant to aminoglycosides, ciprofloxacin, and many cephalosporins
c. *Burkholderia mallei*
   1) Formerly classified as *Pseudomonas mallei*
   2) Closely related to *B pseudomallei* but is a much less common cause of human disease
   3) Causative agent of glanders, a disease of horses, donkeys, and mules
   4) Rare in Europe and North America because of aggressive control of disease in animals
   5) Transmission to humans: through contact with infected equines
   6) Clinical presentation similar to that of melioidosis: pustular skin lesions, cavitary pneumonia, bacteremia, and multiple organ abscesses
   7) Antimicrobial susceptibility and therapy are similar to those of *B pseudomallei*
6. *Haemophilus influenzae*
   a. Pleomorphic gram-negative coccobacillus
   b. Colonizes human upper respiratory tract and causes a spectrum of invasive and noninvasive infection
   c. *Haemophilus influenzae* is perhaps the most important of the 8 *Haemophilus* species associated with human disease
   d. Other *Haemophilus* species of importance
      1) *Haemophilus ducreyi*: causes chancroid
      2) *Haemophilus aphrophilus* and *Haemophilus paraphrophilus*: rare causes of infective endocarditis
      3) *Haemophilus influenzae* biogroup *aegyptius*: causes epidemic conjunctivitis and Brazilian purpuric fever
   e. For growth, *H influenzae* requires accessory growth factors: X factor (from iron-containing pigments such as hemin) and V factor (from nicotinamide adenine dinucleotide or nicotinamide adenine dinucleotide phosphate)
   f. Many *H influenzae* strains carry a polysaccharide capsule (types are designated by letters *a* through *f*)
   g. Noninvasive infections caused by *H influenzae*
      1) Otitis media, conjunctivitis, bronchitis, and sinusitis
      2) Often caused by nonencapsulated *H influenzae* strains
   h. Invasive infections caused by *H influenzae*
      1) Leading cause: *H influenzae* type b (Hib)
      2) Meningitis, epiglottitis, bacteremia, pneumonia, periorbital cellulitis, and septic arthritis
      3) Introduction of infant vaccination against Hib in 1991 has significantly decreased the rates of Hib colonization and disease among children
   i. Drugs of choice for treatment
      1) Invasive infection with *H influenzae*
         a) Third-generation cephalosporins (cefotaxime and ceftriaxone)
         b) β-Lactamase production is common among *H influenzae* strains, and ampicillin is no longer adequate empirical therapy for invasive disease
      2) Noninvasive disease: oral antimicrobials such as macrolides, amoxicillin-clavulanate, trimethoprim-sulfamethoxazole, and oral second-generation cephalosporins
7. *Brucella* species
   a. Small, intracellular, gram-negative bacilli endemic to domestic mammal populations in certain geographic areas
   b. *Brucella* species cause abortions in these mammals
   c. Transmitted to humans through unpasteurized dairy products (most commonly raw milk and cheese) and cause the zoonosis brucellosis
   d. Four *Brucella* species (with animal reservoirs) cause human disease

1) *Brucella abortus* (cattle)
2) *Brucella canis* (dogs)
3) *Brucella suis* (pigs)
4) *Brucella melitensis* (goats)
   e. Geographic areas with high prevalence of *Brucella*: Mediterranean, Middle East, Central America, South America, and India
      1) In the United States, most cases involve transmission from unpasteurized dairy products and cheese imported from Mexico
      2) *Brucella* is uncommon in the United States, but natural reservoirs include bison populations in the western United States
   f. Brucellosis is typically a febrile syndrome, often with anemia, leukopenia, malaise, weight loss, and chronic fever
      1) Common sites of involvement
         a) Bones and joints: sacroiliitis and vertebral osteomyelitis
         b) Cardiovascular system: endocarditis is uncommon but accounts for most deaths from brucellosis
         c) Gastrointestinal tract
         d) Genitourinary system
      2) Diagnosis
         a) Recovery of *Brucella* from cultures of bone marrow, blood (less likely to be positive than bone marrow), or localized sites of infection
         b) Serologic diagnosis: helpful, but *B canis* is not detected by currently available serum agglutination tests
      3) Treatment
         a) Doxycycline plus rifampin for 6 weeks, with prolonged therapy (≥6 months) for endocarditis
         b) In addition, trimethoprim-sulfamethoxazole, streptomycin, and gentamicin are used in various treatment regimens against *Brucella*
8. *Francisella tularensis*
   a. Causes tularemia, a zoonosis transmitted to humans through handling infected wild animals, including mammals (especially rabbits), birds, fish, and amphibians, or through the bite of an infected tick
   b. A small, aerobic pleomorphic gram-negative coccobacillus with intracellular localization in human infection
   c. Laboratory instructions and precautions
      1) If tularemia is suspected, notify the microbiology laboratory in advance: *F tularensis* requires special cysteine-enriched media to grow
      2) Biosafety level 3 conditions are required for culture because *F tularensis* can be highly infectious to laboratory personnel
   d. Patients with tularemia can present with several different febrile syndromes
      1) Ulceroglandular tularemia
         a) Most common
         b) Ulcerated, erythematous lesion (Figure 7.5) at the site of entry
         c) Lymphadenopathy of the regional draining lymph nodes
      2) Other presentations
         a) Typhoidal form: hepatosplenomegaly but few localizing symptoms
         b) Pulmonary
         c) Oculoglandular: painful, unilateral conjunctivitis and cervical or preauricular lymphadenopathy
         d) Oropharyngeal: pharyngitis and cervical lymphadenopathy
   e. Possible agent of bioterrorism: presentation of multiple cases of previously healthy persons with acute pulmonary infiltrates and fever should prompt consideration of pulmonary tularemia
   f. Treatment of tularemia: aminoglycosides are drugs of choice

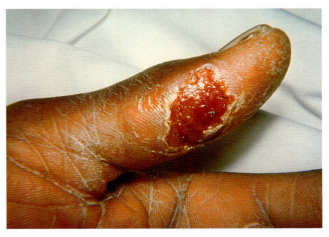

Figure 7.5. Thumb With Skin Ulcer of Tularemia. (Adapted from Centers for Disease Control and Prevention. Public Health Image Library [PHIL]: photographs, illustrations, multimedia files. [cited 2006 Aug 23]. Available from: http://phil.cdc.gov/phil/home.asp.)

9. *Pasteurella* species
   a. Oral flora of various mammals commonly includes *Pasturella multocida*
      1) Bipolar, gram-negative bacillus
      2) Causes rapidly progressive soft-tissue infections after bites from animals, especially cats but also dogs, pigs, and rats
      3) Therapy for infected animal bites
         a) Careful consideration of the need for surgical débridement
         b) Antibacterials with activity against *Pasturella* and anaerobes (these infections are usually polymicrobial)
   b. Respiratory infections such as pharyngitis or pneumonia occur less commonly, often in persons with a history of contact with animals
   c. Penicillin, amoxicillin-clavulanate, and quinolones have activity against *Pasteurella*; cephalexin does not
10. *Bordetella pertussis* and *Bordetella parapertussis*
    a. *Bordetella pertussis*
       1) A small gram-negative respiratory pathogen
       2) Agent of pertussis (also called whooping cough)
       3) Highly transmissible among humans
          a) Before introduction of vaccine for pertussis, this respiratory pathogen was a common cause of illness and death among young children in the United States
          b) Pertussis is increasingly recognized as a potential cause of chronic cough due to waning immunity in previously immunized persons
    b. Pertussis: a prolonged illness with 3 phases
       1) Initial or catarrhal stage
          a) Lasts 1 to 2 weeks
          b) Characterized by upper respiratory symptoms, rhinorrhea, fever, and mild cough
          c) *Bordetella pertussis* is communicable during this stage
       2) Paroxysmal stage
          a) Can last for several weeks
          b) Sudden episodes of severe cough with a characteristic "whoop" and posttussive vomiting
          c) Laboratory analysis frequently shows lymphocytosis during this stage
       3) Convalescent stage
          a) Can last for several months
          b) Involves a gradual resolution of the coughing spells
    c. Diagnosis of pertussis: culture or polymerase chain reaction (PCR) of a swab of nasopharyngeal mucus (but recovery of the organism is uncommon after several weeks of illness)
    d. Antimicrobial therapy for pertussis
       1) Macrolides or trimethoprim-sulfamethoxazole
       2) Treatment generally does not shorten the duration of illness after paroxysms of cough develop
       3) Prophylactic antibiotics are indicated for household and close contacts to decrease the frequency of secondary transmission
11. *Streptobacillus moniliformis* and *Spirillum minus*
    a. Gram-negative branching rods and facultative anaerobes
    b. Part of the normal oral flora of rats
    c. Agents of rat-bite fever
       1) Acquired through the bite or scratch of a rat or consumption of food or water contaminated with rat feces
       2) Systemic febrile illness
       3) Red or purple maculopapular rash on the extremities is common
       4) Asymmetrical, large joint polyarthritis may accompany the fever
       5) Rat-bite fever can progress to a fulminant sepsis with a high mortality rate
       6) Therapy
          a) Antibacterials of choice: penicillin or doxycycline
          b) Quinolones are not active against *S moniliformis* and *S minus*
12. *Legionella pneumophila*, *Legionella micdadei*, and other *Legionella* species
    a. Fastidious, slender gram-negative bacilli
    b. Human legionellosis: *L pneumophila* is the etiologic agent of most cases, but *L micdadei* and other species are also pathogenic
    c. *Legionella* live in environmental and artificial reservoirs of fresh water
    d. Transmission to humans

1) Most likely through inhalation of contaminated aerosols from air conditioners, building water supplies, and evaporation condensers that contain unfiltered warm water
2) Filtration of water in these systems appears to eliminate the amebae that are necessary for the intracellular multiplication of *Legionella* species
e. Two main types of human legionellosis: legionnaires disease and Pontiac fever
   1) Legionnaires disease
      a) Acute pneumonia with systemic manifestations caused by *Legionella* species
      b) May be accompanied by confusion and hyponatremia
      c) Can result in respiratory failure and death
      d) First recognized outbreak occurred during the 1976 American Legion convention in Philadelphia, Pennsylvania, and was linked to the hotel air conditioning system
   2) Pontiac fever
      a) Acute, self-resolving illness with fever, chills, myalgias, headache, fatigue, and upper respiratory symptoms
      b) First recognized in 1968 among persons who worked in a building in Pontiac, Michigan
      c) Pneumonia is not a prominent finding in this illness, which may represent an acute hypersensitivity reaction to *Legionella* infection
f. Diagnostic methods to detect *Legionella* infection
   1) Culture of respiratory secretions on buffered charcoal-yeast extract agar
   2) *Legionella* often grow slowly (3-5 days) and do not grow on blood agar
   3) Serology for *L pneumophila* serotype 1
      a) Available but has limited sensitivity
      b) Comparison of acute and convalescent titers is required, making serology of limited value in diagnosis of acute infection
   4) Diagnosis of acute infection
      a) Direct fluorescent antibody (DFA) testing of *Legionella* in respiratory secretions is highly specific but less than 60% sensitive
      b) Legionella urinary antigen testing to detect *L pneumophila* serogroup 1 is useful
      c) Recent studies have shown that PCR assay is a suitable alternative to culture or DFA testing of respiratory secretions
g. Antibiotic therapy
   1) β-Lactam antibiotics are not active against *Legionella* species
   2) Antibiotics of choice: macrolides and quinolones
   3) For severe disease or Legionellosis in an immunocompromised patient, 1 of the following combinations is recommended
      a) A macrolide plus rifampin
      b) A quinolone plus rifampin
      c) A quinolone plus a macrolide
13. *Capnocytophaga canimorsus*
    a. In normal oral flora of dogs
    b. Facultative gram-negative anaerobe
    c. Causes fulminant sepsis in splenectomized or immunocompromised persons after dog bites, contact between a dog's mouth and a person's broken skin (including licking wounds), or scratches from dogs
    d. Susceptible to penicillins, quinolones, and clindamycin
    e. Resistant to aminoglycosides
14. *Bartonella henselae*, *Bartonella quintana*, and *Bartonella bacilliformis*
    a. *Bartonella* species are gram-negative bacilli with mammalian reservoirs (animal or human)
    b. Grow slowly and are difficult to isolate in blood culture, so that diagnosis is more commonly made with serology or PCR of blood or tissue
    c. Cause various human illnesses
       1) *Bartonella henselae* causes cat-scratch disease
          a) Acute, suppurative lymphadenitis
          b) Most cases occur in children and young persons
          c) Major mode of transmission to humans: scratch, bite, or lick from a young cat
       2) *Bartonella quintana* causes chronic bacteremia or infective endocarditis
          a) Often among persons with poor hygiene and body lice

b) *Bartonella quintana* was the agent of trench fever, recognized in World War I as an illness with periodic fevers occurring approximately every 5 days (thus, *quintana*)
3) Both *B quintana* and *B henselae* can cause bacillary angiomatosis
   a) Occurs in immunodeficient persons (such as persons with human immunodeficiency virus infection)
   b) Angioproliferative condition
      i) Red or purple nodular skin lesions that bleed when punctured
      ii) Vascularized hepatic lesions known as peliosis hepatis
4) *Bartonella bacilliformis* is geographically restricted to the Peruvian and Ecuadorean Andes and causes 2 diseases
   a) Oroyo fever, a chronic febrile illness
   b) Verruga peruana, a skin disease with angioproliferative papular lesions similar to those of bacillary angiomatosis
   d. Antimicrobial therapy for infections caused by *Bartonella* species varies according to the host and the nature of infection
      1) For immunocompetent hosts, treatment of cat-scratch disease is primarily supportive, but a short course of azithromycin may provide some clinical benefit
      2) For other *Bartonella* infections, regimens including macrolides, β-lactams, and doxycycline have been used
15. *Aeromonas* species
    a. Motile gram-negative bacilli
    b. Live in freshwater environments and on fish
    c. Diseases
       1) Diarrhea from ingestion of contaminated water
       2) Severe skin and soft tissue infections of wounds sustained in freshwater
    d. Therapy with medicinal leeches
       1) *Aeromonas hydrophila* infections have been reported after therapy
       2) Prophylaxis: antibacterials active against *Aeromonas* are commonly given during medicinal leech therapy
    e. *Aeromonas* species produce a β-lactamase conferring resistance to many β-lactams and carbapenems
    f. Quinolones, trimethoprim-sulfamethoxazole, and aminoglycosides have been used successfully to treat *Aeromonas* infections
16. HACEK agents
    a. *Haemophilus* (*H aphrophilus*, *H paraphrophilus*), *Actinobacillus actinomycetemcomitans*, *Cardiobacterium hominis*, *Eikenella corrodens*, and *Kingella kingae*
    b. Pleomorphic gram-negative bacilli
    c. Part of normal human oral flora
    d. Uncommon cause of infective endocarditis overall, but owing to their fastidious growth in blood culture they are a common cause of culture-negative infective endocarditis
       1) Blood cultures often require prolonged incubation (5-7 days) for growth
       2) Treatment: 4 to 6 weeks of a third-generation or fourth-generation cephalosporin or ampicillin-sulbactam intravenously

III. Summary of Epidemiologic Associations and Diseases
   A. *Acinetobacter* Species
      1. Intensive care unit patient, wounded soldier with battlefield trauma
      2. Multidrug-resistant nosocomial infection: bacteremia, wound infection, and ventilator-associated pneumonia
   B. *Aeromonas hydrophila*
      1. Laceration sustained in freshwater
      2. Wound infection
   C. *Bartonella henselae*
      1. Person (especially a child) with contact with cats (especially kittens)
      2. Cat-scratch disease (lymphadenitis)
   D. *Burkholderia pseudomallei*
      1. Southeast Asian agricultural worker or rice farmer
      2. Melioidosis: febrile illness, septic shock, nodular pulmonary infiltrates, and splenic abscesses
   E. *Brucella abortus*, *B melitensis*, and *B suis*
      1. Resident of endemic area (Mexico, Middle East, Mediterranean) who ingested raw milk or unpasteurized cheese
      2. Systemic, chronic febrile illness with anemia

F. *Capnocytophaga canimorsus*
   1. Asplenic person who was bitten by a dog
   2. Overwhelming sepsis
G. *Eikenella corrodens*
   1. Intravenous drug abuser who licked needle before injection
   2. Soft tissue abscess at injection site
H. *Escherichia coli* O157:H7
   1. Ingestion of undercooked hamburger or unpasteurized fruit juice
   2. Bloody diarrhea or hemolytic uremic syndrome
I. *Francisella tularensis*
   1. Hunter or trapper who handles wild animals, including rabbits
   2. Febrile illness with ulcerated skin lesion and regional lymphadenopathy
J. *Neisseria meningitidis*
   1. Epidemic outbreaks in sub-Saharan Africa during the dry season, travelers returning from pilgrimage to Mecca, and college students living in dormitories
   2. Meningitis and sepsis
K. *Pasteurella multocida*
   1. Person bitten by cat
   2. Rapidly progressive soft tissue infection resistant to cephalexin
L. *Salmonella typhi*
   1. Traveler to Africa or Asia
   2. Typhoid fever
M. *Vibrio cholerae*
   1. Traveler returning from Peru or other area with cholera epidemic
   2. Profuse diarrhea with volume depletion
N. *Vibrio vulnificus*
   1. Person with cirrhosis who ingests raw oysters from Gulf of Mexico
   2. Gangrenous soft tissue infection with sepsis
O. *Yersinia pestis*
   1. Rancher with contact with prairie dogs in the western United States
   2. Plague: sepsis and buboes

Suggested Reading

Paterson DL, Bonomo RA. Extended-spectrum beta-lactamases: a clinical update. Clin Microbiol Rev. 2005 Oct;18(4):657–86.

Rodriguez-Bano J, Paterson DL. A change in the epidemiology of infections due to extended-spectrum beta-lactamase-producing organisms. Clin Infect Dis. 2006 Apr 1;42(7):935–7. Epub 2006 Feb 27.

Wilson WR, Sande MA, Henry NK, Drew WL, Relman DA, Steckelberg JM, et al. Current diagnosis & treatment in infectious diseases. New York (NY): McGraw-Hill; c2001.

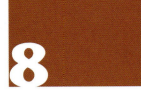

M. Rizwan Sohail, MD

Select Anaerobic Bacteria: *Clostridium tetani* and *Clostridium botulinum*

I. *Clostridium tetani*
   A. Introduction
      1. Tetanus: nervous system disorder characterized by intense, painful muscle spasms
      2. Causative agent: *Clostridium tetani*
      3. Well-known disease from ancient times
      4. Tetanus is prevalent in developing countries, but it is rare in developed nations owing to universal childhood vaccination
      5. Common modes of acquisition: puncture wounds, gunshot wounds, burns, compound fractures, and contaminated or unsterile injections
   B. Microbiology
      1. Obligate anaerobic, gram-positive, spore-forming bacillus
      2. Present in mammalian gut and ubiquitous in soil
         a. Spores are extremely stable in environment
         b. Spores are rendered noninfectious by hydrogen peroxide or autoclaving
   C. Pathogenesis
      1. Entry point into body: damaged skin or mucosa
      2. Conditions promoting bacterial growth
         a. Presence of devitalized tissue
         b. Coinfection with other bacteria
         c. Presence of a foreign body
      3. *Clostridium tetani* releases 2 toxins: tetanospasmin (a metalloproteinase, commonly called tetanus toxin) and tetanolysin
         a. Tetanospasmin causes neurologic manifestations of tetanus
         b. Tetanospasmin exploits retrograde axonal transport to reach spinal cord and brainstem
         c. Toxin causes disinhibition of excitatory neurons, including those in anterior horn cells and autonomic nervous system, resulting in muscle spasms and generalized autonomic dysfunction
         d. Toxin binding: irreversible
   D. Epidemiology
      1. Annual estimates for developing countries: 1 million cases of tetanus and 200,000 to 300,000 deaths
      2. Centers for Disease Control and Prevention reports 35 to 70 cases in the United States annually
         a. Majority are older adults (older than 60 years)

b. Increasing number of cases occur in younger population owing to injection drug use
c. Neonatal tetanus: extremely rare in the United States but accounts for half of tetanus deaths in developing countries
d. Most infections occur in persons who did not receive the complete vaccination series

E. Clinical Manifestations
1. Median incubation period: 7 to 8 days (range, 3-21 days)
   a. Duration of incubation period partially depends on distance of site of infection from central nervous system (longer incubation period with injuries to feet than with trauma to chest or neck)
   b. Shorter incubation period is associated with severe disease
2. Illness can progress for 2 weeks
3. Recovery requires growth of new axonal terminals (usually 4-6 weeks)
4. Generalized tetanus
   a. Most common and severe clinical form
   b. Patients have tonic contraction of skeletal muscles and intermittent, intense, painful muscular spasms (Figure 8.1)
   c. Consciousness is not impaired
   d. Spasms can be triggered by sensory stimuli (eg, loud noises, light, or physical contact)
   e. Clinical features are summarized in Box 8.1
5. Localized tetanus
   a. Occasionally tetanus involves 1 extremity at initial presentation, but it evolves to generalized tetanus in the majority of cases
   b. An example is cephalic tetanus after head and neck injuries: patients present with only cranial nerve involvement at an early stage
6. Neonatal tetanus
   a. Infants at risk: born without protective passive immunity (owing to lack of maternal immunization)
   b. Occurs in first 2 weeks after birth and is mostly caused by unsterile handling of umbilical stump
   c. Clinical features include rigidity, spasms, trismus, inability to suck, and seizures (Figure 8.2)
      1) Can rapidly progress within hours
      2) Mortality exceeds 90% (leading cause of death is apnea)
      3) Developmental delay is frequent among survivors

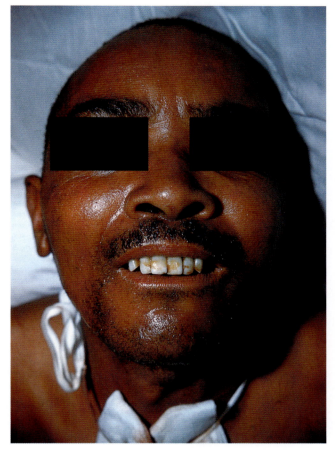

Figure 8.1. Facial Tetany. Note the contraction of the masseter and neck muscles. (Adapted from Centers for Disease Control and Prevention [Internet]. [cited 2010 Apr 13]. Available from: http://www.cdc.gov/vaccines/vpd-vac/tetanus/photos.htm. Content provider: Dr Thomas F. Sellers, Emory University.)

Box 8.1

Clinical Features of Tetanus

Symptoms related to autonomic hyperactivity
  Early phase: irritability, restlessness, sweating, and tachycardia
  Late phase: fever, profuse sweating, labile blood pressure (hypotension or hypertension), and cardiac arrhythmias
Symptoms related to skeletal muscle contractions or spasms
  Trismus (also called lockjaw)
  Stiff neck
  Opisthotonos (muscle spasms causing backward arching of head, neck, and spine)
  Risus sardonicus (sardonic smile) (Figure 8.1)
  Board-like, rigid abdomen
  Laryngospasm with airway obstruction
  Sustained contraction of respiratory muscles, resulting in respiratory failure
  Dysphagia (risk of aspiration pneumonia)
  Fractures of long bones and spine (from prolonged and severe muscle contractions)

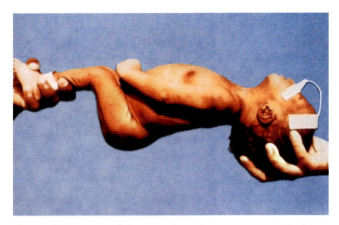

Figure 8.2. Neonatal Tetanus. *Clostridium tetani* caused bodily rigidity. (Adapted from Centers for Disease Control and Prevention [Internet]. [cited 2010 Apr 13]. Available from: http://www.cdc.gov/vaccines/vpd-vac/tetanus/photos.htm.)

Table 8.1
Differential Diagnosis of Tetanus

Condition or Syndrome	Differentiating Features
Trismus (due to dental infection)	May be confused with cephalic form of tetanus
	Presence of dental infection and lack of generalized progression or superimposed muscle spasms distinguish it from tetanus
Malignant neuroleptic syndrome	Fever, change in mental status, and history of a provoking agent
	Patients with tetanus have normal mental status
Drug-induced dystonias	For example, phenothiazine-induced dystonia
	Include eye deviation and writhing movement of head and neck
	Absence of tonic contractions
	Symptoms resolve with anticholinergic antagonists (benztropine)
	Patients with tetanus do not have eye deviation or lateral head turning, and they do not respond to anticholinergic antagonists
Strychnine poisoning	Usually from accidental or intentional ingestion of rat poison
	Clinical distinction is quite difficult
	Assay of blood, urine, and tissue for strychnine may be performed in reference laboratories
Stiff man syndrome	No facial spasms or trismus
	Rapid response to diazepam
	Laboratory identification of autoantibodies against glutamic acid decarboxylase

    F. Differential Diagnosis
       1. Differential diagnosis of tetanus is summarized in Table 8.1
    G. Diagnosis
       1. Diagnosis is based on clinical features (Box 8.1)
       2. No special laboratory tests are necessary or helpful to confirm the diagnosis
       3. Wound cultures are not reliable
    H. Management
       1. Patients should be treated in critical care unit
       2. Supportive care is the cornerstone of managing tetanus (Table 8.2)
       3. Other components of management
          a. Halting toxin production
          b. Neutralizing unbound toxin
          c. Controlling muscle spasms
          d. Managing dysautonomia
    I. Prognosis and Outcome
       1. Mortality in developing countries: 8% to 50%
       2. In developed countries, most patients recover owing to excellent supportive care
       3. Mortality of neonatal tetanus: 10% to 60%
    J. Prevention
       1. Clinical disease does not confer immunity, and tetanus can recur if patient is not immunized
       2. Adequate immunization
          a. Primary vaccination series: provided as diphtheria and tetanus toxoids and acellular pertussis (DTaP) vaccine in childhood followed by adult boosters every 10 years with tetanus and diphtheria toxoids (Td) vaccine
          b. Adults should receive 1 dose of tetanus-diphtheria-acellular pertussis (Tdap) vaccine instead of Td once in their lifetime
       3. Tetanus toxoid: 100% efficacy in immunocompetent patients
       4. Patients with humoral deficiencies should receive passive immunization with human tetanus immunoglobulin (HTIG) after tetanus-prone injuries (wounds contaminated with dirt, saliva, puncture wounds, etc)
       5. Patients who undergo stem cell transplant should be revaccinated after engraftment
  II. *Clostridium botulinum*
    A. Introduction
       1. Botulism: a neuroparalytic syndrome caused by neurotoxin produced by *Clostridium botulinum*
          a. First major documented outbreak occurred in Germany in the 1820s from "sausage poisoning"

Table 8.2
Management of Tetanus

Goal	Action
Halt toxin production	Aggressively débride wound (to eradicate spores and necrotic tissue)
	Administer antibiotics against *Clostridium tetani*: penicillin G and metronidazole are effective against *C tetani*; broad-spectrum antibiotics may be used if polymicrobial wound infection is suspected
Neutralize unbound toxin	Administer HTIG intramuscularly as soon as diagnosis is made (associated with improved survival; intrathecal use has no proven benefit)
	Use equine antitoxin if HTIG is not available
Control muscle spasms	Administer sedatives: benzodiazepine (intravenous infusion of diazepam) or propofol
	Administer neuromuscular blockade if sedation alone is inadequate: pancuronium or vecuronium intravenously (an alternative is baclofen intrathecally)
	Control noise and light (which can provoke muscle spasms)
Manage autonomic dysfunction	Magnesium sulfate: a presynaptic neuromuscular blocker that inhibits catecholamine release (the only drug studied in randomized controlled trials)
	Alternatives include labetalol (both α-blockade and β-blockade) and magnesium sulfate
Provide active immunization	All patients should receive a complete series of tetanus and diphtheria toxoids (Td) vaccination starting at the time of diagnosis (doses should be given at least 2 wk apart)
Provide supportive care	Provide mechanical ventilation
	Consider early tracheostomy since prolonged ventilator dependence is expected for most patients
	Prevent decubital ulcers and ventilator-associated pneumonias
	Administer sucralfate or proton pump inhibitors to prevent gastric ulcers and gastrointestinal tract bleeding
	Provide enteral feeding (preferably PEG tube)
	Administer low-molecular-weight heparin for DVT prevention
	Begin physical therapy when spasms have resolved

Abbreviations: DVT, deep vein thrombosis; HTIG, human tetanus immunoglobulin; PEG, percutaneous endoscopic gastrostomy.

---

      b. The term *botulism* is derived from *botulus*, the Latin word for sausage
  2. The US Food and Drug Administration approved botulinum toxin for treatment of neuromuscular disorders, including blepharospasm, strabismus, and torticollis, and for many cosmetic procedures

B. Microbiology
  1. *Clostridium botulinum*: a motile, spore-forming, anaerobic, gram-positive bacillus
  2. Ubiquitous in environment: may be isolated from fruits, vegetables, meat, seafood, soil, and marine sediment
  3. Ideal growth conditions: warm temperature and anaerobic environment
      a. Spores are heat resistant (can survive at 100°C for >5 hours)
      b. Toxin is heat labile (destroyed by boiling)
      c. Spores are inactivated in chlorinated water in 20 minutes
  4. Seven distinct toxin types (identified by letters *A* through *G*)
      a. Types A, B, E, and F (and occasionally G) cause human illness
      b. Types C and D cause disease in chickens, cattle, and ducks
      c. All cause flaccid paralysis
      d. Toxin itself has no odor or flavor
      e. Strains A and B produce enzymes that spoil food, resulting in unpleasant odor or flavor
      f. Food looks and tastes normal if colonized by other strains
      g. Botulinum toxin is the most potent toxin known: 1 g of aerosolized toxin can kill an estimated 1.5 million people (a concern for potential bioterrorism)

C. Pathogenesis
  1. Organism or toxin enters body by ingestion, wound contamination, or inhalation (eg, a bioterrorism event)
  2. Predisposing factors for colonization of gastrointestinal tract with *C botulinum*: achlorhydria, postoperative status, mucosal disease, or antibiotic use
  3. Toxin is resistant to breakdown by gastric acid or enteric enzymes
  4. Toxin spreads through vascular system
  5. Toxin does not cross blood-brain barrier, so effects are limited to peripheral nervous system
      a. Binds to presynaptic side of peripheral cholinergic synapses at ganglia and neuromuscular junctions

b. Does not bind at adrenergic synapses
   c. Causes irreversible inhibition of acetylcholine release, resulting in muscle paralysis
   d. Return of normal function requires formation of new synapses, a process that may take several months
D. Epidemiology
   1. Average number of cases reported in the United States each year: 110
      a. Infant botulism: 72%
      b. Foodborne botulism: 25%
      c. Wound botulism: 3%
   2. Most foodborne cases occur as small outbreaks, generally from home-canned fish, fruits, or vegetables
      a. Foods associated with recent outbreaks: fermented fish (Alaska), home-canned bamboo shoots (Thailand), carrot juice (several US states and Canada), and home-preserved jalapeno peppers (Michigan)
      b. Other food items implicated in botulism outbreaks: asparagus, green beans, beets, corn, baked potatoes, garlic, chili peppers, and tomatoes
   3. Infant botulism
      a. Classically associated with ingestion of raw honey
      b. In the United States, most cases are caused by ingestion of environmental dust containing *C botulinum* spores
      c. Most patients are 2 to 8 months old
   4. Wound botulism
      a. Increasing number of reports involving injection drug users (intramuscular or subcutaneous injection of "black tar" heroin)
      b. Also reported in patients who inhale cocaine
E. Clinical Manifestations
   1. Clinical manifestations of different forms of botulism are summarized in Table 8.3 and Box 8.2
   2. Hallmark of illness: acute bilateral cranial neuropathies, followed by symmetrical descending paralysis
   3. Other characteristic features
      a. Lack of central nervous system involvement (patients are awake and responsive)
      b. Absence of fever
      c. No sensory deficit
      d. Normal blood pressure and heart rate

> **Box 8.2**
> Clinical Manifestation of Botulism in Adults
>
> Prodromal gastrointestinal tract symptoms: nausea, vomiting, abdominal pain, and diarrhea (only in foodborne botulism)
> Fever and leukocytosis: with contaminated wound infection (only in wound botulism)
> Cranial nerve palsies: diplopia, dysphagia, dysphonia, blurred vision, dysarthria, nystagmus, ptosis, and facial weakness
> Descending muscular weakness: weakness of trunk and upper extremities and then lower extremities
> Smooth muscle paralysis: constipation and urinary retention
> Respiratory failure: from diaphragmatic paralysis or upper airway compromise (or both)

   4. Varies from mild illness to critical condition and death within a day after initial symptoms develop
   5. Wound botulism
      a. Generally associated with puncture wounds, skin and soft tissue abscesses, and deeper infections
      b. Occasional cases from abrasions and surgical incisions
      c. Fever may occur from polymicrobial infection (Figure 8.3)
      d. *Clostridium botulinum* does not penetrate intact skin
F. Differential Diagnosis
   1. Differential diagnosis of botulism is summarized in Table 8.4
G. Diagnosis
   1. Accurate diagnosis of botulism requires a high degree of clinical awareness and a detailed history and physical examination

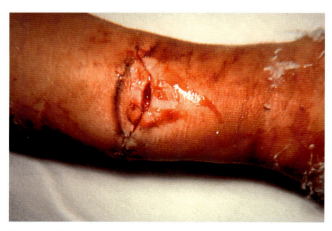

Figure 8.3. Wound Botulism. After a 14-year-old boy fractured his right ulna and radius, wound botulism developed. (Adapted from Centers for Disease Control and Prevention [Internet]. [cited 2010 Apr 13]. Available from: http://phil.cdc.gov/phil/imageidsearch.asp [image number 1936].)

Table 8.3

Clinical Manifestations and Management of Botulism

Syndrome	Acquisition	Incubation Period	Clinical Manifestation	Diagnosis	Management
Infant botulism	Ingestion of spores followed by in vivo toxin production in GI tract	Unknown	Constipation, lethargy, poor feeding, weak cry, drooling, irritability, bulbar palsies, failure to thrive, poor muscle tone (floppy infant syndrome)	Serum toxin assay results may be negative. Diagnosis confirmed by isolation of spores and toxin in stool samples	Supportive care. BIG-IV (BabyBIG)
Foodborne botulism	Preformed toxin in contaminated food	6 h to 8 d (typically 12-36 h)	Prodromal GI tract symptoms (nausea, vomiting, diarrhea, abdominal pain, dry mouth) followed by profound neuromuscular weakness (Box 8.2)	Serum toxin bioassay in mice. Isolation of toxin from stool, vomitus, or suspected food items	Supportive care. Equine serum antitoxin
Adult infectious botulism	In vivo toxin production in GI tract	Unknown	Cranial nerve palsies followed by descending neuromuscular weakness (Box 8.2)	Isolation of spores and toxin in stool samples	Supportive care. Equine serum antitoxin. Avoid antibiotics (can lyse bacteria in GI tract, resulting in further toxin release)
Wound botulism (Figure 8.3)	In vivo toxin production in contaminated wound	4-14 d	Local inflammation at wound (with fever and leukocytosis). Systemic findings similar to other forms (Box 8.2) except no prodromal GI symptoms	Isolation of clostridia from wound. Toxin assays of stool and vomitus are negative	Supportive care. Equine serum antitoxin. Antibiotics for wound infection
Inhalational botulism	Preformed toxin (eg, from a bioterrorism event)	12-48 h (estimated)	Profound neuromuscular symptoms (Box 8.2)	Serum toxin bioassay in mice. Isolation of toxin from suspected sources of bioterrorist attack	Supportive care. Equine serum antitoxin

Abbreviations: BIG-IV, Botulism Immune Globulin Intravenous (human); GI, gastrointestinal.

Table 8.4
Differential Diagnosis of Botulism

Condition or Syndrome	Differentiating Features
Myasthenia gravis	Autonomic symptoms are absent in myasthenia gravis
Guillain-Barré syndrome (GBS)	Usually GBS causes ascending paralysis, sensory abnormalities, and elevated CSF protein, but botulism results in descending paralysis, normal sensory findings, and a normal CSF analysis profile
	GBS does not alter pupillary reactivity
Meningitis or encephalitis	CSF profile is abnormal in meningitis or encephalitis but normal in botulism
Lambert-Eaton myasthenic syndrome	Can be excluded by electromyography or antibody testing
	No autonomic symptoms
Poliomyelitis	Febrile on presentation
	Muscular weakness in polio is generally asymmetric, but botulism causes symmetrical descending flaccid paralysis
Tick (*Dermacentor*) paralysis	Evidence of tick bite or attachment
	Ascending paralysis
Stroke	Clinical presentation and brain imaging
	Patients with botulism have normal findings on computed tomographic or magnetic resonance imaging of the brain and spinal cord
Others (heavy metal intoxication, tetrodotoxism, shellfish poisoning, and antimicrobial-associated paralysis)	Features vary, depending on causative agent

Abbreviation: CSF, cerebrospinal fluid.

2. Diagnostic tests for different forms of botulism are summarized in Table 8.3
   a. Anaerobic cultures may take 5 to 7 days
   b. Mouse neutralization tests for detection of toxin in various body fluid samples can take up to 48 hours
   c. Electromyographic studies may provide supplemental information but are not necessary for diagnosis
3. Fever and leukocytosis: present only in patients with wound botulism
   a. Ask patients about injection drug use
   b. Ask patients about history of trauma and contamination of open wounds with soil

H. Management
  1. Management of patients with botulism is summarized in Table 8.3
  2. Any form of botulism is a medical emergency
     a. Do not delay treatment while awaiting results of confirmatory tests
     b. If botulism is suspected from history and clinical presentation, the patient should be immediately hospitalized
  3. Supportive care is the cornerstone of management
  4. Respiratory failure is the most common cause of death
     a. All patients should be closely monitored for respiratory failure with pulse oximetry and evaluation of arterial blood gases and airway patency
     b. Mechanical ventilation should be initiated if there are signs of impending respiratory failure
  5. Small-volume nasogastric feeding may help to reduce risk of aspiration
  6. Patients with paralytic ileus should receive parenteral nutrition
  7. Laxatives and enemas may be used in patients with foodborne botulism
  8. Two types of antitoxins are available
     a. Equine serum trivalent botulism antitoxin (A, B, and E)
        1) Used to treat all patients older than 1 year
        2) Available through Centers for Disease Control and Prevention
        3) Does not reverse current paralysis
        4) Antitoxin use is associated with decreased mortality, shortened duration of symptoms, and less time with mechanical ventilation
        5) Antitoxin use may result in anaphylaxis (3% of patients) and serum sickness (20% of patients) since it is derived from horse serum
     b. Human Botulism Immune Globulin Intravenous (BIG-IV)
        1) Intravenous administration in infants (younger than 1 year)
        2) If infant botulism is suspected, do not delay use of toxin while waiting for results of confirmatory tests
        3) Allergic reactions are rare

9. Antibiotics are reserved for patients with wound botulism, especially those with fever, leukocytosis, or cellulitis or abscess at the wound
    a. Penicillin G: the most commonly used agent
    b. Metronidazole: an alternative for patients with penicillin allergy
    c. Aminoglycosides: contraindicated because they can worsen neuromuscular blockade in these patients
    d. Antibiotic therapy should be accompanied by aggressive wound débridement (even in the absence of cellulitis or abscess)
    e. Avoid use of antibiotics for infant botulism and adult infectious botulism because lysis of clostridium bacilli in the gut may result in increased toxin release

I. Prognosis and Outcome
    1. Mortality
        a. Overall mortality from botulism in the United States among patients receiving good supportive care: 5% to 10% (<1% among infants)
        b. Higher mortality among patients with shortness of breath at initial presentation
    2. Recovery
        a. Most patients with mild illness fully recover in first 3 months
        b. Patients with severe disease may take longer to recover or have partial recovery

J. Prevention
    1. Food precautions
        a. Do not feed honey to infants (younger than 1 year)
        b. Preserve food properly
        c. Promptly refrigerate food
        d. Discard suspected food
    2. Immunity to botulinum toxin does not develop, even after severe disease
    3. Vaccine is available (limited supplies) for laboratory workers with high risk of exposure

Suggested Reading

American Academy of Pediatrics. Tetanus (Lockjaw). In: Pickering LK, editor. Red book: 2009 Report of the Committee on Infectious Diseases. 28th ed. Elk Grove Village (IL): American Academy of Pediatrics; c2009. p. 655–60. [cited 2010 July 30]. Available from: http://aapredbook.aappublications.org/cgi/content/full/2009/1/3.132.

Infant Botulism Treatment and Prevention Program [Internet]. [cited 2010 Apr 12]. Division of Communicable Disease Control, California Department of Public Health. Available from: http://www.infantbotulism.org.

Reddy P, Bleck TP. *Clostridium botulinum* (Botulism). In: Mandell GL, Bennett JE, Dolin R, editors. Principles and Practice of Infectious Diseases. 7th ed. Philadelphia (PA): Churchill Livingstone/Elsevier; c2010. p. 3097–102.

Sobel J. Botulism. Clin Infect Dis. 2005 Oct 15;41(8):1167–73. Epub 2005 Aug 29.

Thwaites CL, Farrar JJ. Preventing and treating tetanus. BMJ. 2003 Jan 18;326(7381):117–8.

Wassilak SGF, Murphy TV, Roper MH, Orenstein WA. Tetanus toxoid. In: Plotkin SA, Orenstein WA, editors. Vaccines. 4th ed. New York (NY): Saunders; c2004. p. 745–82.

Julio C. Mendez, MD

Borrelia and *Leptospira* Species

I. *Borrelia*
   A. Introduction
      1. *Borrelia* species (except *Borrelia burgdorferi*) cause relapsing fever
      2. Relapsing fever: a zoonosis characterized by cyclic fevers alternating with periods of relative well-being
         a. Endemic or tick-borne relapsing fever
            1) Caused by several *Borrelia* species associated with soft ticks of the genus *Ornithodoros*
            2) Tick-spirochete specificity is useful for identifying *Borrelia* species
         b. Epidemic or louse-borne relapsing fever
            1) Caused by *Borrelia recurrentis*
            2) Transmitted by the human body louse
   B. Etiologic Features
      1. The genus *Borrelia* belongs to the family Spirochaetaceae
      2. Borreliae are helical, actively motile, microaerophilic microorganisms
      3. Have flagellae
      4. Strains cannot be distinguished by morphologic characteristics
      5. Tick-borne borreliae remain viable in their natural tick vectors for up to 12 years
   C. Epidemiology and Transmission
      1. Relapsing fever occurs throughout the world
      2. Louse-borne relapsing fever
         a. Usually occurs in epidemics associated with catastrophic events, such as war or famine, resulting in overcrowding and dissemination of body lice
         b. Humans are the only hosts
         c. Transmission occurs when the louse harboring *B recurrentis* is crushed, resulting in the release of the organism, which then penetrates the skin or mucous membrane
      3. Tick-borne relapsing fever
         a. Each causative *Borrelia* species is associated with a certain tick species
         b. In addition to having the human reservoir, these borreliae have animal reservoirs in rodents and other small animals
         c. Ticks inhabit caves, decaying wood, and animal homes
         d. Ticks feed at night and lack a painful bite
         e. Transmission occurs when saliva or excrement harboring these borreliae is released by the feeding tick
   D. Pathophysiology
      1. Febrile illness: after transmission, borreliae multiply rapidly in the bloodstream

2. Afebrile period: with immune recognition, borreliae are cleared from the bloodstream and sequestered in internal organs
3. Relapsing fever: under further pressure from the immune system, borreliae undergo a cyclic process of antigenic variation alternating with specific antibody production

E. Clinical Manifestations
1. The clinical manifestations of louse-borne and tick-borne relapsing fever are similar
2. Compared with tick-borne disease, louse-borne disease has a longer incubation period, longer febrile periods and afebrile intervals, and fewer relapses
3. Relapsing fever: both types have an acute onset of high fever with rigors, severe headache, myalgias, arthralgias, and lethargy
4. Initial physical findings: variable but may include altered sensorium, conjunctival suffusion, petechiae, and diffuse abdominal tenderness with hepatomegaly and splenomegaly
5. Fever: remittent and accompanied by tachycardia and tachypnea
6. Iritis and iridocyclitis: may permanently impair vision
7. Truncal skin rash of 1 to 2 days' duration: common at the end of the primary febrile episode, and it can be petechial, macular, or papular
8. Neurologic findings
   a. Reported in up to 30% of patients
   b. Include coma, cranial nerve palsies, hemiplegia, meningitis, and seizures
9. Most common causes of death
   a. Myocarditis with associated arrhythmias
   b. Cerebral hemorrhage
   c. Hepatic failure
10. Characteristic course of disease
   a. Primary febrile episode terminates abruptly in 3 to 6 days
   b. After 7 to 10 days, fever and symptoms suddenly recur
   c. Duration and intensity of symptoms progressively decrease with each relapse
      1) Louse-borne relapsing fever: usually a single relapse
      2) Tick-borne relapsing fever: multiple relapses are the rule

F. Diagnosis
1. Definitive diagnosis of relapsing fever
   a. Demonstration of borreliae in the peripheral blood of febrile patients (Figure 9.1)

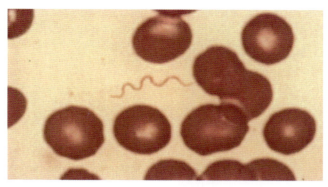

Figure 9.1. *Borrelia* Species. Peripheral blood smear from a patient with relapsing fever (Wright Stain). (Adapted from Rhee KY, Johnson WD Jr. *Borrelia* species [relapsing fever]. In: Mandell GL, Bennett JE, Dolin R, editors. Mandell, Douglas, and Bennett's principles and practice of infectious diseases. Vol 2. 6th ed. Philadelphia [PA]: Elsevier Churchill Livingstone; c2005. p. 2795–8. Used with permission.)

   b. Spirochetes are found in 70% of cases when wet blood smears are examined by darkfield microscopy or when thick and thin smears are examined with Giemsa or Wright stain
2. Diagnostic yield can be increased by examination of acridine orange–stained smears by fluorescence microscopy or buffy coat smears
3. Agglutinating, complement-fixing, borreliacidal, and immobilizing antibodies are detectable in serum
   a. These tests are not generally available
   b. If performed, they are of limited diagnostic value owing to antigenic variation of strains and the complexity of the relapse phenomenon
4. Results of serologic tests for syphilis and Lyme disease may also be positive
   a. Recent data suggest that relapsing fever associated with borreliae may be discriminated from these infections
   b. Distinction is based on presence of detectable titers against the surface protein glycerophosphodiester phosphodiesterase (GlpQ)
5. Spirochetes have been detected in cerebrospinal fluid (CSF) by smear or by animal inoculation in up to 12% of patients with central nervous system signs
6. Differential diagnosis of relapsing fever
   a. Includes malaria, typhoid fever, hepatitis, leptospirosis, rat-bite fever, Colorado tick fever, and dengue

b. Exclude these diagnoses with epidemiologic considerations, occurrence of relapses, and demonstration of spirochetemia
G. Treatment
1. Relapsing fever has been treated successfully with tetracycline, chloramphenicol, penicillin, and erythromycin
    a. Louse-borne relapsing fever
        1) Tetracycline in a single oral dose (500 mg): the preferred therapy except in pregnant women and children younger than 8 years (tooth and bone staining)
        2) Erythromycin in a single oral dose (500 mg): an equally effective alternative therapy
    b. Tick-borne relapsing fever
        1) Often treated with either tetracycline or erythromycin (500 mg) every 6 hours for 5 to 10 days
        2) Higher dosage is used because of the higher rate of treatment failures and relapses in these patients
2. Meningitis or encephalitis: treat with parenteral antibiotics, such as penicillin G, cefotaxime, or ceftriaxone, for 14 days or more
3. Mortality is less than 5% with treated relapsing fever, but mortality is up to 40% with untreated epidemic louse-borne disease
4. Antibiotic treatment typically induces a Jarisch–Herxheimer reaction that coincides with the clearing of spirochetemia
    a. Severe rigors, leukopenia, an increase in temperature, and a decrease in blood pressure
    b. Most severe in louse-borne disease treated with penicillin

II. *Leptospira*
A. Introduction
1. Leptospirosis
    a. A zoonosis of global distribution
    b. Caused by infection with pathogenic spirochetes of the genus *Leptospira*
    c. Greatly underreported, particularly in tropical regions
    d. Maintained in nature by chronic renal infection of carrier animals
        1) Excrete the organism in their urine
        2) Contaminate the environment
2. Human infection
    a. Occurs after direct contact with infected urine or tissues
    b. More commonly, occurs after indirect exposure to the organisms in damp soil or water
    c. Most cases are probably asymptomatic
    d. Extremely wide spectrum of illness: from undifferentiated febrile illness to severe multisystem disease with high mortality rates
B. Etiologic Features
1. Leptospires are thin, tightly coiled spirochetes
2. Their small diameter allows visualization with darkfield microscopy
3. Readily cultured in polysorbate-albumin media
4. Classified into several species
    a. Defined by their degree of genetic relatedness as determined by DNA reassociation
    b. Currently, 13 named species and 4 unnamed genomospecies, which include pathogenic and nonpathogenic strains
    c. Classification is supported by 16S RNA gene sequencing
5. Genome sequence has been determined for 1 strain, *Leptospira interrogans* serovar *lai*, leading to a better understanding of leptospiral pathogenesis
C. Epidemiology and Transmission
1. Leptospirosis is endemic throughout the world
    a. Human infections are endemic in most regions
    b. Peak incidence occurs in the rainy season in tropical regions and in late summer to early fall in temperate regions
    c. In the United States, the highest incidence is in Hawaii (according to active surveillance results, annual incidence in 1992 was approximately 128 per 100,000)
2. Most important reservoirs: rodents and other small mammals, but livestock and companion animals are also important sources of human infection
3. Carrier animals
    a. Usually become infected when young
    b. Infected animals may excrete leptospires in their urine intermittently or continuously throughout life
4. Direct contact: important in transmission to veterinarians, workers in milking sheds on dairy farms, abattoir workers, butchers, hunters, and animal handlers
5. Indirect contact: more common
    a. Responsible for disease after exposure to wet soil or water

b. Most cases are acquired by this route in the tropics
D. Pathophysiology
1. Leptospires enter the body through various routes
   a. Cuts and abrasions
   b. Mucous membranes or conjunctivae
   c. Aerosol inhalation of microscopic droplets
2. Leptospires are carried in the blood throughout the body
   a. Systemic vasculitis facilitates migration of spirochetes into organs and tissues
   b. Accounts for a broad spectrum of clinical illness
3. Severe vascular injury can ensue, with various manifestations
   a. Pulmonary hemorrhage
   b. Ischemia of the renal cortex
   c. Tubular epithelial cell necrosis
   d. Destruction of the hepatic architecture, resulting in jaundice and liver cell injury with or without necrosis
E. Clinical Manifestations
1. Leptospiral infection has a broad spectrum of severity
2. Subclinical illness followed by seroconversion
3. Two clinically recognizable syndromes
   a. A self-limited systemic illness (approximately 90% of infections)
   b. A severe, potentially fatal illness accompanied by any combination of renal failure, liver failure, and pneumonitis with hemorrhagic diathesis (Figure 9.2)
      1) Mean incubation period is 10 days (range, 5-14 days)
      2) May have 2 distinct phases
         a) Initial septicemic phase (also called the acute stage)

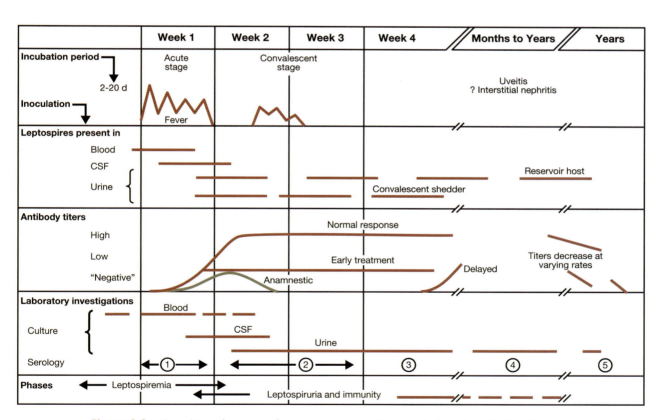

Figure 9.2. Clinical Manifestations of Leptospirosis Over Time. Circled numbers (1-5) indicate specimen numbers for serology: 1 and 2 are acute-stage samples; 3 is convalescent-stage sample, which may facilitate detection of a delayed immune response; and 4 and 5 are follow-up samples, which may provide epidemiologic information, such as the presumptive infecting serogroup. CSF indicates cerebrospinal fluid. (Adapted from Levett PN, Haake DA. Leptospira species [Leptospirosis]. In: Mandell GL, Bennett JE, Dolin R, editors. Mandell, Douglas, and Bennett's principles and practice of infectious diseases. Vol 2. 7th ed. Philadelphia [PA]: Churchill Livingstone/Elsevier; c2010. p. 3059–66. Used with permission.)

i) Begins abruptly
ii) High, remittent fever (38°C-40°C) and headache, chills, rigors, and myalgias
iii) Conjunctival suffusion without purulent discharge
iv) Abdominal pain, anorexia, nausea, vomiting, and diarrhea
v) Cough and pharyngitis
vi) Lasts 5 to 7 days
vii) Leptospires can be recovered from blood, urine, and CSF during this phase
viii) Death is exceedingly rare in the septicemic phase
ix) Defervescence is followed by the immune phase of illness

b) Immune phase (also called convalescent stage)
  i) Generally lasts 4 to 30 days
  ii) Leptospires disappear from blood and CSF
  iii) Disappearance of leptospires coincides with the appearance of IgM antibodies
  iv) Organisms can be detected in almost all tissues and organs and in urine for several weeks, depending on the severity of the disease
  v) Symptoms in the immune phase include those in the acute phase and additional signs and severe symptoms
    (a) Jaundice, renal failure, cardiac arrhythmias, pulmonary symptoms, aseptic meningitis
    (b) Conjunctival suffusion (with or without hemorrhage), photophobia, eye pain
    (c) Muscle tenderness
    (d) Adenopathy
    (e) Hepatosplenomegaly

c) Severe cases may progress directly from the septicemic phase (without the characteristic brief improvement in symptoms) to fulminant illness
  i) Fever greater than 40°C
  ii) Rapid onset of liver failure, acute renal failure, hemorrhagic pneumonitis, cardiac arrhythmia, or circulatory collapse
  iii) Mortality among these patients ranges from 5% to 40%

F. Laboratory Diagnosis
  1. Direct detection methods
    a. Darkfield microscopic examination
      1) Direct visualization of leptospires in blood or urine
      2) Low sensitivity (40.2%) and specificity
    b. Staining methods
      1) Immunofluorescence staining, immunoperoxidase staining, and silver staining
      2) Not widely used because of the lack of commercially available reagents and their relatively low sensitivity
    c. Monoclonal antibody–based dot–enzyme-linked immunosorbent assay (ELISA) for detection of leptospiral antigen in urine assay
      1) Positive results among 75% of patients on the day of hospital admission in 1 study
      2) This assay has not been evaluated widely and is not available commercially
    d. Several polymerase chain reaction (PCR) assays have been developed for the detection of leptospires
      1) Chief advantage of PCR: prospect of confirming the diagnosis during the acute (leptospiremic) stage of the illness, when treatment is likely to have the greatest benefit
    e. Histologic diagnosis has traditionally relied on silver impregnation staining, but immunohistochemical staining offers greater sensitivity and specificity
  2. Isolation and identification
    a. Leptospires can be isolated from blood, CSF, and peritoneal dialysate fluid during the first 10 days of the illness
      1) Urine can be cultured after the first week of illness
      2) Albumin-polysorbate media, such as EMJH or PLM-5
      3) Incubated at 30°C for several weeks
      4) Initial growth may be very slow
    b. Isolated leptospires are identified to the serovar level by either of 2 methods
      1) Traditional serologic methods
      2) Molecular methods, such as pulsed-field electrophoresis

3. Indirect detection methods
    a. Diagnosis is by serology in the majority of leptospirosis cases
    b. Reference standard assay: microscopic agglutination test (MAT)
        1) Live antigens representing different serogroups of leptospires are reacted with serum samples
        2) Examined by darkfield microscopy for agglutination
        3) A serologically confirmed case of leptospirosis is defined by a 4-fold increase in MAT titer to 1 or more serovars between acute-stage and convalescent-stage serum specimens run in parallel
            a) Titer of at least 1:800 in the presence of compatible symptoms is strong evidence of recent or current infection
            b) Suggestive evidence for recent or current infection includes a single titer of at least 1:200 obtained after the onset of symptoms
G. Treatment and Prevention
    1. Antibiotic therapy
        a. Consistently prevents disease or decreases the duration of leptospiruria
        b. Initiate as early in the course of disease as suspicion allows
    2. Specific antibiotics
        a. Severe disease: usually treated with intravenous penicillin
            1) Jarisch-Herxheimer reactions have been reported in patients treated with penicillin
            2) Once-daily ceftriazone has been shown to be as effective as penicillin
        b. Mild disease: treated with oral doxycycline
        c. Chemoprophylaxis for unavoidable exposure to leptospires in endemic environments: doxycycline

Suggested Reading

Barbour AG. Relapsing fevers and other *Borrelia* infections. In: Guerrant RL, Walker DH, Weller PF, editors. Tropical infectious diseases: principles, pathogens, and practice. Philadelphia: Churchill Livingstone; c1999. p. 535–46.

Everard JD. Leptospirosis. In: Cox FEG, editor. The Wellcome Trust illustrated history of tropical diseases. London: The Wellcome Trust; c1996. p. 110–19, 416–8.

Garrity GM, editor. Bergey's manual of systematic bacteriology. 2nd ed. New York: Springer; c2001.

Leptospirosis worldwide, 1999 [English, French]. Wkly Epidemiol Rec. 1999 Jul 23;74(29):237–42.

Levett PN. Leptospirosis. Clin Microbiol Rev. 2001 Apr;14(2):296–326.

Schwan TG, Hinnebusch BJ. Bloodstream- versus tick-associated variants of a relapsing fever bacterium. Science. 1998 Jun 19;280(5371):1938–40.

Alan J. Wright, MD

10

Tick-Borne Infections

I. Introduction
   A. Tick-Borne Infections
      1. Very serious illnesses in healthy children and adults
      2. Clinical presentation is often nonspecific and diagnosis is difficult
      3. Clinicians should have a high index of suspicion for tick-borne infections and begin appropriate empirical antibiotic therapy for the best therapeutic outcome
      4. This chapter reviews the 4 most common tick-borne infections in the United States: Lyme disease, ehrlichiosis, babesiosis, and Rocky Mountain spotted fever
   B. Important Facts About Ticks
      1. Ticks have been known since antiquity: Homer wrote about ticks in 800 BC
      2. Over 840 known species
      3. Present in most parts of world
      4. Obligate blood-sucking arthropods
         a. Common vector for transmitting disease
         b. Can transmit various pathogens
         c. Transmit pathogens during blood meal when they regurgitate or during defecation
      5. Tick bites often go unnoticed: 40% to 50% of persons bitten do not recall being bitten
      6. Ticks have complex feeding behavior
         a. Questing: resting on vegetation while waiting for host
         b. Engagement: clinging to host (<24 hours)
         c. Exploration: crawling to suitable skin
         d. Penetration: inserting mouth parts into skin
         e. Attachment and feeding: sucking blood
         f. Engorgement: acquiring full blood meal
         g. Detachment and disengagement: releasing from host
   C. Tick Classification
      1. Two families
         a. Argasidae: soft ticks (167 species)
            1) No hard dorsal plate
            2) Feed rapidly (over a period of hours)
         b. Ixodidae: hard ticks (670 species)
            1) Have a hard dorsal plate
            2) Found in wooded areas
            3) Feed slowly (over a period of days)
            4) In the United States, ticks in 3 genera transmit most tick-borne infections to humans
               a) *Amblyomma americanum*: Lone Star tick
               b) *Ixodes*
                  i) *Ixodes scapularis*: deer tick; eastern black-legged tick

ii) *Ixodes pacificus*: western black-legged tick
c) *Dermacentor*
i) *Dermacentor andersoni*: wood tick
ii) *Dermacentor variabilis*: American dog tick
D. Tick Life Cycle
1. Four stages (spanning about 2 years)
a. Egg
b. Larva (6 legs)
c. Nymph (8 legs)
d. Adult (8 legs)
2. Each stage requires a blood meal for maturation
3. Each stage may feed on a different animal reservoir

II. Tick-Borne Diseases
A. Definitions
1. *Tick-borne disease*: illness that results after a tick bite and transmission of a microorganism or a toxin
2. The tick is the *vector* transporting a microorganism from its *reservoir*, in a mammalian animal that is usually not harmed by the microorganism, to a human (dead-end host)
B. Tick-Borne Diseases in the United States
1. Most common
a. Rocky Mountain spotted fever
b. Ehrlichiosis
c. Lyme disease
d. Babesiosis
2. Less common
a. Tularemia
b. Tick-borne relapsing fever
c. Tick paralysis
d. Colorado tick fever
3. Uncommon
a. Leptospirosis
b. Q fever
c. Tick-borne encephalitis
d. Typhus
e. Leishmaniasis
f. Mediterranean spotted fever
g. African tick fever
C. Noninfectious Dermatologic or Bite Reactions From Ticks
1. Toxic reactions
2. Erythematous macules, papules, nodules
3. Tissue necrosis
4. Ulcers
5. Bite granulomas
6. Localized alopecia
7. Lichenification
8. Secondary infection: cellulitis
9. Delayed hypersensitivity reaction
10. Fever, pruritus, urticaria
11. Anaphylaxis
12. Paralysis: neurotoxin
13. A skin reaction that occurs within a few days after a tick bite is *not* a tick-borne infection

III. Lyme Disease
A. Introduction
1. Lyme disease was initially described in 1977 from a cluster of persons with oligoarthritis in Connecticut
2. Over 20,000 new cases are reported each year in the United States
3. Now the most common tick-borne disease in the United States
4. Caused by a spirochete
a. *Borrelia burgdorferi*: in the United States
1) A fastidious organism
2) Grows in Barbour-Stoenner-Kelly medium
b. *Borrelia afzelii* or *Borrelia garinii*: in Europe
B. Epidemiology
1. Lyme disease is endemic in the United States, Europe, and Asia
2. In the United States: endemic in about 12 states; reported in 46 states
a. Three primary areas where Lyme disease is endemic
1) Northeast: Maine to Maryland
2) Midwest: Wisconsin and Minnesota
3) West: California and Oregon
3. Regional differences in species of tick that transmits disease
a. Northeast and Midwest: *I scapularis*
b. West: *I pacificus*
4. Reservoirs: white-footed mice and white-tailed deer
5. Seasonal distribution: spring and summer
6. Certain tick stages transmit effectively during certain seasons
a. Nymph ticks feed on mice in spring and summer
b. Adult ticks feed on deer in summer
7. Risk of infection depends on density of ticks and prevalence of infected ticks
C. Clinical Features
1. Lyme disease is a multisystem disease with 3 stages
a. Early local infection
1) Erythema migrans (90% of infected persons)
2) Cerebrospinal fluid (CSF) seeding

b. Early disseminated infection
   1) Multifocal erythema migrans (10%)
   2) Heart (5%)
   3) Musculoskeletal system (10%)
   4) Nervous system (15%)
c. Late-stage infection
   1) Oligoarthritis (50%)
   2) Nervous system effects
2. Erythema migrans
   a. Important clinical feature of Lyme disease
   b. Seen in 90% of cases
   c. Occurs in early infection stage at the bite site
      1) Onset after bite: 7 to 10 days (range, 3-30 days)
      2) A skin lesion that appears or disappears within 24 hours after bite is *not* erythema migrans
   d. Appearance
      1) Usually single lesion: red, round, macular, and expanding (Figure 10.1)
      2) Sometimes irregular, raised, vesicular, and pruritic
      3) Rash center is variable: homogenous (60%), intense (30%), or clearing (10%)
      4) Multifocal lesions can occur in the early disseminated stage
   e. Location: axilla, inguinal or popliteal areas, belt line
   f. Associated symptoms: fever, fatigue, myalgias, arthralgias, headache, stiff neck, lymphadenopathy
   g. Lyme disease serology is often negative when erythema migrans is present
   h. Must rule out other rash diseases that have similar circular appearance
3. Musculoskeletal symptoms
   a. Very common
   b. Occur in early disseminated or late stages
      1) Early disseminated stage: tenosynovitis, unilateral (10%)
      2) Late stage: intermittent attacks of joint swelling and pain (50%)
   c. Joints: oligoarthritis in large joints (eg, knee)
   d. Occasionally chronic, persistent arthritis due to chronic synovitis
   e. Treatment: oral antibiotics
4. Neurologic features
   a. Occur in early disseminated and late stages
   b. Lymphocytic meningitis
   c. Cranial nerve palsies (especially cranial nerve VII)
   d. Radiculoneuritis
   e. Tertiary neuroborreliosis (5%)
      1) Peripheral neuropathy
      2) Encephalopathy
      3) Neurocognitive dysfunction
5. Post-Lyme disease syndrome
   a. Chronic nonspecific symptoms develop in a small percentage of patients
      1) Fatigue
      2) Fibromyalgia
      3) Arthralgias
      4) Forgetfulness
   b. Duration of symptoms: months to years
   c. No documented evidence of active infection
   d. No evidence that antibiotics are effective for treatment
D. Laboratory Findings
   1. Diagnostic tests should be used to confirm suspected cases of Lyme disease
   2. Cultures of skin lesion, joint fluid, and CSF: low sensitivity
   3. Polymerase chain reaction (PCR) testing
      a. Fairly sensitive: skin biopsy, joint fluid
      b. Insensitive: blood, CSF
   4. Serology: best diagnostic test for Lyme disease
      a. Not standardized
      b. Usually negative in early Lyme disease and positive in later infection
      c. Early antibiotic therapy may decrease antibody response
      d. Enzyme-linked immunosorbent assay (ELISA)
         1) Used by most laboratories to screen for Lyme disease

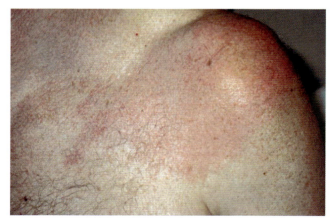

Figure 10.1. Erythema Migrans in Lyme Disease. (Adapted from Tibbles CD, Edlow JA. Does this patient have erythema migrans? JAMA. 2007 Jun 20;297[23]:2617–27. Used with permission.)

a) IgM: usually negative within first 2 weeks but positive by 4 to 6 weeks (70%-80%)
b) IgG: usually positive by 4 weeks
2) Must confirm positive ELISA results with Western blot to detect specific antibodies against *B burgdorferi*
a) IgM bands: 23, 39, 41 kDa
b) IgG bands: 18, 23, 28, 30, 39, 41, 45, 58, 66, 93 kDa
c) Centers for Disease Control and Prevention criteria for diagnosis: 2 IgM bands or 5 IgG bands

E. Diagnosis
1. Diagnosis of Lyme disease can be difficult
2. Early Lyme disease
   a. A clinical diagnosis
   b. Serology results often negative
3. Late Lyme disease
   a. Screen with serology and rule out other diagnoses
   b. When to diagnose late Lyme disease
      1) Exposure to ticks where Lyme disease is endemic
      2) Presence of compatible clinical features
      3) Confirmation with serologic tests (Western blot)
4. Nonspecific symptoms and detection of IgG antibody should *not* be basis for diagnosis
   a. IgM antibody can produce false-positive results
   b. IgG antibody can be from prior infection or cross-reaction

F. Treatment
1. Antibiotic treatment of Lyme disease is effective and follows national guidelines
2. Treatment is based on organ involvement
   a. Erythema migrans (local or disseminated)
      1) First choice: oral doxycycline for 14 to 21 days
      2) Alternative for children and pregnant females: amoxicillin
      3) Second choice: oral cephalosporins (second- or third-generation)
      4) Success rate: greater than 90% (intravenous therapy is not better than oral)
   b. Oligoarthritis: oral doxycycline for 30 to 60 days
   c. Neurologic features
      1) Bell palsy: oral doxycycline for 14 days
      2) Central nervous system (CNS) disease or peripheral neuropathy: intravenous ceftriaxone or penicillin for 14 days
   d. Cardiac features
      1) First degree atrioventricular block: oral doxycycline for 14 days
      2) Second or third degree atrioventricular block: intravenous ceftriaxone for 14 days

G. Prophylaxis After Tick Bite
1. Several prospective trials compared antibiotic therapy with placebo after *Ixodes* bites
   a. Compared risk of acquiring Lyme disease with antibiotic efficacy and adverse effects
   b. Most studies, including meta-analysis with 600 patients, concluded that routine antibiotic therapy is not warranted where disease is *not* endemic
   c. Prospective study compared doxycycline with placebo in area where disease is hyperendemic
      1) Lyme disease incidence: less in antibiotic group (0.4%) than placebo group (3.2%) (P=.04)
      2) Adverse reactions: more in antibiotic group (30.1%) than placebo group (11.1%)
2. Reasonable approach: give single dose of doxycycline (200 mg) when certain conditions are all present
   a. An adult or nymph *I scapularis* is attached for 36 hours or more
   b. Local rate of tick infection with *B burgdorferi* is 20% or more
   c. Prophylaxis can be started within 72 hours of tick removal
   d. Doxycycline is not contraindicated

IV. Ehrlichiosis
A. Introduction
1. Tick-transmitted *Ehrlichia* infections have been known in veterinary medicine since 1910
2. Human *Ehrlichia* infections recognized since 1987
3. *Ehrlichia* are obligate intracellular bacteria
   a. *Ehrlichia* have trophism for hematopoietic cells and grow within membrane-bound vacuoles
   b. *Ehrlichia* is transmitted in a zoonotic cycle involving ticks and mammals
4. Two main *Ehrlichia* infections in humans
   a. Human monocytic ehrlichiosis (HME): discovered in 1987
      1) Agent: *Ehrlichia chaffeensis*
      2) Infects monocytes
   b. Human granulocytic anaplasmosis (HGA): discovered in 1994
      1) Agent: *Anaplasma phagocytophilum*
      2) Infects neutrophils

c. HME and HGA are separate disease entities
B. Human Monocytic Ehrlichiosis
  1. Geographic distribution in United States
     a. Regions: Southeast, mid-Atlantic, South Central
     b. States: North Carolina, Arkansas, Oklahoma, Missouri, California
  2. About 600 cases reported each year in the United States
  3. Ticks: *A americanum* (Lone Star tick) and *D variabilis* (American dog tick)
  4. Reservoir: white-tailed deer and other mammals
  5. Season: spring and summer (peak)
  6. Illness begins 1 to 2 weeks after tick bite
C. Human Granulocytic Anaplasmosis
  1. Geographic distribution in United States
     a. Regions: New England, mid-Atlantic, Upper Midwest
     b. States: Wisconsin, Minnesota, Connecticut, New York, Massachusetts, California, Florida
  2. About 600 cases reported each year in the United States
  3. Ticks: *I scapularis* (deer tick); *I pacificus* (western black-legged tick); *D variabilis* (American dog tick)
  4. Reservoir: white-footed mouse
  5. Season: spring and summer
D. Clinical Features
  1. Wide spectrum of disease among patients with ehrlichiosis: asymptomatic to severe symptoms
  2. Clinical features of symptomatic ehrlichiosis
     a. Usually an abrupt onset: 1 to 2 weeks after tick bite
     b. Nonspecific symptoms
        1) Fever, chills, malaise
        2) Severe headache
        3) Myalgias (severe and diffuse)
        4) Nausea, vomiting, abdominal pain
     c. Rash: macular-papular or petechial
        1) HME: 35% to 40%
        2) HGA: 2% to 5%
  3. No chronic disease documented
  4. Clinical complications can occur
     a. Acute respiratory failure
     b. Acute renal failure
     c. Hypotension
     d. Gastrointestinal tract hemorrhage
     e. Disseminated intravascular coagulation (DIC)
     f. Opportunistic infections (viral and fungal)
     g. CNS disease
     h. Myocarditis and congestive heart failure
     i. Rhabdomyolysis
  5. Clinical differences between HME and HGA
     a. HME: more severe infection
        1) More complications
        2) Higher mortality (2%-3% vs 0.5%-1%)
     b. HME: more rash illness (35%-40% vs 2%-5%)
     c. HME: more neurologic complications (CNS)
E. Laboratory Findings
  1. Leukopenia: in the first week
  2. White blood cells: intracytoplasmic inclusions (morulae) (Figure 10.2)
  3. Thrombocytopenia
  4. Abnormal findings on liver function tests (LFTs): increased levels of alanine aminotransferase (ALT) and aspartate aminotransferase (AST)
  5. CSF: lymphocytic pleocytosis; increased protein level
F. Diagnosis
  1. When to suspect ehrlichiosis
     a. History of tick exposure or bite
     b. Suggestive symptoms
     c. Compatible laboratory test results
        1) Leukopenia
        2) Thrombocytopenia
        3) Abnormal LFT results
  2. Confirmation of diagnosis of ehrlichiosis
     a. Blood smear: morulae
        1) HME: 10% to 20%
        2) HGA: 25% to 75%
     b. Antibody tests: immunofluorescence assay (IFA) positive for IgM or 4-fold increase in IgG titers
     c. PCR: *Ehrlichia* DNA
        1) Sensitivity: 70% to 90%
        2) Specificity: >95%
G. Treatment
  1. Treatment should not be delayed: begin when ehrlichiosis is suspected (before confirming test results)
  2. Drug of choice: doxycycline
     a. Dosage: 100 mg twice daily for 14 days
     b. Response: usually within 24 to 48 hours
  3. Alternative therapy: rifampin (use of chloramphenicol is controversial)
  4. Treatment recommendations are based on empirical data, not comparative studies
V. Babesiosis
  A. Introduction
    1. *Babesia*: an intraerythrocytic parasite
    2. More than 100 species, most of which infect animals

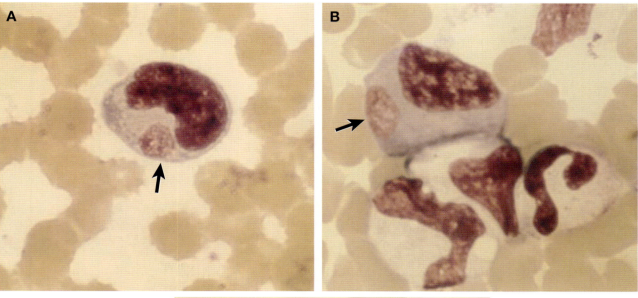

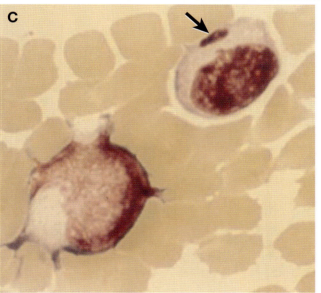

Figure 10.2. Intraleukocytic Inclusion Bodies of *Ehrlichia* Species. These buffy-coat smears are from a 13-year-old girl with fever, encephalitis, neutropenia, and disseminated intravascular coagulation (original magnification ×1,000). A and B, Arrows show the classic mulberry-like structures called morulae. C, Arrow shows an immature inclusion body. (Adapted from Glaser C, Johnson E. Images in clinical medicine. Ehrlichiosis. N Engl J Med. 1995 May 25;332[21]:1417.)

3. Reservoir: animals (cattle and rodents)
4. Two *Babesia* species are important in causing human disease
   a. *Babesia microti*: United States
   b. *Babesia divergens*: Europe
B. Epidemiology
   1. *Babesia* infections are reported worldwide
      a. Europe: Britain, France, Spain, Germany, Yugoslavia, Russia, Sweden
      b. United States
         1) Northeast (disease is endemic): Massachusetts (Cape Cod, Nantucket); New York City (Long Island, Shelter Island); New Jersey; Connecticut; Rhode Island

2) Midwest (disease is sporadic): Wisconsin and Minnesota
3) Other areas: Washington, California, Missouri, Indiana, Georgia, Virginia
2. Transmission of *Babesia*
   a. Tick bites: *Ixodes* (especially *I scapularis*)
      1) Coinfections (Lyme disease, ehrlichiosis) may occur
      2) Seasonality: May to September
   b. Transfusions
      1) More than 40 cases reported
      2) *Babesia* remains viable in stored blood
      3) No seasonality
C. Clinical Features
   1. Babesiosis incubation period: 1 to 9 weeks
      a. After tick bite: 1 to 3 weeks
      b. After transfusion: 6 to 9 weeks
   2. Nonspecific symptoms
      a. Fever, chills, sweats
      b. Fatigue, malaise
      c. Headache, altered mental status
      d. Gastrointestinal tract symptoms: nausea, vomiting
   3. Wide spectrum of disease
      a. Mild to severe or fulminant disease
      b. Severity of illness is dependent on host risk factors
         1) Normal host
            a) Milder disease
            b) Lower mortality (about 5%)
         2) Abnormal host
            a) More severe disease
            b) Can resemble malaria (fever, anemia, organomegaly)
            c) Higher mortality (30%-40%)
         3) Risk factors associated with severe disease
            a) Splenectomy
            b) Older age
            c) Human immunodeficiency virus infection
            d) Cancer
            e) Medical conditions: coronary artery disease, chronic obstructive pulmonary disease, congestive heart failure
      c. Clinical course can be complicated
         1) Severe hemolytic anemia
         2) Congestive heart failure or shock (or both)
         3) Disseminated intravascular coagulation
         4) Acute renal failure
         5) Acute respiratory failure or acute respiratory distress syndrome
         6) Coma
         7) Death
D. Laboratory Findings
   1. Hemolytic anemia
      a. Increased reticulocyte count
      b. Increased lactate dehydrogenase level
      c. Hemoglobinuria
   2. Leukocyte count: normal or decreased
   3. Thrombocytopenia: mild
   4. Abnormal LFT results: increased levels of alkaline phosphatase, ALT, and AST
   5. Polyclonal gammopathy
E. Diagnosis
   1. Thin blood smear (Giemsa or Wright stain)
      a. Intraerythrocytic parasites
         1) Ring forms or Maltese cross (Figure 10.3)
         2) Must distinguish from malaria
      b. Parasitemia
         1) From 1% to more than 80%
         2) Variable and can last for weeks (from 3-12 weeks to 7 months)
   2. Serology (IFA)
      a. IgG: greater than 1:64 is positive
      b. IgM: greater than 1:64 is positive
   3. PCR testing
      a. Detect *Babesia* DNA
      b. Highly sensitive and specific
F. Treatment
   1. Mild babesiosis in a healthy host
      a. Often not diagnosed
      b. Probably resolves without therapy
   2. Moderate or severe babesiosis should be treated

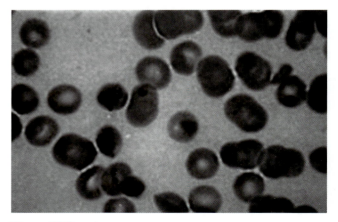

Figure 10.3. *Babesia microti*. Organisms are shown inside human erythrocytes (original magnification ×100). (Adapted from Krause PJ. Babesiosis. Med Clin North Am. 2002 Mar;86[2]:361–73. Used with permission.)

a. Standard treatment: quinine (650 mg every 8 hours) and clindamycin (600 mg every 6 hours) for 7 to 10 days
b. Alternative treatment: atovaquone (750 mg every 12 hours) and azithromycin (500-1,000 mg on day 1 and 250-1,000 mg on days 7-10)
   1) Equal efficacy as standard treatment of nonsevere illness
   2) Less adverse toxicity
3. Exchange transfusion
   a. Adjunctive treatment for certain cases
      1) Use is controversial
      2) No controlled treatment trials
      3) Used to decrease parasitemia rapidly and to decrease cytokines
   b. Recommended for severe, fulminant life-threatening infections
      1) High level of parasitemia (>10% or >5% with complications)
      2) Severe hemolysis
      3) Immunocompromised host
      4) Infections with *B divergens*

G. Prevention
1. No babesiosis vaccine is available and no chemoprophylaxis is recommended
2. Best prevention: personal protective measures
   a. Avoid areas where ticks are endemic
   b. Wear protective clothing
   c. Use tick repellent: diethyltoluamide (DEET) on skin and permethrin on clothing
   d. Examine for ticks and remove promptly

VI. Rocky Mountain Spotted Fever
A. Introduction
1. The most frequently reported rickettsial infection in the United States
2. About 200 cases reported each year
3. First described in late 1800s in northwestern United States (Montana and Idaho)
4. Causative agent, *Rickettsia rickettsii*, discovered in 1906 by Howard Ricketts
   a. Gram-negative
   b. Obligate intracellular organism
   c. Trophism for vascular epithelium
   d. Small mammals (voles, mice, dogs) serve as reservoir for *R rickettsii*

B. Epidemiology
1. Rocky Mountain spotted fever is endemic in the United States, Canada, Central America, and South America
2. Reported from most areas in the United States, but primarily West, South Central, and Southeast (states with the most cases: North Carolina, South Carolina, Tennessee, and Oklahoma)
3. Transmitted by wood ticks and dog ticks
4. Seasonal distribution: April to September (95%)
5. Age-specific incidence: highest in children
6. Risk factors: exposure to wooded areas, dogs, and ticks

C. Clinical Features
1. Incubation period: usually 2 to 5 days (range, 2-14 days)
2. Onset of symptoms: usually abrupt
3. Clinical features
   a. Nonspecific febrile illness
   b. Fever (100%)
   c. Headache (severe) (90%)
   d. Rash (>90%) (Figure 10.4)
   e. Myalgias (intense) (80%)
   f. Malaise and anorexia (95%)
   g. Other
      1) Sore throat
      2) Gastrointestinal tract: nausea, vomiting, abdominal pain, diarrhea

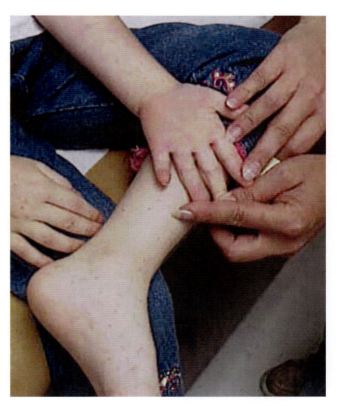

Figure 10.4. Fading Centripetal Rash of Rocky Mountain Spotted Fever. (Adapted from Masters EJ, Olson GS, Weiner SJ, Paddock CD. Rocky Mountain spotted fever: a clinician's dilemma. Arch Intern Med. 2003 Apr 14;163[7]:769–74. Used with permission.)

3) Neurologic: seizures, focal signs, confusion, hallucinations
4) Ocular: conjunctivitis, periorbital edema
5) Cardiac: myocarditis, arrhythmia
6) Extremities: swelling of hand and feet, joint pain
7) Hearing loss

h. Distinctive features of rash
1) Onset: usually 3 to 5 days (range, 1-15 days) after fever
2) Location: begins on ankles and wrists
3) Progression
4) Initially a maculopapular rash
   a) Progresses to petechiae and purpura
   b) Spreads to trunk, palms, and soles: centripetal rash
   c) May become hemorrhagic with skin necrosis and digital gangrene

D. Pathophysiology
1. *Rickettsia rickettsii* has trophism for vascular endothelial cells
2. Replicates and causes damage
   a. Vascular injury
   b. Vascular permeability
   c. Vasculitis and necrosis
3. Pathophysiology: vasculitis
4. Pathology: vasculitis and lymphocytic infiltration

E. Complications
1. DIC and shock
2. Noncardiogenic pulmonary edema
3. Myocarditis and arrhythmias
4. Skin necrosis and extremity gangrene
5. Hemolysis
6. Renal failure
7. Encephalitis and stroke
8. Gastrointestinal tract bleeding

F. Laboratory Findings
1. Leukocyte count: normal or decreased
2. Platelet count: usually decreased
3. Transaminase concentrations: increased
4. CSF findings: usually normal

G. Diagnosis
1. Diagnosis of Rocky Mountain spotted fever can be difficult
   a. Diagnosis often missed initially
   b. Tick bite may be asymptomatic (30%-40%)
   c. Early in the illness, symptoms are nonspecific
   d. Rash may be misdiagnosed as from another disease
2. Diagnostic clues
   a. Patient was in area where disease is endemic
   b. Patient was exposed to ticks
   c. Fever and centripetal, petechial rash
   d. Distinctive features
      1) Edema around eyes, hands, and feet
      2) Relative bradycardia
      3) Calf tenderness
      4) Hearing loss
3. Confirmation of clinical diagnosis
   a. Serologic testing: IFA, ELISA
      1) Early testing: often negative
      2) Positive tests: 7 to 14 days after onset
      3) Requirement: acute and convalescent tests with a 4-fold increase in titer
   b. Immunostaining testing on tissue
      1) Direct fluorescence (70%-90%)
      2) Immunoperoxidase
   c. Molecular tests: detect *R rickettsii* DNA (PCR)

H. Treatment
1. Antibiotic treatment: give early for best outcome
2. Need to have high index of suspicion and begin empirical therapy
3. Goal: begin therapy within 2 to 5 days after onset
4. Drug of choice: doxycycline (100 mg every 12 hours)
5. Alternative treatment: chloramphenicol (if patient is allergic or pregnant)
6. Oral therapy for early, nonsevere cases; intravenous therapy for severe cases
7. Duration of treatment: 7 to 10 days

I. Prognosis
1. Rocky Mountain spotted fever is often a severe disease with variable mortality
   a. Without therapy: 25%
   b. With therapy: 5%
2. Factors for poor prognosis
   a. Older age group
   b. Male
   c. Black race
   d. Nonspecific early presentation
   e. Delayed diagnosis and therapy
   f. Neurologic symptoms and complications
   g. Increased creatinine level, decreased platelet count, increased LFT values

VII. Prevention of Tick-Borne Infections
A. Prevent Tick Bites
1. Best way to prevent infection where disease is endemic
2. Wear protective clothing
   a. Wear long pants and long-sleeve shirt

      b. Keep clothing tight around ankles and wrists
      c. Walk on cleared trails and avoid brushy vegetation
    3. Apply DEET (15%-33%) to exposed skin, with repeated applications
    4. Apply permethrin to clothing
    5. Examine for ticks and remove within 24 hours
  B. Remove Ticks Properly
    1. After an attached tick is found, remove it promptly to decrease transmission of pathogens
    2. Remove tick without causing it to vomit or defecate and without leaving tick mouth parts behind
    3. Best tick removal method
      a. Use tweezers or small forceps
      b. Grasp tick close to skin attachment
      c. Apply gentle traction straight outward
      d. Do not squeeze or twist ticks
      e. Do not remove with unprotected fingers
      f. Do not use petroleum jelly, fingernail polish, isopropyl alcohol, or hot match tip

VIII. Coinfections
  A. Ticks Can Carry Several Infectious Agents
    1. A tick can transmit more than 1 organism, resulting in a coinfection
    2. *Ixodes scapularis* can be infected with *B burgdorferi*, *Ehrlichia*, and *Babesia*
    3. Well-documented cases of coinfections
      a. Lyme disease and *Ehrlichia*
      b. Lyme disease and *Babesia*
      c. *Ehrlichia* and *Babesia*
      d. *Ehrlichia* and Rocky Mountain spotted fever
  B. When to Suspect a Coinfection
    1. There are overlapping clinical features
    2. The clinical features are more severe or not typical of a certain infection

IX. Summary
  A. Ticks Cause Serious Human Diseases
    1. Have a high index of suspicion for tick-borne diseases
    2. When to suspect a tick-borne disease
      a. History of exposure to ticks with or without a tick bite
      b. Compatible illness
        1) Fever and centripetal rash: Rocky Mountain spotted fever
        2) Fever and abnormal results on complete blood cell count and LFTs: Ehrlichiosis
        3) Expanding circular rash: Lyme disease
        4) Fever, abnormal erythrocytes, hemolytic anemia: babesiosis
    3. When a tick-borne disease is suspected, begin treatment before confirming with tests
    4. Empirical drug of choice: doxycycline
  B. Tick-Borne Diseases are Preventable
    1. Wear protective clothing
    2. Use DEET on exposed skin
    3. Apply permethrin to clothing
    4. Inspect for ticks and remove attached ticks early

Suggested Reading

Bakken JS, Dumler S. Human granulocytic anaplasmosis. Infect Dis Clin North Am. 2008 Sep;22(3):433–48.

Krause PJ. Babesiosis. Med Clin North Am. 2002 Mar;86(2):361–73.

Krause PJ, Lepore T, Sikand VK, Gadbaw J Jr, Burke G, Telford SR 3rd, et al. Atovaquone and azithromycin for the treatment of babesiosis. N Engl J Med. 2000 Nov 16;343(20):1454–8.

Masters EJ, Olson GS, Weiner SJ, Paddock CD. Rocky Mountain spotted fever: a clinician's dilemma. Arch Intern Med. 2003 Apr 14;163(7):769–74.

Olano JP, Walker DH. Human ehrlichioses. Med Clin North Am. 2002 Mar;86(2):375–92.

Steere AC. Lyme disease. N Engl J Med. 2001 Jul 12;345(2):115–25.

Vannier E, Gewurz BE, Krause PJ. Human babesiosis. Infect Dis Clin North Am. 2008 Sep;22(3):469–88.

Wormser GP, Dattwyler RJ, Shapiro ED, Halperin JJ, Steere AC, Klempner MS, et al. The clinical assessment, treatment, and prevention of Lyme disease, human granulocytic anaplasmosis, and babesiosis: clinical practice guidelines by the Infectious Diseases Society of America. Clin Infect Dis. 2006 Nov 1;43(9):1089–134. Epub 2006 Oct 2. Erratum in: Clin Infect Dis. 2007 Oct 1;45(7):941.

Irene G. Sia, MD

Mycobacteria

I. Epidemiology
   A. Distribution
      1. Worldwide
      2. Highest incidence in sub-Saharan Africa, India, China, Southeast Asia, Micronesia, and Russia
   B. Risk Factors
      1. Prevalent in populations at risk of human immunodeficiency virus (HIV): inner-city minority populations, intravenous drug users
      2. More than half of all US cases are in foreign-born individuals
      3. Risk factors for reactivation of disease years after infection
         a. HIV infection, AIDS
         b. End-stage renal disease
         c. Diabetes mellitus
         d. Hematologic or reticuloendothelial malignancies
         e. Corticosteroid or other immunosuppressive medications
         f. Decreased cell-mediated immunity with old age
         g. Silicosis
         h. Alcoholism
         i. Gastrectomy, jejunoileal bypass

II. Etiology
   A. *Mycobacterium tuberculosis* Complex
      1. *Mycobacterium tuberculosis*, *Mycobacterium bovis*, *Mycobacterium africanum*, and *Mycobacterium microti*
      2. *Mycobacterium tuberculosis*: humans are the only natural reservoir
      3. *Mycobacterium bovis*
         a. Consumption of unpasteurized milk products from infected cow
         b. Cattle-to-human transmission also occurs
         c. More often causes extrapulmonary diseases
III. Major Clinical Manifestations
   A. Primary Tuberculosis
      1. Patients with tuberculosis (TB) usually present with fever; less commonly, pleuritic chest pain, retrosternal or interscapular pain
      2. Physical examination findings are usually normal
      3. Hilar adenopathy, often resolving in 1 year or more
   B. Reactivation TB
      1. Majority of adult non-HIV TB cases
      2. Cough, weight loss, fatigue, fever, night sweats, chest pain, dyspnea, hemoptysis
      3. Physical examination findings nonspecific; rales may be present

4. Typically, apical posterior segment of upper lobes; less frequently, superior segment of lower lobes or anterior segment of upper lobes
5. Computed tomography (CT): centrilobular lesions, nodules, and branching linear densities ("tree in bud")

C. Endobronchial TB
1. Associated with extensive pulmonary TB
2. Barking cough, sputum production
3. Decreased breath sounds, rhonchi, wheezing on examination
4. Upper lobe infiltrates and cavity with ipsilateral spread to lower lobe and possibly to superior segment of contralateral lower lobe (most common)
5. Complications include endobronchial ulceration or perforation, obstruction, atelectasis, bronchiectasis, tracheal or bronchial stenosis

D. Lower Lung Field TB
1. Uncommon
2. Lower lobe consolidation more extensive; cavitation may be present

E. Tuberculoma
1. Rounded mass lesions; rarely, cavitation

F. Complications of Pulmonary TB
1. Hemoptysis, pneumothorax, bronchiectasis, extensive pulmonary destruction
2. Symptoms: progressive dyspnea, hemoptysis, weight loss

IV. Diagnosis of TB
A. Sputum Examination
1. Smear microscopy
   a. Visualization of acid-fast bacilli
   b. Ziehl-Neelsen or Kinyoun stain
   c. Auramine-rhodamine or auramine O stain with fluorescence microscopy

B. Gastric Aspiration
1. Children: specimen obtained through nasogastric tube on awakening in the morning
2. Acid-fast bacillus (AFB) smears are not useful because of contamination with ingested nonpathogenic environmental mycobacterial species

C. Culture
1. Solid medium
   a. Potato- or egg-based media (Middlebrook 7H10 or 7H11 agar)
   b. Albumin in agar base (Lowenstein-Jensen medium)
2. Liquid medium
   a. BACTEC blood culture system
   b. Septi-Chek AFB system
   c. Mycobacterial Growth Indicator Tube (MGIT): positive results in approximately 8 days

D. Identification
1. Morphologic and biochemical characteristics
   a. Test for pyrazinamidase production
   b. Differentiates *M tuberculosis* from *M bovis*
2. Nucleic acid–based detection method

E. Drug Susceptibility Testing
1. BACTEC system
2. Colorimetric microplate-based method
3. Mycobacteriophage-based system

F. Radiology
1. Chest radiograph
   a. Low sensitivity and low specificity
   b. Unusual findings are common in HIV-positive patients and elderly patients
2. CT scan
   a. More sensitive
   b. Suggestive findings: cluster of nodules, tree-in-bud lesions, or upper lobe or superior segment of lower lobe

V. Extrapulmonary TB
A. Characteristics
1. Higher incidence among HIV-positive persons
2. Skin test results are more often positive than results with pulmonary TB
3. Obtaining tissue is often necessary for diagnosis
4. Other diagnostic methods
   a. Polymerase chain reaction testing
   b. Other nucleic acid amplification tests
   c. Cerebrospinal fluid (CSF) analysis: adenine deaminase may be increased
   d. Bronchoalveolar lavage
   e. Pericardial fluid analysis

B. Miliary TB
1. From uncontrolled hematogenous dissemination of *M tuberculosis*
2. Acute disease may be fulminant, with multiorgan system failure, septic shock, and acute respiratory distress syndrome
3. Lungs, gastrointestinal tract, central nervous system (CNS), skin, cardiovascular system, adrenal gland, bone, eye, larynx, ear

C. Tuberculous Meningitis
1. Complication after primary dissemination: common among children and young adults in countries with high incidence of TB
2. Chronic reactivation disease: adults in countries with low incidence of TB
3. Risks (adults): immunodeficiency due to aging, alcoholism, malnutrition, malignancy, HIV infection
4. Changes most marked at base of brain

5. Clinical stages
    a. Prodrome: insidious onset of malaise, lassitude, headache, low-grade fever, personality changes
    b. Meningitis phase: pronounced neurologic symptoms
    c. Paralytic: rapid progression to stupor, coma, seizure, hemiparesis
6. If untreated: death within 5 to 8 weeks
7. Majority of persons have positive tuberculin skin test (TST)
8. About 50% have abnormalities on chest radiography
9. Diagnosis may be difficult
    a. CSF examination findings
        1) Increased protein (100-150 mg/dL)
        2) Decreased glucose (<45 mg/dL)
        3) Mononuclear pleocytosis: elevated white blood cell count (100-150/μL)
    b. AFB smears
    c. Polymerase chain reaction testing
    d. Neuroradiology
10. Indications for adjunctive corticosteroid
    a. Traditionally indicated for patients with objective neurologic findings or stupor-coma
    b. Newer data indicate improved survival overall, with benefit most evident in patients with less neurologic compromise
11. Surgery: for management of hydrocephalus
D. Tuberculoma of the CNS
    1. Conglomerate caseous foci within the brain
    2. Single or multiple enhancing nodular lesions on CT
    3. Focal neurologic symptoms or signs of intracranial mass lesion
E. Spinal TB Arachnoiditis
    1. Focal inflammatory disease with gradual encasement of spinal cord
    2. Signs and symptoms
        a. Nerve root and cord compression
        b. Spinal or radicular pain, hyperesthesias
        c. Lower motor neuron paralysis
        d. Bladder or rectal sphincter dysfunction
        e. Anterior spinal artery thrombosis and spinal cord infarction
    3. Diagnosis: abnormal levels of protein in CSF, magnetic resonance imaging, tissue biopsy
F. Tuberculous Pericarditis
    1. Four stages: dry, effusive, absorptive, and constrictive
    2. Nonspecific symptoms
        a. Fever, weight loss, night sweats
        b. Cardiopulmonary symptoms: cough, dyspnea, chest pain, orthopnea
        c. Usually insidious onset
        d. Signs and symptoms of cardiac tamponade
        e. Signs and symptoms of constrictive pericarditis
    3. Diagnosis: pericardiocentesis, pericardial biopsy
    4. Adjunctive corticosteroid: decreases mortality and the need for subsequent pericardiocentesis
    5. Pericardiectomy: for recurrent effusion or continued increase in central venous pressure after 4 to 6 weeks of antitubercular and corticosteroid therapy
VI. Tuberculosis in HIV-Infected Patients
    A. Symptoms
        1. Usually similar to symptoms in non–HIV-infected patients
        2. Weight loss, fever of unknown origin, malaise
    B. Incidence
        1. Higher incidence of extrapulmonary TB
        2. Higher incidence of pleural disease
VII. Tests for Latent TB Infection
    A. Tuberculin Skin Test
        1. TST conversion occurs 2 to 12 weeks after primary infection
            a. In the United States: Mantoux test only
            b. Intradermal injection of 0.1 mL (5 IU) of purified protein derivative (PPD) into volar or dorsal surface of the forearm
        2. Targeted testing of high-risk persons
            a. Indications for single TST
                1) Single potential exposure to TB
                2) Incidentally discovered fibrotic lung lesion
                3) Immigrants and refugees from countries with high prevalence of TB
            b. Indications for annual TST for screening
                1) HIV infection
                2) Ongoing potential close contact with active TB cases
                3) Medical condition that increases risk of active TB
        3. Booster phenomenon
            a. Initially false-negative result on TST
            b. Boosted to a true-positive result with 2-step TST in certain patients
                1) History of TB
                2) Decreased delayed-type hypersensitivity reaction
                3) History of BCG vaccination
        4. TST interpretation
            a. Same for persons who have received BCG vaccine and for persons who have not

b. Reaction of 5 mm or more is positive for certain persons
   1) HIV-positive persons
   2) Close contacts of TB patients
   3) Persons with fibrotic changes on chest radiograph consistent with prior TB
   4) Organ transplant patients
   5) Patients receiving prednisone (or equivalent) (≥15 mg daily for ≥1 month)
c. Reaction of 10 mm or more is positive for certain persons
   1) Recent (≤5 years) immigrants from countries with high prevalence of TB
   2) Injection drug users
   3) Residents and employees of high-risk congregates
   4) TB laboratory personnel
   5) Patients with high-risk clinical conditions
d. Reaction of 15 mm or more is positive for certain persons
   1) Low-risk persons
e. Subsequent TST result is considered positive if induration measures 10 mm or more and has increased by 6 mm or more
5. Potential causes of false-negative TST result
   a. Viral, bacterial, or fungal infections
   b. Live virus vaccinations
   c. Metabolic derangements
   d. Low protein levels
   e. Lymphoid diseases
   f. Use of corticosteroids and other immunosuppressive drugs
   g. Older age
   h. Recent or overwhelming TB infection
   i. Stress
B. Whole Blood Interferon-γ Assay
   1. QuantiFERON-TB Gold test (approved by US Food and Drug Administration)
   2. T-SPOT.*TB* test (available in Europe)
   3. Indications
      a. Same as for TST
      b. Targeted testing for individuals at increased risk of TB
         1) Contact investigation
         2) Evaluation of recent immigrants
         3) Surveillance program for infection control
C. Nucleic Acid Amplification Assays
   1. Gen-Probe Amplified MTD test
   2. Amplicor *Mycobacterium tuberculosis* test
   3. Positive test of smear-positive sample is diagnostic

VIII. Treatment of TB
A. Treatment of Latent TB Infection in HIV-Negative Patients
   1. Screen for active TB with chest radiography before treating latent TB infection (LTBI)
   2. Regimens
      a. Preferred regimen: isoniazid (INH) daily for 9 months
         1) Contraindications
            a) Previous INH hepatitis
            b) Serious adverse reaction to INH
            c) Active hepatitis or end-stage liver disease
         2) Add pyridoxine for patients at risk of neuropathy (eg, diabetes, pregnancy)
      b. RIF daily for 4 months (use for exposure to INH-resistant TB)
      c. RIF plus pyrazinamide (PZA): not recommended, as there had been numerous reports of severe liver injury and death with this regimen
   3. Contraindications
      a. Patient receiving other medications associated with liver injury
      b. Excessive alcohol consumption
      c. Underlying liver disease
      d. History of INH-associated liver injury
   4. For multidrug-resistant (MDR)-TB exposure
      a. Individualized treatment based on drug susceptibility pattern of index case
      b. Consider PZA plus ethambutol (EMB) or a quinolone (ciprofloxacin, ofloxacin) for 12 months
   5. Monitoring
      a. Baseline laboratory testing: not routinely indicated
      b. Indications for baseline serum alanine aminotransferase (ALT), aspartate aminotransferase (AST), and total bilirubin
         1) HIV infection
         2) Liver disease (hepatitis B and C, alcohol abuse)
         3) Pregnancy
         4) First 3 months post partum
         5) Suspected or undiagnosed liver disease
      c. Monthly questioning for signs and symptoms of hepatic injury or intolerance
      d. Indications for monthly monitoring of liver enzymes
         1) Concurrent use of medications with possible drug interactions
         2) Daily alcohol use
         3) Previous INH intolerance
         4) Chronic liver disease
         5) Peripheral neuropathy

6) Pregnancy
7) Ongoing injection drug use
8) Young women, particularly minority women
9) HIV infection
B. Treatment of LTBI in HIV-Positive Patients
  1. Indications
    a. TST reaction of 5 mm or more
    b. Recent contact with patient with infectious TB
    c. History of untreated or inadequately treated TB
    d. Unavoidable high-risk exposure (eg, prison)
  2. Regimen
    a. Preferred: INH for 9 months
    b. INH-resistant TB exposure: RIF for 4 months
    c. MDR-TB exposure: rifamycin (RIF, rifabutin) plus PZA for 2 months, or rifamycin for 4 to 6 months
      1) Use at least 2 drugs for 12 months
      2) Close clinical follow-up for 2 years or more
  3. Directly observed therapy (DOT) is mandatory for twice-weekly regimens
C. Treatment of TB in HIV-Negative Patients
  1. Use at least 2 effective drugs (Table 11.1)
  2. DOT ensures completion of appropriate therapy
  3. Initial phase of 2 months is followed by continuation phase for 4 to 7 months
    a. Initial phase: 3 possible dosing schedules
      1) Daily throughout
      2) Daily for 2 weeks and then twice weekly for 6 weeks
      3) Twice weekly throughout
    b. Continuation phase: 3 possible dosing schedules
      1) Daily
      2) Twice weekly by DOT
      3) Three times weekly by DOT
    c. Indications for 7-month continuation phase
      1) Cavitary TB, with positive sputum culture after 2 months of treatment
      2) PZA not given during the initial phase
      3) Once-weekly INH-plus-rifapentine regimen, with positive sputum culture after 2 months of treatment
D. Treatment of TB in HIV-Positive Patients
  1. General principles: same as for treatment of HIV-negative patients
  2. Consider issues related to drug interactions, immune status, and prevention of resistance
  3. Preferred first-line therapy for patients receiving protease inhibitors: rifabutin-based regimen for 6 months
  4. Initiation of antiretroviral therapy: delay for 2 months to avoid paradoxical worsening of TB, unless CD4 cell count is less than $100/\mu L$
  5. Intermittent therapy
    a. Not recommended with low CD4 cell count or severe immunodeficiency
    b. High risk of relapse and RIF resistance

Table 11.1

Treatment Regimens for Drug-Susceptible Tuberculosis in Patients Who Are Not Infected With Human Immunodeficiency Virus

Initial Phase			Continuation Phase		
Regimen	Drugs	Schedule	Regimen	Drugs	Schedule
1	INH + RIF + PZA + EMB	7 d weekly for 56 doses (8 wk); or 5 d weekly for 40 doses (8 wk)	1a	INH + RIF	7 d weekly for 126 doses (18 wk); or 5 d weekly for 90 doses (18 wk)
			1b	INH + RIF	Twice weekly for 36 doses (18 wk)
			1c	INH + RPT	Once weekly for 18 doses (18 wk)
2	INH + RIF + PZA + EMB	7 d weekly for 14 doses (2 wk), then twice weekly for 12 doses (6 wk); or 5 d weekly for 10 doses (2 wk), then twice weekly for 12 doses (6 wk)	2a	INH + RIF	Twice weekly for 36 doses (18 wk)
			2b	INH + RPT	Once weekly for 18 doses (18 wk)
3	INH + RIF + PZA + EMB	3 times weekly for 24 doses (8 wk)	3a	INH + RIF	3 times weekly for 54 doses (18 wk)
4	INH + RIF + EMB	7 d weekly for 56 doses (8 wk); or 5 d weekly for 40 doses (8 wk)	4a	INH + RIF	7 d weekly for 217 doses (31 wk); or 5 d weekly for 155 doses (31 wk)
			4b	INH + RIF	Twice weekly for 62 doses (31 wk)

Abbreviations: EMB, ethambutol; INH, isoniazid; plus sign, in combination with; PZA, pyrazinamide; RIF, rifampin; RPT, rifapentine.

6. INH plus rifapentine once weekly: contraindicated in continuation phase
7. Follow-up
   a. DOT recommended for all
   b. Monthly sputum collection until culture is negative
8. Immune reconstitution inflammatory syndrome
   a. Occurs in 10% to 35%
   b. Risk: initial CD4 cell count of less than 100/µL with subsequent decrease in viral load and large increase in CD4
   c. Self-limited
   d. No treatment alteration or interruption necessary

E. Evaluation
   1. HIV test: recommended for all TB patients
   2. CD4 cell count: for HIV-positive patients
   3. Serology for hepatitis B and C: intravenous drug use, birth in Asia or Africa, HIV positive
   4. Baseline tests: serum AST, ALT, bilirubin, alkaline phosphatase, and creatinine and platelet count
   5. If EMB is used: visual acuity and red-green color discrimination
   6. Follow-up sputum examination: culture monthly until 2 consecutive cultures are negative
   7. Monthly clinical evaluation: identify possible adverse effects and assess adherence
   8. Treatment completion: determined by total number of doses taken
   9. Patients with high risk of treatment failure or relapse: cavitation on initial chest radiograph and positive sputum culture at 2 months
   10. Drug-induced hepatitis
       a. Symptomatic and serum AST level is more than 3 times the upper limit of normal
       b. Asymptomatic and serum AST level is more than 5 times the upper limit of normal

F. Antitubercular Drugs
   1. Summary of side effects and use in pregnancy (Table 11.2)

G. Possible Reasons for TB Treatment Failure
   1. Nonadherence
   2. Drug resistance
   3. Drug malabsorption
   4. Laboratory error
   5. Biologic variation in response

H. Treatment of Drug-Resistant TB
   1. Risk factors
      a. Previous TB treatment
      b. TB treatment failure or relapse in advanced HIV infection, treated with intermittent anti-TB regimen
      c. Exposure or contact with resistant TB
      d. Failure to respond to empirical treatment
   2. Multidrug-resistant TB (Table 11.3)
      a. Use at least 4 effective drugs
      b. Initial empirical therapy: 5 first-line drugs (INH, RIF, EMB, PZA, streptomycin) with or without a fluoroquinolone
         1) Tailor to drug susceptibility
         2) Include a parenteral aminoglycoside (streptomycin, kanamycin, amikacin, capreomycin) and a quinolone (levofloxacin, moxifloxacin)
      c. Second-line therapy
         1) Less clinical experience with these drugs compared with first-line agents
         2) Increased incidence and severity of adverse effects
         3) Unfavorable pharmacokinetic profile
      d. Minimum of 18 to 24 months
      e. DOT mandatory
      f. Examine HIV-positive patients every 4 months for additional 24 months to monitor for relapse
      g. Surgical intervention for localized pulmonary disease
      h. Predictors for successful outcome: surgical intervention, fluoroquinolone use, younger age
      i. Preventive therapy for contacts
         1) INH resistance: rifamycin for 4 to 6 months or rifamycin plus PZA for 2 months
         2) RIF resistance: INH for 9 months
         3) MDR: PZA plus EMB, *or* PZA plus a quinolone for 12 months

I. Treatment of TB in Special Situations
   1. Children
      a. EMB not routinely used
   2. Extrapulmonary TB
      a. Treatment similar to treatment of pulmonary TB
      b. Treat for 6 months; if meningitis, treat for 9 to 12 months
      c. Adjunctive corticosteroid for TB pericarditis and meningitis
   3. Culture-negative pulmonary TB and radiographic evidence of prior TB
      a. Standard 6-month regimen

Table 11.2
Antitubercular Drugs

Drug	Important Side Effects	Use in Pregnancy	Comments
First-line drugs			
Isoniazid	Hepatitis (age dependent), peripheral neuropathy, rash	Safe for fetus, but increased hepatotoxicity in women Postpone preventive therapy until delivery	Pyridoxine supplementation recommended for patients at high risk for neuropathy
Rifampin	Gastrointestinal tract upset, hepatotoxicity, rash, bleeding problems Red-orange secretions	Safe	Induces hepatic microsomal enzymes, resulting in increased hepatic clearance and decreased effectiveness of some drugs Caution for women taking oral contraceptive pills; use supplemental barrier method Reduces effectiveness of most protease inhibitors and nonnucleoside reverse transcriptase inhibitors
Rifapentine	Hyperuricemia, arthralgia, hepatotoxicity Red-orange secretions	Use if necessary	Can be used in once-weekly regimen Not recommended for HIV-positive patients
Rifabutin	Rash, hepatotoxicity, leukopenia, thrombocytopenia, uveitis Red-orange secretions	Safe	Drug interactions with protease inhibitors and nonnucleoside reverse transcriptase inhibitors
Ethambutol	Optic neuritis, peripheral neuropathy	Safe	Test for visual acuity and color vision
Pyrazinamide	Hepatotoxicity, gastrointestinal tract upset, hyperuricemia	Generally not recommended	
Second-line drugs			
Cycloserine	Dose-related psychosis, convulsions, depression, headache	Crosses placenta May be used if necessary	Periodic renal, hepatic, and hematologic tests
Ethionamide	Gastrointestinal tract: metallic taste, nausea, vomiting, abdominal pain Neurotoxicity: perineuritis, optic neuritis, anxiety Endocrine: hypothyroidism, gynecomastia, alopecia, impotence Hepatotoxicity, hypersensitivity reactions	Contraindicated	Pyridoxine supplementation recommended Liver function tests Test for thyrotropin
Levofloxacin, moxifloxacin, gatifloxacin	Gastrointestinal tract upset QT prolongation	Probably safe	
p-Aminosalicylic acid	Gastrointestinal tract intolerance often severe Hypersensitivity reactions: fever, joint pain, rash Malabsorption syndromes, hypothyroidism, hepatotoxicity	Has been used safely	Liver function tests Thyroid function tests Caution: sodium load
Streptomycin	Ototoxicity, neurotoxicity (weakness, circumoral paresthesia), nephrotoxicity	Contraindicated	Audiogram, vestibular testing, Romberg testing Renal function test
Amikacin/kanamycin	Ototoxicity, nephrotoxicity, neurotoxicity	Contraindicated	Audiogram, vestibular testing, Romberg testing Renal function test
Capreomycin	Auditory, vestibular, renal Electrolytes	Avoid	Audiogram, vestibular testing, Romberg testing Renal function test

Abbreviation: HIV, human immunodeficiency virus.

Table 11.3

Treatment Options for Drug-Resistant Tuberculosis

Drug Resistance	Regimen	Treatment Duration, mo
INH ± SM	RIF + PZA + EMB ± FQN for patients with extensive disease or HIV	6-9
INH + RIF ± SM	FQN + PZA + EMB + IA[a] ± alternative agent[b]	18-24
INH + RIF ± SM + EMB or PZA	FQN + EMB or PZA (if active) + IA[a] + 2 alternative agents[b]	24
RIF	INH + PZA + EMB ± streptomycin for 2-3 mo, or ± FQN for patients with extensive disease *or* INH + PZA + streptomycin	9-12
PZA	INH + RIF	9

Abbreviations: EMB, ethambutol; FQN, fluoroquinolone; HIV, human immunodeficiency virus; IA, injectable agent; INH, isoniazid; plus-minus sign, with or without; plus sign, in combination with; PZA, pyrazinamide; RIF, rifampin; SM, streptomycin.

[a] Injectable agent: streptomycin, amikacin, kanamycin, or capreomycin.
[b] Alternative agents: ethionamide, cycloserine, *p*-aminosalicylic acid, clarithromycin, amoxicillin-clavulanate, linezolid.

      b. Alternative: INH-RIF-PZA-EMB for 2 months, followed by INH-RIF for 2 months (4 months total); if HIV positive, treat for 6 months or more
4. Renal insufficiency and end-stage renal disease
      a. Dose adjustments
      b. Administer drugs after dialysis
      c. Monitor serum concentrations of cycloserine and EMB
5. Liver disease
      a. Baseline serum AST greater than 3 times the upper limit of normal
          1) RIF-EMB-PZA for 6 months
          2) INH-RIF for 9 months
          3) RIF-EMB for 12 months with or without another agent (eg, fluoroquinolone) for first 2 months
6. Pregnancy and breast-feeding
      a. INH-RIF-EMB for 9 months; give pyridoxine supplement
      b. PZA probably safe
      c. Contraindicated: streptomycin, capreomycin, *p*-aminosalicylic acid
      d. TST positive and asymptomatic
          1) Perform chest radiography after the 12th week of pregnancy
          2) Postpone preventive therapy until delivery, unless HIV positive or recent TST conversion
          3) If indicated, use INH plus pyridoxine
          4) Breast-feeding is not contraindicated for patients receiving preventive therapy
IX. Nontuberculous Mycobacteria
   A. Epidemiology
      1. Generally, nontuberculous mycobacteria (NTM) are free-living microorganisms
      2. Ubiquitous in the environment: surface water, tap water, soil, domestic and wild animals, milk, food products
      3. Can inhabit body surfaces without causing disease ("contaminants" or "colonizers")
      4. Can cause several diseases (Table 11.4)
      5. Runyon classification of common NTM causing human disease
         a. Four groups: classification according to growth rates, colony morphology, and pigmentation in the presence or absence of light
         b. Slowly growing mycobacteria
            1) Group I (photochromogens)
               a) *Mycobacterium kansasii* (common cause of human disease)
               b) *Mycobacterium marinum*
            2) Group II (scotochromogens)
               a) *Mycobacterium gordonae* (common laboratory isolate; often a contaminant)
               b) *Mycobacterium scrofulaceum*
            3) Group III (nonphotochromogens)
               a) *Mycobacterium avium* complex (MAC) (common cause of human disease)
               b) *Mycobacterium terrae* complex
               c) *Mycobacterium ulcerans*
               d) *Mycobacterium xenopi*
               e) *Mycobacterium simiae*
               f) *Mycobacterium malmoense*
               g) *Mycobacterium szulgai*
               h) *Mycobacterium asiaticum*

Table 11.4
Diseases Caused by Nontuberculous Mycobacteria

Clinical Disease	Etiologic Agent More Common	Etiologic Agent Less Common	Remarks
Pulmonary	MAC M kansasii	M abscessus M fortuitum M xenopi M malmoense M szulgai M simiae M asiaticum	Older persons with or without underlying lung disease; cystic fibrosis
Lymphadenitis	MAC M scrofulaceum M malmoense	M abscessus M fortuitum	Children
Skin and soft tissue	M marinum M ulcerans	Rapidly growing mycobacteria	By direct inoculation
Disseminated		Rapidly growing mycobacteria	Severely immunocompromised hosts

Abbreviations: *M*, *Mycobacterium*; MAC, *Mycobacterium avium* complex.

    c. Rapidly growing mycobacteria
       1) Group IV
          a) *Mycobacterium fortuitum*
          b) *Mycobacterium chelonae*
          c) *Mycobacterium abscessus*
  6. Other NTM
    a. *Mycobacterium genavense*
    b. *Mycobacterium haemophilum*
    c. *Mycobacterium smegmatis*
B. Diagnosis of NTM Disease
  1. Skin test not commercially available
  2. Sputum smear and culture
  3. Bronchoscopy with bronchoalveolar lavage in some cases
  4. Microscopy: Ziehl-Neelsen or Kinyoun stain, fluorochrome stain, Gram stain
  5. Culture
    a. Solid media: growth in 2 to 4 weeks
    b. Liquid media: growth in 10 to 14 days
  6. Species identification
    a. Traditional method
       1) Growth characteristics
       2) Biochemical tests
    b. Rapid method
       1) Specific nucleic acid probes (for *M kansasii*, MAC, *M gordonae*)
       2) High-performance liquid chromatography (for MAC)
       3) Susceptibility testing by proportion method with only 1 critical concentration of drug
  7. Diagnosis requires fulfillment of clinical, radiographic, and microbiologic criteria
    a. Clinical criteria
       1) Cough, fatigue
       2) Fever, weight loss, hemoptysis, dyspnea
    b. Radiographic criteria
       1) Chest radiography: infiltrates with or without nodules, cavitation, multiple nodules
       2) CT scan: multiple small nodules or reticulonodular infiltrates, multifocal bronchiectasis
    c. Microbiologic criteria
       1) At least 3 sputum or bronchial wash samples in 1 year
          a) Three positive cultures with negative AFB smears, *or*
          b) Two positive cultures with 1 positive AFB smear, *or*
       2) One bronchial wash
          a) Positive culture and positive AFB smear (2+, 3+, or 4+), *or*
          b) Positive culture and growth on solid media (2+, 3+, or 4+), *or*
       3) Transbronchial or lung biopsy
          a) Positive for NTM, *or*
          b) Consistent histopathologic features (granulomatous inflammation or AFB or both) and 1 or more sputum or bronchial wash cultures positive for NTM, *or*
          c) Positive culture from pleural fluid or other normally sterile extrapulmonary site

C. *Mycobacterium avium* Complex
1. *Mycobacterium avium* and *Mycobacterium intracellulare*
   a. Most common cause of pulmonary disease worldwide
   b. Acquired through inhalation or ingestion
   c. No human-to-human transmission
   d. Causes pulmonary or disseminated infection
2. Pulmonary disease
   a. Cavitary lung disease
      1) Primarily white, middle-aged or elderly men
      2) Risk factors: underlying lung disease, age, alcoholism, male sex
      3) Variable signs and symptoms: cough, fatigue, malaise, weakness, dyspnea, chest discomfort, occasional hemoptysis
      4) Resembles TB clinically and radiographically
      5) Typically upper lobe cavitary disease
      6) Generally indolent
   b. MAC in areas of bronchiectasis
      1) Older adults
      2) Most commonly in patients previously treated for TB and in cystic fibrosis patients
   c. Mid-lung interstitial disease
      1) No underlying lung disease
      2) Risk factors: nonsmoker, age older than 50 years, female sex
      3) Persistent cough and purulent sputum; usually no fever or weight loss
      4) Interstitial disease on chest radiography
      5) Lady Windermere syndrome: syndrome with right middle lobe or lingular infiltrates in elderly women without predisposing lung disease
   d. Hypersensitivity pneumonitis
      1) Associated with hot tub use
      2) Immunocompetent hosts without underlying lung disease
3. Disseminated disease
   a. Primarily affects severely immunocompromised hosts (eg, persons with AIDS, hematologic malignancy, or history of immunosuppressive therapy)
   b. Risk factor: *Pneumocystis jiroveci* pneumonia
   c. Intermittent or persistent fever, fatigue, malaise, anorexia, weight loss
4. MAC in HIV-positive patients
   a. Increased risks with CD4 cell count less than 50/μL
   b. Risk factor for dissemination: low CD4 cell count, use of indoor swimming pool, previous bronchoscopy, consumption of raw or partially cooked fish or shellfish, treatment with granulocyte colony-stimulating factor, genetic predisposition
   c. Prevention: daily rifabutin, daily clarithromycin, or once-weekly azithromycin
D. *Mycobacterium kansasii*
1. Found in tap water; never in soil or natural water supplies
2. No person-to-person transmission
3. Risk factors: chronic obstructive pulmonary disease, malignancy, immunosuppressive drugs, alcohol abuse, pneumoconiosis, HIV infection, age older than 50 years, male sex, occupation (miner, welder, sandblaster, painter), homelessness, and lower socioeconomic status
4. Clinical syndromes
   a. Pulmonary disease: resembles TB; cavitation in majority of cases
   b. Disseminated disease: rare; occurs in immunocompromised hosts
   c. Extrapulmonary disease: lymph nodes, bone marrow, bone, joints, skin
E. Rapidly Growing Mycobacteria
1. Found in the environment; also found in hospitals, contaminated reagents, and pharmaceuticals
2. Grow readily within 7 days
3. Clinical presentation
   a. Pulmonary disease: cough is a frequent complaint; 3 or more lobes often involved; diagnosis usually delayed
   b. Lymphadenitis: cervical lymphadenopathy in children
   c. Disseminated disease: uncommon; occurs in severely immunocompromised hosts; patients may present with multiple subcutaneous nodules or spontaneously draining abscesses
   d. Skin and soft tissue infection
      1) Nodules, recurrent abscesses, chronic draining sinuses
      2) Associated with nail salon whirlpool footbaths
   e. Musculoskeletal infections: tenosynovitis; may be indolent, slowly progressive, destructive

f. Prosthetic device infection: tympanostomy tube, pacemaker
g. Surgical site infection
    1) Patients present with multiple recurrent abscesses around surgical wound
    2) Augmentation mammoplasty, cosmetic surgical procedures, LASIK (laser-assisted in-situ keratomileusis), heart surgery
h. Catheter-related infections: in cancer patients
4. Rapidly growing mycobacteria in HIV-positive patients
    a. Disseminated disease with pustular or nodular cutaneous lesions
    b. Pulmonary disease
    c. Multifocal osteomyelitis
    d. Lymphadenitis
F. *Mycobacterium marinum*
    1. Aquatic habitat: freshwater and saltwater, swimming pools, fish tanks
    2. Exposure to water, usually associated with trauma: minor abrasion, laceration, puncture wound, bite wound
    3. Causes cutaneous disease: fish tank granuloma
G. Treatment of NTM Disease
    1. Treatment regimens and durations are summarized in Table 11.5
    2. Drug susceptibility testing
        a. *Mycobacterium avium* complex
            1) Routine testing not recommended, with 2 exceptions
                a) Test for clarithromycin if a patient was previously treated with a macrolide or received prophylaxis with a macrolide
                b) Test if treatment with clarithromycin has failed
        b. *Mycobacterium kansasii*
            1) Test for only RIF initially
            2) Test for other drugs (rifabutin, EMB, clarithromycin, quinolones, aminoglycosides) only if RIF-resistant
            3) All isolates are resistant to PZA
        c. Rapidly growing mycobacteria

Table 11.5
Treatment of Nontuberculous Mycobacteria

Organism	Treatment Regimen	Treatment Duration	Remarks
MAC			Newer macrolides are cornerstone of therapy
Pulmonary disease	Clarithromycin (or azithromycin) + RIF *or* Rifabutin + EMB ± streptomycin for 8 wk	Until culture results are negative for 1 y	For HIV-negative patients. Add streptomycin for extensive disease
Disseminated disease	Clarithromycin (or azithromycin) + EMB ± third drug	≥12 mo (possibly for the rest of the patient's life)	Rifabutin: the preferred third drug
Prophylaxis	Rifabutin *or* Clarithromycin *or* Azithromycin *or* Azithromycin + rifabutin		For HIV-positive patients with CD4 cell counts <50/μL or with history of prior opportunistic infection
Lymphadenitis	Excisional surgery *or* Clarithromycin as part of a multidrug regimen. For treatment failure: EMB + rifabutin + ciprofloxacin (or levofloxacin) *or* Amikacin *or* Ciprofloxacin (or ofloxacin) + clofazimine + ethionamide + streptomycin (or amikacin)		Drug susceptibility testing recommended. Optimize HAART. Consider surgical resection for localized disease
Mycobacterium kansasii	INH + RIF + EMB. If RIF resistant: Higher-dose INH + EMB + TMP-SMX + streptomycin *or* Clarithromycin + EMB + INH ± TMP-SMX	18 mo, with negative culture results for ≥12 mo	Substitute clarithromycin or rifabutin for RIF in HIV patients receiving protease inhibitors. Also active: moxifloxacin, ethionamide, linezolid
Rapidly growing mycobacteria	Imipenem, cefoxitin, RIF, ciprofloxacin, clarithromycin, doxycycline, TMP-SMX, amikacin	Minimum 6-12 mo	

(continued)

Table 11.5
(continued)

Organism	Treatment Regimen	Treatment Duration	Remarks
Cutaneous	Amikacin (or tobramycin) + cefoxitin (or imipenem) for ≥2 wk; then switch to oral medication: for *Mycobacterium abscessus*—clofazimine, clarithromycin for *Mycobacterium chelonae*—clarithromycin, clofazimine, ciprofloxacin, doxycycline	Minimum 4 mo	Amikacin for *Mycobacterium fortuitum* and *M abscessus* Tobramycin for *M chelonae* Surgery in some cases
Pulmonary	Drug susceptibility testing is essential for effective therapy	6-12 mo	2-Drug regimen
Mycobacterium marinum	Clarithromycin, minocycline (or doxycycline), TMP-SMX, or RIF + EMB	≥3 mo	Débridement may be necessary

Abbreviations: EMB, ethambutol; HAART, highly active antiretroviral therapy; HIV, human immunodeficiency virus; INH, isoniazid; MAC, *Mycobacterium avium* complex; plus-minus sign, with or without; plus sign, in combination with; RIF, rifampin; TMP-SMX, trimethoprim-sulfamethoxazole.

1) Test all clinically significant isolates
2) Test for amikacin, cefoxitin, imipenem, a sulfonamide, fluoroquinolones, doxycycline, clarithromycin
3) Resistant to all antitubercular drugs
3. Drug toxicity monitoring
   a. Liver: clarithromycin
   b. Kidney: aminoglycoside
   c. Auditory and vestibular function: aminoglycoside, azithromycin
   d. Hematologic indexes: sulfonamides, cefoxitin

Suggested Reading

Blumberg HM, Burman WJ, Chaisson RE, Daley CL, Etkind SC, Friedman LN, et al; American Thoracic Society, Centers for Disease Control and Prevention and the Infectious Diseases Society. American Thoracic Society/Centers for Disease Control and Prevention/Infectious Diseases Society of America: treatment of tuberculosis. Am J Respir Crit Care Med. 2003 Feb 15;167(4):603–62.

De Groote MA, Huitt G. Infections due to rapidly growing mycobacteria. Clin Infect Dis. 2006 Jun 15;42(12):1756–63. Epub 2006 May 11.

Griffith DE, Aksamit T, Brown-Elliott BA, Catanzaro A, Daley C, Gordin F, et al; ATS Mycobacterial Diseases Subcommittee; American Thoracic Society; Infectious Disease Society of America. An official ATS/IDSA statement: diagnosis, treatment, and prevention of nontuberculous mycobacterial diseases. Am J Respir Crit Care Med. 2007 Feb 15; 175(4):367–416. Review. Erratum in: Am J Respir Crit Care Med. 2007 Apr 1;175(7):744–5. dosage error in text.

Targeted tuberculin testing and treatment of latent tuberculosis infection. This official statement of the American Thoracic Society was adopted by the ATS Board of Directors, July 1999. This is a Joint Statement of the American Thoracic Society (ATS) and the Centers for Disease Control and Prevention (CDC). This statement was endorsed by the Council of the Infectious Diseases Society of America. (IDSA), September 1999, and the sections of this statement. Am J Respir Crit Care Med. 2000 Apr;161(4 Pt 2):S221–47.

Christine L. Terrell, MD

Nocardia and Actinomyces

I. *Nocardia*
   A. Organisms
      1. Filamentous, branching, aerobic organisms that are gram-positive and weakly acid-fast (Figure 12.1)
      2. Main species associated with human disease
         a. *Nocardia asteroides*: 80% to 90% of cases in the United States
         b. *Nocardia brasiliensis*: most common cause of cutaneous and lymphocutaneous disease; in the United States, found mostly in the South
         c. *Nocardia farcinica*: tends to be more resistant to antibiotics; tends to result in disseminated disease
         d. *Nocardia nova*: consistently susceptible to ampicillin and erythromycin; causes mainly noncutaneous disease
         e. *Nocardia otitidiscaviarum*: inconsistently susceptible to trimethoprim-sulfamethoxazole (TMP-SMX); causes mainly noncutaneous disease
         f. *Nocardia transvalensis*: a less common cause of noncutaneous disease
   B. Epidemiology
      1. Soilborne
      2. Found worldwide
      3. Mode of entry: mainly inhalation but also direct inoculation of the skin (trauma, surgery, or animal bites)
      4. No reported cases of human-to-human transmission
      5. Nearly 67% of patients have an underlying immunodeficiency, primarily a cell-mediated abnormality
         a. Patients with malignancies (hematologic more than solid organ), especially those who received corticosteroid therapy or chemotherapy
         b. Transplant recipients, particularly kidney or heart transplant recipients
         c. Uncommon in AIDS patients (perhaps related to *Pneumocystis jiroveci* pneumonia prophylaxis with TMP-SMX)
         d. Patients with alcoholism or diabetes mellitus
         e. Patients with alveolar proteinosis, chronic obstructive pulmonary disease, bronchiectasis, chronic granulomatous disease, or tuberculosis
         f. Patients receiving tumor necrosis factor antagonists
      6. More than 33% of patients are immunocompetent

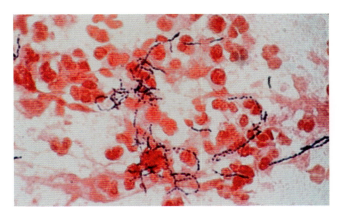

Figure 12.1. *Nocardia*. The filamentous, branching organisms are gram-positive (Gram stain). (Adapted from Pfizer. Used with permission.)

C. Clinical Manifestations
  1. Pulmonary disease
     a. Present in 67% of all cases of nocardiosis
     b. Present in 80% to 90% of cases due to *N asteroides*
     c. Suppurative necrosis and abscess formation is typical; can be granulomatous
     d. Course is acute, subacute, or chronic; symptoms tend to wax and wane
     e. Nonspecific symptoms: fever, night sweats, anorexia, weight loss, cough, dyspnea, hemoptysis, and pleuritic chest pain
     f. Manifests as endobronchial inflammatory masses, pneumonia, lung abscess, or cavitary disease; there may be pleural involvement
     g. Radiographic findings include cavitary or noncavitary lung masses, 1 or more nodules, reticulonodular infiltrates, interstitial infiltrates, lobar consolidation, pleural effusions, and empyema
     h. Common finding: contiguous spread or hematogenous dissemination, particularly to brain and soft tissues
     i. Differential diagnosis includes actinomycosis, other bacterial infections, mycobacterial disease, fungal disease, and malignancy
  2. Disseminated infection
     a. About 50% of all *Nocardia* infections disseminate, usually from pulmonary source
     b. Most frequent site: central nervous system (CNS)
        1) Other sites: cutaneous and subcutaneous tissues, retina, kidneys, bone, joints, and heart (endocarditis)
        2) Virtually any organ

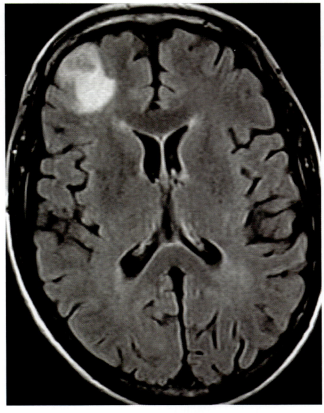

Figure 12.2. Computed Tomographic Scan of Brain Abscess in Patient With Nocardiosis. (Adapted from Greenfield RA. Norcardiosis: multimedia. [cited 2010 Nov 22]. Available from: http://emedicine.medscape.com/article/224123-media. Used with permission.)

  3. CNS disease
     a. Occurs in 20% to 33% of all cases of *Nocardia* and in 45% of disseminated cases
     b. Most frequent: brain abscess (Figure 12.2)
        1) Can occur anywhere in brain
        2) Often multiple and multiloculated
        3) Can manifest insidiously without causing symptoms for months or years, especially in immunocompetent host
        4) Nonspecific symptoms: fever, headache, seizures, meningismus, focal deficits, ataxia, and behavioral changes
        5) Consider the diagnosis in an immunocompromised person with brain and pulmonary masses
        6) Tissue biopsy: not always required with proven *Nocardia* pulmonary infection but recommended with immunocompromised host because of considerable risk of coexisting pathologic changes

7) If *Nocardia* infection is diagnosed at another site, brain imaging should be done to rule out abscess
8) Differential diagnosis: abscess due to anaerobes, aerobes, fungi, or parasites; malignancy
   c. Meningitis
      1) Rare
      2) With or without concomitant brain abscess
      3) Usually subacute or chronic presentation
      4) Cerebrospinal fluid: usually shows neutrophilic pleocytosis with low glucose and elevated protein levels
4. Ophthalmologic disease
   a. As part of disseminated disease: retina is usually involved
   b. Keratitis and endophthalmitis can result from direct inoculation into the eye
   c. Endophthalmitis can occur after cataract surgery
5. Cutaneous disease
   a. Primary cutaneous disease
      1) From direct inoculation (eg, while farming or gardening)
      2) Mainly in immunocompetent patients
      3) Pustules, abscesses, and cellulitis
      4) Similar to staphylococcal or streptococcal infection but more indolent
      5) Usually self-limited but should be treated since disseminated infection cannot always be ruled out
   b. Lymphocutaneous disease
      1) Occurs when primary cutaneous disease spreads to regional lymph nodes, which then suppurate
      2) Sporotrichoid, but tends to be more purulent than *Sporothrix schenckii* (Figure 12.3)
      3) Cutaneous involvement: from disseminated focus
         a) Same type of lesions as in primary cutaneous infections
         b) Occurs in 2% of cases of disseminated nocardiosis
   c. Mycetoma (Madura foot)
      1) Chronically progressive and destructive
      2) Patients initially present with a painless nodule days to months after inoculation
      3) Usually located distally on extremities
      4) Features
         a) Suppurative granulomata

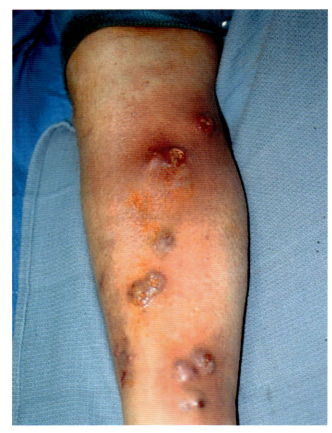

Figure 12.3. *Nocardia brasiliensis* Lymphadenitis Affecting Leg. (Adapted from Wheeler CK, DeCesare GE, Mannari RJ, Payne GW, Robson MC. Diagnostic dilemmas: cutaneous nocardiosis. Wounds. 2005;17[5]:131–6. Used with permission.)

         b) Progressive fibrosis and necrosis
         c) Local destruction
         d) Sinus tracts exuding macroscopic sulfur granules (macrocolonies)
         e) It is the only form of nocardiosis with sulfur granules
      5) Most common cause of mycetoma in the United States
         a) Usually *N brasiliensis*
         b) Less commonly *N asteroides*, *N otitidiscaviarum*, *N transvalensis*
      6) Warm, rural environments
      7) Often unresponsive to antibiotics if muscle and bone have become involved
   d. Agents and diseases to consider in differential diagnosis of cutaneous disease
      1) Fungi
      2) Mycobacteria (especially rapid growers and *Mycobacterium marinum*), *Erysipelothrix*, and tularemia

3) Cutaneous leishmaniasis
            4) Other causes of mycetoma
      6. Colonization
         a. Occasionally: transient colonization of sputum or skin
         b. Sputum colonization: generally in patients who have underlying lung disease and who are not receiving corticosteroids
         c. Some clinicians advocate treating all patients who have pulmonary isolates and immunocompromised patients
         d. Laboratory contamination: thought to be rare
   D. Diagnosis
      1. Definitive diagnosis: isolation and identification of organism from clinical specimen
      2. Isolation of *Nocardia*: most commonly from respiratory secretions, skin biopsy specimens, or aspirates collected from deep sites
      3. Staining
         a. Gram stain: organisms from direct smears may not be visible
         b. Modified acid-fast stain: *Nocardia* organisms are partially acid-fast, so request modified acid-fast stain
      4. Cultures
         a. *Nocardia* organisms grow on many types of routine media
         b. *Nocardia* growth may be obscured by growth of mixed flora if specimens were from nonsterile sites (eg, respiratory secretions)
         c. Buffered charcoal yeast extract agar and modified Thayer-Martin agar: beneficial in decreasing overgrowth of other organisms
         d. Always collect at least 3 sputum specimens for culture
         e. Specimens from bronchoscopy or open lung biopsy may be needed because of relative insensitivity of sputum cultures
         f. Typically growth is seen in 5 to 21 days
      5. Blood isolates are difficult to recover
         a. May grow in 3 to 4 weeks on standard blood culture media
         b. Optimize chances of isolation with blind subcultures to selective media in 2 weeks
         c. If available, polymerase chain reaction testing is sensitive and specific
         d. Speciation and susceptibility testing: important since resistance patterns vary by species
   E. Treatment
      1. General considerations
         a. Drug of choice: TMP-SMX
            1) Excellent tissue penetration
            2) Monitor blood levels
               a) Patients with life-threatening disease
               b) Patients for whom treatment has failed
               c) Patients at risk of dose-related toxicity
               d) Sulfamethoxazole level should be 100 to 150 mg/dL 2 hours after dose
            3) Poorly tolerated by many
            4) Treatment may fail
               a) Especially among immunocompromised hosts and those with CNS disease
               b) Contributing factors
                  i) Primary drug resistance
                  ii) Inadequate penetration into sites of infection (especially with *N otitidiscaviarum*)
                  iii) Presence of undrained pus
                  iv) Overwhelming infection or superinfection
               c) Consider use of TMP-SMX in combination with a parenteral agent for patients at risk of treatment failure, at least until definite response is seen
         b. Alternative agents
            1) Oral: minocycline, amoxicillin-clavulanic acid, extended-spectrum quinolones, macrolides, dapsone, and linezolid (high risk of hematologic side effects if used for >4 weeks)
            2) Parenteral: amikacin, carbepenems, and third-generation cephalosporins
         c. Additional procedures occasionally necessary: surgical drainage or débridement in combination with antibiotics
      2. Treatment of severe pulmonary or disseminated disease in immunocompetent or immunosuppressed host
         a. Consider induction therapy: 2 parenteral agents for 3 to 6 weeks or until clinical improvement is noted
            1) Amikacin (7.5 mg/kg every 12 hours) plus TMP-SMX (5/25 mg/kg in 2-6 divided doses)
               a) In CNS disease: ceftriaxone (2 g daily) or meropenem (1 g every 8 hours) can be

substituted for amikacin; avoid imipenem because of seizure risk
            b) In sulfonamide-resistant disease: replace TMP-SMX with imipenem (500 mg every 6 hours), meropenem (1 g every 8 hours), ampicillin-sulbactam (3 g every 6 hours), ceftriaxone (2 g daily), or cefotaxime (2 g every 6 hours)
        b. After 3 to 6 weeks of induction or after patient improves, switch to oral monotherapy for most patients
            1) TMP-SMX (5/25 mg/kg every 12 hours)
            2) Minocycline (100 mg every 12 hours)
            3) Amoxicillin-clavulanic acid (875 mg every 12 hours)
        c. Mild and moderate cases of pulmonary disease can often be treated with oral medication alone
        d. With CNS disease: surgery
            1) If lesions are large and accessible *or*
            2) If patient's condition deteriorates within 2 weeks *or*
            3) If no improvement within 1 month
        e. Duration of therapy
            1) Immunocompetent host: 6 to 12 months
            2) Immunocompromised hosts and patients with CNS disease: at least 12 months
    3. Treatment of cutaneous or lymphocutaneous disease
        a. Single agent for 2 to 6 months
            1) TMP-SMX (2.5/12.5 mg/kg every 12 hours)
            2) Minocycline (100 mg every 12 hours)
            3) Alternative oral agents if susceptibility is proved
        b. For mycetoma: extend treatment for 6 to 12 months
    4. Suppressive therapy
        a. Consider for patients who receive maintenance dosages of corticosteroids or cytotoxic agents and for patients with AIDS
        b. Low dose administered daily
  F. Summary of When to Consider a Diagnosis of Nocardiosis
    1. Indolent pulmonary disease occurring with cellular immunodeficiency
    2. Soft tissue or CNS disease (or both) occurring with subacute or chronic pulmonary disease
    3. Lymphocutaneous disease resembling sporotrichosis
    4. Presence of modified acid-fast or weakly gram-positive delicately branching bacilli
II. *Actinomyces*
  A. Organisms
    1. Branching, gram-positive, acid-fast–negative, facultative anaerobes
        a. Fastidious and slow growing
        b. Form sulfur granules in infected tissue, pus, and sinus tract drainage
            1) Microscopic or macroscopic, hard, yellow grains of tangled bacterial filaments
            2) No actual sulfur involved; named for yellow color
            3) Can be scanty
            4) Similar granules can be seen with *N brasiliensis*, *Actinomadura madurae* (with mycetoma), and *Staphylococcus aureus* (with botryomycosis)
            5) *Actinomyces odontolyticus* does not form sulfur granules
    2. Multiple species can cause human disease
        a. Cause of most human actinomycosis: *Actinomyces israelii*
        b. Less common causes: *Actinomyces naeslundii*, *Actinomyces viscosus complex*, *Actinomyces odontolyticus*, *Actinomyces meyeri*, and *Actinomyces gerencseriae*
  B. Epidemiology
    1. Reservoir: humans only
    2. Commensals: in oral cavity, gastrointestinal tract (GI), and female genitourinary tract
    3. No human-to-human transmission
  C. Pathogenesis and Pathology
    1. Most actinomycotic infections are polymicrobial
    2. Common copathogens: *Actinobacillus actinomycetemcomitans*, *Eikenella corrodens*, *Fusobacterium* species, *Bacteroides* species, *Capnocytophaga* species, *Haemophilus* species, *Staphylococcus* species, *Streptococcus* species, and members of the Enterobacteriaceae family
    3. Disruption of mucosal barrier is required
        a. Oral and cervicofacial disease is associated with gingivitis, dental procedures, orofacial trauma, cancer, cancer surgery, and radiotherapy
        b. Thoracic infections are often related to aspiration
        c. GI infection is related to GI surgery, diverticulitis, appendicitis, and foreign bodies

                    d. Genitourinary tract infections are often associated with intrauterine devices (IUDs) or surgery
            4. Infection spreads across anatomical barriers; hematogenous spread is infrequent
            5. Microscopic findings
                a. Acute or chronic inflammatory granulation tissue
                    1) Neutrophils, foamy macrophages, plasma cells, and lymphocytes
                    2) Surrounded by dense fibrosis
                b. Both profound fibrosis and acute suppuration can be associated with healing lesions
                c. Multinucleated giant cells: especially in pulmonary disease
                d. Sulfur granules: present but often sparse within tissue and pus
        D. Clinical Manifestations
            1. Orocervicofacial disease
                a. Introduction
                    1) Most common: 50% of cases of actinomycosis
                    2) Mainly *A israelii* and copathogens
                b. Signs and symptoms
                    1) Typically a chronic, slowly progressive, nontender, indurated mass (lumpy jaw) that evolves into multiple abscesses with fistulae and sinus tracts (Figure 12.4)
                    2) Pain: little or none
                    3) Less often: acute, rapidly progressive, suppurative mass with significant pain and trismus
                    4) Constitutional symptoms, including fever, are uncommon but occasionally occur in acute cases
                    5) Regional adenopathy is rare
                    6) Highly recognizable clue to diagnosis: fistulization from perimandibular area
                    7) Overlying skin is often fixed to mass and has red-blue hue
                c. Location
                    1) Periapical and endodontic infection occurs more frequently than is recognized
                    2) Most common site of diagnosed disease: perimandibular area, especially submandibular area; maxillary disease occurs less frequently
                    3) Maxillary and ethmoid sinuses
                    4) Other soft tissues of head and neck
                    5) Underlying osteomyelitis is uncommon
                    6) Extension to any contiguous structure is possible
                d. Differential diagnosis includes malignancy, tuberculosis, and fungal disease
            2. Abdominal disease
                a. Introduction
                    1) Accounts for 20% of cases of actinomycosis
                    2) Diagnosis is made preoperatively in less than 10% of cases since malignancy is often suspected
                    3) Most common predispositions: appendicitis (especially with perforation), diverticulitis, GI surgery, and trauma
                    4) Sources include thoracic disease or hematogenous dissemination
                b. Signs and symptoms
                    1) Fever, abdominal pain, weight loss, change in bowel habits, and palpable abdominal mass
                    2) Usually an abscess or a fixed, hard mass involving only 1 organ
                    3) Very indolent course, with weeks to months passing between onset and diagnosis
                c. Location
                    1) Virtually any organ or space can be involved
                    2) Most frequent (65% of abdominal cases): right-sided disease with ileocecal involvement, usually after appendicitis
                    3) Left-sided disease (7% of cases): diverticulitis or foreign body perforation of left side of colon

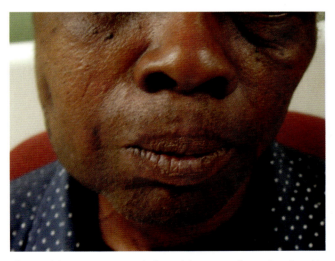

Figure 12.4. Lumpy Jaw. (Adapted from Bartell HL, Sonabend ML, Hsu S. Actinomycosis presenting as a large facial mass. Dermatol Online J. 2006 Feb 28;12[2]:20. Used with permission.)

4) Occasionally: esophageal or gastric cases
5) Fistulas to abdominal wall or perineum (33% of abdominal cases)
6) Less common locations
   a) Perirectal or perianal disease with abscesses or sinus or fistulous tracts
   b) Hepatic disease: generally single or multiple abscesses
   c) Urogenital disease: most commonly ureteral obstruction and hydronephrosis from contiguous abdominal or pelvic disease
   d. Computed tomographic (CT)-guided percutaneous biopsy or endoscopic biopsy with colonoscopy may allow preoperative diagnosis
   e. Differential diagnosis includes malignancy, tuberculosis, inflammatory bowel disease, and diverticular abscess
3. Thoracic disease
   a. Introduction
      1) Accounts for 15% of cases of actinomycosis
      2) Source: aspiration of oropharyngeal organism; uncommonly due to direct extension from other cervicofacial or abdominal disease
   b. Signs and symptoms
      1) Chest pain, fever, and weight loss; occasionally, hemoptysis
      2) Most common manifestation: indolent mass lesion or pneumonia
      3) Pleura involved in more than 50% of cases (thickening, effusion, and empyema)
      4) Consider a diagnosis of actinomycosis if empyema spontaneously drains through chest wall
      5) Pulmonary disease: consider a diagnosis of actinomycosis
         a) If pulmonary disease extends across fissures or pleura *or*
         b) If disease involves mediastinum (most commonly pericarditis) or contiguous bony structures or extends to chest wall (Figure 12.5)
   c. Radiologic findings vary: patchy infiltrates, mass lesions, and cavitary lesions
4. Pelvic disease
   a. Role of IUD
      1) Pelvic actinomycosis: most cases are related to presence of IUD; can also be due to extension of abdominal disease

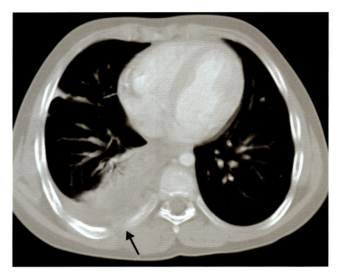

Figure 12.5. Computed Tomographic Scan of Chest Wall Invasion in Actinomycosis. Arrow points to area where thoracic disease has invaded chest wall. (Adapted from Kordes U, Beutel K, Cachovan G, Schafer H, Helmke K, Sobottka I. Gingivitis as probable source of a thoracic actinomycosis due to *Actinomyces israelii* and *Actinobacillus actinomycetemcomitans*. Arch Dis Child. 2004 Oct;89[10]:895. Used with permission.)

      2) Before disease develops, IUDs have been in place for at least 1 year (average, 8 years)
      3) If *Actinomyces* organisms are noted on Papanicolaou test in asymptomatic patient: close follow-up is warranted, not necessarily removal of device
      4) If patient has pelvic pain or vaginal bleeding or discharge not attributable to another cause, IUD should be removed even if *Actinomyces* organisms are not noted on Papanicolaou test
   b. Signs and symptoms
      1) Indolent presentation
      2) Fever, abdominal pain, weight loss, and vaginal bleeding or discharge
      3) Initially, endometriosis progresses to pelvic mass or tubo-ovarian abscesses
      4) Common: genitourinary tract and perirectal involvement
      5) Fistulous tracts to abdominal wall or bowel
   c. Differential diagnosis includes malignancy, pelvic inflammatory disease, and tuberculosis
5. CNS disease
   a. Rare
   b. Hematogenous or contiguous from cervicofacial source

c. Presentation
   1) Most common: brain abscess
      a) Single or multiple
      b) Headache, focal neurologic findings with or without fever
      c) Ring-enhancing, thick-walled lesions
   2) Occasionally: solid nodular lesion (actinomycotic granuloma)
   3) Meningitis: acute or chronic
   4) Infection: cranial or spinal epidural or subdural
6. Musculoskeletal disease
   a. Most common: facial bone osteomyelitis, especially mandible
   b. Vertebral osteomyelitis: less common in antibiotic era
   c. Prosthetic joint infections have been reported
   d. Indolent extremity infections, usually secondary to trauma
7. Disseminated disease
   a. Uncommon: due to hematogenous spread
   b. Most common: *A meyeri*
   c. Any organs: especially lungs and liver
   d. Usually manifests as multiple nodules
   e. Often indolent
E. Diagnosis
   1. Diagnosis is often made at surgery since malignancy is often suspected
   2. Definitive diagnosis
      a. Histology
         1) Typically, acute or chronic inflammatory tissue with neutrophils, macrophages, plasma cells, and lymphocytes with surrounding fibrosis
         2) Can see dense fibrosis alongside areas of acute suppuration and healing lesions
         3) Sulfur granules
            a) Often seen in pus or within microabscesses in tissue sections
            b) Can be rare, especially if significant fibrosis is present, so examine multiple sections of biopsy tissue
            c) Not seen well with hematoxylin-eosin stain
            d) Use Gram stain or silver stain to distinguish from coccal and bacillary bacteria and from fungi
            e) Use acid-fast stain to distinguish from *Nocardia* (*Actinomyces* are acid-fast negative)
      b. Culture
         1) Anaerobic technique
         2) Gram stain: more sensitive than culture
         3) Branching filamentous rods: except *A meyeri*, which is nonbranching
         4) Isolation: rare if antibiotics were given within previous 7 to 10 days
         5) Usually grows in 5 to 7 days; can take 2 to 4 weeks
         6) Best sources: draining sinus tracts, other pus, sputum, and large biopsy specimens, especially if sulfur granules are present
         7) Avoid use of swabs: cotton filaments may be confused with the organism on microscopy
         8) Avoid contamination with other oral GI or genitourinary tract commensals when obtaining specimen
         9) Part of normal flora of oral cavity and female genitourinary tract: therefore, identification of *Actinomyces* from mouth, sputum, bronchoscopy specimen, or cervicovaginal secretions are not meaningful unless sulfur granules were seen or clinical setting is appropriate
F. Treatment
   1. Antibiotics
      a. Minimize relapse: prolonged courses with high doses
         1) Drugs of choice: penicillin intravenously (IV) (3-4 million units every 4 hours), amoxicillin orally (500 mg every 6 hours), *or* penicillin orally (500-1,000 mg every 6 hours)
            a) Prudent to treat copathogens
            b) Treat for 2 to 6 weeks IV; then treat for 6 to 12 months with oral antibiotics
            c) Less intensive therapy if disease is less extensive, especially in cervicofacial area
         2) Alternatives to penicillin
            a) Minocycline (100 mg IV or orally every 12 hours)
            b) Doxycycline (100 mg IV or orally every 12 hours)
            c) Tetracycline (500 mg orally every 6 hours)
            d) Clindamycin (900 mg IV every 8 hours or 300-400 mg orally every 6 hours)

e) If pregnant: erythromycin (500-1,000 mg IV every 6 hours or 500 mg orally every 12 hours)
f) Anecdotal evidence of efficacy: ceftriaxone, ceftizoxime, imipenem, and ciprofloxacin
b. Generally, course of antibiotics is indicated before any surgery, even with extensive disease
c. Monitor response with CT or magnetic resonance imaging
d. Well-defined abscess: consider percutaneous drainage and antibiotics
2. Surgery
a. If disease is in critical location (eg, certain areas of CNS)
b. If severe necrosis and larger abscesses are involved
c. If medical therapy alone fails (eg, persisting sinus or fistulous tracts, refractory fibrotic lesions)
d. Combine with high-dose prolonged antibiotic therapy
G. Summary of When to Consider a Diagnosis of Actinomycosis
1. Chronic pulmonary infection extends through chest wall
2. Pelvic infection in patient with indwelling IUD
3. Firm jaw lump
4. Abdominal mass with draining sinus tracts

Suggested Reading

Bennhoff DF. Actinomycosis: diagnostic and therapeutic considerations and a review of 32 cases. Laryngoscope. 1984 Sep;94(9):1198–217.

Lederman ER, Crum NF. A case series and focused review of nocardiosis: clinical and microbiologic aspects. Medicine (Baltimore). 2004 Sep;83(5):300–13.

Lerner PI. Nocardiosis. Clin Infect Dis. 1996 Jun;22(6):891–903.

Russo TA. Agents of Actinomycosis. In: Mandell GL, Bennett JE, Dolin R. Mandell, Douglas, and Bennett's principles and practice of infectious diseases. Vol 2. 6th ed. Philadelphia (PA): Churchill Livingstone/Elsevier; c2005. p. 2924–34.

Smego RA Jr, Foglia G. Actinomycosis. Clin Infect Dis. 1998 Jun;26(6):1255–61.

Sorrell TC, Mitchell DH, Iredell JR. *Nocardia species*. In: Mandell GL, Bennett JE, Dolin R. Mandell, Douglas, and Bennett's principles and practice of infectious diseases. Vol 2. 6th ed. Philadelphia (PA): Churchill Livingstone/Elsevier; c2005. p. 2916–24.

13

Shimon Kusne, MD
Ann E. McCullough, MD

Candida Species

I. Characteristics
   A. Microbiology
      1. *Candida* are oval yeast: 4 to 6 μm in diameter
      2. Reproduce by budding: usually produce pseudohyphae (budding yeast without full detachment of daughter cell) (Figures 13.1 and 13.2)
      3. Identification
         a. Usually based on morphology and sugar assimilation
         b. Germ tube test–positive species: *Candida albicans* and *Candida dubliniensis*
      4. Species that are human pathogens
         a. Most common (>60%): *C albicans*
         b. Others: *C dubliniensis*, *Candida glabrata*, *Candida parapsilosis*, *Candida tropicalis*, *Candida kefyr* (formerly *Candida pseudotropicalis*), *Candida krusei*, *Candida lusitaniae*, *Candida guilliermondii*
   B. Epidemiology
      1. *Candida* is a common colonizer of the gastrointestinal tract; also commonly found on skin
      2. Most infections originate from the patient's own colonizing *Candida* organisms
      3. *Candida* is also found in the environment
      4. Risk factors for invasive candidiasis include neutropenia, AIDS, abdominal surgery, prolonged courses of antibacterials, immunosuppressive therapy, intravascular catheters, prosthetic devices, long intensive care unit stays, parenteral nutrition, and renal failure
      5. *Candida* is the fifth most common agent to cause bloodstream infection in hospitals
      6. An increase in species other than *C albicans* has been observed

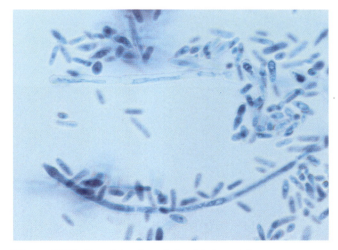

Figure 13.1. Pseudohyphae of *Candida krusei*. Long pseudohyphae are shown with elongate or oval blastoconidia (lactophenol cotton blue, original magnification ×600).

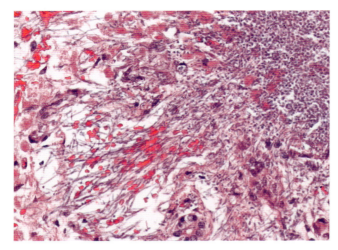

Figure 13.2. Liver. This preparation shows the edge of a hepatic candidal microabscess from a patient who died of disseminated candidiasis. Filamentous pseudohyphae stream through the tissue in the left side of the image; a round yeast cluster is in the upper right corner (hematoxylin-eosin, original magnification ×200).

        a. Centers using fluconazole prophylaxis: increase in *C krusei* and *C glabrata* has been observed
        b. Use of intravenous catheters: association with *C parapsilosis* infection
  II. *Candida* Infection
     A. Clinical Manifestations
        1. *Candida* infection may involve almost any organ (Figures 13.3 and 13.4)

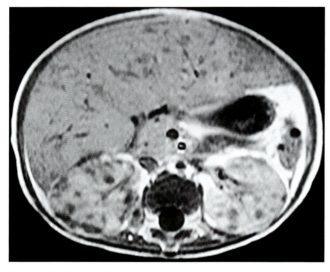

Figure 13.3. *Candida* Abscesses in the Liver Kidney, and Spleen on Magnetic Resonance Imaging. (Adapted from Edwards JE Jr. *Candida* species. In: Mandell GL, Bennett JE, Dolin R, editors. Mandell, Douglas, and Bennett's principles and practice of infectious disease. Vol 2. 7th ed. Philadelphia [PA]: Churchill Livingstone/Elsevier; c2010. p. 3225-40. Used with permission.)

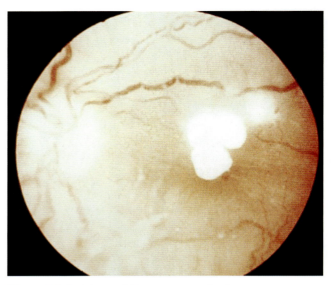

Figure 13.4. Advanced Hematogenous *Candida* Endophthalmitis. (Adapted from Fishman LS, Griffin JR, Sapico FL, Hecht R. Hematogenous *Candida* endophthalmitis: a complication of candidemia. N Engl J Med. 1972 Mar 30; 286[13]:675-81. Used with permission.)

        a. Table 13.1 lists various *Candida* infections by organ involvement
        b. Table 13.2 describes select infection syndromes
        c. Figure 13.5 shows gastric ulcer with invasive candidiasis

Table 13.1

Candida Infections by Organ Involvement

Organ or System	Infection
Gastrointestinal tract	Oral mucositis, esophagitis, gastric and intestinal mucositis
Genitalia	Vulvovaginitis, balanitis
Skin, nails	Folliculitis, disseminated (usually skin nodules), intertrigo, paronychia, onychomycosis, diaper rash, perianal erythema, chronic mucocutaneous candidiasis
Central nervous system	Brain abscesses, meningitis
Respiratory tract	Pneumonia, bronchitis, laryngitis, epiglottitis
Cardiovascular	Myocarditis, pericarditis
Urinary tract	Urethritis, bladder fungus ball, cystitis, pyelonephritis, perinephric abscess, kidney fungus ball
Musculoskeletal	Osteomyelitis, diskitis, arthritis, costochondritis, myositis
Intra-abdominal organs	Peritonitis, hepatosplenic candidiasis, pancreatitis, hepatitis, cholecystitis
Eye	Endophthalmitis
Other	Mediastinitis, candidemia, septic thrombophlebitis

Table 13.2
Select *Candida* Infection Syndromes

Syndrome	Clinical Presentation	Pathogenesis	Treatment
Candida esophagitis	Underlying immunosuppression Painful swallowing, substernal chest pain May be asymptomatic Thrush may not be present	Invasion of esophageal mucosa	Fluconazole Itraconazole Voriconazole Caspofungin Micafungin for 14-21 d
Candida vaginitis	Predisposition: diabetes mellitus, antibiotics, pregnancy, oral contraceptives, immunosuppression Erythema, pruritus, discharge (curd-like)	Caused mostly by *Candida albicans*, but other species are increasingly involved Complications occur with moderate or severe episodes in abnormal host, with recurrences, or with involvement of species other than *C albicans*	Topical antifungal (eg, clotrimazole, miconazole) One dose of oral fluconazole (150 mg) In complicated cases, use longer courses Vaginal suppositories of boric acid with involvement of species other than *C albicans* (especially *Candida glabrata*)
Chronic mucocutaneous candidiasis	Chronic infection of skin, mucous membranes, hair, and nails Patients present in first decade of life Half the patients have endocrine abnormality (adrenal insufficiency, hypoparathyroidism)	Underlying T-cell dysfunction	Azoles long-term
Candida endocarditis	Most common fungal endocarditis Large emboli may move to major vessels Blood cultures are usually positive	Seeding of abnormal native valves or prosthetic valves, heroin addiction	Surgery Amphotericin B plus flucytosine for 6-10 wk Fluconazole for chronic suppressive therapy Monitor for relapse for minimum of 2 y
Candidemia and acute disseminated candidiasis	Fever in neutropenia not responding to antibacterials Sepsis syndrome or evidence of dissemination to eye, skin, bone, brain, and other organs In immunosuppressed host, course may be smoldering	In healthy host, usual source is intravascular lines In neutropenic and other immunosuppressed patients, the source is frequently the gut Hematogenous dissemination to almost every organ Candidemia is detected in only 50% of disseminated cases	Indwelling catheter should be removed Initiate antifungal therapy with echinocandin, fluconazole, or amphotericin B Echinocandin is favored with moderate to severe illness or recent azole exposure (treatment or prophylaxis) and when *C glabrata* is suspected Fluconazole is favored for less critically ill patients who have had no azole exposure and if the isolate is *C albicans* or *Candida parapsilosis*

(Continued)

Table 13.2
(continued)

Syndrome	Clinical Presentation	Pathogenesis	Treatment
Hepatosplenic candidiasis (chronic disseminated candidiasis)	Usually occurs in a leukemic person who recovers from neutropenia with fever and elevated alkaline phosphatase and who has many densities in liver, spleen, kidney, and other organs by computed tomography or magnetic resonance imaging	Hematogenous spread	Intravenous amphotericin B (or liposomal preparation) for 1–2 wk, followed by prolonged oral fluconazole
Endophthalmitis	Ocular pain, blurry vision, floaters White, cotton ball–like lesions	After eye trauma, surgery, or hematogenous seeding (15% in candidemia)	Intravenous amphotericin B Fluconazole Amphotericin B plus flucytosine for refractory cases Vitrectomy in difficult cases
Candida peritonitis	Abdominal pain, fever with peritoneal dialysis or after abdominal surgery or spontaneous bowel perforation	Infection from dialysis catheter or leakage of bowel contents into peritoneal cavity	Removal of dialysis catheter, surgical repair of bowel leak Fluconazole or caspofungin for 2–3 wk
Central nervous system candidiasis	Brain abscess or meningitis Lymphocytic pleocytosis with low glucose levels in 60%	Usually hematogenous	Amphotericin B plus flucytosine
Urinary tract candidiasis	Colony counting not helpful in distinguishing colonization from infection	Predisposition: antibiotics, Foley catheters, diabetes mellitus	Indications for treatment of candiduria: Symptomatic Renal transplant Use of instruments in urinary tract Neutropenia Very low-birth-weight infants Fluconazole Amphotericin B Flucytosine Bladder irrigation usually not recommended but may be indicated in cystitis due to fluconazole-resistant *Candida*

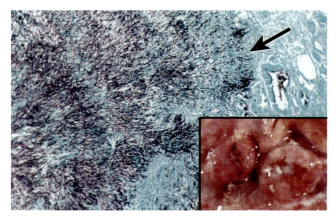

Figure 13.5. Stomach. Inset shows 2 kissing gastric ulcers from a patient who died of AIDS. Photomicrograph shows gastric ulcer section with a radial array of invasive candidiasis. Arrow points to leading edge (Gomori methenamine silver, original magnification ×100).

- B. Diagnosis
  1. Sensitivity of positive blood culture in disseminated candidiasis (diagnosed at autopsy): only 50%
     a. Clinicians should assess patients for invasive candidiasis
     b. Clinicians should consider initiation of empirical antifungals on the basis of known risk factors
  2. Patient who has neutropenia: start empirical antifungal therapy in febrile patients not responding to broad-spectrum antibacterials
  3. Patient who does not have neutropenia but is at risk: typically a febrile intensive care unit patient who has intravascular lines or devices and who has colonies of *Candida* in multiple sites
- C. Laboratory Testing
  1. Superficial candidal infection (mucocutaneous)
     a. Usually documented by scraping the surface and demonstrating hyphal and pseudohyphal elements
     b. Potassium hydroxide, calcofluor white, or silver stain
  2. Deep-seated infection
     a. Usually documented with biopsy and culture of tissue and sterile fluids
     b. Positive culture of nonsterile specimens (urine, sputum, stool) indicates colonization
  3. Antibody and antigen testing
     a. Offered by some laboratories
     b. Usually lacks sensitivity and specificity
     c. Not used for clinical indications
  4. Susceptibility testing (broth microdilution and Etest)
     a. Usually used for species other than *C albicans*, especially in cases of antibiotic failure
     b. Failure of treatment of *C glabrata* and *C krusei* with fluconazole is correlated with high minimum inhibitory concentrations
     c. Resistance to amphotericin B has been observed most commonly with *Candida lusitaniae*
- D. Treatment
  1. Treatment of invasive candidiasis (or candidemia)
     a. Previously, treatment was limited to amphotericin B, which was hampered by significant toxicity
     b. Addition of the azoles, liposomal amphotericin preparations, and echinocandins has considerably improved treatment options
  2. Treatment of candidemia in patients who do not have neutropenia or major immunodeficiency: published findings
     a. Fluconazole was equivalent to amphotericin B
     b. Most of the study patients had renal failure, nonhematologic cancer, or gastrointestinal tract disease
  3. Treatment of invasive candidiasis: published findings
     a. The echinocandin caspofungin was equivalent to amphotericin B
     b. Patients in the study were stratified on the basis of neutropenia and Acute Physiology and Chronic Health Evaluation (APACHE) II score
  4. Initial treatment of candidemia
     a. Based on literature and Infectious Diseases Society of America guidelines
     b. Fluconazole, echinocandin (caspofungin, micafungin, anidulafungin), or amphotericin B preparation (Table 13.2)
  5. Treatment of candidemia in patients who are not neutropenic
     a. Indications for favoring echinocandins (instead of fluconazole)
        1) Moderate to severe illness
        2) Recent azole exposure (treatment or prophylaxis)
        3) Suspected etiologic agent is *C glabrata*
     b. Indications for favoring fluconazole
        1) Less critically ill patients
        2) No recent azole exposure
        3) Isolate is *C albicans* or *C parapsilosis*

6. Treatment of candidemia in patients who are neutropenic
   a. Echinocandin or lipid formulation of amphotericin B is favored for most patients with an unknown *Candida* isolate
   b. Indications for favoring fluconazole
      1) Less critically ill patients
      2) No recent azole exposure
      3) Suspected etiologic agent is not *C glabrata*
7. Duration of treatment: 2 weeks after eradication of *Candida* from bloodstream
   a. If signs and symptoms attributed to fungemia have resolved *and*
   b. If the following have been excluded: persistent fungemia, metastatic complications, and neutropenia
8. Treatment of *Candida* pyelonephritis
   a. If isolates are fluconazole-sensitive: 2-week course of oral fluconazole (400 mg daily)
   b. If isolates are fluconazole-resistant (especially *C glabrata*): amphotericin B (0.6-0.7 mg/kg daily) with or without flucytosine (25 mg/kg every 6 hours) or flucytosine alone

Suggested Reading

Edwards JE Jr. *Candida* species. In: Mandell GL, Bennett JE, Dolin R, editors. Mandell, Douglas, and Bennett's principles and practice of infectious disease. Vol 2. 7th ed. Philadelphia (PA): Churchill Livingstone/Elsevier; c2010. p. 3225–40.

Ostrosky-Zeichner L, Rex JH, Bennett J, Kullberg BJ. Deeply invasive candidiasis. Infect Dis Clin North Am. 2002 Dec;16(4):821–35.

Pappas PG, Kauffman CA, Andes D, Benjamin DK Jr, Calandra TF, Edwards JE Jr, et al; Infectious Diseases Society of America. Clinical practice guidelines for the management of candidiasis: 2009 update by the Infectious Diseases Society of America. Clin Infect Dis. 2009 Mar 1;48(5): 503–35.

Snydman DR. Shifting patterns in the epidemiology of nosocomial *Candida* infections. Chest. 2003 May;123 (5 Suppl):500S–3S.

Shimon Kusne, MD
Ann E. McCullough, MD

Aspergillus Species

I. Microbiology
   A. Characteristics
      1. Ubiquitous molds
      2. In culture
         a. Grow quickly
         b. Fluffy colonies
         c. Usually propagate best at room temperature
      3. Microscopic examination
         a. Erect conidiophore has a swollen vesicle covered with phialides, which give rise to conidia (Figure 14.1)
         b. In tissue, hyphae predominate
   B. Pathogens
      1. Most common: *Aspergillus fumigatus*
      2. Other pathogenic species include *Aspergillus flavus, Aspergillus terreus, Aspergillus niger, Aspergillus ustus,* and *Aspergillus nidulans*
      3. Increasing reports of other rare species causing infection
II. Epidemiology
   A. Spores
      1. Ubiquitous: found in soil, water, food, air, and decaying vegetation
      2. After hospital renovation and construction, dispersed spores have caused clusters of cases of invasive aspergillosis

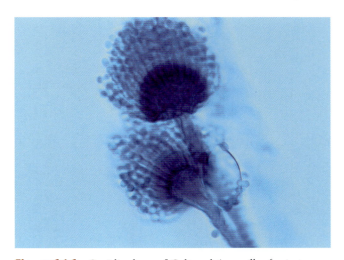

Figure 14.1. Conidiophore of Cultured *Aspergillus fumigatus*. Chains of conidia extend in partial radial array. Such structures are rare in tissue, typically seen only in culture (lactophenol cotton blue, original magnification ×600).

   3. Contaminated hospital water supplies and potted plants in patient rooms have also been implicated in cases of nosocomial invasive aspergillosis
   B. Risk Factors
      1. Primary risk factor for invasive aspergillosis: immunosuppression

a. Neutropenia
b. Corticosteroids
c. Tumor necrosis factor α antagonists
d. Stem cell, bone marrow, and solid organ transplant
2. Inherited and acquired immunosuppressive states (eg, chronic granulomatous disease and AIDS)
III. Pathogenesis
A. Portal of Entry
1. Usually lungs: inhaled conidia transform into hyphae
2. Entry through skin is possible (sites of wounds or intravenous catheters)
B. Vascular Invasion
C. Dissemination
IV. Aspergillosis
A. Angioinvasive
1. Causes thrombosis of vessels and tissue infarcts
2. Disruption of vessels invaded by the fungus, especially in the lung (Figure 14.2), may lead to massive hemorrhage and death
3. In immunosuppressed hosts, mortality from invasive aspergillosis is very high (nearly 100% in some series)
4. Clinical presentation, pathogenesis, and treatment are summarized in Table 14.1
B. Diagnosis
1. Direct identification
a. Gomori methenamine silver stain
b. Septate hyphae branched at approximately 45° (Figure 14.3)

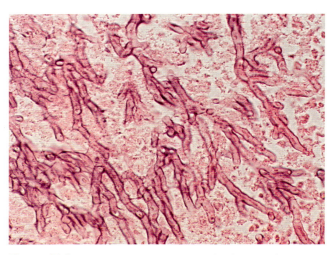

Figure 14.3. Lung. Filamentous, septate hyphae invading tissue, often branching at approximately 45° angles (hematoxylin-eosin, original magnification ×400).

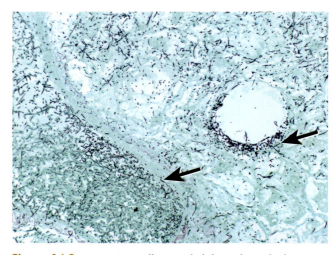

Figure 14.2. Lung. *Aspergillus* invaded throughout the lung in this immunocompromised patient. Arrow on left indicates a vessel wall; hyphae of *Aspergillus* fill the lumen. Arrow on right indicates hyphae concentrated as they invade a capillary wall (Gomori methenamine silver, original magnification ×200).

c. Rarely, fruiting conidia
d. Other filamentous fungi have similar appearances: fungal culture is indicated for confirmation
C. Culture
1. Blood culture results are rarely positive
2. Because *Aspergillus* spores are ubiquitous, the diagnosis of invasive aspergillosis may require histologic confirmation to distinguish invasion from colonization
3. In patients with leukemia or bone marrow transplants, culture alone may be highly indicative of invasive disease
D. Serology
1. Double-sandwich enzyme-linked immunosorbent assay
a. Detects *Aspergillus* circulating antigen galactomannan
b. Has been used successfully by some groups in bone marrow transplant recipients with good sensitivity (95%) for early detection of aspergillosis
c. Results were not promising in solid organ transplant recipients
d. False-positive results from use of piperacillin-tazobactam, laboratory contamination, and cross-reaction with other fungi
2. Polymerase chain reaction techniques
a. Investigational and not standardized
b. May have a role in the future for early diagnosis of aspergillosis
3. Susceptibility testing
a. Offered by many laboratories

Table 14.1
Clinical Features of Aspergillosis

Diagnosis	Clinical Presentation	Pathogenesis	Treatment
Allergic bronchopulmonary aspergillosis	Underlying asthma or cystic fibrosis, central bronchiectasis, transient lung infiltrates, elevated total IgE, high titers for *Aspergillus* (IgG, IgE), eosinophilia	Atopic individuals become sensitized to inhaled *Aspergillus*	Corticosteroids, itraconazole
Fungus ball	Asymptomatic or hemoptysis	Round collection of hyphal elements in an old lung cavity (upper lobe) or in a sinus (usually maxillary)	Antifungals are usually not effective. Surgery for recurrent hemoptysis and considered for immunosuppressed host. In some cases, intracavitary instillation of amphotericin B
Otomycosis	Fungal otitis externa and invasive disease leading to mastoiditis	May colonize only the external canal or invade surrounding tissue	Cleansing the external canal and systemic treatment in invasive disease
Invasive pulmonary aspergillosis	Febrile illness in neutropenia. Nonspecific symptoms (cough, dyspnea, hypoxemia, hemoptysis). Radiology may show pleural effusion, nodules, and cavities. Halo sign of low attenuation area around a nodule is considered early radiologic evidence of invasive disease	Colonizing fungus invading the airway usually in immunosuppressed host. The fungus is angioinvasive and may cause thrombosis of vessels and lung infarcts	Systemic antifungals: voriconazole or amphotericin B (conventional or liposomal), or combination of voriconazole with caspofungin
Tracheobronchitis	Lung transplant recipients with ulcerated and membranous infection at the suture site. AIDS patients	Colonization followed by local invasion may cause disruption of local anastomosis in lung transplant recipients	Systemic antifungals, possibly aerosolized
Sinusitis	Inflammatory signs (eg, facial pain, swelling, fever) or smoldering and silent	Immunosuppressed host, especially with neutropenia, may appear to have rhinocerebral mucormycosis with invasion of surrounding structures (eg, bone, brain)	Débridement of the sinus is important along with use of antifungals
Disseminated aspergillosis	Any organ may be involved in dissemination; commonly, dissemination of pulmonary infection to brain	Hematogenous spread	Systemic antifungals
Cerebral aspergillosis	Most common cause of brain abscess in organ transplant; presenting symptoms of brain space-occupying lesion	Hematogenous spread usually from pulmonary infection or contiguous extension from sinuses	Systemic antifungals and drainage when possible; voriconazole is efficacious
Osteomyelitis	Most common is lumbar vertebral infection in immunosuppressed host, chronic granulomatous disease, drug addicts	Hematogenous spread or contiguous extension from another focus of infection (eg, lung empyema)	Débridement and antifungals (itraconazole)
Skin infection	Ulcerated skin lesions, eschar formation at a wound or intravenous catheter site	Hematogenous dissemination to skin or invasion at wound edges and catheter exit sites	Débridement and antifungals

b. No correlation with clinical outcomes has been established
   c. *Aspergillus terreus* is resistant to amphotericin B and may deserve special attention for treatment options
E. Treatment
   1. Poor outcome in invasive aspergillosis is related to late diagnosis and treatment
   2. Liposomal amphotericin B
      a. Clinicians can use high doses (≥5 mg/kg) with much less nephrotoxicity compared with conventional amphotericin B
      b. Randomized trial results: similar efficacy with either 3 mg/kg daily or 10 mg/kg daily for primary therapy
   3. Voriconazole
      a. Drug of choice for primary treatment of invasive aspergillosis
      b. Randomized trial (most patients had hematologic diseases) compared voriconazole with amphotericin B deoxycholate: better response and better survival with voriconazole
   4. Other triazoles active against aspergillosis: itraconazole and posaconazole
   5. Primary treatment of invasive aspergillosis
      a. Voriconazole: drug of choice
      b. Liposomal amphotericin B: an alternative drug when voriconazole is contraindicated
      c. Amphotericin B deoxycholate: recommended if voriconazole and liposomal amphotericin B are not available
   6. Considerations in salvage therapy when treatment with voriconazole fails
      a. Change to other antifungals such as amphotericin B formulations and echinocandins
      b. Confirm diagnosis
      c. Assess dosage and monitor drug levels
   7. *Aspergillus terreus*
      a. Intrinsic resistance to amphotericin B
      b. Treat with voriconazole, emphasizing the importance of fungal culture in diagnosis and treatment
   8. Echinocandins
      a. Active drugs against invasive aspergillosis
      b. Caspofungin
         1) First approved echinocandin
         2) Efficacy and safety in patients intolerant of other treatments or with disease refractory to other treatments
   9. Combination therapy
      a. Occasionally administered by clinicians
      b. Especially used for salvage therapy (eg, caspofungin plus voriconazole or caspofungin plus amphotericin B)
      c. Utility has not been validated by controlled clinical trials
      d. Initial use of combination therapy is not routinely recommended
   10. Considerations for surgical resection in invasive aspergillosis
       a. Lesions contiguous to heart and great vessels or chest wall involvement
       b. Osteomyelitis, pericardial infection, endocarditis, and others
   11. Aspergillosis prophylaxis
       a. Primary prophylaxis: effective in recipients of hematopoietic stem-cell transplants who received immunosuppressive therapy for graft-versus-host disease and in neutropenic patients with acute myelogenous leukemia or myelodysplastic syndrome
       b. Secondary prophylaxis: use of voriconazole during immunosuppression treatment may prevent recurrence

Suggested Reading

Denning DW. Invasive aspergillosis. Clin Infect Dis. 1998 Apr;26(4):781–803.

Patterson TF. *Aspergillus* Species. In: Mandell GL, Bennett JE, Dolin R. Mandell, Douglas, and Bennett's principles and practice of infectious diseases. Vol 2. 7th ed. Philadelphia (PA): Churchill Livingstone/Elsevier; c2010. p. 3241–56.

Walsh TJ, Anaissie EJ, Denning DW, Herbrecht R, Kontoyiannis DP, Marr KA, et al; Infectious Diseases Society of America. Treatment of aspergillosis: clinical practice guidelines of the Infectious Diseases Society of America. Clin Infect Dis. 2008 Feb 1;46(3):327–60.

15

Histoplasma capsulatum

Janis E. Blair, MD

I. Introduction
   A. Histoplasmosis
      1. Most common endemic mycosis
      2. One of the most common opportunistic infections in persons with AIDS
   B. *Histoplasma capsulatum*: 2 Varieties
      1. *Histoplasma capsulatum* var *capsulatum*
         a. Causes histoplasmosis in Americas, parts of Africa, eastern Asia, and Australia; rarely, in Europe
      2. *Histoplasma capsulatum* var *duboisii* (*Histoplasma duboisii*)
         a. Causes African histoplasmosis
         b. Only in Africa between the Tropic of Cancer and the Tropic of Capricorn and on the island of Madagascar
         c. Manifests as a subacute granuloma of the skin or bone but may disseminate to the skin, lymph nodes, bones, joints, lungs, and abdomen
II. *Histoplasma capsulatum*
   A. Microbiology and Mycology
      1. Dimorphic fungus
         a. Exists as a mold in soil
         b. Exists as a yeast in humans and animals
      2. Varieties are distinguished by size of yeast cells in tissue
         a. *Histoplasma capsulatum* var *capsulatum*: 1-4 µm
         b. *Histoplasma capsulatum* var *duboisii*: 10-12 µm
   B. Ecology
      1. Associated with bird and bat droppings
         a. Birds
            1) Not infected with *Histoplasma*, but droppings provide rich nutrient source for maintaining fungal growth
            2) Birds may serve as vectors for transmission to previously uninfected bird roosts through contamination (eg, beaks, feet, wings)
         b. Bats
            1) May become infected with *Histoplasma*
            2) May drop *H capsulatum* in their feces
      2. Roosts of chickens, pigeons, oilbirds, starlings, and grackles are commonly infected
      3. Other less well-described ecological niches are likely
III. Histoplasmosis
   A. Epidemiology
      1. Geographic distribution (Figure 15.1)
         a. Mainly in the Ohio and Mississippi river valleys

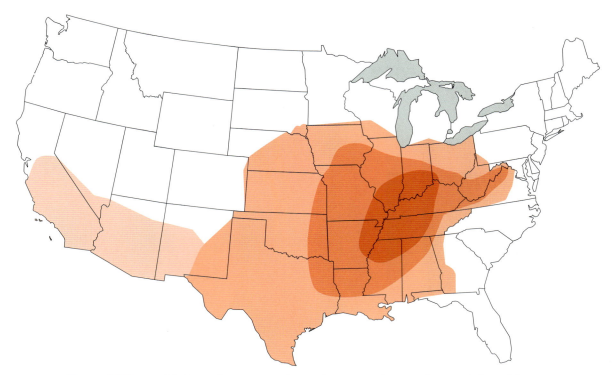

Figure 15.1. Simplified Distribution Map of Histoplasmosis in the United States. (Adapted from Dr Fungus [Internet]. [cited 2010 Mar 18]. Available from: http://www.doctorfungus.org. Used with permission.)

    b. In the United States, histoplasmosis is endemic also in the southeastern central and mid-Atlantic states
2. Environmental risk factors
    a. Disturbed accumulations of bird and bat droppings
        1) Building construction, renovation, or demolition
        2) Soil excavation, spelunking, farming, or cleaning sites that harbor the fungus
    b. Disturbances can send the spores airborne, resulting in infection downwind
3. Other risk factors
    a. Race or sex: no clear predilection
    b. Children: high rate of asymptomatic and mild infections
    c. Persons aged 15 to 34 years: highest incidence of acute histoplasmosis in acute outbreaks (possibly associated with participation in activities that result in greater exposure)
    d. Infants (younger than 1 year) and elderly (older than 54 years): higher risk of disseminated infection
4. Transmission
    a. Main route of acquisition is by inhalation of *H capsulatum* spores from the soil
    b. No transmission of disease from human to human or from animal to human
5. Wide spectrum of clinical illness: from asymptomatic illness to severe, disseminated infection
6. Risk of symptomatic disease
    a. Where histoplasmosis is endemic, symptomatic disease develops in less than 5% of persons exposed to *H capsulatum*
    b. In outbreaks and when exposure to *H capsulatum* is heavy, symptomatic disease develops in 50% to 100% of those exposed
7. Incubation period: 7 to 14 days (mean, 10 days)

B. Acute Histoplasmosis
1. More than 90% of cases are unrecognized
2. Clinical Features
    a. In a small proportion of patients: flulike illness with fever, chills, nonproductive cough, substernal chest discomfort, headache, and generalized malaise
    b. Other less common symptoms: arthralgia, erythema nodosum, erythema multiforme
    c. Uncommon: frank arthritis
    d. In 6% of patients: pericarditis, with precordial chest pain and fever

> **Box 15.1**
>
> **Indications for Treatment of Histoplasmosis**
>
> Treatment indicated
>   Acute pulmonary histoplasmosis with diffuse infiltrates
>   Subacute pulmonary histoplasmosis with focal infiltrates for >1 mo
>   Granulomatous mediastinitis with obstruction
>   Chronic pulmonary histoplasmosis
>   Disseminated histoplasmosis
> Treatment not indicated
>   Acute pulmonary histoplasmosis with mild illness
>   Pericarditis
>   Rheumatologic symptoms
>   Broncholithiasis
>   Histoplasmoma
>   Presumed ocular histoplasmosis
>   Fibrosing mediastinitis[a]
>
> [a] Antifungal treatment has not been proved effective, but a 3-month trial should be considered, especially for patients who have an elevated erythrocyte sedimentation rate or complement fixation titers ≥1:32.
>
> Adapted from Mocherla S, Wheat LJ. Treatment of histoplasmosis. Semin Respir Infect. 2001 Jun;16(2):141-8. Used with permission.

    3. Treatment
        a. Generally, a self-limited infection that does not require therapy
        b. If symptoms are severe or last for more than 1 month, treatment is indicated (Box 15.1 and Table 15.1)

C. Chronic Pulmonary Histoplasmosis
    1. More common in persons with underlying lung disease (eg, emphysema)
    2. Chronic or recurrent pulmonary symptoms include cough, dyspnea, and sputum production, often accompanied by fever, sweats, and weight loss
    3. No mediastinal or hilar lymphadenopathy
    4. Without treatment, progressive illness causes fibrosis, upper lobe cavitation, and loss of pulmonary function
D. Disseminated Histoplasmosis
    1. More likely to occur in persons with defective cell-mediated immunity (patients with AIDS or hematologic malignancies, transplant recipients, and patients receiving corticosteroids or other immunosuppressive therapy)
        a. Immunocompromised hosts: 33% mortality
        b. Disseminated infection in AIDS patients: fatal if untreated
    2. Wide spectrum of clinical illness
        a. Severe multisystem illness involving the bone marrow, liver, spleen, and lungs
        b. Indolent infection localized to the gastrointestinal tract, skin, adrenal glands, brain, meninges, or other extrapulmonary tissue

Table 15.1

Histoplasmosis Treatment Recommendations Summarized From the 2007 Treatment Guidelines of the Infectious Diseases Society of America

Type of Histoplasmosis	Moderately Severe to Severe Manifestations	Mild to Moderate Manifestations
Acute pulmonary	L-AMB[a], then itraconazole[b] for 12 wk total Corticosteroid[c] for respiratory distress	Treatment is usually unnecessary For patients with prolonged symptoms, itraconazole[b] for 6-12 wk
Chronic cavitary pulmonary	Itraconazole[b] for 12-24 mo	Itraconazole[b] for 12-24 mo
Disseminated		
In nonimmunosuppressed patient	L-AMB[a] for 1-2 wk, then itraconazole[b] for ≥12 mo	Itraconazole[b] for ≥12 mo
In immunosuppressed patient[d]	L-AMB[a] for 1-2 wk, then itraconazole[b] for life	Itraconazole[b] for life
Meningitis	L-AMB 5.0 mg/kg daily for 4-6 wk, then itraconazole 200 mg 2-3 times daily for ≥12 mo	L-AMB 5.0 mg/kg daily for 4-6 wk, then itraconazole 200 mg 2-3 times daily for ≥12 mo
Mediastinal lymphadenitis	Itraconazole[b] for 6-12 wk Corticosteroid[e] in severe cases with obstruction or compression of contiguous structures	Treatment is usually unnecessary Itraconazole[b] if symptoms present for >1 mo
Mediastinal granuloma	Itraconazole[b] for 6-12 wk	Treatment is usually unnecessary Itraconazole[b] 6-12 wk for symptomatic cases
Fibrosing mediastinitis	Antifungal treatment is not recommended Itraconazole[b] for 3 mo[f] Intravascular stents if pulmonary vascular obstruction	Antifungal treatment is not recommended Itraconazole[b] for 3 mo[f]

(continued)

Table 15.1
(continued)

Type of Histoplasmosis	Moderately Severe to Severe Manifestations	Mild to Moderate Manifestations
Pericarditis	Corticosteroid[e], then NSAID Pericardial drainage if hemodynamically unstable Itraconazole[b] (only if corticosteroid administered) for 6-12 wk	NSAID
Rheumatologic	Corticosteroid[e], then NSAID Itraconazole[b] (only if corticosteroid administered) for 6-12 wk	NSAID
Broncholithiasis	No antifungal treatment Removal of broncholith	No antifungal treatment Removal of broncholith
Histoplasmoma (pulmonary nodule)	No antifungal treatment	No antifungal treatment

Abbreviations: L-AMB, lipid formulation of amphotericin B; NSAID, nonsteroidal anti-inflammatory drug.

[a] L-AMB dosage is generally 3.0 to 5.0 mg/kg intravenously daily for 1 to 2 weeks. Amphotericin B deoxycholate formulation (0.7-1.0 mg/kg daily intravenously) is an alternative for patients at low risk of nephrotoxicity.

[b] Itraconazole dosage is 200 mg 3 times daily for 3 days, then 200 mg twice daily.

[c] Methylprednisolone (0.5-1.0 mg/kg daily intravenously during the first 1-2 weeks of antifungal therapy) is recommended for patients with respiratory complications, including hypoxemia or significant respiratory distress.

[d] If immunosuppression cannot be reversed.

[e] Prednisone 0.5 to 1.0 mg/kg daily (maximum dosage, 80 mg daily) in tapering doses over 1 to 2 weeks is recommended for patients with hemodynamic compromise or with disease recalcitrant to NSAID therapy; concurrent itraconazole therapy is recommended.

[f] Therapy is controversial and probably ineffective except in cases of granulomatous mediastinitis misdiagnosed as fibrosing mediastinitis. If clinical findings cannot differentiate these 2 manifestations, itraconazole can be administered.

Data from Wheat LJ, Freifeld AG, Kleiman MB, Baddley JW, McKinsey DS, Loyd JE, et al; Infectious Diseases Society of America. Clinical practice guidelines for the management of patients with histoplasmosis: 2007 update by the Infectious Diseases Society of America. Clin Infect Dis. 2007 Oct 1;45(7):807–25. Epub 2007 Aug 27.

E. Fibrosing Mediastinitis
  1. Rare, late manifestation
     a. Characterized by destructive perinodal fibrosis, encompassing and invading adjacent structures of the mediastinum
     b. Results in major airway or vascular occlusion
  2. Must be distinguished from idiopathic mediastinal fibrosis
  3. Fibrosing mediastinitis associated with histoplasmosis is characterized by its focus in lymph nodes, calcification, and invasion into airways and pulmonary vessels
  4. Bilateral involvement is associated with a high mortality rate
  5. Symptoms: hemoptysis, dyspnea, cough, and pleuritic chest pain
     a. Symptoms begin at age 21 to 40 years
     b. Death occurs about 6 years after onset of symptoms
  6. Persons with the most severe histoplasmosis-associated mediastinal adenitis are thought to be at risk of fibrosing mediastinitis
  7. Pharmacologic therapy has no proven role, but if fibrosing mediastinitis cannot be distinguished from granulomatous mediastinitis, some experts suggest itraconazole therapy for 6 to 12 weeks
F. Presumed Ocular Histoplasmosis
  1. Macular involvement and choroiditis causing visual loss have been attributed to histoplasmosis
     a. No proof of association
     b. Attribution is based on rates of histoplasmin skin test reactivity
  2. Not an active infection
  3. Therapy
     a. Antifungal therapy is not indicated
     b. Corticosteroid and laser therapy have been used
G. Diagnosis
  1. Table 15.2 compares diagnostic findings in various forms of histoplasmosis
  2. Diagnosis is sometimes missed or delayed because the disease is not considered
  3. Fungal culture
     a. *Histoplasma capsulatum* grows as a mold on fungal media when incubated at 25°C
     b. Cultures must be maintained at least 1 month to ensure isolation

Table 15.2
Diagnostic Findings in Various Forms of Histoplasmosis

Procedure	Asymptomatic Infection	Acute Pulmonary Histoplasmosis		Chronic Pulmonary Histoplasmosis	Disseminated Histoplasmosis	Fibrosing Mediastinitis
		Low Inoculum	High Inoculum			
Determination of fungal burden	Low	Low	High	Low	High	Low
Chest radiography	Hilar LAN, pulmonary nodules, calcified granuloma, or normal	Mediastinal LAN, focal or patchy infiltrate	Diffuse pulmonary infiltrates	Progressive infiltrate, fibrosis, and cavitation (may mimic tuberculosis)	Generally diffuse infiltrate; may be normal in 25%-39%	Chest radiography may be normal; computed tomography may show focal fibrosis
Antigen testing	Negative	Generally negative (low fungal burden)	Generally positive; 75% have antigen in urine	Negative	Positive	Negative
Measurement of antibody titer	Low-level positive or negative	Generally positive owing to longer interval between infusion and presentation	Generally negative if checked 4 mo after exposure	Generally positive	Positive in 70%	Positive in 67%
Culture	Generally no growth	Rarely positive	Positive respiratory secretions or lung biopsy	Positive in 60%-85% from sputum or bronchoscopy (multiple specimens may be required)	Blood cultures positive in ≥80%; bone marrow positive in 75%; respiratory cultures positive in 70% with diffuse infiltrates	Negative

Abbreviation: LAN, lymphadenopathy.

c. Cultures are most often positive in patients with disseminated or chronic pulmonary histoplasmosis
   1) Yield is higher if multiple specimens are submitted
   2) Sensitivity of culture is low (<10%) with other forms of histoplasmosis
4. Histopathology
   a. Immunocompetent hosts: noncaseating or caseating granulomas
   b. Immunosuppressed hosts: loose granulomas, lymphohistiocytic aggregates, or diffuse mononuclear cell infiltrates
   c. Microscopic appearance
      1) Intracellular yeast seen in macrophages (occasionally extracellular) (Figures 15.2 and 15.3)
      2) Ovoid yeast, 3 to 5 μm in diameter, with narrow-based budding (Figure 15.4)
   d. Sensitivity with surgical specimens: 50%
5. Serology
   a. Positive results for more than 90% of patients with histoplasmosis
   b. Sensitivity: lower among immunocompromised hosts
   c. Cross reactions: common with paracoccidioidomycosis, blastomycosis, aspergillosis, and, less frequently, coccidioidomycosis or candidiasis
   d. Seroconversion occurs 2 to 6 weeks after exposure
      1) In general, antibodies clear after recovery

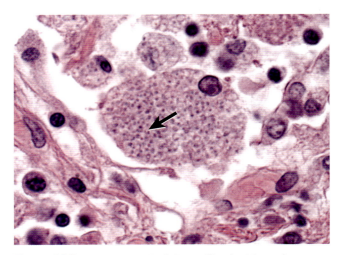

Figure 15.3. Lung Tissue With Large Alveolar Macrophage Filled With *Histoplasma capsulatum*. Arrow indicates individual organism with small clear halo retraction artifact (hematoxylin-eosin, original magnification ×500).

      2) Antibodies persist with chronic progressive infection
      3) Antibodies persist for several years after prolonged exposure
   e. Immunodiffusion
      1) Identifies H and M precipitin bands
      2) Is less sensitive than complement fixation when used for screening
      3) H precipitin clears within 6 months after infection
      4) M precipitin may persist for several years

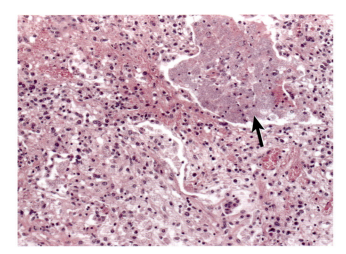

Figure 15.2. Lung Tissue From Patient With Pneumonia and Fatal Disseminated Histoplasmosis. Alveoli are filled with clustered macrophages (arrow) containing bluish punctate *Histoplasma capsulatum* in a background of organizing pneumonia (hematoxylin-eosin, original magnification ×200).

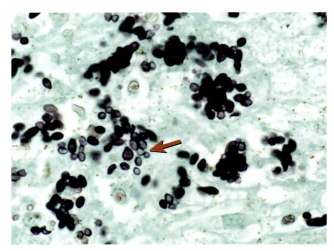

Figure 15.4. Lung Tissue With Clustered, Black-Staining *Histoplasma capsulatum*. The generally round, small, thin-walled organisms are of similar size and lack a capsule (arrow) (Gomori methenamine silver, original magnification ×500).

f. Complement fixation
   1) Results are generally stronger with yeast antigens than mycelial antigens
   2) For about 95% of patients with histoplasmosis, results are positive
6. Antigen Detection
   a. Antigen can be detected in urine, serum, and bronchoalveolar lavage fluid
   b. Antigens may be detected before antibody formation
   c. Antigen disappears with effective treatment
   d. Sensitivity
      1) Sensitivity is higher for antigen in urine than in serum
      2) Acute pulmonary histoplasmosis, when patients present within the first month after exposure: 75%
      3) Disseminated infection: 92% for antigen detected in urine
      4) Subacute pulmonary histoplasmosis: 25%
      5) Chronic pulmonary histoplasmosis: 10%
7. Radiology
   a. Asymptomatic infection may be identified with incidental discovery of calcified or uncalcified hilar lymphadenopathy, pulmonary nodules, or calcified granulomas in spleen
   b. Acute pulmonary histoplasmosis
      1) After low-inoculum infection: mediastinal lymphadenopathy with focal or patchy pulmonary infiltrates on chest radiograph
      2) After high-inoculum infection: diffuse pulmonary infiltrate on chest radiograph
   c. Chronic pulmonary histoplasmosis
      1) Chronic or recurrent pulmonary symptoms, progressive lung infiltrates, fibrosis, and cavitation
      2) Clinically and radiographically similar to tuberculosis
H. Treatment
   1. See Box 15.1 and Table 15.1

Suggested Reading

Cano MV, Hajjeh RA. The epidemiology of histoplasmosis: a review. Semin Respir Infect. 2001 Jun;16(2):109–18.

Hage CA, Wheat LJ, Loyd J, Allen SD, Blue D, Knox KS. Pulmonary histoplasmosis. Semin Respir Crit Care Med. 2008 Apr;29(2):151–65.

Kauffman CA. Histoplasmosis: a clinical and laboratory update. Clin Microbiol Rev. 2007 Jan;20(1):115–32.

Wheat LJ, Freifeld AG, Kleiman MB, Baddley JW, McKinsey DS, Loyd JE, et al; Infectious Diseases Society of America. Clinical practice guidelines for the management of patients with histoplasmosis: 2007 update by the Infectious Diseases Society of America. Clin Infect Dis. 2007 Oct 1;45(7):807–25. Epub 2007 Aug 27.

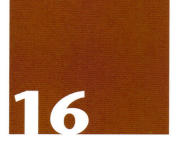

Janis E. Blair, MD

Blastomyces dermatitidis

I. Introduction
   A. Geographic Distribution of *Blastomyces dermatitidis*
      1. *Blastomyces dermatitidis* is a fungus endemic in the central and eastern United States
      2. Coendemic with *Histoplasma capsulatum* in much of the central and southeastern United States, including the Mississippi and Ohio river valleys
      3. Distribution of *B dermatitidis* extends farther north and west than *H capsulatum* and includes northern Wisconsin, Minnesota, Ontario, and Manitoba
   B. Ecology
      1. Fungal growth occurs in nitrogen-rich soils close to streams, rivers, and lakes
      2. Many outbreaks of blastomycosis occur within 100 meters of recreational water
II. Blastomycosis
   A. Epidemiology
      1. Sporadic cases are most common among men with heavy vocational or recreational exposure to woods or streams
      2. Sporadic cases also occur in urban sites where people have little or no recreational or vocational exposure to woods or streams
   B. Clinical Disease
      1. Almost always acquired by inhalation
         a. Portal of entry is the lung
         b. Pulmonary illness may spontaneously resolve or become progressive, requiring medical evaluation and treatment
      2. Infections may be asymptomatic, mildly symptomatic, or highly symptomatic
      3. Relative proportion of asymptomatic infections is not known because there is no skin test to detect asymptomatic infection
      4. Wide spectrum of symptoms and severity of pulmonary infection
         a. Asymptomatic
            1) Detectable only by investigation for outbreak
            2) Most common in healthy persons
            3) True incidence is unknown
         b. Brief flulike illness
            1) Fever, chills, headache, myalgia, nonproductive cough
            2) Resolves spontaneously
         c. Acute pneumonia
            1) Abrupt onset of symptoms
            2) High fever, chills, malaise, myalgia, arthralgia, productive cough, pleuritic chest pain

d. Subacute or chronic progressive pneumonia
   1) Illness resembles tuberculosis (low-grade fever, productive cough, night sweats, weight loss) or lung cancer (pulmonary mass, chronic cough, weight loss)
   2) Accounts for the majority of recognized cases
   3) About 25% of cases have an accompanying skin or bone disease
e. Fulminant respiratory failure
   1) High fever and diffuse infiltrate
   2) Mortality: 50%
f. With AIDS and human immunodeficiency virus (HIV)
   1) Most patients with AIDS and blastomycosis have diffuse infiltrate and widely disseminated infection
   2) In patients with HIV infection, blastomycosis is an opportunistic infection

5. Extrapulmonary illness
   a. May occur after pulmonary symptoms and signs have resolved
   b. Blastomyces can occur in virtually any organ
      1) Skin
         a) Verrucous or ulcerated lesions
         b) Subcutaneous abscesses
      2) Bones
         a) Often a lytic osteomyelitis of vertebrae, pelvic bones, sacrum, skull, ribs, or long bones
         b) Often accompanied by adjacent soft tissue abscess
      3) Genitourinary system
         a) Prostatitis, epididymo-orchitis
         b) Urine culture after prostatic massage improves detection
      4) Central nervous system
         a) Meningitis or cranial abscess
         b) Much higher yield with ventricular fluid than spinal fluid

C. Immunity
   1. Cellular immunity and adequate neutrophil function are important for control
   2. Immunocompromised patients
      a. Blastomyces may cause infection in immunocompromised patients, but other fungal infections (eg, disseminated histoplasmosis or cryptococcosis) are much more likely to cause opportunistic infection
      b. Immunosuppression increases the intensity of the infection and increases the risk of relapse
      c. Mortality among immunocompromised patients: as high as 30%

D. Diagnosis
   1. Blastomyces infection can be diagnosed by culture or pathology because no colonization state exists
   2. Microbiology
      a. *Blastomyces dermatitidis* is easily cultured
      b. Mycelial growth in 5 to 30 days
      c. Ectoantigen testing or DNA probes allow rapid identification
      d. Purulent material (sputum or other specimen)
         1) Usually available for examination because the inflammatory response to blastomyces is a suppurative reaction
         2) Easiest and most rapid diagnostic test is examination of expectorated sputum or aspirated pus after 10% potassium hydroxide digestion
         3) Direct smear of sputum: doubly refractile wall (8-20 μm), multiple nuclei, large single buds with a broad neck of attachment to the parent cell
   3. Serology
      a. Very few cases are identified serologically
      b. Tests are available but have poor sensitivity: enzyme immunoassay, complement fixation, immunodiffusion, Western blot, and radioimmunoassay
      c. Any positive serologic test result has enough specificity to prompt pursuit of appropriate diagnostic procedures (eg, sputum culture, biopsy) to confirm or reject the diagnosis
   4. Radiology
      a. No characteristic radiographic pattern
      b. Chest radiographs show a range of findings
         1) Single or multifocal patchy, lobar, or alveolar infiltrates
         2) Single or multiple nodules
         3) Mass-like lesions
         4) Cavitation is uncommon; cavitation closes with successful therapy
         5) Hilar lymphadenopathy: not as common as in histoplasmosis
         6) Calcifications with healing are rare
   5. Histopathology
      a. Fungal stains
         1) Periodic acid-Schiff, methenamine silver

2) Papanicolaou technique: bronchoscopy washings show organisms
b. Most cases are diagnosed by direct smear or culture of material obtained at bronchoscopy
c. On occasion, histopathology of tissue specimens is diagnostic (Figures 16.1–16.4)

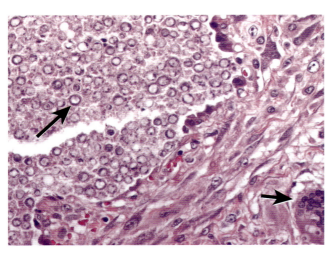

Figure 16.1. Open Lung Biopsy Specimen From Patient With Blastomycotic Pneumonia. The preparation shows numerous round organisms packed in the alveolar space (long arrow) and a Langhans giant cell (short arrow) (hematoxylin-eosin, original magnification ×200).

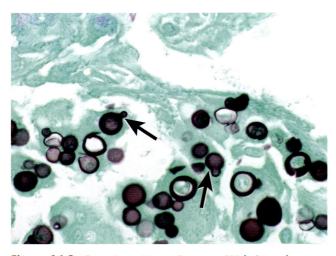

Figure 16.2. Open Lung Biopsy Specimen With Stained *Blastomyces dermatitidis*. Numerous round yeast forms, often with thick walls, stain black. Some show broad-based budding (arrows) (silver chromate with fast green, original magnification ×500).

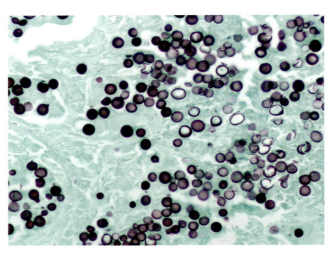

Figure 16.3. Open Lung Biopsy Specimen With Stained *Blastomyces dermatitidis*. The round organisms are usually clear internally (silver chromate with fast green, original magnification ×400).

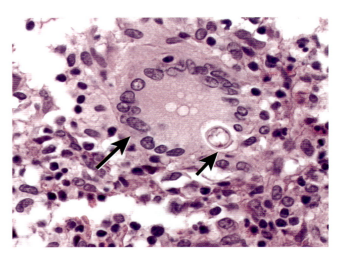

Figure 16.4. Open Lung Biopsy Specimen With Langhans Giant Cell. Langhans giant cell (long arrow) contains a large engulfed blastomycotic yeast form (short arrow). The stained organism shows a thick double-contoured wall with some internal vacuolation (hematoxylin-eosin, original magnification ×500).

E. Treatment
1. Treatment is summarized in Table 16.1
2. In many patients resolution is spontaneous without specific therapy
3. For asymptomatic or mild illness, no therapy is needed—only close follow-up

Table 16.1
Treatment of Blastomycosis

Type of Disease	Preferred Treatment	Alternative Treatment
Pulmonary		
Life-threatening	L-AMB 3-5 mg/kg daily *or* AMB total dose 1.5-2.5 g	Initiate therapy with L-AMB *or* AMB Switch to itraconazole 200-400 mg daily after condition is stabilized
Mild to moderate	Itraconazole 200 mg 3 times daily ×1 d, then 200-400 mg daily	Ketoconazole 400-800 mg daily *or* fluconazole 400-800 mg daily
Disseminated		
CNS	L-AMB 5 mg/kg daily ×4-6 wk, then an oral azole: fluconazole 800 mg daily, itraconazole 200 mg 3 times daily, *or* voriconazole 200-400 mg daily for at least 12 mo	For patients unable to tolerate a full course of AMB, consider fluconazole 800 mg daily
Non-CNS		
Life-threatening	L-AMB 3-5 mg/kg daily *or* AMB total dose 1.5-2.5 g	Initiate therapy with L-AMB *or* AMB Switch to itraconazole 200-400 mg daily
Mild to moderate	Itraconazole 200-400 mg daily	Ketoconazole 400-800 mg daily *or* fluconazole 400-800 mg daily
Immunocompromised host	L-AMB 3-5 mg/kg daily *or* AMB 1.5-2.5 g ×1-2 wk until stabilized Then itraconazole 200 mg 3 times daily × ≥12 mo	After primary course of AMB, suppressive therapy should be continued with itraconazole 200-400 mg daily For patients who have CNS disease or who cannot tolerate itraconazole, consider fluconazole 800 mg daily
Special circumstances		
Pregnancy	L-AMB 3-5 mg/kg daily Avoid azoles	
Pediatrics	L-AMB 3-5 mg/kg daily *or* AMB total dose >30 mg/kg *or* itraconazole 10 mg/kg daily (up to 400 mg daily)	Itraconazole 10 mg/kg daily (up to 400 mg daily)

Abbreviations: AMB, amphotericin B deoxycholate; CNS, central nervous system; L-AMB, liposomal amphotericin B.

4. Chronic blastomycosis does not commonly resolve without treatment
5. Untreated blastomycosis can be associated with mortality rates of nearly 60%
6. All patients with chronic or extrapulmonary blastomycosis should be treated
7. Treatment options
   a. Itraconazole 400 mg daily for 6 months
   b. Amphotericin B is used when aggressive treatment is required

Suggested Reading

Bradsher RW Jr. Pulmonary blastomycosis. Semin Respir Crit Care Med. 2008 Apr;29(2):174–81.

Bradsher RW, Chapman SW, Pappas PG. Blastomycosis. Infect Dis Clin North Am. 2003 Mar;17(1):21–40.

Chapman SW, Dismukes WE, Proia LA, Bradsher RW, Pappas PG, Threlkeld MG, et al; Infectious Diseases Society of America. Clinical practice guidelines for the management of blastomycosis: 2008 update by the Infectious Diseases Society of America. Clin Infect Dis. 2008 Jun 15;46(12):1801–12.

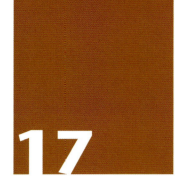

Janis E. Blair, MD

Coccidioides Species

I. Introduction
   A. Geographic Distribution
      1. Coccidioidomycosis is endemic only in the Western Hemisphere (Figure 17.1)
      2. Endemic in southern Arizona, New Mexico, Texas, and much of central and southern California
      3. Highly endemic in northern Mexico
      4. Endemic in small areas in South American countries, including Argentina, Brazil, Colombia, Paraguay, and Venezuela
   B. Ecology
      1. Organism grows in soil
      2. Grows only in semiarid, geographically restricted region: the Lower Sonoran Life Zone
   C. Mycology
      1. Two nearly identical species cause coccidioidomycosis
         a. *Coccidioides immitis*
         b. *Coccidioides posadasii*
      2. Organisms grow in the mycelial phase in the soil
         a. As soil dries, the mycelia disarticulate into environmentally resistant arthroconidia (spores) that are easily aerosolized and dispersed
         b. Upon inhalation, the fungus enters the lungs and converts to the tissue parasitic phase, which consists of alternating spherules and endospores

II. Coccidioidomycosis
    A. Epidemiology
       1. Males more often infected: probably related to occupational or recreational dust exposure
       2. Risk factors for disseminated infection
          a. Certain races (African American, Filipino)
          b. Pregnancy, especially the third trimester
          c. Illnesses that affect T-lymphocyte function
             1) Human immunodeficiency virus infection (particularly with CD4 cell count <100/µL)
             2) Cancer (particularly Hodgkin lymphoma)
             3) Exogenous immunosuppression (eg, transplant recipients)
    B. Clinical Disease
       1. Majority of persons (60%) with primary infections are asymptomatic
       2. Persons with symptomatic infection (40%) have variable presentations
          a. From self-limited pulmonary infection to life-threatening disseminated infection
          b. Erythema nodosum, erythema multiforme, and other transient rashes are seen in about 10% to 50% of persons with acute pulmonary infection
       3. Common symptoms of primary infection include fever, chills, malaise, headache, myalgia, and cough

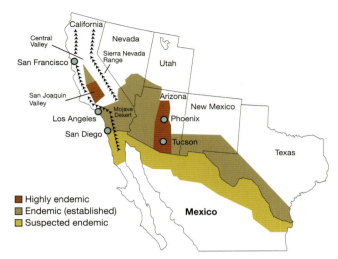

Figure 17.1. Geographic Distribution of Coccidioidomycosis. Map shows southwestern United States and northern Mexico. (Adapted from Blair JE. Coccidioidomycosis in liver transplantation. Liver Transpl. 2006 Jan;12[1]:31–9. Used with permission.)

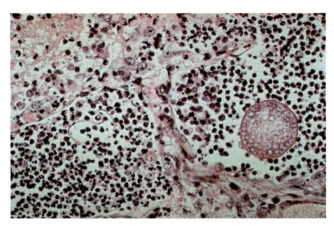

Figure 17.2. *Coccidioides* Spherule. Specimen was from lung (hematoxylin-eosin, original magnification ×400).

4. Extrapulmonary coccidioidomycosis
   a. Occurs at any site
   b. Common locations include skin, meninges, bone, and joints
5. Coccidioidal meningitis
   a. Occurs in less than 1% of patients who have symptomatic coccidioidomycosis
   b. Subacute onset of headache with or without fever, photophobia, nausea, and neurologic deficits
   c. Basilar leptomeningeal involvement is most common and may be complicated by hydrocephalus
   d. Vasculitis due to coccidioidal infection may result in stroke

C. Immunity
1. T-cell–mediated immunity is important in control of infection

D. Diagnosis
1. Symptoms and signs of coccidioidomycosis are nonspecific
   a. A high degree of awareness is needed
   b. Diagnostic studies are helpful in confirming the diagnosis
2. Microbiology
   a. *Coccidioides* species can be isolated from sputum or other specimens (Figures 17.2 and 17.3)
   b. Culture
      1) The organism grows on most laboratory media, but most microbiology laboratories prefer fungal media
      2) Growth typically occurs in 2 to 7 days but may take longer
3. Serology
   a. Enzyme immunoassay
   b. Immunodiffusion: generally the slowest to turn positive, but it is the most specific
   c. Complement fixation: a quantitative assay, allowing comparison of titers over time
   d. Clinical control of infection should be accompanied by a decrease in the titer
   e. Complement fixation titers greater than 1:16 have been associated with extrapulmonary infection
4. Radiology
   a. Chest radiographic findings can be variable: single or multifocal infiltrates, mass, nodules, or nodular infiltrates (Figure 17.4)

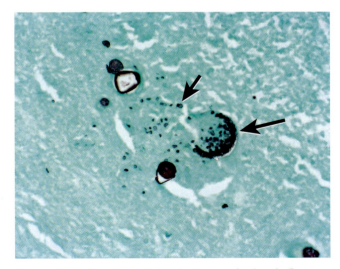

Figure 17.3. *Coccidioides* Spherule. Ruptured spherule (long arrow) is releasing endospores (short arrow) (Grocott-Gomori methenamine-silver stain, original magnification ×400).

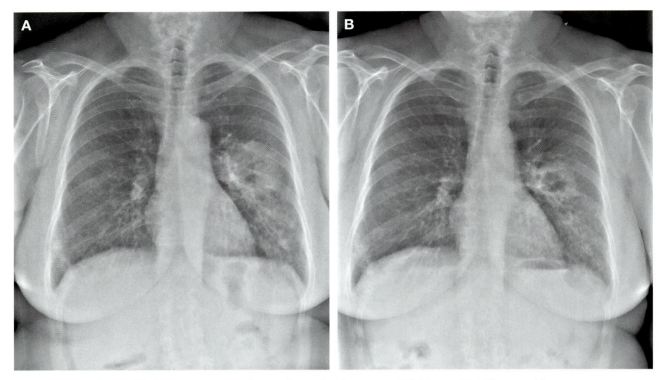

Figure 17.4. Posteroanterior Chest Radiographs of a 62-Year-Old-Woman With Rheumatoid Arthritis and Acute Coccidioidomycosis. A, Radiograph was taken approximately 1 month after presentation and initiation of fluconazole therapy. Nodular infiltrate is apparent in the left mid and lower lung. B, Radiograph taken 2 months later shows a thick-walled cavity in the left lung.

      b. Hilar lymphadenopathy is common
      c. Cavities, seen in the minority of patients, become thin walled with time
      d. Miliary pattern is uncommonly seen
   5. Cerebrospinal fluid (CSF) for meningitis
      a. Lymphocytic meningitis, occasionally with eosinophils
      b. Elevation of protein may resolve more slowly than pleocytosis
      c. Glucose level often less than 40 mg/dL
      d. Culture is rarely positive for fungal growth
      e. Serology is positive in 75%; yield increases with repeated CSF examinations
E. Treatment
   1. For many patients, this infection is self-limited and does not require therapy
   2. Medication
      a. Generally either fluconazole or itraconazole (400 mg daily)
      b. Severe, life-threatening infection may warrant amphotericin B
      c. For meningitis, most patients can be treated with fluconazole 400 mg twice daily indefinitely
   3. Follow-up
      a. Close follow-up is warranted to ensure resolution of clinical symptoms, radiographic abnormalities, and serologic results
      b. Asymptomatic patients with persistently positive serologic results should be monitored but not necessarily treated

Suggested Reading

Anstead GM, Graybill JR. Coccidioidomycosis. Infect Dis Clin North Am. 2006 Sep;20(3):621–43.

Blair JE. Coccidioidal meningitis: update on epidemiology, clinical features, diagnosis, and management. Curr Infect Dis Rep. 2009 Jul;11(4):289–95.

Chiller TM, Galgiani JN, Stevens DA. Coccidioidomycosis. Infect Dis Clin North Am. 2003 Mar;17(1):41–57.

Crum NF, Lederman ER, Stafford CM, Parrish JS, Wallace MR. Coccidioidomycosis: a descriptive survey of a reemerging disease: clinical characteristics and current controversies. Medicine (Baltimore). 2004 May;83(3):149–75.

Galgiani JN, Ampel NM, Blair JE, Catanzaro A, Johnson RH, Stevens DA, et al; Infectious Diseases Society of America. Coccidioidomycosis. Clin Infect Dis. 2005 Nov 1;41(9):1217–23. Epub 2005 Sep 20.

Hector RF, Laniado-Laborin R. Coccidioidomycosis: a fungal disease of the Americas. PLoS Med. 2005 Jan;2(1):e2.

18

Paracoccidioides brasiliensis

Janis E. Blair, MD

I. Introduction
   A. Geographic Distribution
      1. *Paracoccidioides brasiliensis* is found only in Latin America
      2. Endemic in Mexico, Central America, and South America (Figure 18.1)
      3. Most cases (80%) have been reported from Brazil, followed by Venezuela, Colombia, Ecuador, and Argentina
   B. Ecology
      1. Precise ecologic niche is not known
      2. Most cases occur in tropical and subtropical forests, where temperatures are mild and humidity is high throughout the year
   C. Mycology
      1. Dimorphic fungus
         a. Yeast forms at 37°C
         b. Mold at lower temperatures
      2. Yeast
         a. Oval, elongated cells (length, 4-30 µm)
         b. Thick refractile cell wall
         c. Cytoplasm contains prominent lipid droplets
         d. "Pilot's wheel" appearance: multiple budding mother cells surrounded by peripheral daughter cells
      3. Mold grows slowly: 20 to 30 days at 20°C to 26°C

II. Paracoccidioidomycosis
   A. Epidemiology
      1. Transmission
         a. Route of transmission is not clear
         b. No human-to-human transmission
      2. Age: most patients are older than 30 years
      3. Sex: for clinical disease, the male to female ratio is 15:1, but for skin test reactivity, the ratio is 1:1
      4. Latency: very long (>30 years)
   B. Clinical Disease
      1. Most primary infections are asymptomatic
      2. Symptomatic disease ranges from mild and self-limited to severe and progressive
      3. Lungs are primary site of infection, but symptoms do not always reflect this
      4. Symptoms (listed in decreasing frequency)
         a. Mucosal ulcerations in the upper respiratory and digestive tracts
            1) Mucosal lesions are infiltrative, ulcerated, and painful
            2) Involve the mouth, lips, gingiva, tongue, and palate
            3) Less often involve the nose, larynx, and pharynx
         b. Dysphagia and changes in voice
         c. Cutaneous lesions, especially on face and limbs

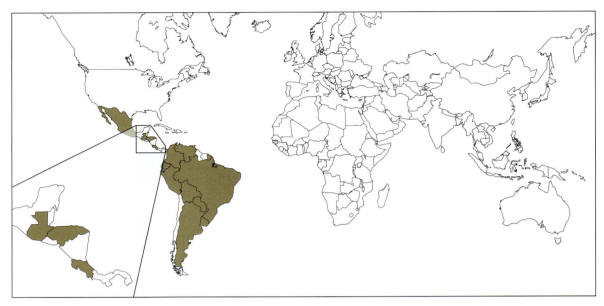

Figure 18.1. Geographic Distribution of *Paracoccidioides brasiliensis*. Shading indicates countries where the fungus is endemic.

       1) Skin lesions appear around orifices and on lower limbs
       2) Lesions are warty, ulcerated, crusted, and granulomatous
    d. Lymphadenopathy, especially in cervical region but also in axillary, mesenteric, and mediastinal lymph nodes
    e. Respiratory symptoms: dyspnea, cough, purulent sputum, and chest pain
    f. Systemic symptoms: weakness, malaise, fever, and weight loss
  5. Draining fistulas may develop
  6. Decreased adrenal function or overt Addison syndrome may occur
C. Immunity
  1. Although cell-mediated immunity is critical, paracoccidioidomycosis is not an opportunistic infection
  2. Few cases have occurred in immunosuppressed hosts
D. Diagnosis
  1. Microbiology
    a. Direct smear of pus or sputum prepared with potassium hydroxide shows organisms in 93% of cases
    b. Calcofluor white stain shows the relatively large cell size, refractile wall, and multiple budding
    c. Culture on fungal media at room temperature for 6 weeks
  2. Serology
    a. Immunodiffusion can detect antibodies for years after infection
    b. Complement fixation is useful for following the response to treatment, but cross-reactions can occur with *Histoplasma*
  3. Skin tests
    a. Not reliable for diagnosis
    b. Many show no reaction during active infection
  4. Chest radiography
    a. Patchy, confluent nodular infiltrate or condensed lesions that are often bilateral and symmetric
    b. Apices are usually spared
    c. Cavities are frequent features
    d. Hilar lymphadenopathy is infrequent feature
    e. Long-term infection shows bullae, fibrosis, and emphysematous areas
    f. Right ventricular hypertrophy is sometimes present
E. Treatment
  1. Medication
    a. Long-acting sulfa medications, 1 to 2 g daily, until response is apparent (days to weeks); then 500 mg daily for 3 to 5 years
    b. Amphotericin B is reserved for severe or unresponsive disease

    c. Ketoconazole, itraconazole, and fluconazole are effective
    d. In small studies comparing imidazoles with sulfadiazine, outcomes were not different
2. Follow-up
    a. Relapses occur frequently
    b. Prolonged treatment courses (up to 2 years) are designed to avoid relapses

Suggested Reading

Bethlem EP, Capone D, Maranhao B, Carvalho CR, Wanke B. Paracoccidioidomycosis. Curr Opin Pulm Med. 1999 Sep;5(5):319–25.

Menezes VM, Soares BG, Fontes CJ. Drugs for treating paracoccidioidomycosis. Cochrane Database Syst Rev. 2006 Apr;19(2):CD004967.

Restrepo A, Benard G, de Castro CC, Agudelo CA, Tobon AM. Pulmonary paracoccidioidomycosis. Semin Respir Crit Care Med. 2008 Apr;29(2):182–97.

Janis E. Blair, MD

19

Sporothrix schenckii

I. Introduction
   A. Geographic Distribution
      1. *Sporothrix schenckii* has a worldwide distribution
      2. The majority of cases of sporotrichosis occur in North America, South America, and Japan
   B. Ecology
      1. Environmental niches include sphagnum moss, decaying vegetation, soil, and hay
   C. Mycology
      1. Dimorphic fungus
         a. In the environment, at 25°C to 30°C, *Sporothrix* grows as a mold
         b. At 37°C, *Sporothrix* grows as a cigar-shaped yeast (length, 4-6 μm)
      2. Readily grows on standard fungal media
II. Sporotrichosis
   A. Epidemiology
      1. Persons at highest risk: those who have outdoor vocations or hobbies and are exposed to environmental conditions in which *Sporothrix* grows best
         a. High-risk activities: rose gardening, topiary production, Christmas tree farming, hay baling, and masonry work
         b. Common portal of entry: punctured skin with primary inoculation
      2. Other routes of transmission
         a. For pulmonary sporotrichosis: inhalation of conidia aerosolized from soil or decaying vegetation
         b. *Sporothrix* can also be transmitted from the bite or scratch of animals, especially cats and armadillos
   B. Clinical Disease
      1. Subacute to chronic cutaneous, subcutaneous, and lymphocutaneous infection
         a. Most common manifestation
         b. After inoculation of conidia into skin or subcutaneous tissue, a primary lesion develops within days to weeks at site of inoculation
         c. A papule enlarges to a nodule and often ulcerates later
         d. Lesions are mildly painful
         e. Drainage is not grossly purulent
         f. Not associated with systemic symptoms
         g. Nodular lesions extend along the lymphatic distribution that is proximal to the initial lesion
         h. Lymphangitic streaking is observed between nodules

2. Fixed cutaneous lesions
   a. No lymphangitic spread
   b. Persist at site of inoculation
   c. May be plaque-like or verrucous, but ulceration is uncommon
   d. Caused by strains that grow best at cooler temperatures (≤35°C)
3. Pulmonary infection
   a. May mimic pulmonary tuberculosis: fever, night sweats, anorexia, weight loss, and fatigue
   b. Cough is productive, with purulent sputum, hemoptysis, or dyspnea
   c. Chest radiographic appearance is similar to that for tuberculosis: cavities are frequently present in upper lobes
4. Osteoarticular sporotrichosis
   a. May follow cutaneous or pulmonary infection, with subsequent fungemia
   b. May be associated with a cutaneous lesion adjacent to or overlying the bone lesion
5. Disseminated visceral lesions
   a. In persons with human immunodeficiency virus infection
   b. May occur with systemic symptoms or meningitis
   c. Skin lesions may be atypical, with punched out ulcerations and minimal inflammation

C. Immunity
   1. Cellular response is both neutrophilic and monocytic
   2. Antibody does not provide protection
   3. T-cell–mediated immunity is important in limiting the extent of infection
   4. Immune status of host
      a. Healthy hosts are just as likely to become infected as immunosuppressed hosts
      b. Immunosuppressed hosts are more likely to have disseminated visceral, osteoarticular, meningeal, or pulmonary infection

D. Diagnosis
   1. For definitive diagnosis, the organism must be isolated from the site of infection
      a. Material can be obtained through swabbing, aspiration, or biopsy
      b. Organisms can grow in samples from sputum, synovial fluid, and cerebrospinal fluid; rarely, blood cultures can grow organisms
   2. Culture
      a. *Sporothrix* grows best on Sabouraud dextrose agar
      b. Culture is kept at room temperature
      c. Growth occurs in days to weeks
   3. Histopathology
      a. Shows a mixed suppurative and granulomatous infection (Figure 19.1)
      b. Multinucleated giant cells may be seen
      c. Periodic acid-Schiff and silver stains show the cigar-shaped yeast forms in tissue (Figure 19.2)
      d. Budding may be seen

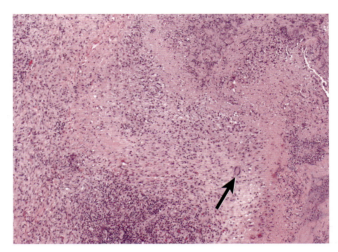

Figure 19.1. Sporotrichosis in Dermis of Left Forearm. Suppurative, necrotizing, partially granulomatous inflammation is present in the dermis. Arrow indicates Langhans giant cell (hematoxylin-eosin, original magnification ×40).

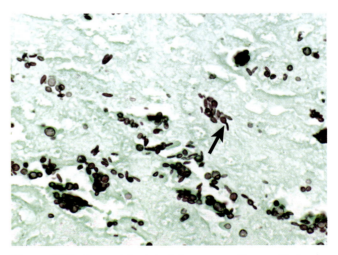

Figure 19.2. Sporotrichosis in Subcutaneous Tissue of Left Forearm. Organisms of various sizes appear black with round, oval, and cigar shapes. Arrow indicates narrow-based "pipe-stem" or "teardrop" budding (Gomori methenamine silver, original magnification ×400).

4. Serology
   a. Available in reference and public health laboratories
   b. Not often used for diagnosis
E. Treatment
   1. All forms of sporotrichosis require treatment
   2. Medication
      a. Itraconazole
         1) More efficacious than ketoconazole or fluconazole
         2) The initial treatment of choice for non–life-threatening sporotrichosis that does not involve the central nervous system
      b. Amphotericin B: treatment of choice for patients who are immunocompromised, have life-threatening or central nervous system disease, or for whom azole treatment has failed
   3. Lymphocutaneous and cutaneous sporotrichosis
      a. Drug of choice: itraconazole 100 to 200 mg daily (nearly 100% resolution with 3-6 months of therapy)
      b. Options for nonresponders
         1) Itraconazole 200 mg twice daily
         2) Terbinafine 500 mg twice daily
         3) Saturated solution of potassium iodide
            a) Gradually increase dosage from 5 drops 3 times daily to 50 drops 3 times daily
            b) Side effects are common
      c. For patients intolerant of other treatments: fluconazole 400 to 800 mg orally daily
   4. Fixed cutaneous lesions
      a. May be treatable with local heat applications (42°C-43°C)
      b. Heat should be applied for at least 1 hour daily for several months
      c. Use a specific device that heats tissues with infrared and far infrared wavelengths
      d. Recommended only for patients who cannot use other forms of treatment
   5. Pulmonary sporotrichosis
      a. Responds poorly to antifungal therapy
      b. Initial choices
         1) Liposomal amphotericin B 3 to 5 mg/kg daily
         2) Amphotericin B deoxycholate 0.7 to 1 mg/kg daily (1-2 g cumulative total)
         3) After infection is stable, amphotericin B preparation can be replaced with itraconazole (200 mg twice daily)
         4) For less severe infections, begin therapy with itraconazole (200 mg twice daily for 12 months)
      c. Response rate with an antifungal regimen: 30%
      d. Definitive treatment when feasible: surgical resection of involved lung tissue
   6. Osteoarticular sporotrichosis
      a. Drug of choice: itraconazole 200 mg twice daily for at least 12 months
      b. Alternatively, liposomal amphotericin B (3-5 mg/kg daily) or amphotericin B deoxycholate (0.7-1 mg/kg daily) can be used initially until infection is stable or if patient cannot tolerate itraconazole
   7. Disseminated sporotrichosis
      a. Treatment usually requires liposomal amphotericin B (5 mg/kg daily for 4-6 weeks)
      b. When patient is clinically stable, medication can be changed to itraconazole (200 mg twice daily)

Suggested Reading

Bustamante B, Campos PE. Endemic sporotrichosis. Curr Opin Infect Dis. 2001 Apr;14(2):145–9.

Kauffman CA. Sporotrichosis. Clin Infect Dis. 1999 Aug;29(2):231–6.

Kauffman CA, Bustamante B, Chapman SW, Pappas PG; Infectious Diseases Society of America. Clinical practice guidelines for the management of sporotrichosis: 2007 update by the Infectious Diseases Society of America. Clin Infect Dis. 2007 Nov 15;45(10):1255–65. Epub 2007 Oct 8.

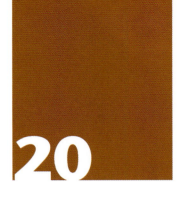

Shimon Kusne, MD
Ann E. McCullough, MD

Cryptococcus neoformans

I. Introduction
   A. Geographic Distribution
      1. Cryptococcosis is caused by 2 varieties of *Cryptococcus neoformans*
         a. *Cryptococcus neoformans* var *neoformans* (serotypes A and D)
         b. *Cryptococcus neoformans* var *gatti* (serotypes B and C)
      2. Serotypes A and D are found worldwide, mostly in avian droppings
      3. Serotypes B and C are found in tropical and subtropical countries in association with eucalyptus trees
   B. Mycology
      1. *Cryptococcus* is an encapsulated yeast
      2. Urease-positive
      3. Colonies are white and mucoid
      4. Grows at 37°C and appears on agar plate after 48 to 72 hours
      5. Main virulence factors
         a. Ability to grow at 37°C
         b. Mucopolysaccharide capsule
         c. Production of melanin owing to the enzyme laccase (a useful property for identifying the pigmented yeast on selective agars)
II. Cryptococcosis
   A. Epidemiology
      1. Risk factors
         a. Having human immunodeficiency virus (HIV) infection, lymphoproliferative malignancies, sarcoidosis, or diabetes mellitus
         b. Being a transplant recipient
         c. Receiving corticosteroid therapy
         d. Can also affect healthy hosts
         e. Age: very uncommon in children
      2. Serotypes A and D mostly affect immunocompromised hosts
      3. Serotypes B and C affect healthy hosts
      4. Nearly all cryptococcal infections in persons positive for HIV are caused by *C neoformans* var *neoformans*
      5. Historically regarded as causing infection in the tropics or subtropics, *C neoformans* var *gatti* has become an emerging cause of infection in the Pacific Northwest of the United States
         a. Primarily infects persons who do not have HIV infection
         b. At least 60 human infections and 15 deaths have been reported
         c. The most common clinical finding was pneumonia
   B. Pathogenesis
      1. Entry into the body: inhalation of yeast

2. Possible outcomes after inhalation of yeast
   a. Eliminated from host
   b. Disseminated to central nervous system (CNS), skin, and other organs
   c. Contained in the body: form a lung–lymph node complex and remain dormant in tissues
3. Severity of illness and dissemination depend on status of immune system: AIDS patients and transplant recipients generally have more serious illness than healthy hosts

C. Clinical Disease
  1. Cryptococcal pneumonia
     a. May be asymptomatic in one-third of healthy hosts
     b. Nonspecific symptoms: fever, cough, chest pain, and weight loss
     c. Chest radiography may show a lung nodule, infiltrates, hilar lymphadenopathy, or cavitation (Figure 20.1)
     d. In severely immunocompromised patients, acute respiratory distress syndrome may develop
     e. Serum cryptococcal antigen test may be negative in disease limited to the lung
     f. A positive serum cryptococcal antigen test for a patient with cryptococcal pneumonia is an indication for lumbar puncture to rule out CNS disease
  2. Cryptococcal CNS disease
     a. CNS involvement includes meningitis, meningoencephalitis, and mass lesions (cryptococcoma)
     b. Manifestation may be smoldering, especially in patients without AIDS
        1) Headache, fever, unstable gait, memory disturbances, and cranial nerve palsies
        2) Nuchal rigidity may be missing
        3) Patient may present with acute hydrocephalus and coma
        4) Computed tomographic scan may be normal in up to 50% of patients
  3. Skin lesions
     a. Cryptococcal skin lesions may be a manifestation of dissemination or, rarely, direct inoculation (eg, laboratory accident)
     b. Various lesions may appear, including papules, ulcers, plaques, and cellulitis
  4. The prostate may provide a sanctuary for the yeast and be involved with a relapse
  5. Eye involvement with cryptococcosis can be direct or indirect
     a. Optic neuritis due to infiltration of the optic nerve
     b. Ophthalmic artery compression due to cerebral edema and high intracranial pressure

D. Diagnosis
  1. Serology
     a. Detects cryptococcal polysaccharide antigen
     b. High sensitivity and specificity (90%-100%) for diagnosis of disseminated disease, including meningoencephalitis
     c. A negative result from only 1 tested specimen does not completely exclude cryptococcal infection, especially if infection is strongly suspected, but a positive result with serum or cerebrospinal fluid (CSF) is highly accurate for the disease
     d. Disseminated infection, especially in otherwise healthy hosts, is usually accompanied by a positive serum cryptococcal antigen test
     e. A CSF antigen titer can be monitored as an indicator of disease response in patients undergoing treatment
     f. Serum cryptococcal antigen is not helpful in management because changes in titer do not correlate with the clinical response
     g. False-positive results can occur rarely in the presence of rheumatoid factor or antigens shared with *Trichosporon beigelii* and *Capnocytophaga canimorsus*
  2. Microscopic examination
     a. India ink preparation of CSF

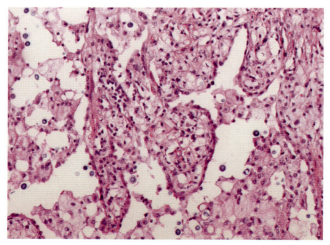

Figure 20.1. Open Lung Biopsy Specimen. Organizing cryptococcal pneumonia with histiocytic reaction. Cryptococci are visible as blue round yeast cells with lightly stained capsules (hematoxylin-eosin, original magnification ×200).

1) Shows the budding yeast (diameter, 3-10 μm) surrounded by the polysaccharide capsule
2) Artifacts and lymphocytes may interfere with its reading
3) Sensitivity ranges from 50% (in patients without AIDS) to more than 80% in patients with AIDS
   b. Organisms can also be seen with several common stains (Figure 20.2)
   c. *Cryptococcus* is unique in having a very thick, mucinous capsule, a feature emphasized with mucicarmine stain (Figure 20.3)
3. Culture
   a. Can grow on routine fungal media
   b. Culture is less sensitive than serology, but blood cultures are positive for 75% of patients who are positive for HIV and have cryptococcal meningitis
   c. White to cream-colored colonies appear in 48 to 72 hours with incubation
   d. Detection in culture in 3 to 7 days
   e. Identification
      1) Biochemical reactions
      2) Molecular methods
   f. Susceptibility testing by broth microdilution
      1) Break points have been adapted from *Candida* testing
      2) *Cryptococcus* may develop resistance to fluconazole and to flucytosine

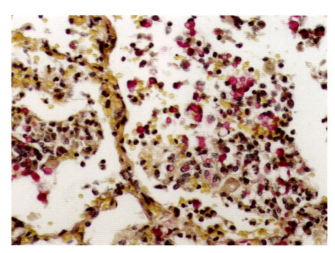

Figure 20.3. Lung Specimen. Disseminated *Cryptococcus* infection in alveolar parenchyma. Cryptococcal polysaccharide capsules stain pink (mucicarmine, original magnification ×200).

E. Treatment
   1. Treatment of cryptococcosis is summarized in Table 20.1
   2. Medication
      a. *Cryptococcus* is usually sensitive to amphotericin B (and its formulations), flucytosine, and azoles
      b. In cryptococcal meningitis, the combination of amphotericin B and flucytosine sterilizes CSF quicker than the azoles do
      c. Compared with amphotericin B alone, the combination of amphotericin B and flucytosine seems to decrease the frequency of relapse
   3. Treatment algorithm for cryptococcal meningoencephalitis in patients positive for HIV
      a. Intravenous amphotericin B (0.7-1.0 mg/kg daily) in combination with oral flucytosine (100 mg/kg daily) divided into 4 doses for 2 weeks (amphotericin B can be replaced by liposomal amphotericin B [3-4 mg/kg daily] or amphotericin B lipid complex [5 mg/kg daily])
      b. Consolidation therapy: oral fluconazole 400 mg daily for 8 weeks
      c. Long-term maintenance therapy
         1) Fluconazole 200 mg daily
         2) Alternative maintenance therapy: itraconazole 200 mg twice daily
         3) If patient cannot tolerate azoles: amphotericin B 1 mg/kg weekly
         4) Consider discontinuation of maintenance therapy when CD4 cell

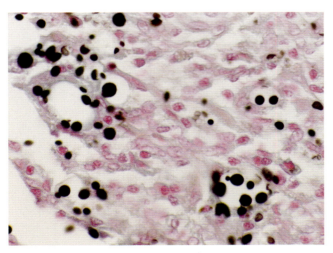

Figure 20.2. Lung Specimen. Cryptococcal granuloma contains round black yeast of various sizes (approximately 2-10 μm) with pinched base budding. The mucinous capsules are not visible with a silver stain (Gomori methenamine silver, original magnification ×400).

Table 20.1
Cryptococcosis: Clinical Features and Treatment

Site	Clinical Presentation	Pathogenesis and Diagnosis	Treatment
Patients Without AIDS			
Non-CNS			
Pulmonary	Patient may present with nonspecific symptoms Radiologic findings vary from single lung nodule to lobar infiltrate and even ARDS	Fungus is inhaled and initially causes lung infection, which may disseminate to other organs Invasiveness is supported by positive serum cryptococcal antigen Lumbar puncture is performed to rule out CNS infection	Severe disease is treated like CNS disease Mild to moderate disease is treated with oral fluconazole (400 mg daily for 6-12 mo) *or* itraconazole (200 mg twice daily) *or* voriconazole (200 mg twice daily) *or* posaconazole (400 mg twice daily)
Extrapulmonary	Examples are skin infection (papules, ulcerated lesions, or cellulitis) and bone infection Prostate may be a sanctuary site	Foci of infection indicate dissemination, but skin infection may result from direct inoculation Lumbar puncture is performed to rule out CNS infection	Generally treated like pulmonary infection, with severity taken into consideration
CNS	Patient may present with meningitis or mass lesion (cryptococcoma)	Usually dissemination from lung infection	Meningitis is treated with induction therapy for ≥4 wk: amphotericin B (0.7-1.0 mg/kg daily) with flucytosine (100 mg daily) Induction therapy is followed by oral fluconazole (200 mg daily for 6-12 mo) Liposomal amphotericin B (3-4 mg/kg daily) or amphotericin B lipid complex (5 mg/kg daily) can be given if patient cannot tolerate amphotericin B Immunosuppressed host may need longer treatments like patients with AIDS
Patients With AIDS			
Non-CNS			
Pulmonary	Patient may present with nonspecific symptoms	Fungus is inhaled Rule out dissemination to CNS with lumbar puncture	Pneumonia associated with CNS disease or dissemination or with ARDS is treated like CNS disease Mild to moderate disease: fluconazole (200-400 mg daily) long-term Alternative treatment: itraconazole (400 mg daily)
Extrapulmonary	As in patients without AIDS	As in patients without AIDS	Similar to treatment of pulmonary disease
CNS	Patients may present with fever, headache, confusion, seizure Classical signs and symptoms of meningitis are usually absent	As in patients without AIDS	Combination treatment: amphotericin B (0.7-1.0 mg/kg daily) with flucytosine (100 mg daily) for ≥2 wk Follow with fluconazole (400 mg daily) for ≥8 wk Maintenance: oral fluconazole (200 mg daily)

Abbreviations: ARDS, acute respiratory distress syndrome; CNS, central nervous system.

Data from Perfect JR, Dismukes WE, Dromer F, Goldman DL, Graybill JR, Hamill RJ, et al. Clinical practice guidelines for the management of cryptococcal disease: 2010 update by the Infectious Diseases Society of America. Clin Infect Dis. 2010 Feb 1;50(3):291–322.

count is more than 100/μL and the HIV viral load is undetectable for at least 3 months
   d. Alternative regimens
      1) Amphotericin B (0.7-1.0 mg/kg daily) or liposomal amphotericin B (3-4 mg/kg daily) or amphotericin B lipid complex (5 mg/kg daily) for 4 to 6 weeks
      2) Amphotericin B (0.7 mg/kg daily) in combination with oral fluconazole (800 mg daily) for 2 weeks, followed by oral fluconazole (800 mg daily) for 8 weeks
      3) Oral fluconazole (≥800 mg daily) in combination with flucytosine (100 mg daily) for 6 weeks
      4) Oral fluconazole (800-2,000 mg daily) for 10 to 12 weeks
      5) Oral itraconazole (200 mg twice daily) for 10 to 12 weeks
4. Treatment algorithm for cryptococcal meningoencephalitis in patients negative for HIV
   a. Similar to treatment of patients positive for HIV, but duration of treatment depends on severity of illness and immunosuppressive state
   b. Induction therapy: amphotericin B (0.7-1.0 mg/kg daily) in combination with flucytosine (100 mg/kg daily) for at least 4 weeks (the minimum of 4 weeks is for patients who have meningitis without complications and, after 2 weeks, a negative CSF fungal culture)
   c. Liposomal amphotericin B (3-4 mg/kg daily) or amphotericin B lipid complex (5 mg/kg daily) can be substituted for amphotericin B (and given in combination with flucytosine)
   d. After induction therapy, oral fluconazole (200 mg daily) is given for 6 to 12 months
5. Treatment of cryptococcal pneumonia in patients positive for HIV
   a. Dissemination and acute respiratory distress syndrome are treated like CNS infection
   b. Options for treatment when there is no dissemination: fluconazole, itraconazole, or fluconazole plus flucytosine
   c. Duration of treatment depends on immune recovery due to antiretroviral therapy
   d. Maintenance fluconazole therapy can be discontinued after 1 year if the CD4 cell count is more than 100/μL and the serum cryptococcal antigen is not increasing and is less than 1:512
6. Treatment of cryptococcal pneumonia in patients negative for HIV is indicated primarily in symptomatic patients
   a. Severe disease is treated like CNS disease
   b. Mild to moderate disease is treated with oral fluconazole (400 mg daily) for 6 to 12 months
   c. Other options: itraconazole (200 mg twice daily), voriconazole (200 mg twice daily), or posaconazole (400 mg twice daily)
   d. Amphotericin B: total dosage of 1 to 2 g
7. Management of increased intracranial pressure (>200 mm water), which is observed in more than 50% of patients who have cryptococcal meningitis
   a. Daily lumbar drainage to remove enough CSF to decrease the opening pressure by 50%
   b. Placement of a lumbar drain may be required

Suggested Reading

Perfect JR. *Cryptococcus neoformans*. In: Mandell GL, Bennett JE, Dolin R, editors. Mandell, Douglas, and Bennett's principles and practice of infectious diseases. Vol 2. 7th ed. Philadelphia (PA): Churchill Livingstone/Elsevier; 2010. p. 3287–304.

Perfect JR, Casadevall A. Cryptococcosis. Infect Dis Clin North Am. 2002 Dec;16(4):837–74.

Perfect JR, Dismukes WE, Dromer F, Goldman DL, Graybill JR, Hamill RJ, et al. Clinical practice guidelines for the management of cryptococcal disease: 2010 update by the Infectious Diseases Society of America. Clin Infect Dis. 2010 Feb 1;50(3):291–322.

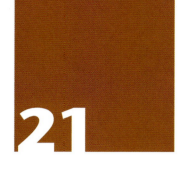

Holenarasipur R. Vikram, MD, FACP, FIDSA

Emerging Fungal Infections

I. Zygomycosis
   A. Microbiology
      1. Phylum Zygomycota, class Zygomycetes, orders Mucorales and Entomophthorales
      2. Saprophytic fungi with a worldwide distribution
      3. Found in soil and decaying organic matter
      4. *Rhizopus* species: most common etiologic agents for human disease, but many other genera are implicated
   B. Epidemiology
      1. Usually acquired through inhalation, ingestion, or cutaneous exposure
      2. Predisposing factors for zygomycosis are listed in Box 21.1
      3. Important modes of transmission for immunocompetent hosts: wound contamination, burns, and trauma
      4. Human-to-human transmission: none reported
      5. Increasing incidence of zygomycosis among patients with hematologic malignancies and bone marrow transplant recipients
         a. Mold infections in solid organ transplant recipients: 27% from non-aspergillus mycelial fungi; 5.7% from zygomycosis
         b. Prophylaxis or therapy with voriconazole, fluconazole, itraconazole, and caspofungin has been associated with breakthrough zygomycosis
      6. Primary site of infection depends on host predisposition
         a. Diabetes mellitus: rhinocerebral, sinus, and sino-orbital disease
         b. Malignancy and bone marrow transplant: pulmonary infection followed by sinus disease
         c. Solid organ transplant: similar frequencies of pulmonary and sinus infections
         d. Deferoxamine therapy: disseminated zygomycosis
         e. Intravenous drug users: cerebral zygomycosis
         f. No underlying condition: cutaneous zygomycosis
         g. Low-birth-weight infants, persons with malnutrition, persons receiving peritoneal dialysis: gastrointestinal zygomycosis
   C. Clinical Features
      1. Rhinocerebral zygomycosis
         a. Nonspecific symptoms such as fever, malaise, headache, and sinus congestion
         b. Serosanguinous or bloody nasal discharge, epistaxis, unilateral facial pain or swelling, black necrotic eschar on the palate or nasal mucosa

Box 21.1

Factors Predisposing Persons to Zygomycosis

Diabetes mellitus
    Diabetic ketoacidosis
    Poorly controlled diabetes mellitus
Chronic metabolic acidosis
    Renal failure
    Chronic salicylate poisoning
Deferoxamine therapy
Iron overload
Immunosuppression
    Neutropenia (due to malignancies or chemotherapy)
    Corticosteroid therapy
    Organ or hematopoietic cell transplant
    Human immunodeficiency virus infection
Skin or soft tissue breakdown
    Burn
    Trauma
    Surgical wound
Miscellaneous
    Intravenous illicit drug use
    Neonatal prematurity
    Malnourishment
    Prolonged use of broad-spectrum antimicrobial agents

Adapted from Chayakulkeeree M, Ghannoum MA, Perfect JR. Zygomycosis: the re-emerging fungal infection. Eur J Clin Microbiol Infect Dis. 2006 Apr;25(4):215–29 as adapted from text from Gonzalez CE, Rinaldi MG, Sugar AM. Zygomycosis. Infect Dis Clin North Am. 2002 Dec;16(4):895–914. Used with permission.

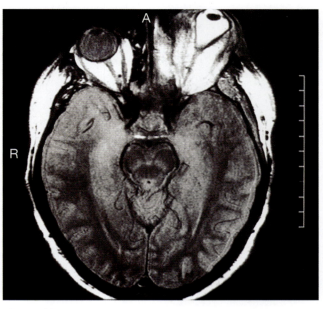

Figure 21.1. Rhinocerebral Zygomycosis. Magnetic resonance image shows orbital extension and diplopia caused by *Rhizopus oryzae*. A indicates anterior; R, right. (Adapted from Dr Fungus [Internet]. [cited 2010 Mar 30]. Available from: http://www.doctorfungus.org/imageban/images/Kaminski006/583.jpg. Used with permission.)

    c. Other conditions seen with progression: periorbital swelling, visual loss, ophthalmoplegia, diplopia, ptosis, proptosis, cranial neuropathies, cavernous sinus thrombosis, and cerebral abscess (Figure 21.1)
  2. Pulmonary zygomycosis
    a. Clinically resembles pulmonary aspergillosis: fever, cough, hemoptysis, pleuritic chest pain, or pleural effusion
    b. Disease may progress to involve contiguous organs such as the mediastinum and pericardium
  3. Cutaneous zygomycosis
    a. Findings include plaques, cellulitis, blisters, nodules, ulcerations, or lesions resembling ecthyma gangrenosum
    b. Deeper involvement may manifest as necrotizing fasciitis, myositis, or osteomyelitis
  4. Gastrointestinal zygomycosis
    a. Acquired through ingestion of contaminated food (fermented milk or bread products)
    b. Stomach is most commonly affected, followed by colon and ileum
    c. Nonspecific abdominal symptoms can progress to bowel perforation, peritonitis, or massive hemorrhage in the gastrointestinal tract
  5. Central nervous system (CNS) zygomycosis
    a. Rhinocerebral infection: 69% of patients
    b. Localized infection: 16% of patients
    c. Part of disseminated infection: 15% of patients
    d. Isolated CNS zygomycosis occurs in intravenous drug addicts
D. Diagnosis
  1. Histopathology
    a. For diagnosis, organism must be seen in tissue
    b. Useful stains include hematoxylin-eosin, Gomori methenamine silver (GMS), periodic acid-Schiff (PAS), calcofluor white
    c. Broad, hyaline, nonseptate fungal hyphae with wide-angled branching (Figure 21.2)
    d. Tissue necrosis and angioinvasion establish the diagnosis

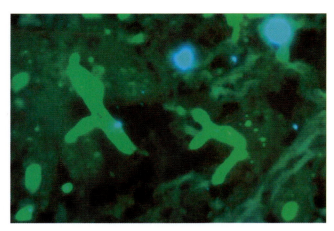

Figure 21.2. *Rhizopus arrhizus*. Fluorescent antibody staining shows broad, thin-walled, nonseptate hyphae. (Adapted from University of South Carolina [Internet]. [cited 2010 Mar 30]. Available from: http://pathmicro.med.sc.edu/mycology/Rhizopus.jpg.)

   2. Culture
      a. Growth in culture does not always indicate active infection
      b. Isolation of Mucorales fungi from a sterile body site or repeated isolation from a nonsterile site is clinically significant, especially for high-risk patients
      c. Blood cultures are seldom positive
      d. Mucorales fungi grow rapidly (1-2 days) on most fungal media (eg, Sabouraud dextrose agar incubated at 25°C-30°C)
      e. Antifungal susceptibility testing is not clinically useful: interpretive minimum inhibitory concentration break points have not been defined for Zygomycetes fungi
   E. Treatment and Prognosis
      1. Mortality rates of 37% to 100% among high-risk, immunocompromised patients
      2. Outcome is a function of the underlying condition, site of infection, and type of therapy (antifungal therapy with or without surgery)
      3. Antifungal agents
         a. Current drugs of choice for zygomycosis: amphotericin B and its lipid formulations
         b. Voriconazole and currently available echinocandins have no activity against Zygomycetes
         c. Posaconazole, a newer azole, has been used as salvage therapy for zygomycosis (reported success rates, 60%-80%)
      4. Adjunctive surgical débridement (whenever feasible) has been associated with better outcomes
      5. Crucial steps: correcting metabolic disturbances (hyperglycemia, acidosis), decreasing immunosuppression, or discontinuing deferoxamine therapy
      6. Used in refractory cases but not routinely recommended: colony-stimulating factors (CSFs), granulocyte transfusion, and hyperbaric oxygen
II. *Fusarium* Infection
   A. Microbiology
      1. *Fusarium* species are filamentous fungi widely distributed on plants and in soil
         a. Most species are common in tropical and subtropical areas
         b. Frequently cause disease in plants
      2. Species most often associated with human disease (fusariosis): *Fusarium solani*, *Fusarium oxysporum*, and *Fusarium chlamydosporum*
   B. Epidemiology
      1. Major predisposing factor: trauma
      2. Disseminated infection tends to develop in neutropenic patients and in bone marrow transplant recipients
      3. Localized infection tends to develop in solid organ transplant recipients
      4. Nosocomial outbreaks of fusariosis: water distribution systems and soil of potted plants in hospitals can lead to disseminated fusariosis in immunocompromised patients
   C. Clinical Features
      1. Keratitis, endophthalmitis, otitis media, cutaneous infections, onychomycosis, burn wound infections, mycetoma, sinusitis, pulmonary infections, endocarditis, peritonitis, intravascular catheter infections, septic arthritis, fungemia, and disseminated infections have been described
      2. Portal of entry: unknown in most cases
      3. Most likely means of exposure: inhalation, ingestion, or skin trauma
      4. Skin involvement in 50% to 70% of patients, contributing to the diagnosis of fusarial infection in the majority
         a. Immunocompromised patients
            1) Most frequent manifestation: multiple painful, erythematous, papular or nodular lesions with or without central necrosis (Figure 21.3)
            2) Necrotic lesions
               a) Resemble ecthyma gangrenosum
               b) Can be seen anywhere, but extremities are most often involved
               c) Tend to progress rapidly and are present in various stages

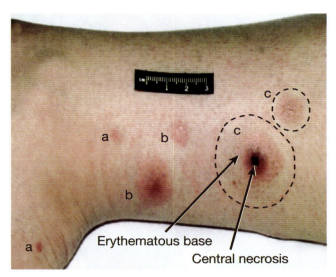

Figure 21.3. *Fusarium* Skin Lesions of Different Types and Ages. Lower extremity involvement in a 32-year-old woman with relapsed leukemia who had undergone allogeneic bone marrow transplant. Disseminated and fatal *Fusarium* infection developed. Lesions included small macular lesions (a), papular lesions of different sizes (b), and 2 target lesions (c) with central necrosis surrounded by an erythematous base, an area of normal skin, and an outer rim of thin erythema (dashed lines). (Adapted from Nucci M, Anaissie E. Cutaneous infection by *Fusarium* species in healthy and immunocompromised hosts: implications for diagnosis and management. Clin Infect Dis. 2002 Oct 15; 35[8]:909–20. Epub 2002 Sep 18. Used with permission.)

- 3) Metastatic skin lesions: associated with fungemia, neutropenia, and death
- 4) Preexisting onychomycosis can lead to local cellulitis and disseminated fusariosis in these patients
  b. Immunocompetent patients
  - 1) Cutaneous infection characterized by skin breakdown, localized involvement, and slow progression
  - 2) Good response to therapy
5. Keratitis
  a. *Fusarium* species are the most common cause of fungal keratitis
  b. A recent outbreak of *Fusarium* keratitis was linked to contaminated contact lens cleaning solution
6. Other clinical findings depend on the site of involvement
D. Diagnosis
  1. Direct examination
     a. Hyaline, septate, randomly branched hyphae in GMS or PAS stains
     b. Appearance resembles *Aspergillus*, *Paecilomyces*, *Acremonium*, and *Pseudallescheria*
  2. Culture
     a. Fungemia in 50% of patients (in contrast to other mold infections in which fungemia is uncommon)
     b. *Fusarium* species grow rapidly on Sabouraud dextrose agar at 25°C and produce cottony, flat colonies
     c. Cylindrical phialides bear characteristic sickle-shaped (or banana-shaped) multiseptate macroconidia (Figure 21.4)
E. Treatment and Prognosis
  1. *Fusarium* species (especially *F solani*) are among the most drug-resistant fungi
  2. Antifungal agents
     a. Drug of choice: amphotericin B (deoxycholate or lipid formulation)
     b. Voriconazole also has been used successfully
     c. *Fusarium* species are intrinsically resistant to currently available echinocandins
     d. Topical natamycin is used to treat *Fusarium* keratitis
     e. *Fusarium* mycetoma may respond to itraconazole
     f. *Fusarium* onychomycosis may be treated with itraconazole and ciclopirox nail lacquer
     g. Adjunctive granulocyte CSF, granulocyte-macrophage CSF, or granulocyte transfusion may be beneficial in some patients with disseminated fusariosis

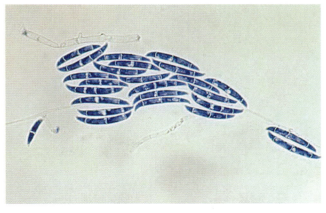

Figure 21.4. *Fusarium solani.* Sickle-shaped (or banana-shaped) multiseptate macroconidia are shown. (Adapted from Dr Fungus [Internet]. [cited 2010 Mar 30]. Available from: http://www.doctorfungus.org/imageban/images/Kaminski005/468.jpg. Used with permission.)

3. Prognosis of disseminated fusariosis: dismal
    a. Predictors of poor prognosis among patients with hematologic malignancies and *Fusarium* infection: persistent neutropenia, disseminated infection, corticosteroid use (therapy for graft-versus-host disease), and stem cell transplant

III. *Pseudallescheria boydii* Infection
   A. Microbiology
      1. A hyaline filamentous fungus
      2. Septate, acute-branching hyphae (resembles aspergillus)
      3. Asexual state: *Scedosporium apiospermum*
   B. Epidemiology
      1. Found worldwide in soil, sewage, polluted water, decaying vegetation, and manure of farm animals
      2. Transmission: inhalation or transcutaneous
   C. Clinical Features
      1. Asymptomatic colonization possible
      2. Chronic subcutaneous infection: mycetoma
      3. Deep or disseminated infection: pseudallescheriasis
         a. Most common sites: lung, bone, joints, and CNS
         b. Sinusitis, keratitis (Figure 21.5), cutaneous infections, lymphadenitis, endophthalmitis, meningoencephalitis, endocarditis, brain abscess, pneumonia, lung abscess, allergic bronchopulmonary disease, bursitis, and urethritis have been described
         c. Disseminated infection
            1) Especially in immunocompromised patients
               a) Most (69%) *Scedosporium* infections develop in hematopoietic stem cell transplant recipients
               b) About half (53%) develop in organ transplant recipients
            2) Predilection to involve the CNS
               a) Brain abscess: 77% (solitary, 41%; multiple, 36%)
               b) Meningitis: 28%
               c) *Scedosporium* infection in 32% to 48% of solid organ transplant patients
      4. Several cases of *P boydii* pneumonia with CNS dissemination have been described after near-drowning events in dirty water (sewage or polluted, stagnant, or muddy water)
      5. Invasive pulmonary pseudallescheriasis
         a. Risk factors
            1) Prolonged neutropenia
            2) Prolonged corticosteroid therapy
            3) Acquired immunodeficiency syndrome
            4) Allogeneic bone marrow transplant
         b. Clinical features include cough, pleuritic chest pain, hemoptysis, and fever
      6. Traumatic implantation of fungus
         a. From activity related to soil or water
            1) Localized disease involving the eye, cutaneous tissue, bone, or osteoarticular areas
            2) Host may be immunocompetent or immunocompromised
         b. From surgery, intravenous drug use, or corticosteroid injections
   D. Diagnosis
      1. Direct examination
         a. Resembles aspergillus
         b. Histopathology may show angioinvasion and thrombosis
      2. Culture
         a. Isolation from sterile site is diagnostic
         b. Grows well in standard mycologic media at 25°C
      3. Serology: not useful
      4. Radiology
         a. Chest radiograph or computed tomographic scan may show nodules, infiltrates, or cavitation
         b. Brain imaging may show solitary or multiple ring-enhancing lesions suggestive of abscesses

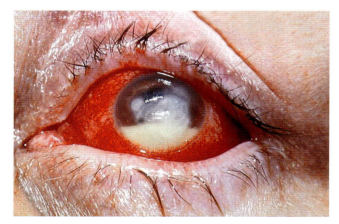

Figure 21.5. *Pseudallescheria boydii* Keratitis. Features include central shaggy corneal ulcer, satellite lesion, and marked hypopyon. (Adapted from Dr Fungus [Internet]. [cited 2010 Mar 30]. Available from: http://www.doctorfungus.org/imageban/images/Kaminski005/464.jpg. Used with permission.)

- E. Treatment and Prognosis
  1. Antifungal agents
     a. *Pseudallescheria boydii* is resistant to amphotericin B
     b. Treatment of choice: voriconazole
     c. Possible synergy between voriconazole and terbinafine
     d. Topical miconazole can be used for keratitis
  2. Adjunctive surgical therapy should be considered for sinusitis, keratitis, brain abscess, or infections of bones, joints, or soft tissues
  3. Prognosis
     a. Mortality for CNS pseudallescheriasis is greater than 75%
     b. For transplant recipients (bone marrow and solid organ), mortality from scedosporiosis is 58%
     c. Disseminated infection predicts shorter survival
     d. Adjunctive surgery independently predicts longer survival
- IV. Dematiaceous Fungal Infection
  - A. Microbiology
    1. A loose grouping of diverse fungi in the family Dematiaceae
    2. Cell walls contain melanin, which may contribute to virulence
    3. Most important human pathogens include *Alternaria* species, *Bipolaris* species, *Cladophialophora bantiana*, *Curvularia* species, *Exophiala* species, *Fonsecaea pedrosoi*, *Madurella* species, *Phialophora* species, *Scedosporium prolificans*, *Scytalidium dimidiatum*, and *Wangiella dermatitidis*
  - B. Epidemiology
    1. Widespread in the environment in soil, wood, and decomposing organic debris
    2. Common in tropical and subtropical countries
  - C. Clinical Features
    1. Various clinical manifestations
    2. Skin and soft tissue infections
       a. Dermatomycosis, onychomycosis, tinea nigra, black piedra, and eumycotic mycetoma
       b. Eumycotic mycetoma: chronic infection of cutaneous and subcutaneous tissues
          1) Adjacent bone can be involved
          2) Abscesses contain large masses of fungal elements that are discharged to the outside as grains through draining sinuses
          3) Most cases involve the feet
    3. Cerebral phaeohyphomycosis
       a. Most common form of systemic phaeohyphomycosis
       b. From hematogenous dissemination after inhalation
       c. Most frequently isolated species include *Cladophialophora bantiana* and *Ramichloridium mackenziei* (Figure 21.6)
       d. Large proportion of patients have no underlying immune deficiency
    4. Disseminated phaeohyphomycosis
       a. Majority of patients have an underlying immune dysfunction
       b. Most common causes: *Scedosporium prolificans* (42%), *Bipolaris spicifera* (8%), and *Wangiella dermatitidis* (7%)
       c. Involves virtually any organ: blood, lung, brain, heart, skin, kidney, liver, spleen, lymph nodes, bone, and joints
    5. Fungal keratitis: dematiaceous molds are the third most common etiologic agents (after *Fusarium* species and *Aspergillus* species)
  - D. Diagnosis
    1. Direct examination
       a. Branching, septate hyphae that appear brown with potassium hydroxide preparation or hematoxylin-eosin stain
       b. Special stain for melanin: Fontana-Masson
    2. Culture
       a. Growth of fungus in tissue specimens
       b. Blood cultures positive for 50% of patients with disseminated disease (especially with *Scedosporium prolificans*)
  - E. Treatment and Prognosis
    1. Treatment is summarized in Table 21.1
    2. No effective antifungal therapy for *Scedosporium prolificans* infection
    3. Cerebral phaeohyphomycosis and disseminated phaeohyphomycosis carry a poor prognosis
- V. Other Emerging Fungal Infections
  - A. *Malassezia* Infection
    1. *Malassezia* species, especially *Malassezia furfur*
    2. Yeasts: part of normal human skin flora
    3. Require long-chain fatty acids for growth in vitro
    4. Cause catheter-related sepsis in patients receiving parenteral lipids through a central venous catheter
    5. Causative agent of pityriasis versicolor (also called tinea versicolor)
    6. Can also cause folliculitis
    7. Catheter-related infections: treated with amphotericin B, itraconazole, or voriconazole

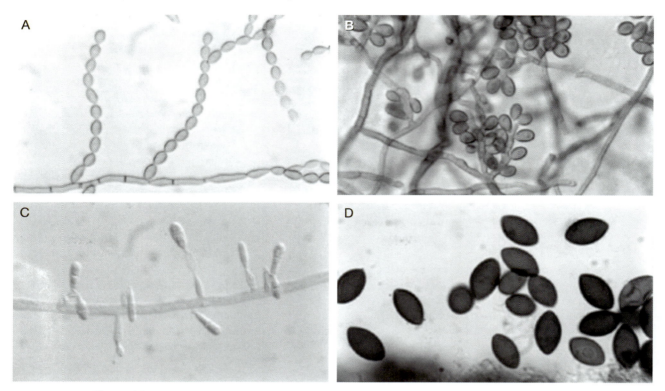

Figure 21.6. Fungi That Are Common Etiologic Agents of Central Nervous System Phaeohyphomycosis. A, *Cladophialophora bantiana*; B, *Ramichloridium mackenziei*; C, *Ochroconis gallopavum*; and D, *Chaetomium strumarium* (original magnification ×920). (Adapted from Revankar SG, Sutton DA, Rinaldi MG. Primary central nervous system phaeohyphomycosis: a review of 101 cases. Clin Infect Dis. 2004 Jan 15;38[2]:206–16. Epub 2003 Dec 19. Used with permission.)

Table 21.1
Treatment of Infections Caused by Dematiaceous Fungi

Infection	Treatment	Comments
Tinea nigra	Topical antifungals	
Dermatomycosis	Itraconazole	
Onychomycosis	Itraconazole	
Keratitis	Débridement Topical natamycin Clotrimazole Miconazole Ketoconazole	Discontinue use of oral corticosteroids Corneal transplant may be required
Mycetoma	Débridement followed by long-term therapy with itraconazole or ketoconazole	
Allergic fungal sinusitis	Surgical removal of impacted mucin followed by oral corticosteroids	Recurrence is common Uncertain role for antifungals
Invasive fungal sinusitis	Extensive surgical débridement followed by amphotericin B	Role of newer antifungal agents is unclear Voriconazole and posaconazole have in vitro activity
Cerebral phaeohyphomycosis	Amphotericin B alone or in combination with flucytosine and itraconazole	Role of newer antifungal agents is unclear High mortality
Disseminated phaeohyphomycosis	Amphotericin B and surgical débridement (if feasible)	Role of newer antifungal agents is unclear Voriconazole and posaconazole have in vitro activity High mortality

B. *Trichosporon* Infection
1. *Trichosporon* species are pathogenic yeasts that inhabit skin and respiratory tract
2. Superficial infection of hair shafts is known as white piedra
3. *Trichosporon beigelii* causes catheter-associated fungemia and disseminated infection in neutropenic patients
   a. Resembles disseminated candidiasis
   b. Endocarditis, peritonitis, esophagitis, endophthalmitis, cholangitis, and hepatitis have been reported
   c. Itraconazole, voriconazole, and posaconazole appear to be potent in vitro
C. *Paecilomyces* Infection
1. *Paecilomyces* species are asexual fungi related to *Penicillium*
2. Frequent airborne contaminants in clinical specimens
3. Contamination of extended-wear contact lenses and ocular surgery can result in corneal ulcer, keratitis, or endophthalmitis
4. Disseminated infection in immunocompromised patients can involve any organ system
5. Human disease is caused by 2 species: *Paecilomyces varioti* and *Paecilomyces lilacinus*
   a. *Paecilomyces varioti* is thermophilic and can grow at 50°C to 60°C
   b. Amphotericin B: *Paecilomyces varioti* is susceptible, but *Paecilomyces lilacinus* is resistant
   c. Voriconazole and posaconazole: appear to be active against *Paecilomyces lilacinus*
D. *Saccharomyces cerevisiae* Infection
1. *Saccharomyces cervisiae* fungemia: 60 cases reported
   a. Probiotics were being used by 50%
   b. Other risk factors: stay in intensive care unit, presence of a central venous catheter, and enteral or parenteral nutrition
   c. Clinical features: fungemia, endocarditis, disseminated disease, liver abscess, and esophageal ulcer
   d. Mortality: 28%
2. Antifungal Agents
   a. Drug of choice: amphotericin B
   b. Fluconazole and itraconazole: strains may show resistance
   c. Voriconazole and posaconazole: good in vitro activity

Suggested Reading

Brandt ME, Warnock DW. Epidemiology, clinical manifestations, and therapy of infections caused by dematiaceous fungi. J Chemother. 2003 Nov;15 Suppl 2:36–47.

Chayakulkeeree M, Ghannoum MA, Perfect JR. Zygomycosis: the re-emerging fungal infection. Eur J Clin Microbiol Infect Dis. 2006 Apr;25(4):215–29.

Ender PT, Dolan MJ. Pneumonia associated with near-drowning. Clin Infect Dis. 1997 Oct;25(4):896–907.

Fleming RV, Walsh TJ, Anaissie EJ. Emerging and less common fungal pathogens. Infect Dis Clin North Am. 2002 Dec;16(4):915–33.

Husain S, Alexander BD, Munoz P, Avery RK, Houston S, Pruett T, et al. Opportunistic mycelial fungal infections in organ transplant recipients: emerging importance of non-Aspergillus mycelial fungi. Clin Infect Dis. 2003 Jul 15; 37(2):221–9. Epub 2003 Jul 9.

Husain S, Munoz P, Forrest G, Alexander BD, Somani J, Brennan K, et al. Infections due to *Scedosporium apiospermum* and *Scedosporium prolificans* in transplant recipients: clinical characteristics and impact of antifungal agent therapy on outcome. Clin Infect Dis. 2005 Jan 1; 40(1):89–99. Epub 2004 Dec 8.

Munoz P, Bouza E, Cuenca-Estrella M, Eiros JM, Perez MJ, Sanchez-Somolinos M, et al. *Saccharomyces cerevisiae* fungemia: an emerging infectious disease. Clin Infect Dis. 2005 Jun 1;40(11):1625–34. Epub 2005 Apr 25.

Nesky MA, McDougal EC, Peacock Jr JE. *Pseudallescheria boydii* brain abscess successfully treated with voriconazole and surgical drainage: case report and literature review of central nervous system pseudallescheriasis. Clin Infect Dis. 2000 Sep;31(3):673–7. Epub 2000 Sep 27.

Nucci M, Anaissie E. Cutaneous infection by *Fusarium* species in healthy and immunocompromised hosts: implications for diagnosis and management. Clin Infect Dis. 2002 Oct 15; 35(8):909–20. Epub 2002 Sep 18.

Nucci M, Anaissie EJ, Queiroz-Telles F, Martins CA, Trabasso P, Solza C, et al. Outcome predictors of 84 patients with hematologic malignancies and *Fusarium* infection. Cancer. 2003 Jul 15;98(2):315–9.

Revankar SG, Patterson JE, Sutton DA, Pullen R, Rinaldi MG. Disseminated phaeohyphomycosis: review of an emerging mycosis. Clin Infect Dis. 2002 Feb 15;34(4):467–76. Epub 2002 Jan 9.

Revankar SG, Sutton DA, Rinaldi MG. Primary central nervous system phaeohyphomycosis: a review of 101 cases. Clin Infect Dis. 2004 Jan 15;38(2):206–16. Epub 2003 Dec 19.

Roden MM, Zaoutis TE, Buchanan WL, Knudsen TA, Sarkisova TA, Schaufele RL, et al. Epidemiology and outcome of zygomycosis: a review of 929 reported cases. Clin Infect Dis. 2005 Sep 1;41(5):634–53. Epub 2005 Jul 29.

van Burik JA, Hare RS, Solomon HF, Corrado ML, Kontoyiannis DP. Posaconazole is effective as salvage therapy in zygomycosis: a retrospective summary of 91 cases. Clin Infect Dis. 2006 Apr 1;42(7):e61–5. Epub 2006 Feb 21. Erratum in: Clin Infect Dis. 2006 Nov 15;43(10):1376.

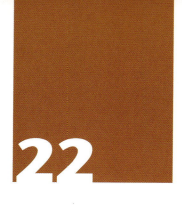

Jon E. Rosenblatt, MD
Bobbi S. Pritt, MD

Parasitic Infections

I. Introduction
   A. Protozoa
      1. Protozoa are single-celled, microscopic eukaryotic organisms (eg, amebae, *Giardia*)
      2. Intestinal protozoa
         a. Usually confined to the gastrointestinal (GI) tract (eg, *Giardia, Cryptosporidium, Cyclospora*) and cause secretory or watery diarrhea
         b. However, some are invasive (*Entamoeba histolytica, Balantidium coli*), producing ulceration of the GI tract or abscesses in other organs (liver, kidney, and lung)
         c. Have both cysts (transmissible form that survives outside the GI tract) and trophozoites (motile invasive or "attachment" form)
      3. Extraintestinal protozoa
         a. Some invade the bloodstream (eg, *Plasmodium, Babesia*)
         b. Some invade cells of various organs, including the central nervous system (CNS) (eg, *Leishmania, Trypanosoma, Toxoplasma, Acanthamoeba, Naegleria, Balamuthia*)
   B. Helminths
      1. Helminths are parasitic worms
         a. Nematodes (roundworms)
         b. Cestodes (tapeworms)
         c. Trematodes (flukes)
      2. Multicellular organisms
      3. Some are microscopic (eg, microfilaria, *Strongyloides* larvae, roundworm eggs)
      4. Some are visible grossly, with lengths from many centimeters (eg, adult ascarids) to many meters (eg, adult tapeworms)
      5. Adults do not multiply in the definitive host
   C. Arthropods
      1. Arthropods (eg, ticks, mites) are generally considered parasites since diagnostic parasitology laboratories are usually responsible for their identification
II. Intestinal Protozoa
   A. *Giardia lamblia* (also called *Giardia duodenalis*)
      1. Microscopic morphology
         a. Trophozoites have flagella and the appearance of 2 eyes (Figure 22.1)
         b. Cysts are football shaped and can be difficult to detect
      2. *Giardia* is the most common intestinal parasite in the United States
      3. Worldwide distribution
      4. Infection through contaminated food or water, including streams, lakes, and municipal surface water supplies

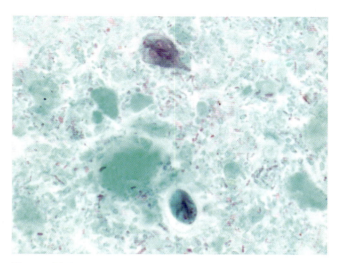

Figure 22.1. *Giardia lamblia* trophozoite (top) and cyst (bottom) (modified trichrome, original magnification ×1,000).

contaminated by wild animals such as beavers
  a. Hikers and campers are at risk
  b. Potentially contaminated water should be treated by boiling, iodine purification, or filtration (≤2 μm filter)
5. Fecal-oral transmission from infected children occurs frequently in child care settings (eg, from unsanitary handling of diapers)
6. Symptoms include watery diarrhea, cramping, bloating, and sulfuric belching and flatulence
  a. Diarrhea is usually self-limited
  b. Diarrhea can cause chronic syndrome of weight loss and malabsorption
7. Diagnosis
  a. Antigen detection with enzyme immunoassay (EIA) or direct fluorescent antibody (DFA)
  b. Microscopic examination of stool for ova and parasites
    1) Multiple examinations may be necessary since the parasite resides in the small intestine and is excreted intermittently
    2) Duodenal aspirates may also be diagnostic but are not more sensitive than multiple stool examinations
8. Treatment
  a. Metronidazole: most commonly used and effective, although it has never been approved by the US Food and Drug Administration (FDA) for this purpose
  b. Tinidazole: an alternative imidazole
  c. Nitazoxanide
  d. Paromomycin: may be a choice for pregnant women
  e. Quinacrine: also effective but not available in the United States
  f. Other agents: albendazole and furazolidone (often used in children)

B. *Cryptosporidium*
  1. Classification: subclass Coccidia, phylum Apicomplexa (also includes *Toxoplasma* and *Plasmodium*)
  2. Microscopic morphology (Figure 22.2)
    a. Sporozoite within a *Cryptosporidium* cyst
    b. Cysts are 4 to 6 μm in diameter
    c. Identified with acid-fast stain
  3. *Cryptosporidium hominis* and *Cryptosporidium parvum* are the 2 species that most commonly infect humans
  4. Outbreaks
    a. Associated with drinking water contaminated from agricultural (cattle) runoff or human fecal contamination of swimming pools, water parks, or day care centers
    b. Largest waterborne disease outbreak in the United States was in 1993 in Milwaukee: 403,000 were infected
    c. Usual chlorination methods may be ineffective in eliminating organism
  5. Clinical disease
    a. Main symptom is secretory watery diarrhea, which may be accompanied by abdominal pain, fever, and vomiting
    b. Diarrhea may be more severe and prolonged in patients with AIDS

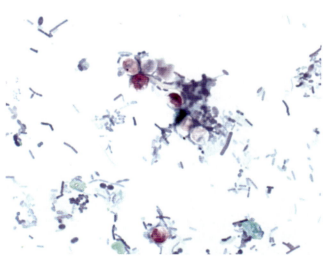

Figure 22.2. *Cryptosporidium* species (modified acid-fast, original magnification ×1,000).

c. Organism is found in upper small intestine (occasionally in stomach and biliary tree), where it adheres to intestinal cells and is covered by a layer of parasitic (or host) material but does not penetrate into the cytoplasm of the intestinal cell
6. Diagnosis
   a. By acid-fast staining or by antigen detection with DFA or EIA methods
   b. May be difficult to see in routine microscopic examination for ova and parasites
7. Treatment
   a. Disease is self-limited in immunocompetent persons
   b. Nitazoxanide, 500 mg orally twice daily for 3 days, may shorten duration
   c. No proven effective therapy for patients who have AIDS or who are otherwise immunosuppressed, but nitazoxanide or paromomycin (alone or in combination with azithromycin) may alleviate some symptoms

C. *Cyclospora cayetanensis*
1. Microscopic morphology
   a. Characteristics are similar to those of *Cryptosporidium*, but cysts are twice as large (diameter, 8-12 μm) (originally called "crypto grande")
   b. Stains with acid-fast or safranin
   c. Cannot be seen in usual ova and parasites examination without special stains
2. Clinical disease
   a. Outbreaks associated with produce (snow peas) and fresh fruit (raspberries) imported from Guatemala
   b. Causes secretory watery diarrhea, often accompanied by prolonged systemic symptoms (eg, malaise, weakness, fatigue)
3. Treatment: diarrhea responds well to trimethoprim-sulfamethoxazole, 1 double-strength tablet twice daily for 7 to 10 days

D. *Isospora belli*
1. Microscopic morphology
   a. Characteristics are similar to those of *Cryptosporidium*, but cysts are 4 times as large (diameter, 16-25 μm), are often binucleate, and are oblong or egg-shaped
   b. Visible with acid-fast stain, but usually are large and characteristic appearance can be seen on ova and parasites examination without special stains
2. Clinical disease
   a. Can penetrate intestinal cells into the cytoplasm
   b. Causes secretory watery diarrhea
   c. Much less common than other protozoan infections
   d. Causes sporadic cases of diarrhea, probably by person-to-person transmission, most often in immunosuppressed patients
3. Diagnosis: routine microscopic examination for ova and parasites
4. Treatment: diarrhea usually responds well to trimethoprim-sulfamethoxazole, 1 double-strength tablet twice daily for 10 days

E. Microsporida
1. An order of protozoa-like intracellular organisms (recent genetic evidence and presence of chitin suggest these may be fungi)
2. Very small (diameter, 1-2 μm, which is the approximate size of bacteria)
3. Clinical disease
   a. Watery diarrhea primarily in patients who have AIDS or who are otherwise immunosuppressed
      1) *Enterocytozoon bieneusi* and *Encephalitozoon intestinalis* are the primary agents of diarrheal disease
      2) Other *Encephalitozoon* species can cause disseminated infections
   b. Invasion of enterocytes (Figure 22.3): spores extrude polar tubules that penetrate cells and inject contents followed by multiplication within the cell
4. Diagnosis
   a. Organisms are detected in stool with trichrome-blue stain
   b. Also stains with calcofluor white because of chitinous surface

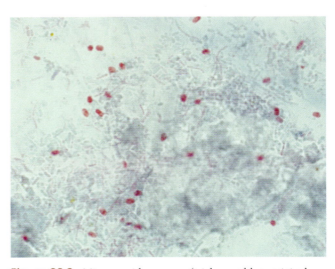

Figure 22.3. Microsporidan spores (trichrome blue, original magnification ×1,000).

c. Difficult to recognize because of small size and morphologic similarity with bacteria and yeasts
d. Not detected with routine microscopic examination for ova and parasites
5. Treatment: albendazole 400 mg orally twice daily for 2 to 4 weeks
a. Effective against *Encephalitozoon* but only variable activity against *E bieneusi*

F. *Dientamoeba fragilis*
1. Pathogenicity
a. Debated in the past but now seems certain that organism is a somewhat infrequent cause of diarrhea both sporadically and in localized outbreaks, especially in children
b. Causes mild to moderate mucosal inflammation and shallow ulcerations with no deep penetration into or beyond intestinal wall
2. Microscopic morphology
a. Small ameba (diameter, 5-15 μm) related to the trichomonads
b. Characterized by binucleate trophozoites with no recognizable cyst form
c. Definitive identification requires permanent stains such as trichrome or iron hematoxylin
3. Diagnosis: microscopic examination of stool for ova and parasites with use of permanently stained smears for specific identification
4. Mode of transmission
a. With absence of cyst form, fecal-oral route is questioned
b. Some evidence points to association with pinworms as a vehicle
5. Treatment
a. Effective therapy of choice: iodoquinol, 650 mg orally 3 times daily for 20 days
b. Alternatives: paromomycin, tetracycline, and metronidazole

G. *Blastocystis hominis*
1. Taxonomy: uncertain
2. Pathogenicity
a. Observed in up to 50% of stools from healthy patients
b. There is no definitive evidence that it is a pathogen or is associated with clinical disease
3. Treatment
a. There is no proven effective therapy
b. There are reports of responses to metronidazole
1) Metronidazole, however, is active against a wide spectrum of bacterial and parasitic organisms
2) *Blastocystis* often persists in the stools of many patients who seem to respond to metronidazole

H. *Entamoeba histolytica*
1. An intestinal protozoan primarily of humans
2. Causes as many as 50 million infections worldwide
3. Transmission: wherever poor sanitation allows for fecal contamination of food and water
4. Microscopic morphology
a. Cyst diameter: 10-15 μm (Figure 22.4)
b. Trophozoite diameter: 10-50 μm (Figure 22.5)

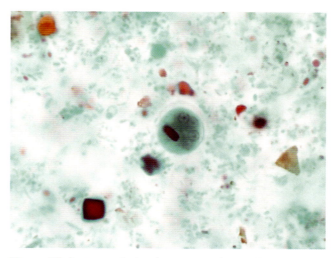

Figure 22.4. *Entamoeba histolytica* cyst with 4 nuclei and a large chromatoid bar (modified trichrome, original magnification ×1,000).

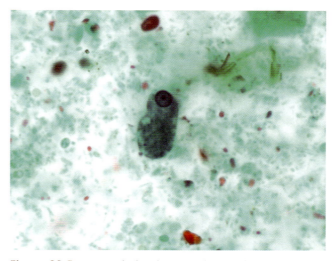

Figure 22.5. *Entamoeba histolytica* trophozoite (modified trichrome, original magnification ×1,000).

5. Pathogenicity
   a. Cysts
      1) Survive outside the body for prolonged periods
      2) Resistant to stomach acidity after ingestion
   b. Trophozoites
      1) Excyst in the terminal ileum or colon
      2) Invade the intestinal mucosa (secretes cytolytic cysteine proteinases)
      3) Produce characteristic undermined ulcers, which may lead to perforation or to dissemination to the liver (or other organs, especially the lung and brain)
      4) Liver abscess is the most frequent complication of disseminated amebiasis
6. *Entamoeba dispar*
   a. Morphologically indistinguishable from *E histolytica*
   b. Nonpathogenic and may be responsible for many of the asymptomatic carriers of amebae
   c. Can only be identified by molecular or immunologic methods
7. Morbidity and mortality
   a. An estimated 40,000 to 100,000 people die annually from amebiasis (death from colitis, liver abscesses, or other complications)
   b. Infection is most prevalent in developing countries
      1) Mexico: about 8% of the population is infected
      2) Vietnam: 21 cases of liver abscess per 100,000 population in city of Hue
      3) Bangladesh: 2.2% of schoolchildren have amebic dysentery
   c. Most cases in the United States occur in immigrants or travelers
8. Diagnosis
   a. Suspected from microscopic examination for ova and parasites, especially if elongated trophozoites with ingested erythrocytes are present
   b. Definitive identification of *E histolytica*: confirmed with specific stool EIA (detects galactose/*N*-acetylgalactosamine lectin)
   c. Serology
      1) May be useful in the diagnosis of abscesses (in liver or other organs), especially if stool examination results are negative
      2) Seroreactivity may persist, however, from a prior infection and should be evaluated with caution in patients from endemic areas
9. Treatment
   a. Noninvasive intestinal amebiasis: iodoquinol or paromomycin
   b. Invasive intestinal or extraintestinal infection: metronidazole (500-750 mg 3 times daily for 7-10 days) or the longer-acting tinidazole (2 g daily for 5 days)
   c. Intestinal amebae may persist after invasive disease is treated, so treatment of invasive disease should be followed by treatment to eradicate the intraluminal infection (paramomycin or iodoquinol)

I. *Balantidium coli*
1. Microscopic morphology (Figure 22.6)
   a. A ciliate
   b. The largest and least common protozoan pathogen
   c. Diameter of oval trophozoite: 10 to 15 μm or as large as 200 μm
2. Pathogenicity
   a. After ingestion of cysts, trophozoites are released and colonize the large intestine, where multiplication and cyst formation occur
   b. Pigs are the main reservoir for human infection, which is often acquired from the ingestion of food or water contaminated with pig feces

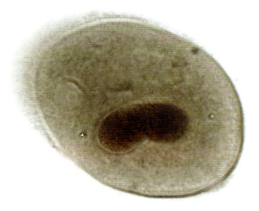

Figure 22.6. *Balantidium coli* trophozoite in unstained wet mount. Note circumferential cilia and kidney bean–shaped nucleus (original magnification ×1,000).

c. Most infections are asymptomatic, but clinical manifestations may include chronic diarrhea and abdominal pain or, rarely, a fulminant colitis resulting in intestinal perforation
3. Diagnosis: the motile trophozoites are found in fresh stool or in stained, fixed specimens
4. Treatment
   a. Treatment of choice: tetracycline (500 mg 4 times daily for 10 days)
   b. Also effective: iodoquinol, metronidazole, and paromomycin

III. Extraintestinal Protozoa
  A. Free-living Amebae: *Acanthamoeba*, *Balamuthia*, and *Naegleria*
    1. Protozoan amebae that are ubiquitous in the environment, especially in water or warm, moist soil
    2. They infect humans when cysts contact mucosal surfaces (eg, when people swim or jump into water) or lacerated or abraded tissue (eg, scratched cornea)
       a. Cysts evolve into trophozoites that are locally invasive
       b. Trophozoites may produce ulcers in the mucosa of the mouth and nose or on the cornea
       c. Trophozoites may migrate to the CNS and cause meningitis or encephalitis
    3. *Acanthamoeba*
       a. Causes granulomatous amebic encephalitis and amebic keratitis
       b. Causes cutaneous lesions and sinusitis in immunocompromised persons
       c. Ample opportunities for persons (healthy or immunocompromised) to have contact with these organisms
          1) Found in different soil and environmental water sources
          2) Found in swimming pools, air conditioning units, dental and dialysis treatment units, eyewash stations, and contact lenses (and contact lens solutions and containers)
       d. Granulomatous amebic encephalitis
          1) A chronic infection progressing slowly over several weeks or months
          2) Multifocal hemorrhagic necrosis, edema, and an inflammatory exudate composed mainly of leukocytes
          3) Trophozoites can be seen in brain tissue and can be detected in cerebrospinal fluid (CSF) by microscopy and culture
          4) There is no standard therapy, but several agents have been used in patients
             a) Trimethoprim (or pyrimethamine) in combination with a sulfa
             b) Ketoconazole or fluconazole
       e. Amebic keratitis
          1) Diagnosis: microscopy and culture of corneal scrapings (typical hexacanth-shaped cysts are seen) (Figure 22.7)
          2) Various topical treatments have been successful
             a) Propamidine plus neomycin-polymyxin-gramicidin ophthalmic solution
             b) Polyhexamethylene biguanide or chlorhexidine ophthalmic solution
    4. *Balamuthia mandrillaris*
       a. A recently described soil ameba
       b. Causes encephalitis in immunocompromised and healthy hosts, especially children
       c. Pathogenesis
          1) Infection is thought to be acquired by invasion of cysts through the respiratory tree or through breaks in the skin
          2) Organism is then transported hematogenously to the CNS, where it causes a granulomatous encephalitis
       d. Diagnosis
          1) Most diagnoses are made at autopsy by identifying the cysts in brain tissue sections

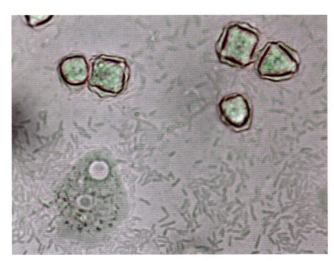

Figure 22.7. *Acanthamoeba* species in unstained culture preparation showing cysts with double wall (upper right) and single trophozoite (bottom left). Bacteria in background are a food source for the trophozoites (original magnification ×40).

2) Specific indirect immunofluorescence has been used to identify *Balamuthia mandrillaris* in tissue but is not generally available
  e. Therapy
    1) There is no recommended therapy
    2) Two patients who survived were reported to have been treated with combinations of pentamidine, flucytosine, fluconazole, sulfadiazine, and a macrolide antibiotic (clarithromycin or azithromycin)
5. *Naegleria fowleri*
  a. Causes primary amebic meningoencephalitis, a severe and most frequently fatal CNS infection, often associated with swimming in warm water ponds, small lakes, or rivers
  b. Infection progresses rapidly and responds poorly to therapy, although amphotericin B (intravenously and intrathecally) plus rifampin may have some benefit
  c. Diagnosis
    1) Amebic trophozoites can be seen on microscopy of fresh, unstained CSF
    2) Trophozoites may be overlooked, however, because of the many similarly appearing polymorphonuclear neutrophils that are usually present
    3) Trichrome-stained smears can help identify the amebae, which can be cultured on ordinary agar plates seeded with *Escherichia coli*
B. *Plasmodium*
  1. Malaria
    a. Four species cause most malaria in humans: *Plasmodium falciparum*, *Plasmodium vivax*, *Plasmodium malariae*, and *Plasmodium ovale*
    b. A fifth species, *Plasmodium knowlesi*, has recently been found to infect humans in Indonesia and other parts of Southeast Asia
    c. Malaria is the most important human parasitic infection: each year approximately 500 million people become infected worldwide and 1.5 to 2.7 million die
      1) Ninety percent of deaths are due to *P falciparum* and occur in sub-Saharan Africa
      2) Most deaths occur among children younger than 5 years—malaria is the leading cause of death in this age group
      3) Malaria is also widespread in Central America, South America, the Caribbean, the Indian subcontinent, the Middle East, and Southeast Asia
    d. Failure to control or significantly diminish malaria (especially severe forms caused by *P falciparum*) is due to several factors
      1) Persistence of the *Anopheles* mosquito vector because of lack of or inadequate use of effective insecticides (especially DDT)
      2) Unavailability of personal protective measures such as insect repellants and treated bed nets
      3) Development of resistance to affordable antimalarials, especially chloroquine
      4) Failure to develop an effective vaccine
      5) Political instability and population migration due to armed conflicts
    e. Life cycle: key to understanding malaria (Figure 22.8)
      1) After the mosquito injects the *sporozoite* into the human host, the parasite multiplies through asexual reproduction
      2) Initially, through the *exoerythrocytic cycle* in the liver, hepatocytes are infected
        a) This phase can persist with *P vivax* and *P ovale*, leading to relapses, if treatment does not include primaquine and does not eradicate these *hypnozoites*
        b) After multiplication in hepatocytes, the resulting *merozoites* enter the bloodstream and infect red blood cells (RBCs)
      3) In the RBCs, merozoites multiply and develop into *schizonts* containing multiple merozoites
      4) The RBCs rupture, liberating the merozoites, which infect other RBCs
      5) A certain number of multiplying parasites are genetically predetermined to develop into sexual cells (male and female *gametocytes*), which do not infect other RBCs
      6) Gametocytes are picked up by a biting mosquito, where sexual reproduction occurs, infectious sporozoites develop, and the cycle continues when the mosquito bites again
    f. Malaria may also be transmitted by blood transfusions from infected donors
  2. *Plasmodium falciparum* (Figures 22.9 and 22.10)

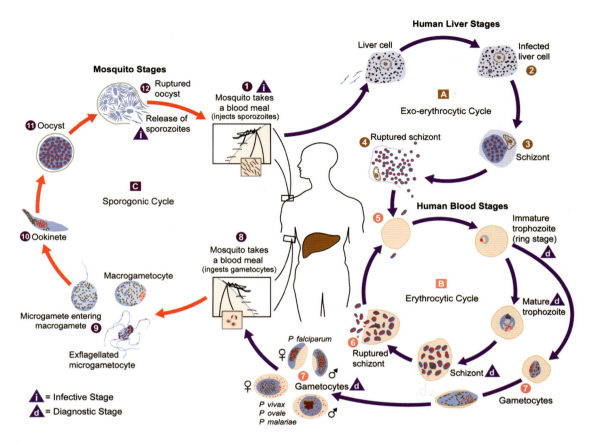

Figure 22.8. Life Cycle of *Plasmodium* Species. *P* indicates *Plasmodium*. (Adapted from Centers for Disease Control & Prevention [Internet]. [cited 2010 Aug 27]. Available from: http://www.dpd.cdc.gov/dpdx/HTML/Malaria.htm).

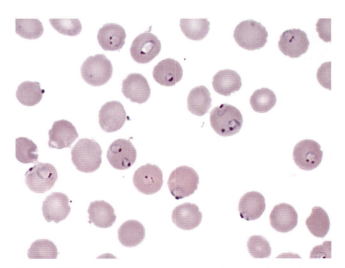

Figure 22.9. *Plasmodium falciparum* ring forms within red blood cells (RBCs). Thin blood film shows small rings, multiply infected RBCs, and high degree of parasitemia (Giemsa, original magnification ×1,000).

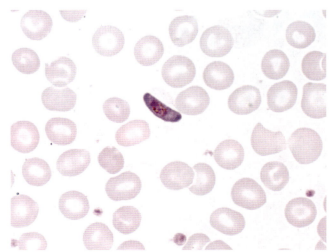

Figure 22.10. *Plasmodium falciparum* banana-shaped gametocyte in thin blood film (Giemsa, original magnification ×1,000).

a. The only species that causes disease (falciparum malaria) that results in significant mortality
b. Infects RBCs of all ages (other species infect primarily young RBCs), resulting in high rates of parasitemia (10%-30%)
   1) Infected RBCs develop surface "knobs" that allow infected RBCs to adhere to endothelial surfaces and to other RBCs
   2) Ultimately, thrombotic obstruction of small vessels occurs throughout the body
   3) This process also seems to activate the release of tumor necrosis factor α, which is involved in the pathogenesis of the disease
c. Severe malaria
   1) Characterized by hemolysis with anemia and hematuria (blackwater fever), renal failure, acute respiratory distress syndrome, hypoglycemia, and cerebral edema
   2) Any of these clinical findings carries a poor prognosis with significant mortality
   3) Hepatosplenomegaly may also be prominent
   4) Mortality rate from falciparum malaria is decreased by 50% among persons with thalassemia or glucose-6-phosphate dehydrogenase (G6PD) deficiency and by 90% among persons with sickle cell trait
d. Relative immunity develops among natives of areas where *P falciparum* is endemic
   1) Increased tolerance of high parasitemias
   2) Decreased likelihood of severe malaria developing
   3) No protection from repeated infections
3. *Plasmodium vivax*
   a. Causes a common form of malaria (vivax malaria)
   b. Produces nonfatal infection characterized by high fever occurring every other day (*tertian fever*)
      1) Tertian fever is related to synchronous cycles of parasite multiplication and RBC rupture
      2) Contrasts with falciparum malaria in which the high fever is persistent and without regular cycles
      3) Rare deaths have occurred from vivax malaria due to rupture of engorged spleens in prolonged infections
   c. Most members of the native populations of western and central Africa are refractory to infection with *P vivax* because they do not have the Duffy blood group antigen on their RBCs
4. Diagnosis of malaria
   a. Microscopic examination of thick and thin Giemsa-stained blood smears
      1) Thick smears are essentially concentrates of blood drops
         a) Can detect the presence of parasites for rapid screening
         b) Cannot identify species because the RBCs are lysed during staining
      2) Thin smears are monolayers of cells similar to those used for differential blood counts
         a) Species of *Plasmodium* are identified by parasite morphology within infected RBCs
         b) Rate of parasitemia is determined by comparing the number of infected RBCs to the total number of RBCs counted ($\geq$200)
   b. Various rapid, simple antigen detection immunochromatographic dipstick tests have been developed in recent years
      1) Rapid and easy to use for screening purposes, especially in resource-poor locations
      2) Have relatively low sensitivity
      3) Are subject to misinterpretation by inexperienced laboratory personnel
      4) Do not differentiate all *Plasmodium* species
5. Prevention of malaria
   a. Prevention should be focused on protection from mosquito bites
      1) Avoidance, barrier clothing, insect repellant containing 30% to 80% DEET (diethyltoluamide), and permethrin-impregnated bed nets
      2) Use of bed nets with insecticide spraying of dwellings is an effective strategy where malaria is endemic
   b. Travelers to areas where malaria is endemic may also receive chemoprophylaxis
      1) Mefloquine, Malarone (atovaquone-proguanil), or doxycycline where *Plasmodium* is resistant to chloroquine (mostly *P falciparum* but some *P vivax* in Papua New Guinea and other islands in the South Pacific)

2) Chloroquine where *Plasmodium* is susceptible (mostly *P vivax* but some *P falciparum* in Central America, the Caribbean, and the Middle East)
6. Treatment of falciparum malaria
   a. Considered a medical emergency, especially in nonimmune persons
      1) Severe malaria may develop within a few hours
      2) High mortality rate
      3) Rates of parasitemia should be monitored to determine prognosis and response to therapy
   b. Exchange transfusion should be considered in nonimmune patients who have parasitemia of 10% or more and clinical signs of severe malaria
   c. Chemotherapeutic regimens are complex, and a current authoritative reference should be consulted (eg, *Drugs for Parasitic Infections*, published by The Medical Letter, Inc)
      1) In the United States, falciparum malaria should be treated with a combination of quinine and doxycycline or clindamycin, or with sulfadoxine-pyrimethamine (Fansidar)
      2) Alternatively, Malarone or mefloquine may be used, although therapeutic doses of mefloquine may cause neuropsychiatric side effects
      3) Quinidine may be used for parenteral therapy
      4) Where available, combinations of artemisinin agents (eg, artesunate, artemether) and mefloquine are widely used
      5) Chloroquine may be used for susceptible malaria (mostly caused by species other than *P falciparum*) and should be followed with a course of primaquine for infections due to *P vivax* and *P ovale* to eradicate the latent liver forms (hypnozoites) and prevent relapses
         a) Test for G6PD deficiency before giving primaquine
         b) Primaquine should not be used in patients with G6PD deficiency because it will induce hemolysis
C. *Babesia microti*
   1. Babesiosis: a tick-borne, malaria-like infection caused by *Babesia microti*, an intraerythrocytic protozoan (a piroplasm)
   2. Babesiosis has been described as a disease that "looks like malaria but acts like Lyme disease"
      a. *Babesia* life cycle (Figure 22.11) is similar to that of *Borrelia*, involving rodents as intermediate host and reservoir and involving ixodid ticks in transmission to humans (in a few cases, transmission has been by blood transfusion)
      b. In the United States, the disease is endemic in New England and focal areas in Wisconsin, Minnesota, and Washington
      c. Babesiosis causes a systemic febrile illness similar to malaria with anemia and a spectrum from asymptomatic to chronic severe disease and death
      d. Babesiosis is worse in asplenic patients and the elderly
   3. Diagnosis
      a. Examination of thick and thin blood smears, as with malaria
         1) Intraerythrocytic parasites may resemble ring forms of *P falciparum* but are more irregular and distorted
         2) Presence of tetrads and "Maltese cross" forms is diagnostic (Figure 22.12)
      b. Serology is available
      c. Molecular detection by polymerase chain reaction (PCR) is available in some reference laboratories
         1) Useful in differentiating malaria from babesiosis
         2) Useful when parasitemia is too low to detect on blood smears
   4. Treatment
      a. Babesiosis is usually a self-limited infection, and mild cases resolve spontaneously
      b. Moderate or severe infections
         1) Treated with a combination of clindamycin 600 mg in combination with quinine 650 mg 3 times daily for 7 to 10 days
         2) Atovaquone plus azithromycin has also been effective
D. Hemoflagellates
   1. Bloodborne flagellated protozoa responsible for leishmaniasis and trypanosomiasis
   2. The organisms have similar life cycles and biologic forms
      a. *Trypomastigote*: an extracellular motile flagellated stage often found in blood
      b. *Amastigote*: a nonmotile intracellular stage located in macrophages and end-organ tissue cells

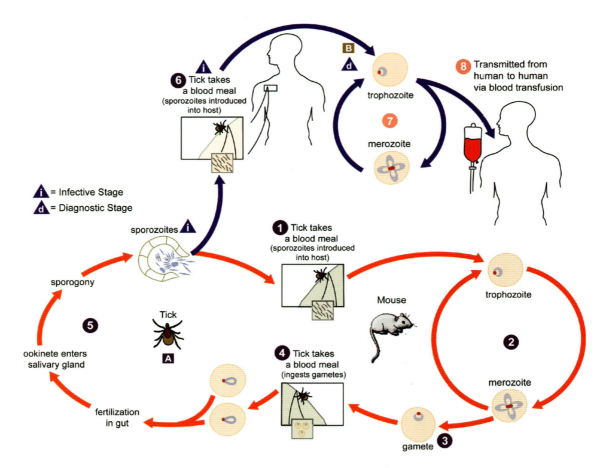

Figure 22.11. Life Cycle of *Babesia microti*. (Adapted from Centers for Disease Control & Prevention [Internet]. [cited 2010 Aug 27]. Available from: http://www.dpd.cdc.gov/dpdx/HTML/Babesiosis.htm).

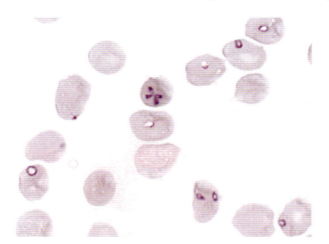

Figure 22.12. Classic tetrad or "Maltese cross" of *Babesia microti* in thin blood film (Giemsa, original magnification ×1,000).

3. *Leishmania* protozoa cause visceral, cutaneous, and mucocutaneous leishmaniasis
4. *Trypanosoma* protozoa cause African trypanosomiasis (sleeping sickness) and American trypanosomiasis (Chagas disease)
5. American trypanosomiasis (Chagas disease)
   a. Caused by *Trypanosoma cruzi*
   b. Each year, 11 to 18 million people are infected and 13,000 die
   c. Endemic in many areas of Latin America, especially rural
      1) Reservoirs: wild and domestic animals around homes
      2) Vector: the reduviid bug (also called kissing bug) lives in cracks and crevices of adobe or stucco dwellings
         a) Bug emerges at night, bites sleeping person, and defecates
         b) Person self-inoculates by scratching the bite
      3) Transmission can also occur congenitally and by blood transfusion and organ transplant
      4) Oral transmission by ingestion of food or drink contaminated with insect parts has been documented
   d. Acute infection

1) Fever, rash, and edema, often of the face (chagoma or Romaña sign), with parasites present in blood
2) Lasts 1 to 2 months with progression to chronic phase, which is lifelong but asymptomatic for 70% to 85% of infected persons
3) In 15% to 30%, disease progresses to invasion and significant organ damage, including heart (muscle and conduction defects) and gastrointestinal tract (megaesophagus and megacolon)

e. Diagnosis
1) Acute phase: *C*-shaped trypomastigotes can be found in peripheral blood smears or buffy coats (Figure 22.13)
2) Chronic phase: serology is positive and intracellular amastigotes may be seen in tissue biopsy specimens
   a) Serologic testing of all blood and organ donors is mandated in the United States
   b) Positive serologic results indicate ongoing infection and infectivity

f. Therapy
1) Effective antiparasitic therapy is limited to acute infections
   a) Benznidazole and nifurtimox are both active
   b) Given 2 to 3 times daily for 30 to 60 days
2) Treatment of progressive chronic infection is limited to management of involved organ dysfunction

6. Human African trypanosomiasis (sleeping sickness)
   a. Each year, approximately 500,000 people are infected with human African trypanosomiasis and 50,000 die
   b. Two subspecies of *Trypanosoma brucei* are responsible: *T brucei rhodesiense* causes East African trypanosomiasis and *T brucei gambiense* causes West African trypanosomiasis
      1) Transmission: bite of the tsetse fly (*Glossina*)
      2) Tsetse flies are relatively resistant to insect repellants, but use of permethrin-impregnated clothing may help prevent bites
      3) Reservoirs: cattle and other ungulates
      4) The disease occurs in wide areas of rural forests and savannahs, including national parks in Kenya and Tanzania (such as the Serengeti National Park) frequented by tourists
   c. Successive generations of parasites produce antigenically distinct *variable surface glycoproteins*, which allow them to avoid specific antibody responses and persist within the host
   d. Human African trypanosomiasis has 2 clinical stages
      1) First stage
         a) Develops 1 to 3 weeks after inoculation
         b) General systemic symptoms: fever, headache, and malaise
         c) A chancre at the bite site and posterior cervical lymph node swelling (Winterbottom sign) may develop
      2) Second stage
         a) CNS symptoms develop
         b) Symptoms are more severe and progress more rapidly (within weeks rather than months) in infection due to *T brucei rhodesiense* (East African trypanosomiasis)
         c) Gait and speech disturbances, mental status changes, and reversal of the normal sleep-wake pattern may progress to coma and seizures
   e. Diagnosis
      1) Blood or buffy-coat smears
         a) Elongated serpentine *trypomastigotes* can be detected (Figure 22.14)

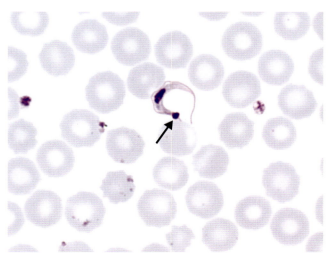

Figure 22.13. *Trypanosoma cruzi* trypomastigote in thin blood film. Note large kinetoplast (arrow) (Giemsa, original magnification ×1,000).

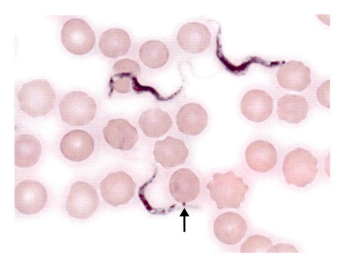

Figure 22.14. *Trypanosoma brucei* trypomastigote in thin blood film. Note large kinetoplast (arrow) (Giemsa, original magnification ×1,000).

- b) Characteristically, they divide frequently in the blood, and duplicate structures can be observed
- 2) CSF analysis: white blood cell counts are elevated, but organisms are rarely found
- 3) *Mott cells* (plasma cells with globular inclusions) are characteristic and may suggest the diagnosis
- 4) Serology
  - a) Useful to confirm the diagnosis
  - b) Available only from the Centers for Disease Control and Prevention or reference laboratories in Europe
- f. Treatment
  1) First-stage infections respond to treatment with suramin or pentamidine
  2) Second-stage (CNS) infections due to *T brucei gambiense* respond to eflornithine, but the drug is difficult to obtain
  3) CNS infections with *T brucei rhodesiense* must be treated with prolonged courses of melarsoprol, an arsenical that causes significant neurotoxicity
     - a) Melarsoprol decreases the high mortality rate to 2% to 7%, but the therapy itself is associated with an 18% rate of reactive encephalopathy and a 4% to 6% mortality rate
     - b) Concurrent use of prednisone can decrease the severity of these adverse effects
7. Leishmaniasis
   a. Leishmaniasis includes visceral, cutaneous, and mucocutaneous infections caused by various species of the protozoan hemoflagellate *Leishmania*
      1) Distribution: primarily in the Mediterranean, Middle East, Africa, and India (Old World forms) and South America (New World forms)
      2) As with trypanosomes there are both amastigotes and trypomastigotes
         - a) Trypomastigotes are rarely seen
         - b) Intracellular amastigotes are the diagnostic and pathogenic forms
      3) Transmission: bite of the sandfly (Figure 22.15)
         - a) After sandflies inoculate the skin, organisms are picked up by macrophages in which amastigotes develop and multiply (Figure 22.16)
         - b) Most infections remain localized to skin and lymph nodes
           - i) In some cases, though, the organism is ultimately transported to cells of the reticuloendothelial system (liver, spleen, and bone marrow)
           - ii) Clinical disease is then characterized by fever, wasting, hepatosplenomegaly, and pancytopenia
   b. Visceral leishmaniasis (called kala-azar in India)
      1) Caused by *Leishmania donovani* (Old World forms) and *Leishmania chagasi* or *Leishmania amazonensis* (New World forms)
      2) Each year, there are 500,000 new cases and 60,000 deaths
      3) Most cases (90%) are in India, Bangladesh, Nepal, Sudan, and Brazil
      4) Reservoirs: infected humans or animals (primarily dogs)
      5) Immunity: T-cell–mediated immunity is suppressed in visceral leishmaniasis, allowing parasites to proliferate in macrophages and disseminate
         - a) Recovery of helper T-cell function is associated with a better prognosis
         - b) Suppression of helper T-cell activity in AIDS patients in Spain and Italy

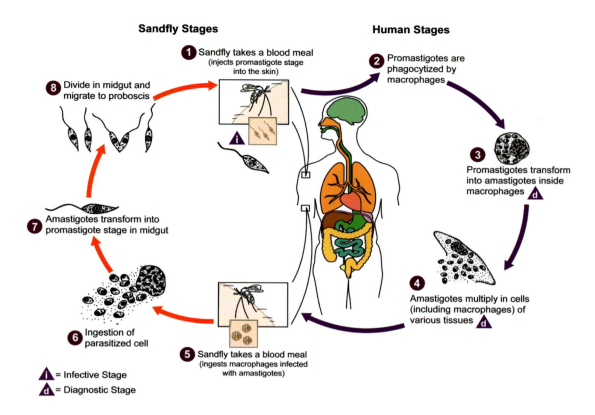

Figure 22.15. Life Cycle of *Leishmania* species. (Adapted from Centers for Disease Control & Prevention [Internet]. [cited 2010 Aug 27]. Available from: http://www.dpd.cdc.gov/dpdx/HTML/Leishmaniasis.htm).

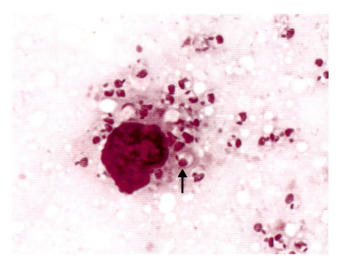

Figure 22.16. Ruptured macrophage containing *Leishmania* species amastigotes in a touch preparation. Arrow points to a single amastigote with a visible nucleus and rod-shaped kinetoplast (Giemsa, original magnification ×1,000).

has been associated with development of visceral leishmaniasis in those who had latent or quiescent infection acquired in childhood

6) Diagnosis
   a) Culture and microscopic examination of bone marrow, splenic aspirates, or liver biopsy specimens
   b) PCR testing may also be done on these specimens
   c) Seroreactivity to the rk39 antigen is indicative of active visceral leishmaniasis
7) Treatment
   a) Liposomal amphotericin B is the drug of choice when it is practical to administer it and the cost of administration is acceptable

b) In many areas, the antimony compound sodium stibogluconate is affordable and effective (cure rate, up to 90%)
c) Miltefosine, the first available oral agent, is as effective as stibogluconate
c. Cutaneous and mucocutaneous leishmaniasis
1) Caused by many species but primarily *Leishmania major* and *Leishmania tropica* (Old World forms) and *Leishmania mexicana* and *L amazonensis* (New World forms)
2) Cutaneous lesions may begin as papules or nodules and resolve spontaneously or progress to punched out ulcers with heaped up borders ("pizza-like")
3) Diagnosis: microscopy and culture of scrapings or impression smears from the edge of the ulcers
4) Treatment
a) Ulcers may resolve on their own
b) Ulcers may respond to various local physical treatments (heat, cold)
c) Ulcers may require chemotherapy with antimony compounds or various other agents (topical paromomycin, miltefosine, pentamidine, itraconazole, ketoconazole, or amphotericin)
d) Mucocutaneous leishmaniasis often causes progressive, disfiguring ulceration in the mouth and nose (*espundia*) and requires aggressive, prolonged treatment with amphotericin or 1 of the other agents listed above
d. Viscerotropic leishmaniasis
1) Described in US soldiers during the First Persian Gulf War
2) Mild form of viscerotropic leishmaniasis is caused by *L tropica*, which usually causes only cutaneous disease
3) The limited dissemination of this parasite beyond the skin probably occurs when patients have no acquired immunity
4) Treatment: responds well to various antiparasitic agents
E. *Trichomonas vaginalis*
1. *Trichomonas vaginalis* is a flagellated protozoan responsible for 180 million sexually transmitted diseases annually
2. Vaginal trichomoniasis
a. Prevalence in women is 3% to 48%, but in some areas (South Africa) it is as high as 65%
b. *Trichomonas vaginalis* has been isolated from 14% to 60% of male partners of infected women and from 67% to 100% of female partners of infected men
c. Infection is usually confined to the vaginal epithelium but may spread to the urethra and fallopian tubes
d. Diagnosis
1) Most often established by microscopic detection of trophozoites in vaginal exudate (Figure 22.17), but the sensitivity is rather low
2) Sensitivity can be significantly increased by culture, but culture delays the diagnosis
3) Molecular hybridization kits are also available but are more expensive than other methods
e. Treatment
1) Metronidazole is the drug of choice, but it has never been approved by the FDA for this indication
2) Metronidazole-resistant strains can be treated with higher doses of metronidazole or with tinidazole
F. *Toxoplasma gondii*
1. *Toxoplasma gondii* is a ubiquitous intracellular protozoan that infects humans and various domestic, agricultural, and wild animals including rodents
a. Reservoirs: rats, mice, and birds

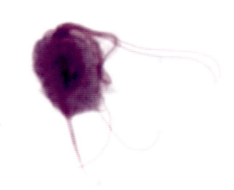

Figure 22.17. *Trichomonas vaginalis* trophozoite (Giemsa, original magnification ×1,000).

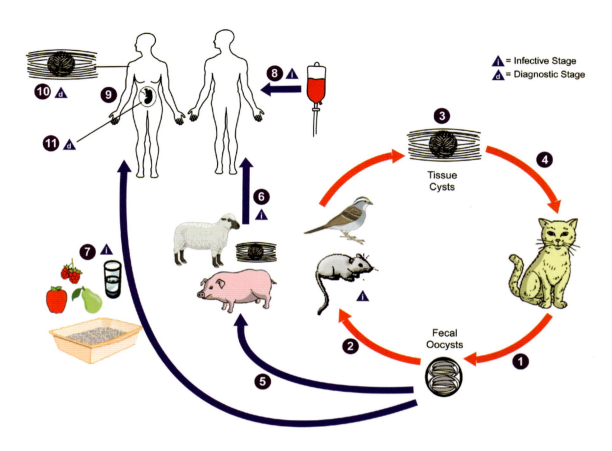

Figure 22.18. Life Cycle of *Toxoplasma gondii*. (Adapted from Centers for Disease Control & Prevention [Internet]. [cited 2010 Aug 27]. Available from: http://www.dpd.cdc.gov/dpdx/HTML/Toxoplasmosis.htm).

b. Infected adults: 20% to 70% in the United States; 90% in France
2. Toxoplasmosis
   a. Transmission
      1) Ingestion of food contaminated by cysts (in undercooked meats or animal feces, especially cat feces) (Figure 22.18)
      2) Congenital infection
   b. Infection
      1) Most infections are asymptomatic, but they may cause acute, self-limited lymphadenitis
         a) Infection can then become latent and eventually manifest as chorioretinitis, encephalitis, or other pathologic condition (Figure 22.19)
         b) Alternatively, infection may reactivate and disseminate if the patient becomes immunosuppressed

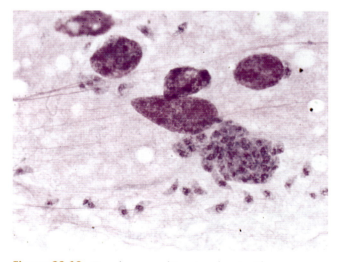

Figure 22.19. *Toxoplasma gondii* ruptured cyst with tachyzoites in touch preparation from brain (Giemsa, original magnification ×1,000).

(eg, toxoplasma encephalitis may develop in AIDS patients with low CD4 cell counts)
2) Congenital infection
   a) Causes significant neurologic deficits or chorioretinitis in 20% of infected children if untreated
   b) As many as 1 in 500 pregnant women may become infected, with fetal infection occurring in 30% to 50% of them
   c) Congenital infection develops least commonly in the first trimester (17% of cases), but the infection is most severe at that time
c. Diagnosis
   1) Primarily by serology
   2) Documentation of recent infection is compromised
      a) Large segment of normal population is IgG positive
      b) IgM may remain positive for a year after acute infection
      c) Immunosuppressed may not produce IgM
      d) Excess false-positive IgM results occur with some commercial assays
      e) IgG avidity testing (high value suggests old infection) may help but is not generally available
      f) Poses significant problem in pregnancy: it is often difficult to demonstrate seroconversion or recent appearance of IgM in time to treat or prevent congenital infection
   3) Alternatives for resolving diagnostic questions
      a) Testing at Centers for Disease Control and Prevention or Toxoplasma Serology Laboratory (Palo Alto, California)
      b) PCR testing on amniotic fluid
      c) PCR testing on CSF or on tissues such as lymph nodes in suspected cases of toxoplasmosis
d. Treatment
   1) Treatment of choice for toxoplasmosis: pyrimethamine in combination with sulfadiazine
   2) For complex clinical situations, an authoritative reference should be consulted (eg, *Drugs for Parasitic Infections*, published by The Medical Letter, Inc)
      a) Treatment of immunocompromised patients
      b) Women infected during pregnancy (spiramycin is used)
      c) Fetal infection and congenitally infected infants

IV. Helminths
   A. Nematodes
      1. Intestinal nematodes
         a. Distribution: 3 billion people are infected worldwide
         b. Clinical disease: worm burden and host state determine disease extent
         c. Diagnosis
            1) Eggs, larvae, or adults in stool
            2) Eosinophilia may be present but is more common when larvae migrate through tissues
         d. Adults live 2 to 3 years
         e. Treatment: albendazole, mebendazole, ivermectin
         f. *Ascaris lumbricoides*
            1) Large, resembling earthworm without annular (circumferential) striations
            2) Infection by ingestion of embryonated eggs where sanitation is poor (worldwide)
            3) Clinical disease
               a) Heavy infection may cause undernutrition or intestinal obstruction
               b) Larvae migrate to lungs, causing eosinophilic pneumonitis (Löffler syndrome)
         g. *Trichuris trichiura* (whipworm) (Figure 22.20)

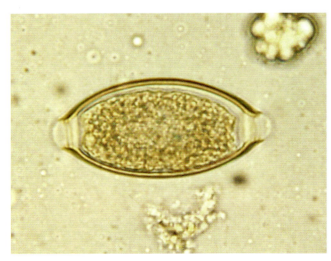

Figure 22.20. *Trichuris trichiura* egg in unstained wet preparation. Bipolar plugs are easily recognized (original magnification ×400).

1) Major intestinal worm of developing countries
2) Whiplike worms live in cecum and colon
3) Clinical disease: abdominal discomfort, malnutrition, anemia, rectal prolapse

h. *Enterobius vermicularis* (pinworm)
1) Endemic worldwide, especially in 5 to 10 year olds
2) Irritation of anal, perianal, and vulvovaginal areas with scratching and trauma; may migrate to appendix or fallopian tubes
3) Diagnosis
   a) Small adult worms are found in perianal area or eggs are found on sticky tape or with paddle sampling
   b) Eggs: typically asymmetrical and flattened on 1 side (Figure 22.21)
4) Recurrences and spread through family with young children are common
5) Management: sterilize pajamas and bedsheets

i. Hookworms (*Ancylostoma duodenale*, *Necator americanus*)
1) Transmission: infection by skin penetration of larvae that are in soil contaminated with eggs from human feces
2) Clinical disease
   a) Larval migration through lungs may cause fever, wheezing, and shortness of breath with abnormal chest radiograph
   b) Anemia in children with heavy infestations
   c) Eosinophilia
3) Diagnosis: eggs in stool
4) Dog and cat hookworms
   a) Infect the skin and migrate through the dermis but penetrate no deeper
   b) This creeping eruption (called *cutaneous larva migrans*) produces migratory serpiginous, erythematous, and intensely pruritic skin lesions
   c) Treatment: albendazole, ivermectin, or *topical* thiabendazole

j. *Capillaria philippinensis*
1) Distribution: endemic in Southeast Asia
2) Transmission: larvae ingested with raw freshwater fish
3) Clinical disease
   a) Larvae are localized in small intestine
   b) Diarrhea and generalized abdominal symptoms
   c) Autoinfection from eggs hatching in intestine (larvae in intestine penetrate mucosa)
4) Diagnosis
   a) Eggs (flattened bipolar plugs), larvae, and adult worms can be found in stool
   b) Small, filamentous worm (3 mm long × 6 μm wide)

k. *Strongyloides stercoralis*
1) Distribution: endemic throughout tropical and subtropical areas, including southeastern United States, wherever sanitation is poor
2) Transmission: skin penetration of filariform larvae that are in soil contaminated with human feces
3) Clinical disease
   a) Larvae migrate through lungs (causing coughing and wheezing) into trachea and are swallowed into the GI tract
   b) Adults mature in small intestine and produce larvae that are passed in stool
   c) Adults may invade intestinal mucosa but not penetrate
   d) Autoinfection
      i) Occurs when larvae mature within intestine and penetrate mucosa

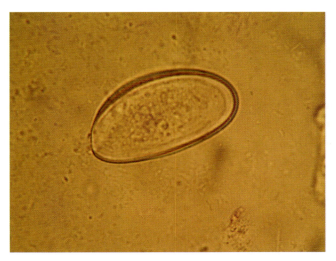

Figure 22.21. *Enterobius vermicularis* egg in unstained tape preparation (original magnification ×400).

ii) Responsible for persistence of infection decades after patient has left area where disease is endemic
iii) May become accelerated (hyperinfection) in immunosuppressed person with disseminated parasites (in CSF, lungs, etc) with accompanying bacterial sepsis and high mortality (especially with corticosteroids)
e) Chronic infection
i) May be asymptomatic
ii) May cause nonspecific GI, skin (rash, urticaria, larva currens), or pulmonary symptoms
4) Diagnosis
a) Eosinophilia is common in all infections
b) Larvae can be found in stool but may require multiple examinations (up to 7) for ova and parasites or specialized procedures (agar plate culture or Baermann method) (Figure 22.22)
c) Serology may be useful but may be positive from prior exposure or infection
5) Treatment: ivermectin is most effective therapy
l. *Anisakis* species (herring worm) and *Pseudoterranova decipiens* (codworm)
1) Anisakiasis

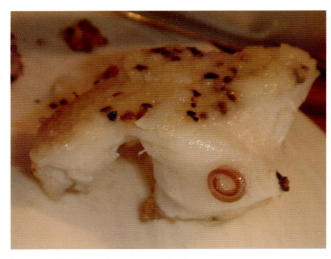

Figure 22.23. Codworm in Fish Flesh.

a) Occurs most commonly in Asia, but can occur anywhere from ingestion of raw or undercooked fish
b) Adult worms are present in fish muscle (Figure 22.23)
2) Clinical disease
a) Worms can penetrate stomach or intestinal mucosa, with local inflammation, and then migrate through peritoneum
b) Symptoms after penetration (including abdominal pain and vomiting) may mimic acute appendicitis or enteritis
3) Diagnosis
a) Endoscopy or peritoneoscopy
b) No eosinophilia
c) No eggs or worms in stool
4) Treatment
a) Endoscopic extraction of worms
b) Surgery if obstruction or peritonitis is present
2. Nematodes that cause disease outside the GI tract (usually from larval migration in tissues; no eggs or worms are found in stool)
a. *Angiostrongylus cantonensis* (rat lungworm)
1) Distribution
a) Mostly in Asia after ingestion of raw or undercooked snails or slugs, which are intermediate hosts (rat is primary host)
b) Recent outbreaks after eating salad in Jamaica
2) Clinical disease

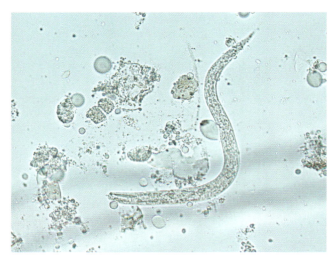

Figure 22.22. *Strongyloides stercoralis* rhabditiform larvae in unstained wet preparation (original magnification ×200).

- a) Primary cause of eosinophilic meningitis
- b) Larvae migrate from GI tract into CNS via bloodstream
- c) Symptoms of meningitis, visual disturbances, and coma
3) Diagnosis
- a) CSF: pleocytosis with eosinophilia; no organisms
- b) Serology: useful but limited availability
4) Treatment: albendazole in combination with corticosteroids may help

b. *Gnathostoma spinigerum*
1) Distribution: endemic in Southeast Asia and Latin America
2) Transmission
- a) Ingestion of larvae in raw or undercooked freshwater fish, including eating ceviche
- b) Adult worms are found in the GI tract of dogs and cats
- c) Eggs are passed in feces
- d) Larvae are found in water
3) Clinical disease
- a) Larvae migrate from GI tract through tissues and can cause migratory subcutaneous swellings similar to skin manifestations from *Loa loa* and *Strongyloides stercoralis* (larva currens)
- b) May cause eosinophilic meningitis
4) Diagnosis: serology is useful but availability is limited
5) Treatment: albendazole and ivermectin are effective, but success is limited in meningitis

c. *Dracunculus medinensis* (guinea worm)
1) Transmission: ingestion of freshwater copepods
2) Clinical disease
- a) Larvae migrate through intestinal wall and peritoneum to tissues of abdominal wall and thorax
- b) Adults mature and mate in tissues
- c) Females migrate to skin, forming blisters that burst on water exposure and liberate larvae into water
3) Diagnosis: see worm emerge from blister
4) Treatment: mechanical removal of adult worm (winding it around matchstick); no effective antiparasitic

d. *Trichinella spiralis*
1) Trichinosis
- a) Ingestion of inadequately cooked pork, bear, or meat of other carnivorous animals
- b) Now rare in US farm-raised pork
2) Clinical disease
- a) Larvae from meat migrate from GI tract to primarily striated muscle tissue, where they encyst and evoke an inflammatory reaction (Figure 22.24)
- b) Fever, headache, diarrhea, myalgias, arthralgias, facial swelling
3) Diagnosis
- a) Eosinophilia is prominent
- b) Serology is confirmatory
- c) Muscle biopsy shows larvae
4) Treatment: corticosteroids in combination with albendazole is effective

e. *Toxocara canis* and *Toxocara catis* (dog and cat ascarids)
1) Transmission
- a) Ingestion of eggs from infected dog or cat feces contaminating soil
- b) Most common in young children with a history of pica
2) Clinical disease
- a) Larvae hatched from eggs penetrate intestine and migrate through tissues, especially liver, but may be found in eye, CNS, skin, lung, and other sites
- b) Persons may be asymptomatic or have fever, cough, abdominal pain,

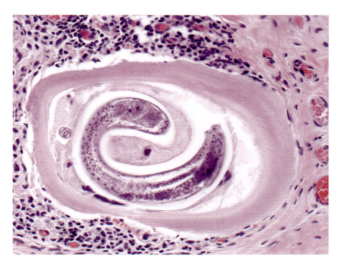

Figure 22.24. Encysted *Trichinella* larvae (hematoxylin-eosin, original magnification ×400).

hepatomegaly (ie, *visceral larva migrans*)
            3) Diagnosis
                a) Eosinophilia is prominent
                b) Serology is useful
            4) Treatment: albendazole (with corticosteroids in severe cases)
        f. *Baylisascaris procyonis* (raccoon roundworm)
            1) Transmission
                a) Ingestion of eggs from raccoon feces contaminating the ground where raccoons eliminate
                b) Young children with pica or geophagia are especially at risk
            2) Clinical disease
                a) Larvae excyst from eggs in intestine and migrate through tissues with a predilection for the brain
                b) *Neural larva migrans* can cause severe and often fatal encephalitis, especially in children; eye may also be involved
            3) Diagnosis
                a) CSF eosinophilia and peripheral eosinophilia are prominent
                b) Serology is useful but availability is limited (possibly available at state veterinary laboratories or Centers for Disease Control and Prevention)
            4) Prognosis
                a) Grave for CNS infection
                b) Most cases are fatal or have severe neurologic residua
            5) Treatment
                a) Albendazole: drug of choice but has not been shown to alter course of encephalitis
                b) May try prophylactic use in children with pica near raccoon areas
    3. Filarial nematodes (macroscopic adults reside in lymphatics or subcutaneous tissues; microscopic offspring [microfilariae] are found in blood or skin)
        a. Lymphatic filariasis
            1) Agents
                a) *Wuchereria bancrofti*
                    i) Wide distribution in tropics and subtropics including Asia, Africa, and Latin America
                    ii) Causes 90% of cases of filariasis
                b) *Brugia malayi*, *Brugia timori*: limited to southern Asia
            2) Transmission: various mosquito species pick up microfilariae from blood of infected human and transmit larval form to new host
            3) Clinical disease
                a) Adult worms develop in lymphatics and evoke inflammatory response that leads eventually to narrowing, calcification, and obstruction
                b) Lymphadenitis and lymphedema develop (elephantiasis in legs and scrotum)
                c) Cholera may occur
                d) Tropical pulmonary eosinophilia may occur, especially in young males (paroxysmal asthma with pulmonary infiltrates and high level of eosinophilia)
            4) Diagnosis
                a) Find microfilariae by examination of thick and thin blood films (as in malaria) or by membrane filtration of blood (Figure 22.25)
                b) Worms moving in lymphatics can be demonstrated by ultrasonography (filarial dance sign)
                c) Antigen and antibody detection in blood can be helpful, but availability is limited
                d) Serology cannot identify specific genus and species
            5) Treatment
                a) Established elephantiasis: treated with conservative measures
                b) Microfilariae: eliminated with diethylcarbamazine citrate (DEC), ivermectin, or albendazole (adult worms have only partial response)

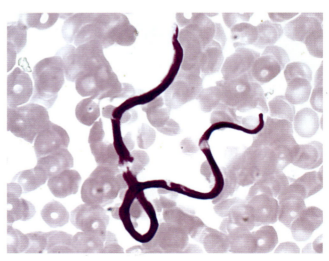

Figure 22.25. Microfilariae in peripheral blood (Giemsa, original magnification ×400).

c) Doxycycline
   i) Eliminates *Wolbachia* (related to *Ehrlichia*), a bacterial endosymbiont of all filariae except *Loa loa*
   ii) Prevents filariae from producing microfilariae
b. *Loa loa* (eyeworm)
   1) Transmission: bloodsucking *Chrysops* fly picks up microfilariae in host blood and transmits larvae to new host
   2) Clinical disease
      a) Adult worms develop and migrate in subcutaneous tissues, producing transient migratory subcutaneous Calabar swellings with severe urticaria
      b) Adult may migrate through conjunctiva (thus the name *eyeworm*) and can be extracted from eye with minimal damage
   3) Diagnosis
      a) See microfilariae in blood smears or by membrane filtration
      b) See adults in swellings or eye
      c) Serology is not species specific
   4) Treatment of choice for eliminating microfilariae and adult worms: DEC
c. *Onchocerca volvulus*
   1) Causes onchocerciasis (African river blindness)
      a) Thirteen million are infected, primarily in equatorial Africa and Latin America
      b) Second leading cause of infectious blindness worldwide
   2) Transmission
      a) Black fly (*Simulium*) picks up microfilariae from skin (not blood) and injects infectious larvae into new host
      b) Black flies breed along free-flowing streams and rivers
         i) Control measures are difficult
         ii) Flies have access to people in villages located close to water sources
   3) Life cycle
      a) Infective larvae develop into adults in subcutaneous nodules
      b) Adults survive an average of 9 years
      c) Adult female worms liberate thousands of microfilariae that migrate through skin, especially to eyes if adult nodules are located on the face, head, or neck
   4) Clinical disease
      a) Dermatitis with pruritus can be chronic and severe, with resultant loss of elasticity and other damage
      b) Ocular manifestations
         i) Neovascularization and corneal scarring lead to corneal opacities and blindness (sclerosing keratitis)
         ii) Uveitis, chorioretinitis, and optic atrophy occur in 5% of infected persons
         iii) Punctate keratitis from dying microfilariae usually resolves without complications (seen most often in younger age groups)
      c) *Onchocerca* are infected with *Wolbachia* symbionts (see the "Lymphatic filariasis" section above), which may have a role in pathogenesis
      d) High-grade eosinophilia is present
   5) Diagnosis
      a) Traditionally by microscopy of skin snips to detect microfilariae (which are *not* present in blood)
      b) Serology may be useful, but it has limited availability and is not species specific
   6) Treatment
      a) Nodules may be surgically removed to detect adult worms and lessen worm burden
      b) Ivermectin kills microfilariae but not adult worms
         i) Repeated courses eventually sterilize adult females
         ii) Additional use of doxycycline (to eliminate *Wolbachia*) may improve outcome, but its use is not well studied
B. Cestodes
  1. Intestinal tapeworms: adults live in GI tract of humans, are composed of segments (proglottids), and may be several meters in length
      a. *Taenia solium* (pork tapeworm), *Taenia saginata* (beef tapeworm), and *Diphyllobothrium latum* (fish tapeworm)
         1) Common names (eg, pork tapeworm) are misnomers since humans, not animals, harbor these tapeworms

a) The tapeworms are acquired by eating inadequately cooked meat or fish containing encysted larvae
b) Found where poor sanitation allows contamination of animal food or in lakes with human feces containing proglottids or eggs
2) Clinical disease
   a) Nonspecific GI complaints associated with minimal morbidity and mortality
   b) *Diphyllobothrium latum* may cause vitamin B_{12} deficiency and a syndrome resembling pernicious anemia (Figure 22.26)
   c) Infected persons may contaminate food with eggs, resulting in larval cestode infection in others (see "Cysticercosis" section below)
   d) Immigrants from areas where intestinal tapeworms are endemic and who work as cooks and domestics pose a special hazard
3) Diagnosis
   a) Observation of tapeworm segments or proglottids in stool
   b) Detection of eggs by microscopic examination of stool for ova and parasites
4) Treatment
   a) Praziquantel results in expulsion of tapeworm
   b) Tapeworm should be examined for presence of scolex (head with attachment hooks) to ensure that entire worm was passed
   c) Retention of scolex in GI tract allows regeneration of tapeworm

5) Prevention and control: thorough cooking of meat and fish, good hand washing, and good personal hygiene
2. Larval cestode infections (infection of humans with the larval form of tapeworm after ingestion of eggs passed by another person harboring the adult tapeworm)
   a. Cysticercosis: infection with the larval form of *T solium*
      1) Clinical disease
         a) Larvae commonly lodge in and form cysts in the brain but are also frequently found in other visceral or subcutaneous tissues (Figure 22.27)
         b) Most symptoms are related to presence of cysts in brain parenchyma, meninges, subarachnoid space, or ventricles
            i) Seizures, headache, hydrocephalus, and other neurologic phenomena are related to number, size, and location of cysts
            ii) Symptoms are exacerbated when dying cysts elicit a local inflammatory response (can occur as a result of therapy)
            iii) Eventually cysts die, contract, fibrose, and calcify on their own, but neurologic symptoms may persist
      2) Diagnosis: suspected on epidemiologic and clinical grounds
         a) In the United States, 90% of cases are in persons who live in or have immigrated from areas where

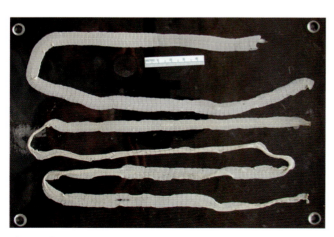

Figure 22.26. *Diphyllobothrium latum*.

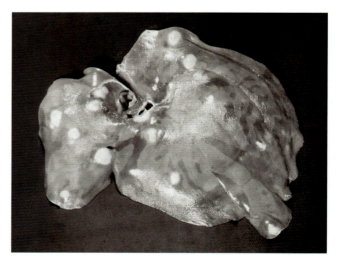

Figure 22.27. Cysticercosis in lung (autopsy specimen).

T solium is endemic, primarily Latin America
  b) Diagnosis is established with computed tomographic (CT) scan showing calcifications or with magnetic resonance imaging (MRI) scan showing typical cysts
  c) Western blot serology may be helpful in confirming the diagnosis
  d) Finding *Taenia* eggs in stool may be useful, but most patients with cysticercosis do not harbor a tapeworm because they have acquired the infection from others
3) Treatment
  a) Albendazole kills cysts
  b) Utility of treatment is debated for several reasons
    i) Cysts die on their own
    ii) Treatment may exacerbate symptoms
    iii) Neurologic residua may not differ between treated and untreated patients
    iv) Limited data suggest that outcomes may be somewhat better in treated patients
  c) Corticosteroids should be added if symptoms worsen with treatment
b. Echinococcosis: hydatid cysts due to infection with larval form of *Echinococcus granulosus*; alveolar cysts due to larval form of *Echinococcus multilocularis*
  1) Life cycle
    a) Small (3-8 mm) adult tapeworm resides in small intestine of carnivorous animals such as dogs, foxes, wolves, and coyotes that became infected by eating cysts from cattle, sheep, and deer
    b) Tapeworm eggs are shed in feces of carnivores
      i) Contaminate food, water, or hands of humans in close contact with these animals
      ii) Hydatid cysts were most common in sheepherders and others who had contact with dogs who had eaten animal viscera
    c) Eggs hatch in human small intestine, liberating larval oncospheres that penetrate mucosa and migrate in the circulation to liver, lung, brain, bone, or most any other organ
    d) Larvae exvaginate in tissues, forming cysts that gradually enlarge and form a germinal layer on the internal cyst wall, from which daughter cysts (plerocercoids) bud off into cyst fluid (hydatid sand)
      i) Single large cysts develop with a defined capsule and multiple septae
      ii) Each daughter cyst can develop into an adult tapeworm or form additional hydatid cysts if spilled into peritoneum
  2) Clinical disease
    a) Most common presentation is large hydatid cyst of liver that develops slowly over many years (Figure 22.28)
      i) Large mass produces pressure
      ii) More cysts occur in liver (50%-70%) than in lungs (20%)
    b) Alveolar cysts from *E multilocularis* enlarge rapidly
      i) Composed of multiple, rapidly forming individual cysts
      ii) Behave like a malignancy
  3) Diagnosis
    a) Visualization of cysts: radiography, ultrasonography, CT, or MRI
    b) Western blot serology
    c) Microscopic detection of daughter cysts in aspirated hydatid sand or in tissue biopsy samples
  4) Treatment
    a) Depends on state of cyst

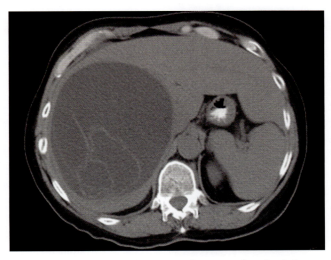

Figure 22.28. Computed Tomographic Scan of Hydatid Cyst in Liver.

b) Albendazole with or without surgical excision of cyst or puncture and aspiration of cyst with injection and reaspiration of cysticidal agents (PAIR)
c) Alveolar cysts
i) Not amenable to surgery or PAIR
ii) Treated with albendazole alone
C. Trematodes
1. Life cycles
a. Recalling the complex life cycles of the various flukes and thereby understanding the epidemiology and sources of infection can be difficult
b. Common features
1) Transmission cycle of all flukes begins by contamination of freshwater with feces or urine containing eggs from infected humans
2) Snails act as intermediate hosts, in which infectious larval forms (cercariae) develop and are released into the water
3) Transmission
a) Skin penetration: *Schistosoma*
b) Ingestion of fish or watercress: liver flukes *Fasciola* and *Clonorchis*
c) Ingestion of crabs or crayfish: lung fluke *Paragonimus*
4) Diseases are perpetuated by the cycle of water being contaminated with feces and then being used for food, bathing, or recreation
2. *Schistosoma*
a. Schistosomiasis
1) Most human disease is caused by *Schistosoma mansoni*, *Schistosoma japonicum*, and *Schistosoma haematobium*
2) Most cases (85%) occur in Africa, but the disease also occurs in Latin America and Asia
b. Life cycle
1) Skin-penetrating cercariae (the larval form) in freshwater infect humans, mature to schistosomula, and migrate to portal blood vessels (Figure 22.29)

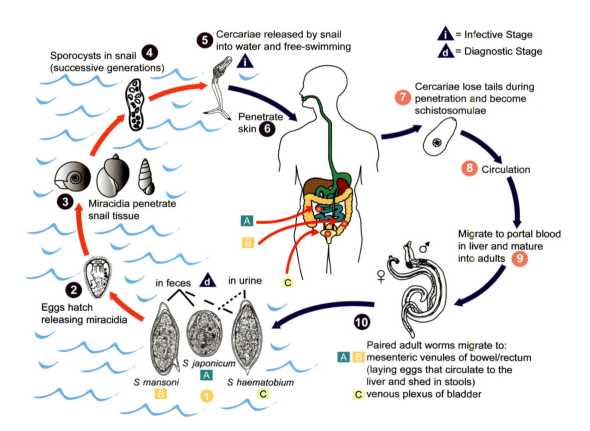

Figure 22.29. Life Cycle of *Schistosoma* Species. S indicates *Schistosoma*. (Adapted from Centers for Disease Control & Prevention [Internet]. [cited 2010 Aug 27]. Available from: http://www.dpd.cdc.gov/dpdx/HTML/Schistosomiasis.htm).

- a) Male and female adults develop in portal blood vessels
- b) Other flukes are hermaphroditic (ie, each organism contains male and female organs, and there are no separate sexes)
2) Adults migrate to mesenteric venules of bowel or rectum (*S mansoni* and *S japonicum*) or to venous plexus of bladder (*S haematobium*)
  - a) Adults mate and persist "in copula" for many years (Figure 22.30)
  - b) Adults do not evoke an inflammatory or immune response
  - c) Each day, adults produce 200 to 2,000 eggs that disseminate to various organs
    - i) Primarily the liver and intestine: *S mansoni* and *S japonicum*
    - ii) Primarily the bladder: *S haematobium*
    - iii) Eggs also penetrate these organs and are shed in stool or urine
    - iv) Eggs provoke granulomatous inflammatory response in tissues, which contributes to disease syndromes
- c. Clinical disease
  1) Acute clinical syndromes
     - a) Pruritic dermatitis at time of cercarial penetration (swimmer's itch)
     - b) Fever, cough, and eosinophilia (Katayama fever) 4 to 8 weeks after exposure
  2) Chronic infection with *S mansoni* and *S japonicum*
     - a) Presinusoidal granulomas and periportal fibrosis in liver cause portal hypertension
     - b) Parenchymal liver function is preserved
  3) Chronic infection with *S haematobium*
     - a) Bladder granulomas, scarring, calcification, and cancer in some instances
     - b) Hematuria and bacterial urinary tract infections are common
  4) Occasionally, *Schistosoma* eggs migrate to brain or spinal cord (transverse myelitis)
- d. Diagnosis
  1) Clinical findings in areas where disease is endemic and identifying eggs by microscopic examination of stool and urine
  2) Rectal "snips" may increase sensitivity of egg detection (Figure 22.31)
  3) Species-specific serology is available
- e. Treatment: praziquantel is specific antiparasitic therapy
3. *Paragonimus westermani* (lung fluke)
  - a. Distribution: endemic primarily in India, China, and Japan
  - b. Life cycle
    1) Ingestion of uncooked crabs or crayfish
    2) Larvae (metacercariae) excyst in small intestine and migrate through diaphragm to pleural cavity

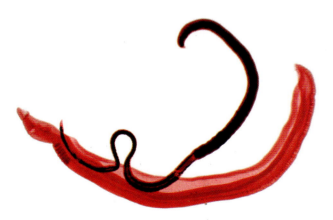

Figure 22.30. Adult *Schistosoma* coupled "in copula" (hematoxylin-eosin, original magnification ×400).

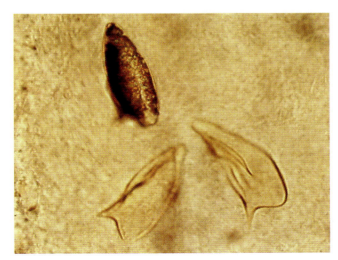

Figure 22.31. *Schistosoma mansoni* eggs in unstained rectal snip preparation (original magnification ×400).

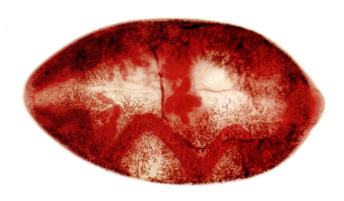

Figure 22.32. Adult *Paragonimus* Fluke.

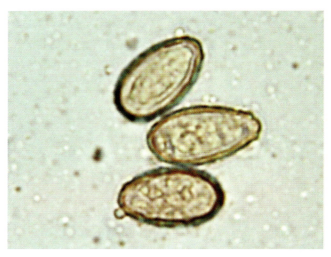

Figure 22.33. Small operculated eggs of *Clonorchis sinensis* in unstained preparation (original magnification ×5,000).

      3) Adult flukes encapsulate in lung and cause inflammation, cavitation, cough, and hemoptysis (Figure 22.32)
    c. Diagnosis
      1) On chest radiograph, lesions may mimic tuberculosis
      2) Microscopic detection of eggs: eggs are excreted in sputum and stool (if swallowed)
    d. Treatment: praziquantel is drug of choice
4. Liver flukes (*Clonorchis sinensis* [also called *Opisthorchis sinensis*] and *Fasciola hepatica*)
    a. *Clonorchis sinensis*
      1) Distribution: widely distributed in Southeast Asia (4 million cases in China)
      2) Life cycle
        a) Infection from ingesting larvae in raw freshwater fish
        b) Larvae migrate to bile ducts, where they develop into adult worms
      3) Clinical disease: heavy infection may lead to obstructive jaundice, liver cirrhosis, and cholangiocarcinoma
      4) Diagnosis
        a) Eosinophilia
        b) Ultrasonographic, MRI, or CT findings, or radiographic signs of intraductal organisms and biliary dilatation
        c) Microscopic detection of eggs in stools (Figure 22.33)
      5) Treatment: praziquantel is drug of choice
    b. *Fasciola hepatica*
      1) Distribution: occurs where sheep and cattle are raised (they serve as reservoirs)
      2) Life cycle
        a) Infection by ingestion of larvae with contaminated watercress
          i) Larvae migrate from intestine through peritoneum
          ii) Larvae penetrate Glisson capsule and enter liver parenchyma, producing acute hepatic damage with fever and eosinophilia
        b) Adult flukes mature in bile ducts over months to years and excrete eggs
      3) Clinical disease: right upper quadrant abdominal pain
      4) Diagnosis
        a) Eosinophilia
        b) MRI or CT scans may show liver lesions with migration tracts
        c) Microscopic detection of eggs in stool (Figure 22.34)
      5) Treatment
        a) Triclabendazole is drug of choice
        b) Praziquantel is *not* effective against *F hepatica*
5. Intestinal flukes (*Fasciolopsis buski*)
    a. Distribution: human infection with this large intestinal fluke occurs in the Far East, where pigs are the major reservoir
    b. Life cycle
      1) Infection by ingestion of larval forms encysted on various types of aquatic vegetation

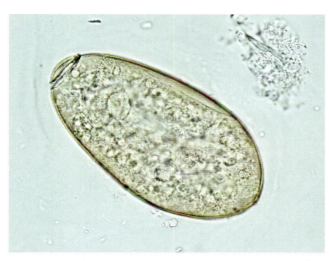

Figure 22.34. Large operculated egg of *Fasciola hepatica* in unstained preparation (original magnification ×1,000).

2) When raw or poorly cooked plants are ingested, the larvae (metacercariae) excyst in the intestines
3) Within 3 months the parasites develop into mature worms that survive 6 months or more
4) Adult worms inhabit the duodenum and jejunum, where they produce large operculated eggs
5) Adults attach to the mucosa and produce local inflammation, ulceration, and abscesses
  c. Clinical disease
   1) Infection with *F buski* is mostly subclinical, although eosinophilia is marked in some persons
   2) With heavy infections, flukes may cause transient obstruction and ileus
  d. Diagnosis: microscopic detection of eggs in stool or duodenal aspirates
  e. Treatment
   1) Praziquantel
   2) Triclabendazole is also effective

Suggested Reading

Guerrant RL, Walker DH, Weller PF. Tropical infectious diseases: principles, pathogens, & practice. 2nd ed. Philadelphia (PA): Elsevier Churchill Livingstone; c2006.

Jong EC, Sanford C. The travel and tropical medicine manual. 4th ed. Philadelphia (PA): Saunders/Elsevier; c2008.

Mandell GL, Bennett JE, Dolin R. Mandell, Douglas, and Bennett's principles and practice of infectious diseases. Vol 2. 6th ed. Philadelphia (PA): Elsevier Churchill Livingstone; c2005.

Peters W, Pasvol G. Tropical medicine and parasitology. 5th ed. London: Mosby; c2002.

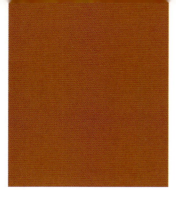

Etiologic Agents

Questions and Answers

Questions

Multiple Choice (choose the best answer)

1. A 67-year-old Cambodian woman sustained a deep laceration on her leg while gardening. The wound was visibly contaminated with soil. She immigrated to the United States 5 years ago and lives with her son and family. She is not aware of having any vaccinations as a child. She takes no medications and has no medication allergies. Which of the following should you recommend for tetanus prophylaxis?
   a. Human tetanus immunoglobulin (HTIG)
   b. Primary series of tetanus toxoid (T)
   c. Primary series of tetanus and diphtheria toxoids (Td)
   d. Primary series of diphtheria and tetanus toxoids and pertussis (DTaP) vaccine
   e. HTIG and primary series of Td

2. A 35-year-old male construction worker sustained a compound fracture of the left femur in a car accident. His thigh wound was grossly contaminated with soil. He underwent débridement of soft tissues and open reduction with internal fixation of fractured bone. Postoperatively, his leg was wrapped in a bulky dressing. Tetanus toxoid and human tetanus immunoglobulin were administered. Forty-eight hours later, the patient complained of blurred vision and weakness in his upper extremities. On examination, he was fully awake, alert, and afebrile. On neurologic examination, he had diplopia, slurred speech, and motor weakness of the upper extremities. His pupils were equal in size and reactive to light. Deep tendon reflexes were decreased symmetrically in the upper extremities. His thigh wound was opened and serosanguineous fluid was drained. Which of the following should be administered?
   a. Vancomycin and clindamycin
   b. Botulism antitoxin and penicillin
   c. Additional human tetanus immunoglobulin and intravenous penicillin
   d. Metronidazole and diazepam
   e. Rabies immunoglobulin and rabies vaccine

3. A 42-year-old homeless man is seen in the emergency department with intermittent, intense, and painful muscular spasms of 2 days' duration. On examination, he is fully awake but irritable. Vital signs include the following: temperature 37°C, pulse rate 110 beats per minute, blood pressure 140/90 mm Hg, and respiratory rate 22 breaths per minute. Examination findings are otherwise unremarkable for the head and neck, chest, heart, and abdomen. A small puncture wound is noted in the left foot with serosanguineous drainage, surrounding erythema, and induration of the skin and soft tissues. No purulence or fluctuation is noted. The patient appears to be quite sensitive to loud noise in the emergency

department. Which of the following statements is true about this illness?
   a. It is caused by an infection with a gram-negative spore-forming rod.
   b. The toxin produced by this organism binds reversibly to nerve endings.
   c. Muscular spasms are caused by a toxin that prevents release of inhibitory neurotransmitters.
   d. The reported penicillin resistance in the causative pathogen is approximately 10%.
   e. If the illness is untreated, the patient's level of consciousness will probably progressively decrease.

4. Which of the following would *not* be included in the optimal management of the patient in the previous question?
   a. Administration of antibiotics to inhibit further toxin production
   b. Surgical consultation for wound débridement
   c. Administration of immunoglobulins to neutralize unbound toxin
   d. Use of penicillin as the drug of choice, with use of metronidazole in patients who are allergic to penicillin
   e. Use of intravenous magnesium sulfate to inhibit catecholamine release

5. A 10-year-old girl presented to her primary care physician with a severe sore throat, headache, nausea, and abdominal pain. On examination, the back of her throat was covered with a purulent exudate with white pus-filled nodules. Culture of the exudate on sheep blood agar produced β-hemolytic colonies composed of gram-positive cocci in chains. The colonies were bacitracin-susceptible. Which organism characteristic is most consistent with this result?
   a. Effectively prevented from causing infection through vaccination
   b. Capable of causing rheumatic fever
   c. Catalase-positive
   d. Optochin-susceptible
   e. Penicillin-resistant

6. An infectious diseases fellow in a program offering medical care in Afghanistan examined an 18-month-old child who had cold symptoms for the past 10 days. Four days earlier, when another physician examined the child, the child had a fever, exudate on his pharynx, and enlarged cervical lymph nodes. His chest was clear. A specimen for a throat culture was taken and the child was given a course of penicillin. On the tenth day of illness, the child's condition worsened. He became increasingly lethargic, with respiratory distress, and was admitted to a hospital. On examination, the child had exudate (resembling a yellowish, thick membrane) in the posterior pharynx. A non–spore-forming, gram-positive rod with a palisade arrangement was recovered. Which process produced the factor that killed him?
   a. Spontaneous point mutation
   b. Generalized transduction
   c. Conjugation
   d. Lysogenic conversion
   e. Transformation

7. Nausea, vomiting, and diarrhea developed in a 24-year-old woman and her husband 5 hours after they ate fried rice at a restaurant. Which organism was most likely involved?
   a. *Clostridium difficile*
   b. Enterotoxigenic *Escherichia coli*
   c. *Bacillus cereus*
   d. *Salmonella enterica* serovar Typhi
   e. *Shigella* species

8. A 25-year-old woman presents with a skin lesion on her left thigh of 6 weeks' duration. It started as a pimple but enlarged over 3 weeks to a mass 4 cm in diameter. It continued to increase in size to 6 cm in diameter despite a 10-day course of cephalexin. On physical examination, a 6-cm-diameter tender fluctuant soft tissue abscess is present over the left anterior thigh. A Gram stain of the aspirate shows gram-positive cocci in clusters and many leukocytes. Which of the following is most likely?
   a. Methicillin-susceptible *Staphylococcus aureus*
   b. Methicillin-resistant *Staphylococcus aureus*
   c. Methicillin-susceptible *Staphylococcus lugdunensis*
   d. Methicillin-resistant *Staphylococcus lugdunensis*
   e. Methicillin-susceptible *Staphylococcus epidermidis*

9. Which of the following statements does *not* describe epidemic relapsing fever?
   a. It is a louse-borne disease.
   b. It is caused by *Borrelia recurrentis*.
   c. It is associated with catastrophic events.
   d. The clinical manifestations are similar to those of endemic relapsing fever.
   e. It is a tick-borne disease.

10. Which of the following is used to establish the definitive diagnosis of relapsing fever?
    a. Serologic tests
    b. Blood culture
    c. Urine culture
    d. Demonstration of the organism in peripheral blood
    e. Animal inoculation

11. A previously healthy 30-year-old man is evaluated because of a 2-day history of fever, chills, myalgia, nausea, and headache. Ten days ago he kayaked on a rain-swollen stream that flows alongside a pig farm. On physical examination, the patient appears moderately ill. His temperature is 38.8°C. Minimal scleral icterus

is noted. Urinalysis shows proteinuria (1+), 35 leukocytes per high-power field, and few granular casts. Other laboratory test results are the following:

Component	Value
Hemoglobin, g/dL	14.2
Leukocytes, ×10⁹/L	8.0
Platelets, ×10⁹/L	167
Serum creatinine, mg/dL	1.8
Aspartate aminotransferase, U/mL	95
Alanine aminotransferase, U/mL	72
Serum total bilirubin, mg/dL	3.8
Serum creatine kinase, U/L	740

Which of the following is the most likely diagnosis?
a. Brucellosis
b. Salmonellosis
c. Leptospirosis
d. *Aeromonas hydrophila* infection
e. Hepatitis A

12. Which of the following statements does *not* describe leptospirosis?
a. It is a disease of global distribution.
b. It is greatly underreported.
c. It is maintained in nature by chronic renal infection of carrier animals.
d. It is maintained in nature by chronic intestinal infection of carrier humans.
e. Most human infections are probably asymptomatic.

13. Which of the following does *not* describe antibiotic therapy for leptospirosis?
a. It decreases the duration of leptospiruria.
b. Doxycycline is the drug of choice for severe disease.
c. Ceftriaxone is as effective as penicillin.
d. Therapy should be initiated as early as possible.
e. Jarisch-Herxheimer reactions have been reported with penicillin.

14. A 55-year-old woman with lymphoma undergoes autologous stem cell transplant. She is hospitalized for 3 weeks afterward with febrile neutropenia; cultures of urine and blood grow *Klebsiella pneumoniae*. She receives treatment with ceftazidime, and after the neutrophil count returns to the reference range, she is dismissed to her home. Two weeks later she is hospitalized with fever and hypotension. Vancomycin and ceftazidime are administered, but after 24 hours of antibacterial therapy, she remains febrile and has worsening hypotension, urine output, and respiratory failure. Cultures of blood grow gram-negative bacilli. While you await results of antimicrobial susceptibility testing, what change in antimicrobial therapy would be appropriate?
a. Add gentamicin to her regimen.
b. Add ciprofloxacin to her regimen.
c. Replace ceftazidime with meropenem.
d. Replace ceftazidime with piperacillin-tazobactam.
e. Replace vancomycin with linezolid.

15. A 59-year-old man presents with a history of intermittent fever and malaise for 3 weeks. He reports that 2 weeks ago he thought he had a cold, and he used an old antibiotic prescription. He does not recall the name of these pills but he reports that they seemed to help temporarily. On examination he is febrile, with poor dentition and a faint diastolic murmur. Endocarditis is suspected, and the patient is referred to the hospital. After blood cultures are drawn, vancomycin and ceftriaxone are administered. Transesophageal echocardiography identifies an aortic valve vegetation and aortic regurgitation. His fever resolves after 3 days. Blood cultures do not grow an organism, and he is dismissed and will continue to receive vancomycin and ceftriaxone through a peripherally inserted central catheter (PICC) line. Just before the blood cultures are to be discarded at 7 days of incubation, the laboratory reports that a single blood culture bottle has turned positive. On Gram stain, the isolate is a small, pleomorphic gram-negative bacillus. The laboratory continues incubation of the remaining blood cultures. Two days later, another bottle turns positive for the same organism. While you await identification of this organism, what would be included in optimal antimicrobial management?
a. Continue administration of ceftriaxone and vancomycin.
b. Add low-dose gentamicin for synergy.
c. Add gentamicin, continue use of ceftriaxone, and stop use of vancomycin.
d. Remove the PICC line, and administer oral amoxicillin-clavulanate.
e. Stop use of vancomycin, but continue use of ceftriaxone.

16. A 23-year-old veterinary technician presents to the emergency department for evaluation of a hand injury. She was handling a cat when it bit her. The cat has been immunized against rabies and was in good health. Two small wounds on her thenar eminence are explored. Radiography shows no disruption of the bone cortex. The wound is washed, and cephalexin 500 mg orally every 6 hours is prescribed. The next day, the patient returns to the emergency department with progressive swelling and pain in her hand. She is febrile, with swelling of the hand and lymphangitic streaking up her forearm. What is the most likely reason for the progression to infection after the cat bite?

a. Suboptimal dose of cephalexin
   b. Failure to treat for *Candida* species present in feline oral flora
   c. Community-acquired methicillin-resistant *Staphylococcus aureus* (CA-MRSA) soft tissue infection
   d. Lack of activity of cephalexin against the predominant infecting bacteria
   e. Poor adherence to the prescribed antibacterial

17. A 48-year-old man is brought to the emergency department with confusion. He has a past history of treatment of alcohol abuse but has continued to drink alcohol. He is febrile and hypotensive. His wife reports that they returned from a trip to New Orleans the previous day. After eating at a seafood restaurant, he had watery diarrhea. He became progressively weaker and confused on the trip home. He is admitted to the intensive care unit, and goal-directed therapy for sepsis is begun. On examination, he has jaundice and ascites. His lower extremities are mottled, with large bullous skin lesions and dusky fingers and toes. What is the most likely cause of his current illness?
    a. *Clostridium difficile* enterocolitis
    b. Overwhelming sepsis due to *Vibrio vulnificus*
    c. Enterotoxigenic *Escherichia coli* with hemolytic uremic syndrome
    d. Meningococcemia
    e. Salmonellosis

18. Which of the following statements is *false* about the diagnosis of Lyme disease?
    a. Early Lyme disease is a clinical diagnosis based on the appearance of skin lesions.
    b. Serology results are often negative in early Lyme disease.
    c. Diagnosis of late Lyme disease is primarily based on confirming serology with a positive Western blot for IgM.
    d. The history of exposure to a tick where Lyme disease is endemic is important for the diagnosis of Lyme disease, but the history of a tick bite may not be known.
    e. Skin lesions within 24 hours of a tick bite are not erythema migrans.

19. Which of the following statements is *false* about Ehrlichiosis?
    a. There are 2 main forms of infection in humans: monocytic ehrlichiosis and granulocytic anaplasmosis.
    b. The 2 forms of ehrlichiosis have different regional endemicity.
    c. Ehrlichiosis has an abrupt onset with nonspecific symptoms, including fever, headache, myalgias, and gastrointestinal tract symptoms.
    d. Early abnormal laboratory findings include leukocytosis and thrombophilia.
    e. A diffuse rash is seen more commonly in monocytic ehrlichiosis.

20. Which of the following statements is *false* about babesiosis?
    a. Babesiosis can be transmitted by a tick bite or a blood transfusion.
    b. The clinical features of babesiosis are variable, and the severity of illness is dependent on the host risk factors.
    c. The treatment of choice is atovaquone and azithromycin, which is more effective than quinine and clindamycin.
    d. Babesiosis can have a complicated clinical course and may need to be treated with exchange transfusions.
    e. The primary laboratory finding is hemolytic anemia.

21. Rocky Mountain spotted fever can be difficult to diagnose. Which of the following is *not* a unique clinical feature of Rocky Mountain spotted fever?
    a. Edema around the eyes or hands and feet
    b. Hearing loss
    c. Centripetal rash
    d. Calf tenderness
    e. Petechial rash

22. A 45-year-old man who has been receiving total parenteral nutrition (TPN) has new-onset blurry vision and pain in his left eye. After a funduscopic examination, which of the following treatments may be considered?
    a. Intravenous liposomal amphotericin B
    b. Fluconazole
    c. Amphotericin B in combination with flucytosine
    d. Vitrectomy
    e. All of the above

23. *Candida* species was recovered from blood culture. After 2 hours of incubation, a germ tube was produced. Which *Candida* is most likely?
    a. *Candida glabrata* or *Candida tropicalis*
    b. *Candida krusei* or *Candida parapsilosis*
    c. *Candida albicans* or *Candida dubliniensis*
    d. *Candida lusitaniae* or *Candida guilliermondii*
    e. All of the above

24. For the syndrome of candidemia and acute disseminated candidiasis, which of the following is a treatment consideration?
    a. Indwelling catheter should be removed.
    b. Initiate treatment with echinocandin, fluconazole, or amphotericin B.
    c. Echinocandin is favored with moderate to severe illness or recent fluconazole use or when *Candida glabrata* is suspected.

d. Fluconazole is favored for less critically ill patients who have had no recent azole exposure or if *Candida albicans* or *Candida parapsilosis* is suspected.
e. All of the above are considerations.

25. Which statement is true regarding *Candida* esophagitis?
    a. Most patients with *Candida* esophagitis have underlying medical conditions.
    b. Patients may have *Candida* esophagitis without oral mucositis (thrush).
    c. Endoscopy demonstrates white patches covering the mucosa.
    d. Esophageal perforation due to *Candida* esophagitis may occur rarely.
    e. All statements are correct.

26. Which of the following is recommended for the initial phase of treating tuberculosis in human immunodeficiency virus (HIV)-positive patients who are receiving an antiretroviral regimen including protease inhibitors or nonnucleoside reverse transcriptase inhibitors?
    a. Isoniazid, rifampin, pyrazinamide, and ethambutol
    b. Isoniazid, ethambutol, pyrazinamide, and streptomycin
    c. Isoniazid, rifabutin, pyrazinamide, and ethambutol
    d. Isoniazid, rifampin, pyrazinamide, and ethambutol
    e. Isoniazid, rifampin, pyrazinamide, and clarithromycin

27. A 30-year-old drug addict with AIDS was evaluated for a 1-cm slightly tender, erythematous draining skin nodule on his right thigh. Pus from the lesion was negative with Gram stain but showed unbranched bacilli with acid-fast stain. Eight weeks later, 3 more lesions appeared on the same extremity. Mycobacterial cultures at 35°C on Middlebrook 7H11 agar and radiometric broth medium had been negative for growth. On routine bacterial culture, few coagulase-negative staphylococci grew. Which of the following is the most likely organism?
    a. *Mycobacterium genavense*
    b. *Mycobacterium chelonae*
    c. *Mycobacterium haemophilum*
    d. *Mycobacterium marinum*
    e. *Mycobacterium malmoense*

28. A 10-year-old boy from Mexico has painless, enlarged cervical lymph nodes. He was healthy otherwise. Biopsy demonstrates granuloma; culture was positive and the agent was identified as *Mycobacterium tuberculosis* by Gen-Probe Amplified MTD test. Which of the following is the most likely organism?
    a. *Mycobacterium tuberculosis*
    b. *Mycobacterium bovis*
    c. *Mycobacterium scrofulaceum*
    d. *Mycobacterium genavense*
    e. *Mycobacterium marinum*

29. On routine testing, a 65-year-old woman working as an interpreter in an AIDS clinic has a tuberculin skin test reaction of 5 mm at 48 hours. On repeat testing 2 weeks later, the skin test reaction is 10 mm. A chest radiograph is normal. Which of the following is true?
    a. All household contacts should have a tuberculin skin test.
    b. She should receive isoniazid prophylaxis.
    c. Induced sputum specimens should be cultured for mycobacteria.
    d. She should take time off from work.
    e. No further follow-up is needed.

30. A 30-year-old man went camping and boating with friends in northern Minnesota. Three weeks later, he had an abrupt onset of fever, chills, malaise, myalgia, headache, and productive cough with purulent sputum. The chest radiograph showed a patchy infiltrate in the left lower lobe. Gram stain of expectorated sputum did not show any predominant organisms, but a potassium hydroxide preparation showed yeast with broad-based budding. Assume that a decision has been made to treat the patient. Which is the most appropriate treatment?
    a. Clarithromycin
    b. Fluconazole
    c. Itraconazole
    d. Ampicillin-clavulanate
    e. Voriconazole

31. A 44-year-old man with no known previous medical history presents to a local emergency department in Wisconsin with a rash. On examination, he has stable blood pressure and heart rate, and he is not in acute distress, although there is evidence of moderate weight loss. A localized purplish nodular eruption is limited to his lower left ankle. Test results for human immunodeficiency virus (HIV) are positive; the CD4 cell count is 114/µL. His chest radiograph is unremarkable. Biopsy of the skin lesion shows granulomatous inflammation with a few round yeast but no budding. Culture eventually grows *Blastomyces dermatitidis*. Results from what other diagnostic test are needed before the culture result?
    a. Cerebrospinal fluid (CSF) examination
    b. Blastomyces serology
    c. Blastomyces urinary antigen testing
    d. Serum cryptococcal antigen testing
    e. Both *a* and *d* are correct.

32. For the patient in the previous question, what is the best therapy?
    a. Itraconaozle 200 mg orally 3 times daily
    b. Itraconazole 400 mg orally 2 times daily

c. Voriconazole 200 mg orally 2 times daily
   d. Amphotericin B deoxycholate 50 mg every other day
   e. Liposomal amphotericin B 3-5 mg/kg daily until condition is stabilized and then itraconazole

33. The role of voriconazole or posaconazole in the treatment of blastomycosis is best summarized by which statement below?
    a. These agents are acceptable alternative therapy for mild to moderate pulmonary infection, according to the current guidelines of the Infectious Diseases Society of America.
    b. Intravenous voriconazole is the treatment of choice for patients with life-threatening blastomycosis who cannot tolerate oral treatment.
    c. These newer triazoles appear to have activity against *Blastomyces*, but their role in treatment has not been determined.
    d. These agents are first-line treatment for life-threatening, disseminated blastomycosis that does not involve the central nervous system.
    e. These agents are acceptable alternative therapy for pregnant patients with severe pulmonary blastomycosis.

34. Which of the following is true about paracoccidioidomycosis?
    a. The precise ecologic niche is not known.
    b. This opportunistic infection commonly occurs in patients infected with human immunodeficiency virus who have low CD4 cell counts (<50 cells/μL).
    c. This infection was originally described in southeastern Asia and parts of Africa.
    d. A self-limited pulmonary infection is the most common clinical presentation.
    e. Multiple randomized controlled studies show that the drug of choice is itraconazole.

35. Which of the following is *true* for paracoccidioidomycosis but *false* for coccidioidomycosis?
    a. The organism is endemic in Brazil.
    b. The clinical spectrum of disease ranges from asymptomatic to severe and life-threatening.
    c. Treatment options include itraconazole, ketoconazole, or fluconazole.
    d. A yeast form is the most common finding in vivo for this dimorphic fungus.
    e. Both choices *a* and *d* are correct.

36. The appearance of multiple buds of yeast surrounding the mother cell of *Paracoccidioides* resembles which of the following?
    a. Ferris wheel
    b. Pilot's wheel
    c. Tuberculin skin test wheal
    d. Windmill
    e. Film reel

37. Which of the following statements about paracoccidioidomycosis is *false*?
    a. Infectious Diseases Society of America (IDSA) treatment guidelines list sulfonamides as the drug of choice.
    b. Paracoccidioidomycosis has been diagnosed in many countries other than those of Latin America; however, in each case the afflicted person previously lived in Latin America.
    c. A long latency period of decades often separates the original infection from the clinical disease.
    d. The most important infection in the differential diagnosis of paracoccidioidomycosis is tuberculosis; coinfection occurs in 15% of cases.
    e. Prompt diagnosis is often hindered by lack of physician awareness.

38. Which of the following situations would most likely result in a respiratory infection characterized by bilateral pulmonary infiltrates with hilar lymphadenopathy and a bronchoscopy washing notable for ovoid yeast forms (2-4 μm) identified by silver stain?
    a. Traveling through a dust storm in Arizona
    b. Cleaning out a chicken coop on a farm in southern Illinois
    c. Boating on a lake in Wisconsin
    d. Camping in Madagascar
    e. Being imprisoned in a federal penitentiary in central California

39. A 20-year-old man who is otherwise healthy presented with a history of fever and night sweats for 3 weeks after a barn remodeling project. Computed tomography of the chest showed mediastinal lymphadenopathy (1-1.5 cm). Biopsy specimens showed organisms that resembled *Histoplasma capsulatum*. While the patient waited for further testing, his symptoms resolved. Which of the following is appropriate treatment?
    a. Liposomal amphotericin B for 2 weeks while making sure that symptoms do not recur
    b. Careful observation with monitoring of *Histoplasma* antigen levels
    c. Itraconazole 200 mg orally twice daily for 30 days
    d. Fluconazole 400 mg orally once daily for 30 days
    e. Choices *b* and *c* above

40. Which of the following statements is true for the *Histoplasma* antigen test?
    a. Serum antigen testing is more sensitive than urinary antigen testing.
    b. In general, urinary antigen testing is more sensitive in acute pulmonary histoplasmosis (low inoculum) than in disseminated histoplasmosis.

c. It is a sensitive assay for suspected fibrosing mediastinitis.
d. False-positive test results can occur with aspiration pneumonia.
e. False-positive test results can occur with pulmonary coccidioidomycosis.

41. Which of the following manifestations of histoplasmosis is typically an indication for antifungal therapy?
    a. Acute pulmonary histoplasmosis with bilateral or diffuse infiltrates
    b. Presumed ocular histoplasmosis
    c. Fibrosing mediastinitis
    d. Mild pericarditis
    e. Yeast of *Histoplasma* identified within a granuloma of calcified mediastinal lymph nodes

42. A patient is referred to your office for a nodular rash that began on the distal forearm and is spreading proximally. Which of the following organisms has caused the infection?
    a. *Sporothrix schenckii*
    b. *Coccidioides posadasii*
    c. *Mycobacterium marinum*
    d. *Nocardia brasiliensis*
    e. *Francisella tularensis*

43. At 14 weeks of gestation, a 24-year-old woman scraped her leg against a wooden fence post, resulting in an extensive abrasion. The abrasion healed nearly completely, but a large, localized ulcerated nodule remained in part of the injured area. Biopsy findings from the lesion were consistent with sporotrichosis. Which is the best treatment option that would not be expected to harm the fetus?
    a. Itraconazole 200 mg twice daily
    b. Fluconazole 200 mg twice daily
    c. Liposomal amphotericin B 3 mg/kg daily
    d. Localized hyperthermia
    e. Supersaturated solution of potassium iodide (SSKI)

44. Classic sporotrichosis has been most commonly associated with disruption of skin and contact with soil or vegetative matter colonized with *Sporothrix*. A large outbreak of sporotrichosis that began in 1998 in Rio de Janeiro, Brazil, resulted in hundreds of human cases that were associated with traumatic or atraumatic contact with animals. Which animals were involved?
    a. Armadillos
    b. Moles
    c. Ground squirrels
    d. Cats
    e. Dogs

45. Which of the following has *not* been described as a cause of sporotrichosis?
    a. Contaminated hay bales used as props in a Halloween spook house in Oklahoma
    b. Florida tree farm workers producing sphagnum moss topiaries
    c. Palm tree thorn injuries in landscapers in Arizona
    d. Sleeping in an old, rust-stained camping tent in Mexico
    e. Human-to-human transmission from a mother's cheek lesion to her infant

46. A 65-year-old woman, an Arizona native with a 50-pack-year history of tobacco use, traveled to Indiana to attend the funeral of her recently deceased sister. While cleaning her sister's old house, the patient encountered bats in the attic. Three weeks after returning from the Midwest, she experienced fever, myalgia, headache, and a dry cough. A chest radiograph showed a pulmonary mass. Serologic results for *Coccidioides*, *Histoplasma*, and *Cryptococcus* were negative. While she waited for the scheduled diagnostic test, her symptoms resolved. When her chest radiograph did not improve, she underwent a transthoracic biopsy of the mass; the histopathologic findings were adenocarcinoma of the lung and a small granulomatous focus with spherules. She underwent partial lobectomy of the affected lung. No other abnormalities were observed on computed tomographic scan or at surgery. What is the treatment of choice for this infection?
    a. Fluconazole
    b. Liposomal amphotericin B
    c. Itraconazole
    d. Observation only
    e. Follow-up with *Coccidioides* serology and observation

47. A 50-year-old man visited Arizona for 3 weeks in the winter. He returned home with a headache, fever, and cough. In the ensuing months, the fever and cough resolved, but the headache progressed. Cerebrospinal fluid (CSF) examination indicated chronic meningitis with elevated protein level, low glucose level, and leukocytosis with a predominance of lymphocytes. The intraventricular pressure was 140 mm water. The CSF fungal culture was negative, but serology was positive for *Coccidioides* species in the serum and the CSF. What is the best treatment at this time?
    a. Liposomal amphotericin B 5 mg/kg daily
    b. Fluconazole 800 mg intravenously daily
    c. Fluconazole 800 mg orally daily
    d. Ventriculoperitoneal shunting
    e. Intrathecal amphotericin B deoxycholate

48. Which organism is most likely to cause coccidioidomycosis in Tucson, Arizona?
    a. *Coccidioides immitis*
    b. *Coccidioides tucsonii*

    c. *Coccidioides galgianii*
    d. *Coccidioides posadasii*
    e. *Coccidioides pappagianisii*

49. An 18-year-old white, pregnant, hypertensive woman recently received a diagnosis of gestational diabetes. She has been unsuccessful in her attempts to stop smoking cigarettes during her 7 months of pregnancy. Which risk factor most likely accounts for dissemination of coccidioidomycosis in this patient?
    a. Smoking cigarettes during pregnancy
    b. Third trimester of pregnancy
    c. Race
    d. Age
    e. Gestational diabetes

50. A 65-year-old man with poorly controlled diabetes presents with progressive left eye proptosis. He is urgently taken to the operating room and undergoes left eye enucleation with extensive débridement. Frozen section examination of tissue specimens shows broad, hyaline, nonseptate hyphae with right-angled branching. Which of the following azoles has activity against this mold?
    a. Fluconazole
    b. Voriconazole
    c. Posaconazole
    d. Itraconazole
    e. Ketoconazole

51. A 45-year-old woman from Arizona with relapsed acute myeloid leukemia underwent allogeneic stem cell transplant. In the pre-engraftment period, neutropenic fever developed. On physical examination, she has a 2×3-cm plaque-like erythematous, nontender lesion on her right forearm. Biopsy specimens show septate, branching, filamentous hyphae invading cutaneous blood vessels. Three days later, the same fungus is growing in her blood culture. What is the most likely pathogen?
    a. *Aspergillus* species
    b. *Rhizopus* species
    c. *Fusarium* species
    d. *Coccidioides immitis*
    e. *Histoplasma capsulatum*

52. Which mold appears as septate, branching hyphae in tissue sections?
    a. *Aspergillus* species
    b. *Paecilomyces* species
    c. *Fusarium* species
    d. *Pseudallescheria* species
    e. All of the above

53. Which of the following is the causative agent of pityriasis versicolor (also called tinea versicolor)?
    a. *Saccharomyces cerevisiae*
    b. *Paecilomyces varioti*
    c. *Trichosporon beigelii*
    d. *Malassezia furfur*
    e. *Cladophialophora bantiana*

54. Which statement is *false* about the virulence and pathogenicity of *Cryptococcus neoformans*?
    a. The polysaccharide capsule is an important virulence factor, and in animal models *Cryptococcus* with a reduced capsule or without any capsule is significantly less virulent.
    b. Melanin production is a virulence factor, and in animal models a mutant *Cryptococcus* that loses the ability to produce melanin is less virulent.
    c. When *Cryptococcus neoformans* mutants lose the ability to grow at 37°C, the yeast loses its virulence.
    d. In mice models, when mutant *Cryptococcus* loses the ability to produce large amounts of urease, its virulence is attenuated.
    e. *Cryptococcus* isolate, which has all 3 characteristics of virulence (presence of capsule, melanin production, growth at 37°C) will always cause invasive disease in an exposed host.

55. Which statement is *false* about lung involvement with cryptococcal infection?
    a. Finding *Cryptococcus neoformans* in the sputum always means that invasive disease is present because cryptococcal colonization is never found.
    b. An immunosuppressed host may present with acute respiratory disease syndrome associated with cryptococcal lung infection.
    c. The radiologic findings in cryptococcal lung infection include nodules, infiltrates, hilar lymphadenopathy, cavitation, and pleural effusion.
    d. Patients may present with symptoms that are nonspecific (such as fever, cough, chest pain, and weight loss), or they may not have any symptoms.
    e. The sensitivity of cryptococcal antigen testing is very low; therefore, patients may present with significant lung infection and negative results on serum *Cryptococcus* antigen testing.

56. Which statement is *false* about the treatment of cryptococcal meningoencephalitis in patients without human immunodeficiency virus infection?
    a. The duration of treatment depends on the severity of illness and the immunosuppressive state.
    b. Induction therapy is usually given for at least 4 weeks with amphotericin B 0.7-1.0 mg/kg daily in combination with flucytosine 100 mg/kg daily.
    c. Amphotericin B lipid complex (5 mg/kg daily) can be given instead of conventional amphotericin B and given in combination with flucytosine.

d. Administration of flucytosine with amphotericin B with fluconazole, or with itraconazole will sterilize the cerebrospinal fluid (CSF) after 2 weeks of combination therapy.
e. After induction therapy, oral fluconazole (200 mg daily) is given for 6 to 12 months.

57. Which statement is true for infection caused by *Cryptococcus neoformans* var *gatti*?
    a. It usually involves immunosuppressed hosts.
    b. Antifungal susceptibility testing results are completely different between *Cryptococcus neoformans* var *neoformans* and *C neoformans* var *gatti*, therefore, treatment is different.
    c. Cryptococcoma formation in the brain is much more common with *C neoformans* var *neoformans* than with *C neoformans* var *gatti*.
    d. The following computed tomographic findings in the brain may all be secondary to *C neoformans* var *gatti* infection: single mass lesion, multiple ring-enhancing lesions, and hydrocephalus.
    e. Brain cryptococcoma due to *C neoformans* var *gatti* is known to respond promptly to antifungal medications.

58. Which of the following is *false* about *Cryptosporidium*?
    a. Intestinal infection occurs primarily in the upper small intestine.
    b. It can be readily killed by chlorination.
    c. It causes a secretory type of diarrhea.
    d. It is not easily detected by routine ova and parasites examination.
    e. It adheres to intestinal mucosal cells but does not invade the cytoplasm.

59. Which of the following is true about Microsporida?
    a. They are morphologically similar to *Cryptosporidium* but larger.
    b. They can usually be detected by routine ova and parasites examination.
    c. Metronidazole is effective treatment of intestinal infections.
    d. Infection occurs primarily in immunocompromised patients.
    e. Fecal leukocytes are frequently present.

60. Which of the following is *false* about free-living amebae?
    a. *Acanthamoeba* have caused severe keratitis in contact lens users.
    b. *Acanthamoeba* are the cause of primary amebic meningoencephalitis.
    c. Infections due to *Naegleria* are poorly responsive to antiparasitic agents.
    d. Organisms are commonly present in moist soil and warm ponds.
    e. The cerebrospinal fluid (CSF) examination is useful in granulomatous amebic encephalitis for microscopic detection and culture of organisms.

61. Which of the following is *not* important in the pathogenesis of severe infection due to *Plasmodium falciparum*?
    a. Ability to infect erythrocytes of all ages
    b. Adherence of infected erythrocytes to vascular endothelium
    c. Persistence of parasites in liver cells as hypnozoites
    d. "Rosetting" of normal erythrocytes around parasite-containing erythrocytes
    e. Release of tumor necrosis factor α and other cytokines during parasitemia

62. Which of the following statements about microscopy of Giemsa-stained peripheral blood smears is *false*?
    a. Early ring forms of *Plasmodium* and *Babesia* may be similar in appearance.
    b. *Plasmodium* species identification is usually accomplished by examination of thick blood films.
    c. Amastigote forms of *Leishmania* are not detectable in thin blood films.
    d. *Trypanosoma cruzi*, which causes Chagas disease, usually assumes a *C* shape in thin blood films.
    e. Tachyzoite (trophozoite) forms of *Toxoplasma gondii* are generally not detectable in thick blood films.

63. Which parasite causes infection that is *not* characterized by significant eosinophilia?
    a. *Strongyloides stercoralis*
    b. *Entamoeba histolytica*
    c. *Trichinella spiralis*
    d. *Toxocara canis*
    e. *Ancylostoma duodenale*

64. Which of these adult tapeworms does *not* reside in the human intestinal tract?
    a. *Echinococcus granulosus*
    b. *Taenia solium*
    c. *Diphyllobothrium latum*
    d. *Taenia saginata*
    e. *Hymenolepis nana*

65. Which of these parasites infects humans through ingestion of helminth eggs?
    a. *Ascaris lubricoides*
    b. *Schistosoma mansoni*
    c. *Strongyloides stercoralis*
    d. *Ancylostoma duodenale*
    e. *Necator americanus*

66. Which of the following is *not* characteristic of infection with *Strongyloides stercoralis*?
    a. Chronic infection can be caused by autoinfection.
    b. Significant eosinophilia is often present.
    c. Acute infection can cause respiratory symptoms and pulmonary infiltrates.
    d. Hyperinfection may be accompanied by bacterial sepsis in immunocompromised persons.
    e. The diagnosis can be made by finding parasitic eggs in the stool of infected patients.

67. Which of the following would *not* cause infection if a person ate raw or undercooked aquatic animals (eg, fish, crabs, snails)?
    a. *Anisakis*
    b. *Gnathostoma*
    c. *Clonorchis*
    d. *Schistosoma*
    e. *Angiostrongylus*

68. Which of the following is *not* caused by both herpes simplex virus and varicella-zoster virus?
    a. Facial paralysis
    b. Acute retinal necrosis in healthy hosts
    c. Encephalitis
    d. Granulomatous vasculitis of intracranial arteries
    e. Disseminated vesicular eruption in immunocompromised hosts

69. Which of the following does *not* help to control hospital spread of adenovirus conjunctivitis?
    a. Decontamination of instruments and environmental surfaces with 10% bleach
    b. Handwashing
    c. Goggles
    d. Gloves
    e. Contact isolation

70. A young woman has polyarticular arthritis in the smaller joints of the hands and feet but no fever, rash, or other local symptoms. Which of the following is she most likely to have?
    a. Mumps virus
    b. Epstein-Barr virus
    c. Human parvovirus B19
    d. Coxsackievirus B
    e. Gonorrhea

71. A 45-year-old male physician (born in 1964) who had recently volunteered at a summer camp in Iowa for teenagers presents with fever, malaise, headache, and unilateral testicular pain with scrotal swelling and erythema. An examination of cerebrospinal fluid (CSF) shows pleocytosis, fewer than 500 white blood cells per microliter (mostly lymphocytes), and a slightly low glucose level, but the culture is negative. What is the most likely reason for this person's acquisition of this infection?
    a. Lack of vaccination and no prior native infection
    b. A new strain of pathogen not covered by prior vaccines
    c. A tick bite
    d. Benign prostatic hypertrophy (BPH)
    e. Community-acquired methicillin-resistant *Staphylococcus aureus* (CA-MRSA) infection

72. Which of the following statements is *false* about the epidemiology of aspergillosis?
    a. *Aspergillus* is ubiquitous, found in soil, water, food, air, and decaying vegetation.
    b. Clusters of invasive aspergillosis have been described after hospital renovation and construction.
    c. Nosocomial invasive aspergillosis cases have been related to contaminated hospital water supplies and potted plants in patient rooms.
    d. The primary risk factor for invasive aspergillosis is immunosuppression, which can be inherited or acquired.
    e. Solid organ transplant recipients are usually not neutropenic and therefore are not at risk of invasive aspergillosis.

73. A liver transplant recipient presented with pulmonary invasive aspergillosis 3 months after his transplant operation. Treatment with amphotericin B will most likely fail if fungal culture yields which of the following *Aspergillus* species?
    a. *Aspergillus flavus*
    b. *Aspergillus terreus*
    c. *Aspergillus fumigatus*
    d. *Aspergillus nidulans*
    e. *Aspergillus ustus*

74. Which of the following statements is *false* regarding invasive aspergillosis?
    a. The fungus is angioinvasive and may cause thrombosis of vessels and infarcts.
    b. A kidney or liver transplant recipient who presents with wheezing and dyspnea 30 days after transplant most likely has the syndrome of *Aspergillus* tracheobronchitis.
    c. Voriconazole is usually recommended as a drug of choice for initiation of treatment of invasive aspergillosis.
    d. Although combination therapy for invasive aspergillosis has been used by many clinicians, no controlled clinical trials have validated this approach.
    e. The finding of aspergillus in the airway of an immunosuppressed patient should trigger an evaluation for invasiveness, and *Aspergillus* species

should not be assumed a colonizer unless proved to be so.

75. Which of the following conditions of invasive aspergillosis is *not* considered a relative indication for surgery?
    a. Osteomyelitis of the distal tibia after trauma and local drainage
    b. Maxillary sinusitis and headache
    c. Multiple small bilateral lung cavitary lesions and hemoptysis
    d. Endocarditis of the mitral valve and atrial fibrillation
    e. Frontal lobe brain lesion and a seizure

76. A 40-year-old man presents with cough and malaise. He had undergone a renal transplant 8 months before and is receiving prednisone. In the right lower lobe, a chest radiograph shows a consolidated lesion that increased in size over the previous month. A Gram-stained specimen from bronchoalveolar lavage is shown. In addition to administering appropriate antibiotics, what should you do?

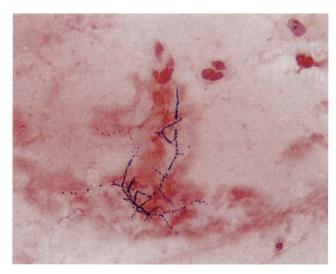

(The photo belongs to Niels Olson's photostream. Used with permission.)

   a. Order computer tomography (CT) or magnetic resonance imaging of the brain.
   b. Order CT of the abdomen.
   c. Draw blood samples for fungal serologic tests.
   d. Obtain a transesophageal echocardiogram.
   e. Consult a thoracic surgeon for more definitive treatment.

77. A 50-year-old gardener presents with subcutaneous nodules of the hand and forearm (as shown in the photograph). The lesions are located along the regional lymphatic vessels and are draining purulent material. Gram stain of the drainage material shows gram-positive filamentous branching organisms. What is the treatment of choice for this infection?

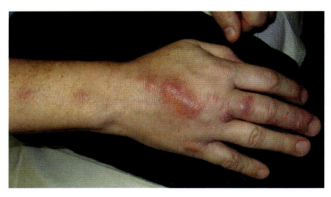

(Adapted from Giordano CN, Ikalb RE, Brass C, Lin L, Helm TN. Nodular lymphangitis: report of a case with presentation of a diagnostic paradigm. Dermatol Oncol J. 2010 Sep 15;16[9]:1. Used with permission.)

   a. Itraconazole
   b. Trimethoprim-sulfamethoxazole
   c. Penicillin
   d. Clarithromycin
   e. Cephalexin

78. A 60-year-old man is referred to you by his dentist. Several weeks after a tooth extraction, a relatively painless mass developed over the patient's mandible. Thick yellow material is draining from the lesion. Gram stain of the drainage shows branching filamentous rods. Past medical history is remarkable for an anaphylactic reaction to penicillin in the remote past. How would you treat this patient?
   a. Trimethoprim-sulfamethoxazole
   b. Doxycycline
   c. Ceftriaxone
   d. Cephalexin
   e. Metronidazole

79. A 65-year-old alcoholic with a long history of smoking presents with weight loss and cough. Chest radiographs show a large mass in the right lower lobe. Physical examination findings include erythema and an apparent sinus tract of the chest. Yellowish debris can be expressed from the sinus tract. His teeth are in poor condition. How would you treat this patient?
   a. Cefazolin
   b. Vancomycin
   c. Penicillin
   d. Nafcillin
   e. Trimethoprim-sulfamethoxazole

Answers

1. Answer e.
Assume that the patient did not have a primary vaccination series as a child in Cambodia. Therefore, she needs to receive the primary series for active immunization and the hyperimmune globulin for rapid passive immunization while antibodies to the vaccine develop.

2. Answer b.
The patient has clinical symptoms of botulism. He needs to receive antitoxin and penicillin to eradicate the organism colonization at the thigh wound.

3. Answer c.
The patient's clinical presentation is compatible with a clinical diagnosis of tetanus. *Clostridium tetani* is a gram-positive bacillus. Tetanospasmin, a powerful neurotoxin produced by *C tetani*, binds to presynaptic nerve endings and causes disinhibition of excitatory neurons. Toxin binding to nerve endings is irreversible, and recovery requires growth of new axonal terminals (which takes 4-6 weeks). The *C tetani* organism is universally susceptible to penicillin. Tetanus does not impair the level of consciousness.

4. Answer d.
Metronidazole is now considered the drug of choice owing to its better safety profile and improved outcomes. Penicillins and other antimicrobials, such as clindamycin, macrolides, and tetracycline, are considered alternative agents for treatment of *C tetani*.

5. Answer b.
This is a case of *Streptococcus pyogenes* pharyngitis. Unfortunately, there is no Food and Drug Administration–approved vaccine for *S pyogenes*. Antibodies against M protein confer protective immunity, but there are many M protein types. *Streptococcus pyogenes* can cause rheumatic fever and acute glomerulonephritis. It is catalase-negative and optochin-resistant. (*Streptococcus pneumoniae* is optochin-susceptible.) Penicillin resistance has not been reported in this organism.

6. Answer d.
This is a case of diphtheria. *Corynebacterium diphtheriae* produces a phage-encoded toxin (diphtheria toxin).

7. Answer c.
Bacillus cereus causes 2 food-borne illnesses: a short-incubation illness and a long-incubation illness. In the short-incubation illness, as in this case, nausea, vomiting, and abdominal cramps follow an incubation of 1 to 6 hours, similar to the course of *Staphylococcus aureus* food poisoning. The illness is caused by a preformed, heat-stable emetic toxin and is most often associated with rice dishes that have been cooked and then held at warm temperatures for several hours.

8. Answer b.
This skin and soft tissue infection is most likely to be caused by *Staphylococcus aureus*. With the lack of response to cephalexin and the overall clinical presentation, methicillin-resistant *Staphylococcus aureus* should be suspected.

9. Answer e.
Epidemic relapsing fever is not a tick-borne disease. It is a louse-borne disease caused by *B recurrentis*, it is associated with catastrophic events, and the clinical manifestations are similar to those of endemic relapsing fever.

10. Answer d.
The definitive diagnosis of relapsing fever is established by the demonstration of the organism in peripheral blood. The other choices are of limited diagnostic value and will not provide a definitive diagnosis.

11. Answer c.
The patient's history and exposure are compatible with leptospirosis. Human infection can occur during water activities, such as kayaking, by indirect exposure to organisms in the water from the urine of carrier animals.

12. Answer d.
Leptospirosis is maintained in nature by chronic renal infection of carrier animals—not by chronic intestinal infection of carrier humans. Leptospirosis is a disease of global distribution, it is greatly underreported, and most human infections are probably asymptomatic.

13. Answer b.
Penicillin is the drug of choice for severe disease, and ceftriaxone has been shown to be as effective as penicillin. Doxycycline is indicated for mild disease. Antibiotic therapy should be initiated as early as possible, and it decreases the duration of leptospiruria. Jarisch-Herxheimer reactions have been reported when penicillin is used.

14. Answer c.
Klebsiella pneumoniae is a gram-negative pathogen that produces extended spectrum β-lactamase (ESBL), conferring resistance to third-generation cephalosporins and other β-lactams. Gram-negative bacteremia in a patient with prior exposure to antibiotics and hospital environments, particularly with a lack of response to initial appropriate empirical therapy, should prompt consideration of infection with an ESBL-producing strain. ESBL-producing organisms have resistance to various β-lactam antibacterials and often to aminoglycosides and quinolones. Now ESBL-producing organisms frequently produce multiple ESBLs, and a corresponding decrease in activity of piperacillin-tazobactam against ESBL-producing gram-negative bacilli has been seen. Combinations of β-lactam and β-lactamase inhibitor are not recommended for use in serious infections with ESBL-producing organisms. Empirical therapy for a suspected ESBL infection should include imipenem or meropenem,

carbapenems with reliable activity against most ESBL-producing strains.

15. Answer e.
A common cause of culture-negative endocarditis is prior antimicrobial therapy, which this patient received. The HACEK gram-negative bacilli (*Haemophilus aphrophilus, Haemophilus paraphrophilus, Actinobacillus actinomycetemcomitans, Cardiobacterium hominis, Eikenella corrodens,* and *Kingella kingae*) cause approximately 3% of the cases of community-acquired endocarditis. Owing to their slow growth in culture, they are a common cause of culture-negative endocarditis. These fastidious bacteria typically take 5 days or more to grow in blood culture. Recommended therapy of HACEK group infective endocarditis involves 4 to 6 weeks of intravenous third- or fourth-generation cephalosporin or ampicillin-sulbactam. Routine addition of an aminoglycoside is no longer recommended.

16. Answer d.
Pasteurella multocida is a predominant organism in infections after feline bites, which often become infected. Proper treatment includes surgical exploration and débridement, evaluation of the need for prophylaxis against rabies and tetanus, and antibacterial therapy directed against *P multocida* and anaerobes. Recommended antibacterials include amoxicillin-clavulanate (or doxycycline in the penicillin-allergic patient). *Pasteurella multocida* is resistant to cephalexin, clindamycin, and often erythromycin; use of these antibiotics alone is inadequate therapy after an animal bite.

17. Answer b.
Vibrio vulnificus is a gram-negative bacterium that can cause severe infection after ingestion of contaminated shellfish or after contact of open wounds with contaminated marine saltwater. This organism should be suspected as a cause of severe sepsis in immunocompromised persons or those with chronic liver disease and recent shellfish ingestion or saltwater contact. Hemorrhagic bullae and skin necrosis can occur. Recommended treatment includes a third-generation cephalosporin and doxycycline.

18. Answer c.
The diagnosis of late Lyme disease is based on exposure to a tick where Lyme disease is endemic, a compatible clinical syndrome, and positive Lyme screening and confirming serology (IgG).

19. Answer d.
Notable abnormal laboratory findings in early ehrlichiosis include thrombocytopenia, leukopenia, and abnormal liver function test results.

20. Answer c.
For treatment of non–life-threatening babesiosis, the combination of atovaquone and azithromycin is as effective as the combination of quinine and clindamycin and is associated with fewer adverse reactions.

21. Answer e.
Rocky Mountain spotted fever can be difficult to diagnose in early disease. Unique clinical features include edema around the eyes, ankle, or hands; hearing loss; centripetal rash; relative bradycardia; and calf tenderness. Although a petechial rash is common, it can be seen in a number of other medical conditions.

22. Answer e.
The diagnosis is *Candida* endophthalmitis, which may be a complication of TPN administration. All choices are correct treatment considerations for *Candida* endophthalmitis. In severe cases, vitrectomy may be offered.

23. Answer c.
After incubation, *C albicans* and *C dubliniensis* may produce a germ tube (a short hypha is formed directly from the yeast cell). The other *Candida* species do not. Incubation is usually in serum for 2 to 3 hours at 37°C.

24. Answer e.
All these statements describe correct treatment considerations for candidemia and acute disseminated candidiasis.

25. Answer e.
All 4 statements correctly describe *Candida* esophagitis.

26. Answer c.
The general principles of tuberculosis therapy are the same as for patients without HIV, including 4-drug therapy in most cases. In addition, careful consideration of drug interactions is essential when choosing antitubercular therapy for patients receiving antiretroviral therapy. Because of the extensive interactions between rifampin and many antiretroviral drugs, most experts prefer a rifabutin-based regimen for 6 months as first-line therapy for HIV-infected patients who are also being treated with protease inhibitors.

27. Answer c.
Patients with *M haemophilum* disease commonly present with painful, erythematous, ulcerating skin nodules and human immunodeficiency virus infection. The organism requires ferric ions (eg, chocolate agar, supplemented media, BACTEC) to grow in culture, and it grows best at 30°C to 35°C.

28. Answer b.
In humans, consumption of unpasteurized milk products such as fresh cheese from infected cows can cause *M bovis* infection. The disease is similar to that caused by other species of the *M tuberculosis* complex, although the anatomical site of *M bovis* disease is more often extrapulmonary. In the United States, *M bovis* disease is more common among Hispanics of Mexican origin. Typically, *M bovis* is resistant to pyrazinamide.

29. Answer e.
Two-step tests are used to avoid interpreting the boost as a new infection. Two-step testing is especially important when initially testing persons who have not had a test in the prior

12 months and who may be subject to regular testing in the future, such as health care workers and employees. For individuals with low risk who enter into a work site where a high risk of exposure to tuberculosis is expected, a positive response is at least 15 mm of induration. This patient otherwise had no significant history of tuberculosis contact.

30. **Answer c.**

Itraconazole is used to treat blastomycosis.

31. **Answer e.**

When a patient infected with HIV has a low CD4 cell count, the differential diagnosis of a round yeast, including especially *Cryptococcus*, is important. Because a disseminated fungal infection is present in an immunosuppressed patient, a CSF examination is indicated.

32. **Answer e.**

According to the updated 2008 Infectious Diseases Society of America guideline, the best therapy for immunocompromised patients with disseminated blastomycosis, such as in this patient, is a few weeks of liposomal amphotericin B followed by itraconazole.

33. **Answer c.**

The role of these newer triazoles, voriconazole and posaconazole, has not been determined, although they appear to have antifungal activity against *Blastomyces*.

34. **Answer a.**

The precise ecologic niche is not known, but the infection is only encountered in persons who have visited or lived where *Paracoccidioides brasiliensis* is endemic (ie, in Latin America and South America, from Mexico to Argentina). The largest number of cases has been reported from Brazil. The infection has not been recognized as opportunistic, and few cases have occurred in immunosuppressed persons. Lungs are the primary site of infection, but complaints resulting from mucosal ulcerations of the upper respiratory and digestive tracts are the most common clinical presentations, followed by cutaneous lesions of the face and limbs.

35. **Answer d.**

Although both fungi are dimorphic, the in vivo form of *Paracoccidioides brasiliensis* is a yeast, whereas the in vivo form of *Coccidioides* species is a spherule. Both fungi are endemic in many parts of Central America and South America, including Brazil. Despite some similarities as noted above, there is no mycologic similarity between the 2 organisms, as the genus names seem to suggest.

36. **Answer b.**

The characteristic appearance of the multiple budding of daughter yeast cells from the mother cell of *Paracoccidioides* has been likened to a pilot's wheel.

37. **Answer a.**

IDSA guidelines do not exist for the treatment of paracoccidioidomycosis. Paracoccidioidomycosis is the only fungal infection that responds to sulfonamide treatment. The dosage for adults is 2 g daily, which can be decreased after a few months when improvement has begun. Treatment should be continued for 3 to 5 years to avoid relapse, which is as high as 25%. Amphotericin B can be used when life-threatening illness is present, and its use has resulted in improvement in up to 70% of patients. Ketoconazole and itraconazole have been found to be effective. Fluconazole is effective only in high doses and has been avoided. Newer azoles such as voriconazole and posaconazole have been shown to be effective but not superior to itraconazole.

38. **Answer b.**

Histoplasma capsulatum var *capsulatum* (1-4 μm) is distinguished from *H capsulatum* var *duboisii* (10-12 μm) by size. *Histoplasma capsulatum* var *duboisii* is the causative agent of histoplasmosis in Africa (reported only between the Tropic of Cancer and the Tropic of Capricorn) and on the island of Madagascar. Exposure to a dust storm in Arizona may result in coccidioidomycosis, and outdoor recreation associated with bodies of water in the Midwest may result in blastomycosis.

39. **Answer b.**

In an otherwise healthy person without symptoms, close observation without treatment is recommended.

40. **Answer e.**

False-positive test results for urinary *Histoplasma* antigen have occurred with active blastomycosis, paracoccidioidomycosis, and coccidioidomycosis.

41. **Answer a.**

Antifungal treatment is not generally administered to patients with presumed ocular histoplasmosis, mild pericarditis, or histoplasmosis identified in old lesions or lymph nodes. Acute infection with diffuse infiltrates warrants antifungal treatment. Antifungal therapy directed at fibrosing mediastinitis has not been successful, although guidelines allow for a 3-month trial of itraconazole.

42. **Answer a.**

The described situation is the most common manifestation of *S schenckii*. The other 4 choices are all in the differential diagnosis of sporotrichosis. An additional consideration in an epidemiologically appropriate situation would be cutaneous leishmaniasis. Some patients with sporotrichosis do not manifest lymphangitic spread but instead have fixed cutaneous lesions that persist at the site of inoculation.

43. **Answer c.**

The azoles are potentially teratogenic and should not be used in pregnancy. SSKI has toxic effects on the fetal thyroid. Localized hyperthermia could be an option, but since the lesion is large, treatment should be liposomal amphotericin B.

44. **Answer d.**

Beginning in 1998, a long-lived outbreak of sporotrichosis (primarily lymphocutaneous) began in the metropolitan and surrounding areas of Rio de Janeiro, Brazil. The outbreak was associated with traumatic (bites and scratches) or atraumatic contact with cats. Professional or household contact with cats was the primary risk factor for this infection. Transmission was thought to be from direct contact with the cats' skin lesions.

45. Answer c.
Although contact with roses and thorns is commonly associated with sporotrichosis, contaminated hay (often baled) and sphagnum moss have been described as sources of *Sporothrix* in outbreaks. No associations have been described with palm or cactus thorn injuries. Farmers, florists, and horticulturalists are at occupational risk.

46. Answer e.
The patient has an asymptomatic coccidioidal lung infection, apparently resected without any residual disease. No treatment is warranted. Another serologic study is needed because early studies may be insensitive.

47. Answer c.
Standard treatment is fluconazole. With nearly 100% oral bioavailability, there is no need to administer parenterally unless there is a contraindication to oral administration. Ventriculoperitoneal shunt is not required at this time, but monitoring for evidence of hydrocephalus is needed.

48. Answer d.
Coccidioides posadasii is the organism responsible for coccidioidomycosis east of California. This species is nearly identical to *Coccidioides immitis*, the organism present in California.

49. Answer b.
Pregnancy, especially the third trimester, is a well-recognized risk factor for disseminated coccidioidomycosis. Pregnant women who contract coccidioidomycosis should be treated with amphotericin B to control infection and (presumably) to decrease the risk of disseminated infection. Cigarette smoking confers a higher risk of severe respiratory disease but not a higher risk of disseminated coccidioidomycosis. Diabetes mellitus, particularly if not well controlled, can increase the risk of cavitary or relapsing pulmonary infection, but diabetes mellitus was a risk factor for dissemination in only 1 of several studies. Age and race are less likely to be predictive of dissemination, which occurs more commonly in older persons, especially those with Filipino or African ancestors.

50. Answer c.
Patients with poorly controlled diabetes or diabetic ketoacidosis, hematologic malignancy, bone marrow or solid organ transplant, or iron chelation therapy with deferoxamine are at risk of rhinocerebral zygomycosis. Presentation can be nonspecific and include nasal congestion, unilateral facial pain, epistaxis, or necrotic eschar with potential progression to proptosis, cranial neuropathies, cavernous sinus thrombosis, or cerebral abscess. *Rhizopus* species are the most common etiologic agents. The fungus can be found in tissue sections at the time of surgical débridement. Amphotericin B and its lipid formulations are the current drugs of choice. None of the azoles (except posaconazole) have activity against zygomycetes. Posaconazole has been successfully used as salvage therapy in patients with zygomycosis.

51. Answer c.
Disseminated *Fusarium* infection (fusariosis) is an uncommon but serious infection in neutropenic patients after chemotherapy or bone marrow transplant. *Fusarium* species are widely distributed in the environment. The fungus is a known cause of onychomycosis and keratitis. Morphologically it resembles *Aspergillus*, with septate, branching hyphae. Two unique aspects of disseminated fusariosis are skin involvement in 50% to 70% of patients and positive blood cultures in 50% of patients. Medical therapy is challenging since *Fusarium* species are frequently resistant to antifungal therapy. *Aspergillus* species and *Rhizopus* species are seldom isolated in blood cultures. *Rhizopus* species are distinct morphologically, with broad-based nonseptate hyphae. This patient is at risk of coccidioidomycosis since she lives in Arizona, and skin is a common site of extrapulmonary coccidioidomycosis. However, *Coccidioides* species and *Histoplasma* species are dimorphic fungi and appear as spherules and yeasts, respectively, in involved tissue specimens.

52. Answer e.
Although encountered most often in immunocompromised patients, *Aspergillus* is only 1 of several molds with septate branching hyphae in tissue specimens. All of the above molds (plus *Acremonium* species) have a similar morphologic appearance. Their antifungal susceptibility and response to medical therapy can be quite variable. Hence, in addition to histopathologic examination, tissue samples for fungal culture are needed for accurate identification of the mold in question.

53. Answer d.
Malassezia is a lipophilic yeast that colonizes humans as early as the neonatal period, and it is part of the normal skin flora in up to 90% of adults. In addition to causing pityriasis versicolor, *M furfur* can cause neonatal pustulosis, blepharitis, folliculitis, seborrheic dermatitis, and white piedra. Owing to its lipophilic nature, *M furfur* has also been associated with catheter-related bloodstream infections, fungemia, and sepsis, especially in patients receiving parenteral nutrition with lipids.

54. Answer e.
Whether invasive disease develops in a patient depends on other factors, including the patient's immunologic status (ie, normal or immunocompromised).

55. Answer a.
Cryptococcus is a saprobe in nature and may also be a colonizer of the airway, especially in patients with chronic lung abnormalities.

56. Answer d.
Sterilization of CSF has been reported with induction therapy with flucytosine in combination with amphotericin B only.

57. Answer d.
Disease is more common in hosts with normal immunologic status. Susceptibility testing results are similar to those with *C neoformans* var *neoformans*. Cryptococcoma formation is more common with *C neoformans* var *gatti*. Response to antifungal agents is usually slow.

58. Answer b.
Cryptosporidium cysts are very resistant to usual chlorination methods. Outbreaks have occurred in cities with modern, well-functioning municipal water treatment systems, especially among immunocompromised persons exposed to small numbers of viable cysts. Contaminated swimming pools require drainage, vigorous cleaning, and superchlorination to become disinfected.

59. Answer d.
Microsporida are tiny organisms about the size of bacteria (2-3 μm) and can be recognized only with special stains. They primarily infect immunocompromised patients, especially those with AIDS, and cause a secretory diarrhea without a significant inflammatory response. Metronidazole is not effective treatment.

60. Answer b.
The free-living amebae are ubiquitous in moist soil and natural water sources. *Acanthamoeba* cause keratitis and chronic granulomatous encephalitis, whereas *Naegleria* cause rapidly fatal meningitis unresponsive to treatment. CSF examination of central nervous system infections often shows motile amebic trophozoites and leukocytes.

61. Answer c.
Each of the responses illustrates a pathogenetic mechanism of *P falciparum* except that parasites do not persist sequestered in liver cells. Sequestration occurs with *Plasmodium vivax* (and *Plasmodium ovale*) and is responsible for relapses if primaquine is not used in initial treatment to eradicate the hypnozoites.

62. Answer b.
Species identification of *Plasmodium* is done with thin blood films because the intracellular morphology of intact erythrocytes is important. Preparation of thick blood films lyses erythrocytes. *Leishmania* and *Toxoplasma* are primarily tissue infections and are not generally found in peripheral blood smears. The *C* rule of American trypanosomiasis (Chagas disease, *T cruzi*) is a reminder that these organisms assume a *C* shape in blood smears.

63. Answer b.
Eosinophilia is not a feature of protozoan infections (such as amebiasis), but it is rather common in helminth infections. It is especially prominent when there is tissue migration of larval forms of the worms, as in strongyloidiasis or trichinellosis.

64. Answer a.
The adult tapeworm of *Echinococcus* resides in the intestines of carnivorous animals (dogs, wolves, coyotes, etc), not in humans. Humans ingest eggs shed in the feces of those animals, and hydatid cysts then develop in humans. The common terms *fish tapeworm* (*Diphyllobothrium*), *pork tapeworm* (*T solium*), and *beef tapeworm* (*T saginata*) are misnomers since the adult tapeworms reside in the intestinal tracts of humans, not in animals.

65. Answer a.
Ascaris is the only one of these helminths that is acquired by the fecal-oral route. The others infect by skin penetration of larval forms found in the soil (hookworms and *Strongyloides*) or water (*Schistosoma*).

66. Answer e.
Strongyloides larvae (not eggs) are found in the stool of infected patients because the eggs hatch (liberating the larvae) while still in the adult female worm or soon thereafter within the intestinal tract. The larvae may be difficult to detect on routine examinations of stool for ova and parasites, and specific procedures such as the agar-plate method may be necessary.

67. Answer d.
Schistosoma is the only one of these parasites that does not infect through ingestion of aquatic animals. It infects through skin penetration of fork-tailed cercariae, which are liberated from freshwater snails.

68. Answer d.
Varicella-zoster virus but not herpes simplex virus has been associated with this complication, which causes a stroke syndrome.

69. Answer b.
The lack of a lipid envelope makes adenoviruses resistant to the lipid-based detergents used in handwashing. Although handwashing is standard practice in all patient care, use of gloves for patient contact with adenovirus is required to prevent transmission.

70. Answer c.
Mumps arthritis is more likely to affect males and larger joints. Joint symptoms in acute Epstein-Barr virus infection generally are not associated with synovitis. Coxsackievirus arthritis is rare. Patients with gonorrhea can present with

arthritis as a solitary symptom, but it is usually monoarticular.

71. Answer a.
Vaccination of mumps did not become available until 1967. Sporadic episodes are usually caused by strains covered by the vaccine. A camper may have presented to the camp physician (ie, this patient) with less specific symptoms and transmitted the virus to the physician by the usual respiratory route. Lyme disease could be a cause of CSF pleocytosis but would not cause the orchitis symptoms. Bacterial epididymitis, as would be associated with BPH, would not cause this patient's CSF abnormalities. CA-MRSA infections are being reported at an increasing frequency, and group residence settings, such as camps, have been implicated as potential sources for the infections. Patients with CA-MRSA infections usually present with skin and soft tissue infections, unlike the presentation in this question.

72. Answer e.
Statement *e* is the only incorrect one. All the other statements are correct regarding the epidemiology of aspergillosis.

73. Answer b.
Aspergillus terreus may be resistant to amphotericin B preparations and therefore would not be a good choice for initial treatment of invasive aspergillosis. The treatment of *A terreus* is voriconazole or other new azoles.

74. Answer b.
All the statements are correct except *b*. The syndrome of *Aspergillus* tracheobronchitis is typically seen after lung transplant.

75. Answer c.
A single lung lesion (not multiple bilateral cavitary lesions) and persistent hemoptysis is a relative indication for surgery.

76. Answer a.
This patient has *Nocardia* pneumonia, which can occur in patients receiving corticosteroids. In this situation, *Nocardia* brain abscess must be ruled out since the presence of a brain abscess would mandate a longer course of treatment.

77. Answer b.
This patient has lymphocutaneous nocardiosis, which is usually caused by *Nocardia brasiliensis*. The Gram stain findings are not consistent with *Sporothrix schenckii* or *Mycobacterium marinum*, 2 other organisms that can cause lymphocutaneous infection. The Gram stain findings also rule out *Staphylococcus* as a cause of this purulent infection. Actinomycosis occurs only under anaerobic conditions and is not a cause of this entity. The drug of choice for lymphocutaneous nocardiosis is trimethoprim-sulfamethoxazole.

78. Answer b.
This patient has cervicofacial actinomycosis (also called lumpy jaw). Because he had an anaphylactic reaction to penicillin, ceftriaxone should be avoided. Trimethoprim-sulfamethoxazole, cephalexin, and metronidazole are ineffective against actinomycosis.

79. Answer c.
This patient has chronic pulmonary actinomycosis, which is often seen in alcoholics with poor dentition. Although the disease may mimic lung cancer, involvement of the chest wall is typical for actinomycosis. The drug of choice is penicillin. The other antibiotics are not effective against actinomycosis.

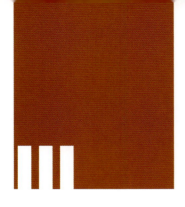

Select Major Clinical Syndromes

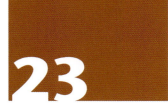

Mary J. Kasten, MD

23

Fever of Unknown Origin

I. Introduction
   A. Definition
      1. Classic definition of *fever of unknown origin* (FUO)
         a. Fever for more than 3 weeks
         b. Temperature of 38.3°C or higher on several occasions
         c. No definitive diagnosis after 1 week of hospital evaluation
      2. Recent series have used other criteria instead of 1 week of hospital evaluation: 1 week of intensive outpatient evaluation, 3 outpatient visits, or a battery of laboratory tests
   B. Preliminary Diagnostic Evaluation
      1. A comprehensive history should be obtained and a physical examination and basic laboratory and radiographic testing should be performed before stating that a patient has FUO (Box 23.1)
      2. There is no clear consensus in the literature for defining the minimal diagnostic evaluation
II. Fever of Unknown Origin
   A. Causes
      1. Box 23.2 lists the major categories of FUO and the illnesses and agents that are most commonly involved in each category
      2. Infections are more common in older FUO series and in series from developing countries where typhoid fever, tuberculosis, and malaria are particularly problematic

---

Box 23.1

Early Testing to Consider in an Evaluation of Fever of Unknown Origin

Complete blood cell count with differential blood count
Routine blood chemistry, including lactate dehydrogenase, bilirubin, and liver enzymes
Urinalysis, including microscopic examination
Chest radiograph
Erythrocyte sedimentation rate
Antinuclear antibodies
Rheumatoid factor
Angiotensin-converting enzyme
Routine blood cultures (3 times) while patient is not receiving antibiotics
Fungal blood cultures
Cytomegalovirus IgM or virus detection in blood
Heterophile antibody testing in children and young adults
Tuberculin skin testing (purified protein derivative tuberculin)
Computed tomography of abdomen and radionuclide scan
Human immunodeficiency virus antibodies or virus detection assay
Further evaluation of any abnormalities detected with testing, history, and physical examination

Adapted from Arnow PM, Flaherty JP. Fever of unknown origin. Lancet. 1997 Aug 23;350(9077):575–80. Used with permission.

Box 23.2
Causes of Fever of Unknown Origin[a,b]

Infection (25%)
  Localized bacterial infection: **cholangitis**, empyema of gallbladder, **hepatic abscess**, **intra-abdominal abscess**, **pelvic abscess**, pelvic inflammatory disease, prostatic abscess and chronic prostatitis, prosthetic joint infection
  Systemic infection and infection caused by a specific organism
    Bacterial: *Bartonella* infection (including cat-scratch disease), **brucellosis endocarditis**, Q fever, rat-bite fever, *Salmonella* infection, **tuberculosis**,[c] Whipple disease, *Yersinia* infection
    Fungal: blastomycosis, coccidioidomycosis, cryptococcosis, **histoplasmosis**
    Parasitic: amebic liver abscess, leishmaniasis, **malaria**, toxoplasmosis, trichinosis, trypanosomiasis
    Spirochete: leptospirosis, Lyme disease, relapsing fever, syphilis
    Viral infections: **cytomegalovirus**, Epstein-Barr virus, hepatitis, **human immunodeficiency virus**, parvovirus
Cancer (15%)[d]
  Hematologic: lymphoma (most frequent diagnosis in many series)
  Solid: atrial myxoma, **colon cancer**, hepatoma, hepatocellular carcinoma, lung, **metastatic disease** (particularly to liver), neuroblastoma, pancreas, **renal**, sarcoma
Rheumatologic or autoimmune (20%)
  Behçet syndrome, cryoglobulinemia, gout, hypersensitivity vasculitis, polyarteritis nodosa, pseudogout, **Reiter syndrome**, rheumatic fever, rheumatoid arthritis, **Still disease**, **systemic lupus erythematosus**, Takayasu arteritis, **temporal arteritis** (occurs in up to 17% of patients older than 65 years), serum sickness, Wegener granulomatosis
Miscellaneous (20%)
  Castleman disease, cholesterol emboli, Crohn disease, cirrhosis (uncertain whether fever occurs from cirrhosis alone or from complications), cyclic neutropenia, **drug fever** (can occur with any medication administered for any duration), Fabry disease, **factitious fever**, **familial Mediterranean fever**, granulomatous hepatitis, habitual hyperthermia, **hematoma**, hyperthyroidism, hypertriglyceridemia, hyperimmunoglobulinemia D syndrome, Kikuchi disease, pancreatitis, pericarditis (postpericardiotomy syndrome or post–myocardial infarction syndrome), pheochromocytoma, pseudotumor, sarcoidosis, systemic lupus erythematosus, **thrombosis** (pulmonary embolism, deep vein thrombosis, cerebral thrombosis), tumor necrosis factor receptor–associated periodic syndrome, thrombotic thrombocytopenic purpura
No diagnosis (20%)

[a] The percentages are estimates of how frequently certain illnesses occur in current series of patients with fever of unknown origin.
[b] Boldface type indicates illnesses and conditions that occur fairly regularly in recent series.
[c] *Mycobacterium tuberculosis* is the most commonly cultured organism from patients with classic fever of unknown origin.
[d] Nearly every cancer has been reported to cause fever of unknown origin.

Box 23.3
Important Historical Elements in Fever of Unknown Origin

Detailed history of present illness
Details of past medical illnesses
Surgical history
Medication use (including prescription drugs, over-the-counter drugs, herbs, vitamins, and supplements)
Alcohol use
Recreational drug use
Occupational exposures
Animal exposure
Travel history
Family history
Sexual history (including history of previous sexually transmitted illness and current and past sexual practices)
Detailed review of systems

    3. FUO is most frequently caused by common diseases with uncommon presentations and less frequently by exotic diseases
B. Diagnosis
  1. History
    a. Clues that may lead to the diagnosis are often identified from a thorough history, physical examination, and routine laboratory testing
    b. Box 23.3 lists historical elements of importance
    c. Table 23.1 lists historical clues related to diagnoses that one should consider in the evaluation of a patient with FUO
    d. Pattern of fever is not usually helpful
      1) Fever higher than 38.9°C suggests an infectious cause, lymphoma, or vasculitis
      2) Intermittent, high spiking fever suggests an abscess, miliary tuberculosis, Still disease, malaria, or lymphoma
      3) Lower temperatures are common in the elderly even with serious infection
      4) Periodic or relapsing fever is common with cyclic neutropenia, lymphoma, malaria, *Borrelia* infection, or *Streptobacillus* infection (rat-bite fever)
      5) Recurrent or episodic FUO with multiple episodes of fever separated by weeks or months is unlikely to be from infection
        a) The cause of recurrent fever often remains undiagnosed
        b) Recurrent fever can be caused by the illnesses listed in Box 23.4
      6) The longer a fever persists, whether recurrent or continuous, the less likely the causative illness is infectious

Table 23.1

Historical Clues in Fever of Unknown Origin

Historical Clue	Related Disease
Travel	
Area where malaria is endemic	Malaria
Prolonged contact with people in developing countries	Tuberculosis, typhoid fever
All travelers without usual sexual partner or single	HIV infection
Southwestern United States	Coccidioidomycosis
Mississippi River Valley	Histoplasmosis
Animal contact (direct or indirect through products or droppings)	
Cats	Cat-scratch disease, toxoplasmosis
Horses, cows, sheep, or goats	Brucellosis, Q fever
Birds	Psittacosis
Bats	Histoplasmosis
Rodents	Rat-bite fever
Sexually active and not monogamous or with new partner	Cytomegalovirus infection, hepatitis, HIV infection
Injection drug use	Hepatitis, HIV infection, right-sided endocarditis
Alcohol use	Alcoholic hepatitis, cirrhosis and its complications
Tick exposure	Babesiosis, ehrlichiosis, Lyme disease, relapsing fever
Family history of similar illness	FMF, Fabry disease, hypertriglyceridemia, TRAPS
Recent colonoscopy, sigmoidoscopy, or abdominal procedure	Abdominal abscess
Recent surgical procedure	Deep vein thrombosis, pulmonary embolism, hematoma
Recent trauma	Hematoma
History of inflammatory bowel disease, diverticulitis, or other abdominal pathology	Abdominal abscess
Known valvular heart disease	Endocarditis
Review of systems	
Abdominal pain	Polyarteritis nodosa, FMF
Back pain	Endocarditis, brucellosis, vertebral osteomyelitis
Headache	Psittacosis, malaria, brucellosis, Q fever, rickettsial illness, relapsing fever, chronic meningitis
Flank pain or hematuria	Renal cell carcinoma
Jaw claudication	Temporal arteritis
Neck or throat pain	Subacute thyroiditis, Still disease
Testicular pain	Polyarteritis nodosa, brucellosis, TRAPS
Pleurisy	FMF, pulmonary embolism, tuberculosis, systemic lupus erythematosus
Rash (transient)	Still disease or other collagen vascular disease
Scalp pain	Temporal arteritis

Abbreviations: FMF, familial Mediterranean fever; HIV, human immunodeficiency virus; TRAPS, tumor necrosis factor receptor–associated periodic syndrome.

2. Physical examination
   a. Physical examination clues are reviewed in Table 23.2
   b. Careful examination of the skin, lymph nodes, mouth, abdomen, genitalia, and eyes can provide important clues to the diagnosis
   c. An ophthalmoscopic examination by an ophthalmologist can be particularly helpful with rheumatologic illness and some infections
   d. Repeated careful cardiac auscultation may detect fleeting murmurs of endocarditis or rheumatic fever
   e. Subsequent examination with attention to new findings has been helpful in providing clues to the eventual diagnosis in several series
3. Laboratory evaluation
   a. Interpretation of routine laboratory test results (Box 23.1) may provide important clues about the cause of FUO

Box 23.4
Causes of Recurrent Fever of Unknown Origin

Still disease
Atrial myxoma
Castleman disease
Crohn disease
Chronic prostatitis
Colon cancer
Cyclic neutropenia
Dental abscess
Drug fever
Subacute bacterial endocarditis (when inadequate empirical antibiotics are given)
Fabry disease
Factitious fever
Fever, aphthous ulcers, pharyngitis, and adenitis syndrome
Familial Mediterranean fever
Granulomatous hepatitis
Hyperimmunoglobulinemia D syndrome
Hypersensitivity pneumonitis
Hypertriglyceridemia
Malignancy (particularly with lymphoma but also with solid tumors)
Pulmonary embolism
Subacute cholangitis
Tumor necrosis factor receptor–associated periodic syndrome

b. Table 23.3 summarizes some of the more helpful abnormal results from routine laboratory testing that should prompt consideration of a specific diagnosis

4. Diagnostic approach
   a. The frequency of the causes of FUO varies from less than 1% for the majority of diagnostic possibilities to 17% for temporal arteritis in patients older than 65 years
   b. There is a high likelihood of false-positive test results: all test results need to be interpreted with caution
   c. An algorithm that fits every patient is impossible to create: the diagnostic approach needs to be individualized
   d. Patients with clues are much more likely to have a diagnosable condition
      1) For example, if a patient had FUO and a history of possibly eating unpasteurized cheese in Greece, brucellosis should be considered, with an evaluation that includes appropriate cultures and serology

Table 23.2
Physical Examination Clues in the Evaluation of Fever of Unknown Origin

Clue	Disease
Cerebellar ataxia	Whipple disease, malignancy
Conjunctival suffusion	Leptospirosis, relapsing fever
Decayed teeth	Dental abscess
Erythema nodosum	Idiopathic erythema nodosum, sarcoidosis, tuberculosis, histoplasmosis, Crohn disease, drug fever
Heart murmur	Endocarditis, atrial myxoma, acute rheumatic fever
Hepatomegaly	Lymphoma, metastatic cancer, alcoholic hepatitis, granulomatous hepatitis, Q fever, typhoid fever
Joint effusion or pain	Rheumatoid arthritis, SLE, pseudogout, gout, familial Mediterranean fever, Lyme disease, Whipple disease, hyperimmunoglobulinemia D syndrome, rheumatic fever, Still disease
Livedo reticularis	PAN, SLE, cryoglobulinemia
Relative bradycardia	Typhoid fever, malaria, leptospirosis, psittacosis, drug fever, factitious fever, lymphoma
Mononeuritis	PAN, sarcoidosis
Myoclonus	Whipple disease
Palpable purpura	Vasculitis, meningococcemia, rickettsial infection
Papules that are dome-shaped and skin-colored on face and neck	Sarcoidosis
Roth spots	Subacute bacterial endocarditis (occasionally occur with other infections, diabetes mellitus, and leukemia)
Splenomegaly	Cytomegalovirus infection, Epstein-Barr virus infection, hematologic malignancy, sarcoidosis, brucellosis, tuberculosis, typhoid fever
Spinal tenderness	Vertebral osteomyelitis, endocarditis, brucellosis, typhoid fever
Sternal tenderness	Leukemia, metastatic cancer
Temporal artery tenderness	Temporal arteritis
Thyroid enlargement or tenderness	Thyroiditis
Testicular tenderness	PAN, brucellosis, TRAPS
Vitiligo	Autoimmune illness

Abbreviations: PAN, polyarteritis nodosa; SLE, systemic lupus erythematosus; TRAPS, tumor necrosis factor receptor–associated periodic syndrome.

Table 23.3

Clues to Fever of Unknown Origin from Results of Routine Laboratory Tests

Result	Possible Diagnosis or Agent
Erythrocytosis	Renal cell cancer
Neutropenia	Tuberculosis, lymphoma, leukemia, brucellosis, typhoid fever, psittacosis, drug reaction, SLE, cyclic neutropenia, Whipple disease
Lymphopenia	Ehrlichiosis, HIV, SLE, tuberculosis, Whipple disease, sarcoidosis, malignancy (especially Hodgkin lymphoma)
Monocytosis	Tuberculosis, PAN, temporal arteritis, brucellosis, sarcoidosis, leukemia, typhoid fever, malaria, leishmaniasis, SLE, subacute bacterial endocarditis
Eosinophilia	Trichinosis or other parasitic infection, lymphoma, drug fever, PAN, SLE, hypersensitivity vasculitis, myeloproliferative disease Bacterial infection is unlikely
Lymphocytosis	CMV, EBV, toxoplasmosis, tuberculosis, lymphoma, drug hypersensitivity (particularly phenytoin)
Basophilia	Leukemia, myeloproliferative disease, lymphoma
Atypical lymphocytes	CMV, EBV, acute HIV, toxoplasmosis, syphilis, brucellosis, drug reactions (including serum sickness), leukemia
Thrombocytopenia	Hematologic malignancy, myeloproliferative diseases, HIV, SLE, vasculitis, EBV, drug fever
Iron deficiency anemia	Colon cancer, Crohn disease, Whipple disease
Erythrocyte sedimentation rate >100 mm/h	Vasculitis, hematologic malignancy, metastatic cancer, endocarditis
Elevated transaminase levels with AST:ALT >2	Alcoholic hepatitis
Elevated alkaline phosphatase level	Hepatic infiltration from infection or cancer, osteomyelitis, biliary disease
Elevated bilirubin level	Cholangitis, cholecystitis
Hematuria	Renal cell cancer, SLE, tuberculosis
Rheumatoid factor	Rheumatoid arthritis, subacute bacterial endocarditis, malaria, hypersensitivity vasculitis
Blood cultures	Factitious fever (unexplained polymicrobic bacteremia)
Hepatitis B surface antigen	PAN
Elevated lactate dehydrogenase level	Malignancy (particularly lymphoma), pulmonary embolism, SLE
Elevated angiotensin-converting enzyme level	Sarcoidosis, tuberculosis, leprosy, deep vein thrombosis, bronchogenic cancer

Abbreviations: ALT, alanine aminotransferase; AST, aspartate aminotransferase; CMV, cytomegalovirus; EBV, Epstein-Barr virus; HIV, human immunodeficiency virus; PAN, polyarteritis nodosa; SLE, systemic lupus erythematosus.

    e. Drug-related fever
       1) Should be ruled out early by discontinuing use of all drugs that are not imperative
       2) Drugs that are commonly associated with FUO are listed in Box 23.5
    f. Habitual hyperthermia should be ruled out early in patients who do not appear ill
    g. Factitious fever should be considered: fever should be documented where the patient cannot alter the reading
    h. Table 23.4 lists tests to consider when clues to the underlying diagnosis from the history, physical examination, and initial laboratory testing have been nondiagnostic
    i. Repeating the history, physical examination, and simple laboratory tests may be more helpful than ordering additional imaging when the first series of tests is uninformative

Box 23.5

Drugs Associated With Fever of Unknown Origin[a]

Allopurinol
Aminoglycosides
Angiotensin-converting enzyme inhibitors
Antihistamines
β-Lactam antibiotics
Clindamycin
Heparin
Hydralazine
Hydrochlorthiazide
Iodides
Isoniazid
Macrolides
Methyldopa
Nitrofurantoin
Phenytoin
Procainamide
Quinidine
Sulfonamides
Vancomycin

[a] Many other drugs have been reported besides those in this list.

Table 23.4

Additional Imaging and Invasive Tests for Investigating Fever of Unknown Origin

Testing	Comments
CT scan of the abdomen and pelvis	A retrospective case series of an abdominal CT in the work-up of FUO reported a yield of 19%
	This test should be considered early; some investigators believe it should be performed before calling a prolonged fever an FUO
	Subsequent CT scans have a much poorer chance of being helpful
CT scan of the chest	Can identify nodules indicative of fungal, mycobacterial, or nocardial infection or malignancy
	Hilar and mediastinal lymphadenopathy may not be evident on chest radiography but may be seen on CT and be amenable to biopsy
Ultrasonography of the abdomen and pelvis	Safe and less expensive than CT
	Helpful when positive but often misses pathologic conditions (follow-up CT would then be indicated)
Cryoglobulins	In at least 1 study, early testing for cryoglobulins in patients who did not have FUO clues was cost-effective compared with other testing
QuantiFERON testing for tuberculosis	Purified protein derivative tuberculin testing was positive in less than 50% of patients with miliary tuberculosis in several FUO series
	QuantiFERON testing appears to be more sensitive but false-negative results occur
Echocardiogram	Subacute bacterial endocarditis is a relatively common cause of FUO (1%-5% of all cases)
	An echocardiogram to look for vegetations and atrial myxoma is reasonable when clues point to the possibility of subacute bacterial endocarditis or the diagnosis remains obscure
Temporal artery biopsy	Temporal artery biopsy is a safe surgical procedure that should be performed in elderly patients who have FUO unless clues point to another diagnosis
Indium scan	Most helpful when localized infection is suspected
Gallium scan	Low sensitivity and specificity but can be helpful when no FUO clues are present
	Low specificity can be helpful since scan can be positive not only with infection but also with some cancers, sarcoidosis, and occasionally aortitis
Technetium scan	Better specificity than gallium
	Best for bone and muscular inflammation or infection
Positron emission tomography	In small case series, has shown promising results with respect to sensitivity and specificity for inflammation
	Like gallium, can be positive with infection, malignancy, and other causes of inflammation
	More information is needed to determine its role in the evaluation of FUO
Duplex ultrasonography of the temporal, occipital, subclavian, and cervical arteries	Helpful when vasculitis is suspected
Magnetic resonance imaging of the aortic arch and the proximal cervical arteries	Has been used successfully in the diagnosis of large vessel vasculitis when clues to an alternative diagnosis were not present and ultrasonographic findings were negative
Liver biopsy	Diagnostic yield of 14% to 17% in carefully chosen patients with FUO
	Controversy exists over how early to consider liver biopsy
	Liver biopsy is indicated when the diagnosis remains elusive and evidence of liver inflammation is present or when a patient's condition is deteriorating and the diagnosis is critical
	High yield with miliary tuberculosis
Muscle biopsy	Helpful when electromyographic findings are abnormal
Bronchoalveolar lavage	Low yield even when chest radiographic findings are abnormal
Sinus radiography	Often positive but abnormalities are only rarely related to FUO
Doppler ultrasonography of the lower extremities	Safe; occasionally identifies a treatable cause
Colonoscopy	Diagnostic for colon cancer, which occasionally manifests only with fever
	Unless clues suggest colon pathology, other diagnoses and testing should usually be considered first
Small bowel radiography	Rarely, a patient with Crohn disease has no symptoms that point to the abdomen as the source of fever
	Carefully reviewed CT often shows the abnormality
Small bowel biopsy	Indicated when intestinal lymphoma or Whipple disease is being considered
Bone marrow biopsy	Abnormalities in the complete blood cell count or blood smear usually suggest that a bone marrow biopsy may be helpful
	Bone marrow cultures have a low diagnostic yield when the bone marrow does not show granulomas or other changes that suggest infection; therefore, bone marrow cultures are not routinely recommended for immunocompetent patients with FUO

Table 23.4
(continued)

Testing	Comments
Skin biopsy	Any rash or unusual skin lesion should be biopsied and cultured early for bacteria, mycobacteria, and fungus
Lumbar puncture	Cerebrospinal fluid examination is not usually helpful unless the patient has symptoms suggesting meningitis or encephalitis
Exploratory laparotomy	Early series of FUO patients (before the routine availability of CT) reported a high yield for exploratory laparotomy
	Currently, exploratory laparotomy is rarely helpful unless imaging findings point to an underlying abdominal process

Abbreviations: CT, computed tomographic; FUO, fever of unknown origin.

C. Treatment
 1. Empirical therapy
  a. Empirical therapy is not recommended for clinically stable patients who have prolonged fever that has defied diagnosis
   1) These patients have a favorable long-term prognosis
   2) They should be monitored closely, and any new symptom should prompt reevaluation
   3) Periodic repeating of the history, physical examination, and basic laboratory tests should be done while the patient is febrile
   4) In many patients, the fever eventually resolves spontaneously
 2. Therapeutic trials
  a. Tetracycline: may be reasonable when a patient appears to have an atypical bacterial infection that has defied diagnosis and the patient's condition is not improving
  b. Antitubercular agents: indicated when the suspicion for tuberculosis is high but the organism has not been detected
  c. Corticosteroids: rarely indicated; reserved for a patient whose clinical condition is deteriorating and who has undergone an exhaustive evaluation and is believed to have a steroid-responsive illness

Suggested Reading

Armstrong W, Kazanjian P. Fever of unknown origin in the general population and in HIV-infected persons. In: Cohen J, Powderly WG, Berkley SF, Calandra T, Clumeck N, Finch RG, et al, editors. Infectious diseases. Vol 1. 2nd ed. Edinburgh: Mosby; c2004. p. 871–80.

Cunha BA. Fever of unknown origin. Infect Dis Clin North Am. 1996 Mar;10(1):111–27.

Knockaert DC, Vanderschueren S, Blockmans D. Fever of unknown origin in adults: 40 years on. J Intern Med. 2003 Mar;253(3):263–75.

Lisa M. Brumble, MD

24

Infections of the Oral Cavity, Neck, and Head

I. Odontogenic Infections
   A. Primary Source of Mouth, Head, and Neck Infections
      1. The origin of many infections of the oral cavity, head, and neck is odontogenic
         a. Typically polymicrobial, with obligate anaerobes and facultative anaerobes
         b. Most of these microbes are part of the indigenous flora of the oral cavity
         c. A microbial shift toward obligate anaerobes occurs as the infection spreads deeper into oral, facial, and neck spaces
      2. The pathway of spreading is anatomically predictable
         a. Initially infection invades the gingiva or other periodontal tissues or tooth enamel
         b. Then infection spreads into surrounding tissues along paths of least resistance (Figure 24.1)
            1) Drainage in combination with parenteral antibiotic therapy is usually required to resolve these infections
      3. Certain microbes are associated with specific anatomical sites during normal colonization and during infection
         a. Common colonizers of tooth surfaces: *Streptococcus sanguinis*, *Streptococcus mutans*, *Streptococcus mitis*, and *Actinomyces viscosus*
         b. Strongly associated with dental caries formation: *S mutans*
      4. Plaque
         a. Normally, plaque formation is disrupted by the cleaning action of the tongue and buccal membranes and by brushing and flossing
         b. Antimicrobial defenses
            1) Buffering effects of saliva and its lysozymes, lactoferrin, β-lysin, lactoperoxidase, and IgA immunoglobulins
            2) Keratinocyte secretions (β-defensin, histatin)
            3) Cell-mediated immunity
         c. An acellular, bacteria-free pellicle largely composed of these salivary components normally covers the teeth, but a lack of brushing or flossing allows this pellicle to become colonized with bacteria, thereby forming plaque
         d. After plaque forms, bacteria erode pits and fissures into the tooth enamel
            1) Enamel, dentin, and pulp are destroyed as the infection spreads deeper into the tooth

a. Suppurative periapical abscesses are polymicrobial: *Fusobacterium nucleatum*, *Bacteroides* species, *Peptostreptococcus* species, *Actinomyces* species, and *Streptococcus* species
b. Infection usually penetrates the bone at certain periapical tooth junctions where the bone is weakest and thereby most susceptible to the increasing pressure of accumulated pus
   1) Mandible: typically near the lingual aspect of the molars
   2) Maxilla: bone is weakest throughout the buccal aspect
7. Periodontal disease
   a. Microbes
      1) In healthy gingival tissue, the flora consists of gram-positive organisms
         a) *Streptococcus oralis*
         b) *Streptococcus sanguinis*
         c) *Actinomyces* species
      2) In gingivitis, a shift occurs toward gram-negative anaerobic rods
         a) *Prevotella intermedia*
         b) *Peptostreptococcus* species
         c) *Capnocytophaga* species
      3) Plaques that develop below the gingival margin are characterized by a preponderance of gram-negative anaerobes and motile organisms such as spirochetes
      4) In advanced periodontitis, additional gram-negative anaerobes and spirochetes are frequently isolated
         a) *Porphyromonas gingivalis*
         b) *Actinobacillus actinomycetemcomitans*
         c) *Bacteroides forsythus*
         d) *Treponema denticola*
   b. Unlike pulpal infections, periodontal infections drain freely; thus, patients have little discomfort
   c. Unlike dentoalveolar infections, periodontal infections are usually limited to the soft tissues in the mouth and rarely spread to deeper facial or neck structures
      1) More often, patients describe itchy gums, vague jaw pain, a bad taste in their mouth, and hot and cold sensitivity
      2) Frank pus can be expressed with mild digital pressure at the site
   d. Acute necrotizing ulcerative gingivitis (Vincent disease or trench mouth) results from necrosis of the gingiva

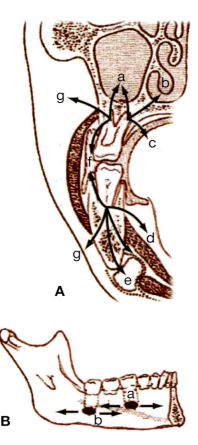

Figure 24.1. Routes of Spread of Odontogenic Orofacial Infections Along Planes of Least Resistance. A, Coronal section in the region of the first molars. In illustration A, a indicates maxillary antrum; b, nasal cavity; c, palatal plate; d, sublingual space (above the mylohyoid muscle); e, submandibular space (below the mylohyoid muscle); f, intraoral manifestation with infection spreading through the buccal plates inside the attachment of the buccinator muscle; g, extraoral manifestation to buccal space with infection spreading through the buccal plates outside the attachment of the buccinator muscle. B, Lingual aspect of the mandible. In illustration B, a indicates apices of the involved tooth above the mylohyoid muscle, with spread of infection to the sublingual space; b, apices of involved tooth below the mylohyoid muscle, with spread of infection into the submandibular space. (From Chow AW, Roser SM, Brady FA. Orofacial odontogenic infections. Ann Intern Med. 1978 Mar;88[3]:392-402. Used with permission.)

   2) Infection can progress to involve the periapical region or alveolar bone
5. Pulpitis
   a. Early pulpitis: tooth is transiently sensitive to heat, cold, and percussion
   b. Advanced pulpitis: tooth is very sensitive to heat; sensitivity resolves with cold
6. Periapical abscess

1) Acute onset of gingival pain that interferes with chewing
2) Frequently associated with fever, regional lymphadenopathy, halitosis, and altered taste
3) Penicillin or metronidazole in conjunction with local débridement is highly effective therapy
8. Management of dentoalveolar and periodontal infections
   a. Surgical drainage and débridement of necrotic tissues
   b. Lavage with oxidizing agents and other antiseptic agents
   c. Tooth extraction, if necessary
   d. Antibiotic support is especially important if drainage is inadequate or if the infection has spread into surrounding soft tissues
   e. In most cases, early dental intervention can resolve odontogenic infections and confine them to the oral cavity
B. Face, Head, and Neck Infections in Deeper Spaces
   1. Failure to resolve odontogenic infections can result in infections spreading into deeper tissues of the face, head, or upper neck
      a. Infection sites in spaces of the face: masticator (including masseteric, temporal, and pterygoid spaces), buccal, canine, and parotid spaces (Figure 24.2)
      b. Infection sites in the suprahyoid region: submandibular, sublingual, and lateral pharyngeal spaces (Figure 24.1)
      c. Infection sites in the neck or infrahyoid region: retropharyngeal, "danger," and pretracheal spaces (Figure 24.3)
   2. Sources of microbes associated with these infections
      a. Mostly odontogenic
      b. Other sources include paranasal sinuses, tonsils and pharynx, and infections of the upper respiratory tract
      c. Organisms of the *Streptococcus milleri* group (SMG) (*Streptococcus anginosus*, *Streptococcus constellatus*, and *Streptococcus intermedius*) often spread from a paranasal sinus or throat infection but are common in oral cavity infections as well
         1) SMG microbes are microaerophilic
         2) SMG microbes can coinfect with anaerobes but often form exclusively SMG-cultured abscesses of the head and neck
         3) Possible routes of spread of infection are summarized in Figure 24.4
      d. Masticator space infections usually arise from infections of the third molars
         1) Patients typically present with trismus and pain in the body of the mandible
         2) Minimal swelling
         3) Spread toward the lateral pharyngeal wall may cause dysphagia
      e. Infections of the deep temporal space usually arise from the posterior maxillary molars

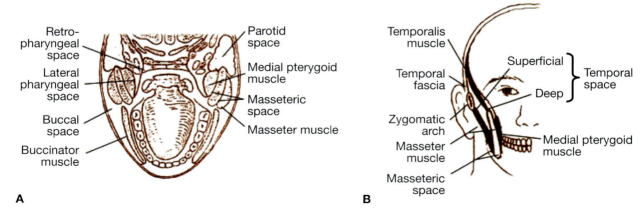

Figure 24.2. Fascial Spaces Around the Mouth and Face. A, Horizontal section at the level of the occlusal surface of the mandibular teeth. B, Frontal view of the face. (From Chow AW, Roser SM, Brady FA. Orofacial odontogenic infections. Ann Intern Med. 1978 Mar;88[3]:392-402. Used with permission.)

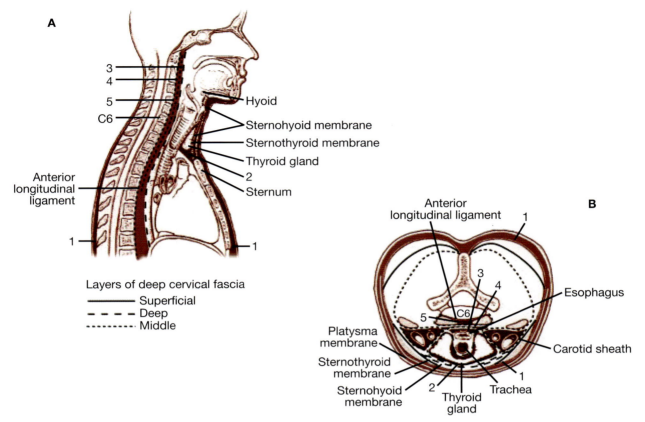

Figure 24.3. Anatomical Relations of Spaces. Lateral pharyngeal, retropharyngeal, and prevertebral spaces are indicated in relation to the posterior and anterior layers of the deep cervical fascia. A, Midsagittal section of the head and neck. B, Cross section of the neck at the level of the thyroid isthmus. In both illustrations, 1 indicates superficial space; 2, pretracheal space; 3, retropharyngeal space; 4, danger space; 5 prevertebral space. (From Chow AW. Infections of the oral cavity, neck, and head. In: Mandell GL, Bennett JE, Dolin R. Mandell, Douglas, and Bennett's principles and practice of infectious diseases. Vol 1. 7th ed. Philadelphia [PA]: Churchill Livingstone/Elsevier; c2010. p. 855-71. Used with permission.)

1) Progression of infection can cause swelling of the eyelid, cheek, and side of the face
2) Infection that spreads into the orbit may cause proptosis, optic neuritis, and abducens nerve palsy

f. Buccal space infections produce marked cheek swelling but minimal trismus or systemic symptoms
   1) Drainage should be superficial and extraoral if required
   2) These infections frequently respond to antibiotic therapy

g. Canine space infections usually originate from maxillary canine or incisor infections
   1) Typically cause upper lip, canine fossa, and even periorbital swellings
   2) May spread into the maxillary sinus
   3) Treatment: intraoral surgical débridement and antibiotics

h. Parotid space infections produce swelling at the angle of the jaw without trismus
   1) Pain may be intense and associated with fever
   2) Especially problematic because of their proximity to the lateral pharyngeal space
      a) Risk of spreading to the lateral pharyngeal space
      b) Risk of spreading from the lateral pharyngeal space to the danger space, visceral space, and posterior mediastinum

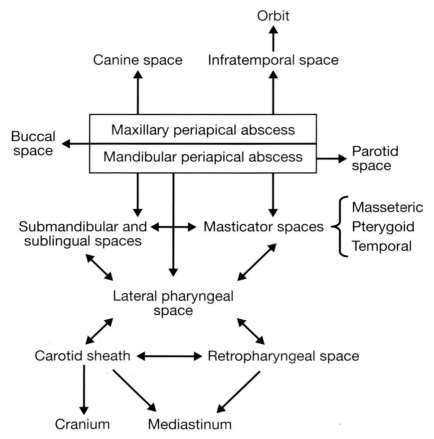

Figure 24.4. Potential Pathways of Extension in Infections of the Deep Fascial Space. (From Chow AW. Infections of the oral cavity, neck, and head. In: Mandell GL, Bennett JE, Dolin R. Mandell, Douglas, and Bennett's principles and practice of infectious diseases. Vol 1. 7th ed. Philadelphia [PA]: Churchill Livingstone/Elsevier; c2010. p. 855-71. Used with permission.)

i. Sublingual and submandibular spaces are separated by the mylohyoid muscle
j. Mandibular molar infections may spread into the submandibular spaces
   1) Swelling is present with little trismus since major mastication muscles are not involved
   2) If molar infection is not apparent, submandibular sialadenitis or lymphadenitis should be suspected
   3) Treatment: antibiotics, dental extraction, and surgical drainage
k. Sublingual space infections typically result from mandibular incisor infections
   1) Patients with sublingual infections present with erythematous, tender, extensive swelling of the mouth floor that may elevate the tongue (see description of Ludwig angina below)
   2) Drainage should be intraorally through the mucosa and parallel to the Wharton duct
   3) If submandibular drainage is required as well, a submandibular approach should reach both spaces
l. Lateral pharyngeal space infections can be odontogenic in origin or arise from pharyngitis, tonsillitis, parotitis, otitis, or mastoiditis
   1) The carotid sheath (containing the common carotid artery, internal jugular vein, and vagus nerve) is dangerously close to the medial wall of the lateral pharyngeal space
   2) Computed tomography (CT) and magnetic resonance imaging (MRI) are the best diagnostic tools to assess the extent of the infection
   3) The lateral pharyngeal space is divided into 2 functional compartments by the styloid process
      a) Anterior (muscular) compartment
         i) Fever or chills, marked pain, and dysphagia

ii) Unilateral trismus and swelling below the angle of the mandible
iii) Medial displacement of the pharyngeal wall
iv) Swelling of the adjacent parotid gland
    b) Posterior (neurovascular) compartment
        i) Infection here is potentially life threatening since the nearby carotid sheath and its contents are at risk of compression or direct infection
        ii) Posterior compartment swelling can be easily missed because it is behind the palatopharyngeal arch, with little pain or trismus
        iii) Complications of infection in the posterior compartment
            (a) Respiratory obstruction due to laryngeal edema
            (b) Internal jugular vein thrombosis (see description of Lemierre syndrome below)
            (c) Erosion of the internal carotid artery (described below)
            (d) Cranial nerve palsies or Horner syndrome
            (e) Suppuration may rapidly advance into the retropharyngeal and danger spaces, mediastinum (inferiorly), or base of the cranium (superiorly)
            (f) Careful airway monitoring is required
            (g) Administration of high doses of antibiotics and prompt surgical drainage are recommended
    m. Retropharyngeal space infections
        1) Retropharyngeal space: posterior part of the visceral compartment that bounds the esophagus, trachea, and thyroid gland with deep cervical fascia and extends inferiorly into the superior mediastinum
        2) Infections may spread to the retropharyngeal space from the adjacent lateral pharyngeal space or result from lymphatic spread from distant sites or penetrating trauma
        3) Clinical signs and symptoms
            a) High fever, chills, dysphagia, dyspnea, neck stiffness, and emesis
            b) Bulging of the posterior pharyngeal wall
            c) Widening of the retropharyngeal space may be seen on lateral neck soft tissue radiographs
        4) Infection is potentially life threatening and necessitates prompt surgical drainage
        5) Complications: hemorrhage, rupture into the airway, laryngeal spasm, bronchial erosion, and jugular vein thrombosis
    n. Danger space
        1) Lies posterior to the retropharyngeal space
        2) Descends directly into the posterior mediastinum to the diaphragm
    o. Pretracheal space infections
        1) Occur from perforations in the anterior esophageal wall
        2) Occasionally a direct extension from an infection of the adjacent retropharyngeal space
        3) Symptoms
            a) Severe dyspnea
            b) Hoarseness may be the initial symptom
            c) Dysphagia and regurgitation of fluids through the nose may occur
        4) Prompt surgical drainage of pretracheal infections is required to prevent spread of infection into the mediastinum
C. Specific Syndromes of Odontogenic Infections in Deeper Spaces
    1. Ludwig angina
        a. Life-threatening, rapidly spreading, indurated cellulitis
        b. No abscess formation or lymphatic involvement
        c. Submandibular and sublingual spaces involved bilaterally
        d. Typically spreading from concomitant mandibular molar infection
        e. Clinical signs and symptoms
            1) Tense, brawny, bilateral swelling of submandibular tissue and enlarged protruding tongue
            2) Drooling, dysphonia, tachypnea, trismus, and dysphagia (odynophagia)
            3) Fever, toxic appearance

f. Pathogens: viridans and other streptococci, *Staphylococcus* species, *Bacteroides*, and other anaerobes
g. Treatment
   1) Monitor airway, and intubate or place tracheostomy if necessary
   2) Parenteral ampicillin-sulbactam, penicillin G in combination with metronidazole, or clindamycin
   3) Surgical drainage
2. Lemierre syndrome
   a. Septic thrombophlebitis of internal jugular vein
   b. Spreads from lateral pharyngeal space and may continue to disseminate
   c. Clinical signs and symptoms
      1) High fever, rigors, pain, swelling at jaw angle and sternocleidomastoid muscle or lateral neck
      2) Subtle to pronounced nuchal rigidity, dysphagia, and dysphonia
   d. Important complications: dissemination of infection can lead to cavitating septic pulmonary emboli or abscesses in brain, kidney, or joints
   e. Pathogens: *Fusobacterium necrophorum* and anaerobic *Streptococcus* and *Bacteroides* species
   f. Further diagnostics: contrast-enhanced CT scan or MRI to demonstrate jugular thrombosis
   g. Treatment
      1) Extended course of antibiotics: ampicillin-sulbactam, clindamycin, or metronidazole
      2) May not require surgical intervention
3. Erosion of carotid artery
   a. Clinical disease
      1) Rare infection, with inflammation of carotid sheath and artery
      2) High mortality (20%-40%) regardless of treatment
      3) Spreads from lateral pharyngeal space, Ludwig angina, or deep cervical lymph nodes
      4) Creates false aneurysm
   b. Clinical signs and symptoms
      1) Small recurrent episodes of bleeding from nose, mouth, or ear ("herald" bleeding)
      2) Carotid artery rupture
   c. Further diagnostics and treatment: surgical consultation to determine need for carotid artery ligation
4. Septic cavernous sinus thrombosis
   a. Clinical disease
      1) Probably spreads from maxillary molar infections, purulent paranasal sinusitis, or facial furuncle
      2) High mortality (15%-30%)
   b. Clinical signs and symptoms
      1) Acute onset of fever, ptosis, proptosis, chemosis, and oculomotor paralysis (midposition fixed pupil, loss of corneal reflex)
      2) Decreased blood return from retina results in papilledema, retinal hemorrhage, and decreased visual acuity
   c. Pathogens
      1) *Staphylococcus aureus* and *Streptococcus* species, including *Streptococcus pneumoniae*
      2) Less frequent: gram-negative bacteria and anaerobes
      3) Rare: *Aspergillus* and Zygomycetes
   d. Further diagnostics: MRI and high-resolution contrast CT scan
   e. Treatment
      1) High doses of intravenous antibiotics while awaiting culture results: vancomycin, ceftriaxone, or metronidazole
      2) Anticoagulants are not required
      3) Surgical decompression of infection source (sinusitis or maxillary molar)
      4) Rarely need to drain cavernous sinus
5. Osteomyelitis
   a. Clinical disease
      1) Mandible with thin cortical plates and poor vascularization is especially vulnerable
      2) Increased intramedullary pressure decreases blood flow
         a) Causes accelerated necrosis and lifting or perforation of periosteum
         b) Results in cutaneous and mucosal abscesses and fistulas
      3) Radiation necrosis and actinomycosis frequently cause chronic sclerosing osteomyelitis
   b. Clinical signs and symptoms: numbness at affected site and mandibular trismus
   c. Treatment
      1) Prolonged antibiotics (weeks to months), especially with actinomycosis
      2) Surgical débridement or resection of infected jaw as determined by oral surgeon

II. Nonodontogenic Orofacial Infections
   A. Oral Mucosal Infections
      1. Noma (also called gangrenous stomatitis)
         a. Clinical disease
            1) Acute rapid destruction of oral and facial tissue
            2) Typically occurs in children with severe malnutrition and debilitation
         b. Clinical signs and symptoms
            1) Inflamed mucosa leads to necrotic ulcers, which develop into painful cellulitis of the lips and cheeks
            2) Result is necrotic sloughing that exposes teeth, bone, and deeper tissues
         c. Pathogens: unknown but thought to be infectious agents
            1) *Borrelia vincentii* and *Fusobacterium nucleatum* are frequently isolated
            2) *Prevotella melaninogenica* may also be cultured
         d. Treatment: high doses of intravenous penicillin
      2. Aphthous stomatitis
         a. Clinical disease
            1) Aphthous ulcers are the most common cause of recurrent oral lesions
            2) Thought to be an autoimmune disorder
            3) Three types: minor, major, and herpetiform
         b. Diagnostics and treatment
            1) Must distinguish from coxsackievirus or herpes simplex virus infection, Behçet syndrome, and agranulocytosis
            2) Symptomatic and supportive treatment: good oral hygiene and use of antiseptic mouthwash
            3) Topical or systemic corticosteroids in extensive cases
         c. Immunocompromised patients
            1) Frequently present with mucositis or stomatitis (eg, from chemotherapy, radiotherapy, bone marrow or solid organ transplant, human immunodeficiency virus infection [HIV] or AIDS, or autoimmune disorders)
            2) Mucosal breakdown is often associated with latent viral reactivation (herpes simplex virus, cytomegalovirus, or varicella-zoster virus) and superinfection with bacteria or fungi (*Candida*)
         3) Treatment
            a) Supportive treatment: good oral hygiene, saline rinse, coating agents, topical antiseptics, and analgesics (systemic analgesics if necessary)
            b) Antiviral prophylaxis can reduce reactivation of latent virus
            c) Secondary infections require correct microbial diagnosis and choice of appropriate antimicrobial
               i) Thalidomide has been reported to be effective in HIV/AIDS patients
   B. Salivary Gland Infections
      1. Suppurative parotitis
         a. Associated with the following groups of patients: immunocompromised, elderly, those receiving radiotherapy, dehydrated, debilitated, postoperative
         b. Clinical signs and symptoms
            1) High fevers and chills
            2) Acute onset of firm, tender or painful, erythematous swelling in preauricular and postauricular areas and in the jaw angle
         c. Important complications
            1) Swelling of neck may lead to respiratory obstruction
            2) Spread into adjacent facial bones may develop into osteomyelitis
         d. Pathogens
            1) Most common: *Staphylococcus aureus*
            2) Possible: Enterobacteriaceae and other gram-negative bacilli
            3) Less frequent: anaerobes such as *Peptostreptococcus* and *Bacteroides*
         e. Treatment
            1) Prompt surgical drainage and decompression are frequently required
            2) Antibiotics: include an antistaphylococcal agent
      2. Chronic bacterial parotitis
         a. Clinical disease
            1) Constant low-grade bacterial infection causing abnormal salivary gland function
            2) Differentiate from Sjögren syndrome
               a) Sjögren syndrome: dry mouth, keratoconjunctivitis, and autoimmune disorder (rheumatoid arthritis, scleroderma, lupus erythematosus, polymyositis, or periarteritis nodosa)

b) Temporomandibular arthritis or arthralgia suggest Sjögren syndrome
    b. Pathogens: usually *Staphylococcus* species or mixed oral aerobes and anaerobes
    c. Treatment
      1) Saline irrigation with or without systemic antibiotics in combination with ductal antibiotics
      2) Parotidectomy in severe cases
  3. Viral parotitis
    a. Clinical disease
      1) Mumps
      2) Parotitis develops in 30% to 40% of mumps virus infections
    b. Clinical signs and symptoms
      1) Rapid onset of tender, swollen parotid glands (unilateral or bilateral) 2 to 3 weeks after exposure
      2) Prodromal phase: fever, chills, headache, preauricular pain, malaise, myalgia, and anorexia
    c. Pathogens
      1) Mumps virus
      2) Other viruses: enteroviruses, influenza virus, HIV
    d. Treatment
      1) Supportive (usually resolves in 5-10 days): prevent dehydration and watch for secondary bacterial infection
      2) HIV parotitis: usually not painful and otherwise asymptomatic
  4. Tuberculous parotitis
    a. Clinical signs and symptoms: chronic nontender swelling of parotid gland
    b. Pathogen: *Mycobacterium tuberculosis*
    c. Treatment: standard tuberculous therapy regimen
III. Miscellaneous Infections of the Head and Neck
  A. Cervical Adenitis
    1. Etiology
      a. Unilateral presentation suggests bacterial
      b. Acute bilateral presentation suggests viral, toxoplasmosis, or group A *Streptococcus*
      c. Chronic or recurrent presentation suggests mycobacteria (typical or atypical), HIV, cytomegalovirus, Epstein-Barr virus, actinomycosis, or *Bartonella henselae* (cat-scratch fever)
    2. Diagnosis: rule out noninfectious causes such as sarcoidosis and malignancies
  B. Infected Embryologic Cysts
    1. Clinical disease
      a. Three embryologic abnormalities
        1) Cystic hygroma or lymphangioma of the neck
        2) Pharyngeal or bronchial cleft cysts
        3) Thyroglossal duct cysts
      b. Hygromas
        1) Evident by 2 years of age
        2) If they enlarge suddenly, suspect bleeding or infection
        3) Can block upper airway
      c. Pharyngeal cleft cysts
        1) Masses or fistulas posterior to the angle of the mandible along the anterior sternocleidomastoid muscle
        2) Can enlarge during an upper respiratory tract infection
      d. Thyroglossal duct cysts
        1) Most common of these 3 abnormalities
        2) A fistula forms during an infection and can block the airway
    2. Treatment
      a. Broad-spectrum antibiotic (eg, cephalosporin)
      b. Surgical excision to prevent recurrence is recommended after resolution of infection
  C. Suppurative Thyroiditis
    1. Clinical disease
      a. Thyroid gland infections are rare but life threatening
      b. Preexisting condition (eg, goiter) is typical
      c. Caused by adjacent deep facial infection, hematogenous dissemination, or anterior esophageal perforation
    2. Clinical signs and symptoms: fever; local pain, tenderness, or warmth; dysphonia or hoarseness; pharyngitis or dysphagia
    3. Pathogens
      a. Most common: *S aureus*, *S pneumoniae*, and *Streptococcus pyogenes*
      b. Others that have been isolated: *Haemophilus influenzae*, *Eikenella corrodens*, viridans streptococci, *Peptostreptococcus* species, *Bacteroides*, and *Actinomyces* species
    4. Diagnostics and treatment
      a. Needle aspiration
      b. Culture to determine specific pathogen for appropriate antibiotic regimen
      c. Surgical drainage
  D. Human and Animal Bites
    1. Clinical disease
      a. Can be serious
      b. Oral flora, not skin flora, are primary infectious organisms
    2. Pathogens

a. Human bites: common pathogens *S aureus*, *Streptococcus* species, *E corrodens*, *H influenzae*, *Bacteroides* species, *Peptostreptococcus* species
  b. Animal bites: *Pasteurella multocida*
 3. Treatment
  a. Initial therapy for animal or human bites: amoxicillin-clavulanate
  b. Penicillin-allergic patient: trimethoprim-sulfamethoxazole in combination with clindamycin, or fluoroquinolone in combination with clindamycin
  c. *Pasteurella multocida*: second- or third-generation cephalosporin
 E. Maxillofacial Trauma
  1. Automobile and motorcycle accidents produce fractures that cross through or penetrate sinus cavities and displace tooth-bearing areas of lower and upper jaws
  2. Careful evaluation of these fracture paths is needed
  3. Secondary infection rates in these areas are high
 F. Radiotherapy and Postsurgical Wounds
  1. Infectious complications arise from common treatments, including radiotherapy, chemotherapy, and surgical resection
  2. Complications: osteonecrosis of mandible, radionecrosis of laryngeal cartilage, and pharyngocutaneous fistulas
  3. Pathogens: *S aureus* and *Pseudomonas aeruginosa* are frequently cultured
  4. Treatment
   a. Prolonged administration of intravenous antibiotics as appropriate for the pathogen
   b. Surgical débridement
IV. Clinical Considerations for Infections of the Head, Neck, and Face
 A. Specimen Acquisition and Diagnosis
  1. Needle aspiration
   a. Thorough surface disinfection before needle aspiration of an abscess decreases specimen contamination
   b. An extraoral approach is preferred
   c. Evacuating air from the syringe, removing the needle for safety, and sealing any syringe openings decreases the chance of oxygen poisoning
   d. Specimen should be transported promptly to the laboratory under anaerobic conditions
   e. Immediately alerting the laboratory personnel to test for anaerobes should ensure optimal culture results and allow for correct antibiotic management
  2. Swab specimens
   a. Less desirable
   b. Difficult to maintain an anaerobic environment
   c. Greater chance of contamination with normal flora
  3. Abscess surgically opened for drainage
   a. Quickly obtain syringe aspirate of the fluid
   b. Place in an anaerobic transporter for a good specimen
  4. Poor management of specimens
   a. Leads to poor diagnostics
   b. Exposes the patient to inappropriate, costly, and undesirable antimicrobial agent decisions
  5. Bone infections
   a. Cultures of sinus tracts are misleading because they are frequently colonized with bacteria that do not reflect the microbiology of the infected bone
   b. Definitive diagnosis frequently necessitates bone biopsies with culture
  6. Imaging techniques to identify and localize deep fascial space infections of the head and neck
   a. Lateral neck radiographs
    1) May show air within necrotic tissue
    2) May show abnormalities in the tracheal air column (eg, deviation or compression)
   b. CT and MRI
    1) Preferred for determining the location and extent of deep fascial space infections of the head and neck
    2) MRI is more sensitive than CT for detecting bone involvement
    3) MRI is useful for identifying vascular lesions (eg, thrombophlebitis of the internal jugular vein)
 B. General Management
  1. Two-part therapy required for suppurative odontogenic infections and nearly all infections of the deep spaces of the face, head, and neck
   a. Prompt surgical drainage with débridement of necrotic tissue
   b. Antibiotic therapy
    1) Penicillin with metronidazole
    2) Amoxicillin or ticarcillin with a β-lactamase inhibitor
    3) A carbapenem, clindamycin, a cephalosporin (cefoxitin, ceftizoxime, cefotetan), or a newer-generation fluoroquinolone (moxifloxacin)

Table 24.1
Initial Empirical Antimicrobial Regimens for Suppurative Infections of the Head and Neck

Infection	Usual Causative Organisms	Antibiotic Regimens[a]
Suppurative orofacial odontogenic infections, including Ludwig angina	Viridans and other streptococci, *Peptostreptococcus* species, *Bacteroides* species, and other oral anaerobes	Penicillin G 2-4 MU IV q 4-6 h *plus* metronidazole 0.5 g IV q 6 h *or* Ampicillin-sulbactam 2 g IV q 4 h *or* Clindamycin 600 mg IV q 6 h *or* Cefoxitin 1-2 g IV q 6 h
Lateral pharyngeal or retropharyngeal space infections		
Odontogenic	Viridans and other streptococci, *Staphylococcus* species, *Peptostreptococcus* species, *Bacteroides* species, and other oral anaerobes	Penicillin G 2-4 MU IV q 4-6 h *plus* metronidazole 0.5 g IV q 6 h *or* Ampicillin-sulbactam 2 g IV q 4 h *or* Clindamycin 600 mg IV q 6 h
Rhinogenic	*Streptococcus pneumoniae*, *Haemophilus influenzae*, viridans and other streptococci, *Bacteroides* species, *Peptostreptococcus* species, and other oral anaerobes	One of the following: 1) Penicillin G 2-4 MU IV q 4-6 h *or* levofloxacin 500 mg IV q 24 h *or* ciprofloxacin 750 mg IV q 12 h *plus* Metronidazole 0.5 g IV q 6 h *or* clindamycin 600 mg IV q 6 h *or* 2) Moxifloxacin 400 mg IV q 24 h
Otogenic	Same as for rhinogenic space infections	Same as for rhinogenic space infections
Suppurative cervical adenitis and infected embryologic cysts	*Streptococcus pyogenes*, *Peptostreptococcus* species, *Fusobacterium* species, oral anaerobes	One of the following: 1) Penicillin G 2-4 MU IV q 4 h *plus* metronidazole 500 mg IV q 6 h *or* 2) Ampicillin-sulbactam 2 g IV q 4 h *or* 3) Clindamycin 600 mg IV q 6 h *or* 4) Cefoxitin 1-2 g IV q 6 h
Suppurative thyroiditis	*Staphylococcus aureus*, *S pyogenes*, *S pneumoniae*, *H influenzae*, viridans and other streptococci, oral anaerobes	Nafcillin 2 g IV q 4-6 h *or* vancomycin 1 g IV q 12 h *plus either* Metronidazole 500 mg IV q 6 h *or* Clindamycin 600 mg IV q 6 h
Cervicofacial actinomycosis	*Actinomyces israelii*, *Arachnia propionica*, *Actinobacillus actinomycetemcomitans*	One of the following: 1) Penicillin G 2-4 MU IV q 4-6 h *or* 2) Doxycycline 200 mg PO or IV q 12 h *or* 3) Clindamycin 450 mg PO q 6 h or 600 mg IV q 6 h
Human or animal bites	*S pyogenes*, *S aureus*, *Eikenella corrodens*, oral anaerobes, *Pasteurella multocida*	One of the following: 1) Ampicillin-sulbactam 2 g IV q 4 h *or* 2) Amoxicillin-clavulanate 500 mg PO q 8 h *or* 3) Moxifloxacin 400 mg IV or PO q 12 h
Maxillofacial trauma, postsurgical wound infections	*S aureus*, *S pyogenes*, *Peptostreptococcus* species, other oral anaerobes, *Pseudomonas aeruginosa*, Enterobacteriaceae	Nafcillin 2 g IV q 4 h *or* vancomycin 1 g IV q 12 h *plus 1 of the following*: 1) Ticarcillin-clavulanate 3.1 g IV q 4 h *or* 2) Piperacillin-tazobactam 3.375 g IV q 6 h *or* 3) Imipenem-cilastatin 500 mg IV q 6 h *or* 4) Meropenem 1 g IV q 8 h *or* 5) Moxifloxacin 400 mg IV or PO q 24 h *or* 6) Tigecycline 100 mg IV, then 50 mg IV q 12 h

Table 24.1
(continued)

Infection	Usual Causative Organisms	Antibiotic Regimens[a]
Suppurative jugular thrombophlebitis (Lemierre syndrome)	*Fusobacterium necrophorum*; same as for odontogenic space infections	Same as for odontogenic space infections
Suppurative cavernous sinus thrombosis	Same as for odontogenic, rhinogenic, or otogenic space infections	Same as for odontogenic, rhinogenic, or otogenic space infections
Mandibular osteomyelitis	Same as for odontogenic space infections	Clindamycin 600 mg IV q 6 h *or* Moxifloxacin 400 mg IV q 24 h
Extension of osteomyelitis from prevertebral space infection	*Staphylococcus aureus*,[b] facultative gram-negative bacilli	Nafcillin 2 g IV q 4 h *or* vancomycin 1 g IV q 12 h *plus either* Tobramycin 1.7 mg/kg IV q 8 h *or* Ciprofloxacin 400 mg IV q 12 h

Abbreviations: IV, intravenously; MU, million units; PO, orally; q, every.

[a] For immunocompromised hosts, consider replacing penicillin G with 1 of the following: cefotaxime 2 g IV q 4 h; ceftriaxone 1 g IV q 12 h; or cefepime 2 g IV q 12 h. Other regimens to consider are ticarcillin-clavulanate 3.1 g IV q 4 h; piperacillin-tazobactam 3.375 g IV q 6 h; imipenem 500 mg IV q 6 h; meropenem 1 g IV q 8 h; moxifloxacin 400 mg IV q 24 h; or tigecycline 100 mg IV, then 50 mg IV q 12 h.

[b] For *Staphylococcus aureus* infections in which methicillin-resistant *S aureus* (MRSA) is suspected, replace nafcillin with vancomycin 1 g IV q 12 h; in immunosuppressed hosts, cefotaxime or ceftriaxone or imipenem, as described in the Table, can be added.

From Chow AW. Infections of the oral cavity, neck, and head. In: Mandell GL, Bennett JE, Dolin R. Mandell, Douglas, and Bennett's principles and practice of infectious diseases. Vol 1. 7th ed. Philadelphia (PA): Churchill Livingstone/Elsevier; c2010. p. 855-71. Used with permission.

    4) Treatment of outpatients with less serious dental infections
        a) Amoxicillin with or without a β-lactamase inhibitor
        b) Penicillin with metronidazole
  2. Table 24.1 summarizes the most likely organisms encountered in specific infection sites and lists recommended antibiotics
C. Prophylaxis of Odontogenic Infections
  1. Meticulous oral hygiene: the best strategy to prevent dental caries and treat periodontitis
  2. Additional steps
    a. Reducing intake of carbohydrate-rich snacks and drinks
    b. Use of fluoride rinses
    c. Brush and floss teeth after each meal
    d. Chlorhexidine oral rinse effectively reduces the number of dental plaque bacteria
      1) Can stain teeth
      2) May induce resistance with prolonged use
  3. Topical antibiotics such as minocycline are sometimes used in adults with periodontitis

Suggested Reading

Brook I. Anaerobic bacteria in upper respiratory tract and other head and neck infections. Ann Otol Rhinol Laryngol. 2002 May;111(5 Pt 1):430–40.

Chow AW. Infections of the oral cavity, neck, and head. In: Mandell GL, Bennett JE, Dolin R, editors. Principles and practice of infectious diseases. Vol 1. 7th ed. Philadelphia (PA): Churchill Livingstone/Elsevier; c2010. p. 855–71.

Ebright JR, Pace MT, Niazi AF. Septic thrombosis of the cavernous sinuses. Arch Intern Med. 2001 Dec 10-24;161(22):2671–6.

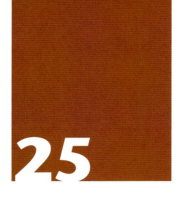

Priya Sampathkumar, MD

Pneumonia[a]

I. Community-Acquired Pneumonia
   A. Introduction
      1. *Community-acquired pneumonia* (CAP): acute infection of the pulmonary parenchyma acquired while the patient was in the community rather than in a hospital
         a. Common illness with considerable morbidity and mortality
         b. Approximately 20% of cases result in hospitalization
      2. Older or immunosuppressed patients with CAP
         a. May present with nonrespiratory symptoms: confusion, failure to thrive, worsening of an underlying chronic illness, or falls
         b. Fever may be absent, but tachypnea is usually present, along with abnormal findings on chest examination
   B. Epidemiology
      1. Age
         a. No age-specific predisposition, but incidence increases with older age
         b. Most patients are older than 50
      2. Most patients have chronic obstructive pulmonary disease, cardiovascular disease, or another chronic disease
   C. Etiology
      1. Common pathogens that cause CAP are listed in Table 25.1
      2. History may suggest specific organisms
      3. *Streptococcus pneumoniae*
         a. A major cause of illness in children
         b. Causes illness and death among persons who are elderly or who have underlying disease
         c. Mortality
            1) An estimated 40,000 deaths in the United States each year
            2) Vaccination might prevent approximately half of these deaths
         d. Racial differences
            1) Alaskan Natives and American Indians: rates of invasive pneumococcal disease are high
            2) Black adults: overall incidence of pneumococcal bacteremia is 3-fold to

---

[a] The "Nosocomial Pneumonia" section of this chapter was adapted from Sampathkumar P. Nosocomial pneumonia. In: Bland KI, Buchler MW, Csendes A, Sarr MG, Garden OJ, Wong J, editors. General surgery: principles and international practice. 2nd ed. Vol 1. London: Springer; c2009. p. 287–95. Used with permission.

Table 25.1

Common Pathogens in Community-Acquired Pneumonia

Patient Type	Etiologic Agent
Outpatient	*Streptococcus pneumoniae*
	Mycoplasma pneumoniae
	Haemophilus influenzae
	Chlamydophila pneumoniae
	Influenza A and B viruses
	Parainfluenza virus
	Respiratory syncytial viruses
Non-ICU inpatient	*S pneumoniae*
	M pneumoniae
	C pneumoniae
	Legionella species
	Influenza A and B viruses
	Parainfluenza virus
	Respiratory syncytial viruses
ICU patient	*S pneumoniae*
	Staphylococcus aureus
	Legionella species
	Gram-negative bacilli

Abbreviation: ICU, intensive care unit.

        5-fold higher than among other racial groups
- e. Concomitant pneumococcal bacteremia
    1) In approximately 10% to 25% of adult patients
    2) Among adults who receive antimicrobial therapy and intensive medical care, the overall case-fatality rate is 15% to 20%
4. *Staphylococcus aureus*
    a. *Staphylococcus aureus* infections are most common in certain groups
        1) Intravenous drug users
        2) Elderly persons
        3) Persons who have had a recent influenza virus infection
        4) Persons who have cystic fibrosis
    b. Community-acquired methicillin-resistant *S aureus* (CA-MRSA) infections, especially with the USA300 strains
        1) Cause necrotizing pneumonia in previously healthy persons
        2) Clues to CA-MRSA infection
            a) Rapidly progressive lung infection in a previously healthy young adult or child
            b) Often accompanied by pulmonary necrosis and shock
    c. When to suspect *S aureus*
        1) Patients have influenza and a bacterial superinfection
        2) Patients have clinical characteristics of staphylococcal toxic shock syndrome
        3) Patients have the unique features of pneumonia caused by USA300 strains (ie, pulmonary necrosis, shock, and neutropenia)
5. Gram-negative organisms
    a. *Pseudomonas aeruginosa*
        1) Not a common cause of CAP
        2) Infects patients who have cystic fibrosis and patients who have severely compromised respiratory defenses
    b. *Neisseria meningitidis*: occasionally involved in epidemics among military recruits
    c. *Yersinia pestis*: infections occur after exposure to an infected rat population
    d. *Burkholderia pseudomallei*: infections occur after exposure to contaminated soil in Southeast Asia
6. Viral pneumonia
    a. Influenza virus: the most common viral pathogen that causes pneumonia
    b. Influenza
        1) Should be recognized early so that appropriate infection control measures can be instituted in the health care setting
        2) Patients commonly present with worsening respiratory symptoms if they have underlying pulmonary and cardiac disease
    c. True influenza pneumonia is rare: occurs in less than 1% of patients
7. Atypical pneumonia
    a. A form of pneumonia in which systemic symptoms are usually more pronounced than respiratory symptoms
    b. Clinical features
        1) Pneumonia of gradual onset
        2) Dry cough
        3) Extrapulmonary symptoms (eg, fatigue, nausea, vomiting, diarrhea, sore throat)
        4) Minimal signs of pulmonary involvement
    c. Most frequently isolated pathogens: *Mycoplasma pneumoniae*, *Chlamydophila pneumoniae*, and *Legionella* species (Table 25.2)
    d. Considerable overlap between typical and atypical pneumonia syndromes
        1) Atypical infection may manifest as typical pneumonia
        2) Pneumococcal infection may manifest as atypical pneumonia

Table 25.2

Features of Atypical Pneumonia

Agent	Incubation Period, d	Seasonality	Exposure	Underlying Chronic Disease	Clinical Features
Mycoplasma pneumoniae	14-21	Year-round	None	None	Adolescents and young adults Upper respiratory tract symptoms Bullous myringitis Meningoencephalitis Myocarditis Hemolytic anemia
Legionella species	2-10	Year-round Summer peak	Cooling towers Hot tubs	Smoking Chronic lung disease Long-term use of corticosteroids Organ transplant	Relative bradycardia Abdominal pain Vomiting and diarrhea Hematuria Confusion Hyponatremia Abnormal liver function test results Mortality: 5%-25% among immunocompetent hosts; higher among immunosuppressed patients
Chlamydophila pneumoniae	14-28			None	Typically in elderly patients Biphasic illness: pharyngitis followed in 1-2 wk by pneumonia May be associated with arthritis and myocarditis

3) Diagnostic tests for the pathogens are not very sensitive
4) Since distinction between typical and atypical pneumonia is difficult, initial treatment regimens for all patients with CAP should include agents directed against the atypical pneumonia pathogens

D. Diagnosis
1. Chest radiography
   a. For all patients with CAP
   b. To establish the diagnosis
   c. To evaluate for complications (eg, pleural effusion, multilobar disease)
2. Assessment of disease severity
   a. For all outpatients
   b. Sputum culture and Gram stain are not required
3. Assessment of all hospitalized patients with CAP
   a. Gas exchange (oximetry or arterial blood gas)
   b. Routine blood chemistry and blood counts
   c. Two sets of blood cultures
4. When causative agent is thought to be a drug-resistant pathogen or resistant to usual empirical therapy
   a. Sputum culture
   b. Gram stain to guide interpretation of culture results
5. When patients have severe CAP
   a. *Legionella* urinary antigen should be measured
   b. An etiologic diagnosis should be made
   c. Diagnosis may require bronchoscopic samples of lower respiratory secretions

E. Treatment
1. Initial treatment
   a. Empirical and based on likely pathogens (Table 25.3)
   b. Organism-specific therapy may be possible after culture results are available
   c. First dose of antibiotic therapy should be given to all hospitalized patients within 8 hours of arrival at the hospital
2. All patients with CAP should be treated for atypical pathogens
   a. Outpatients: a macrolide (or tetracycline) alone
   b. Inpatients: an intravenous macrolide alone if there are no risk factors for drug-resistant *S pneumoniae* (DRSP), gram-negative bacteria, or aspiration
   c. Regimens for outpatients or non–intensive care unit (ICU) inpatients who have risk factors for DRSP or gram-negative bacteria
      1) Either a β-lactam–macrolide combination or an antipneumococcal fluoroquinolone alone

Table 25.3

Empirical Antibiotic Therapy for Community-Acquired Pneumonia

Clinical Setting	Recommended Empirical Treatment
Outpatient: healthy patient with no risk factors for DRSP	Macrolide alone (azithromycin, clarithromycin, or erythromycin) *or* Doxycycline (weak recommendation)
Outpatient: patient with comorbidities, immunosuppression, diabetes mellitus, alcoholism, or other risk factor for DRSP or patient in a region with high (>25%) rate of infection with macrolide-resistant *Streptococcus pneumoniae*	Respiratory FQ alone (moxifloxacin, gemifloxacin, or levofloxacin) *or* β-Lactam[a] + macrolide *or* β-Lactam[a] + doxycycline
Inpatient: non-ICU treatment	Respiratory FQ *or* Respiratory FQ + macrolide *or* Ertapenem + macrolide or doxycycline
Inpatient: ICU treatment	β-Lactam[a] + macrolide *or* β-Lactam[a] + FQ
Inpatient: ICU treatment in patient with risk factors for pseudomonal infection (structural lung disease or failure of outpatient antibiotic therapy)	Antipseudomonal β-lactam[b] + FQ *or* Antipseudomonal β-lactam[b] + aminoglycoside + macrolide *or* Antipseudomonal β-lactam[b] + aminoglycoside + FQ
Inpatient: ICU treatment in patient with suspected MRSA	β-Lactam[a] + macrolide or FQ + vancomycin or linezolid

Abbreviations: DRSP, drug-resistant *Streptococcus pneumoniae*; FQ, fluoroquinolone; ICU, intensive care unit; MRSA, methicillin-resistant *Staphylococcus aureus*.

[a] Cefotaxime, ceftriaxone, or ampicillin-sulbactam.
[b] Piperacillin-tazobactam, cefepime, imipenem, or meropenem.

    2) Between these 2 therapeutically equivalent regimens, the fluoroquinolone may be more convenient for outpatients
  d. ICU patients
    1) Data do not support the use of an antipneumococcal fluoroquinolone alone
    2) β-Lactam antibiotic should be given in combination with either a macrolide or a quinolone
    3) If appropriate, a regimen with 2 antipseudomonal agents should be used for at-risk patients
  e. For patients with risk factors for *P aeruginosa*: antipseudomonal β-lactam antibiotics (eg, cefepime, imipenem, meropenem, piperacillin-tazobactam)
3. Clinical response
  a. Usually an adequate clinical response is apparent within 3 days
  b. For most patients with CAP, the initial antibiotic therapy should not be changed in the first 72 hours unless the patient's clinical condition worsens
  c. CAP patients who do not have a response to initial therapy (≤10% of patients) need additional diagnostic evaluation
    1) Drug-resistant or unusual (or unsuspected) pathogen
    2) Alternative diagnosis (eg, inflammatory disease, pulmonary embolus)
    3) Pneumonia complication
4. Criteria for switching therapy to oral route
  a. Improvement in cough and dyspnea
  b. Afebrile (<37.8°C) on 2 occasions 8 hours apart
  c. Decreasing white blood cell count
  d. Functioning gastrointestinal tract with adequate oral intake
  e. If patient is febrile but other clinical features are favorable, therapy can be switched to oral route
5. Criteria for hospital dismissal
  a. Patient has met criteria for oral therapy

b. Oral therapy has been started
c. Other medical and social factors permit dismissal
6. Duration of therapy
   a. Minimum of 5 days
   b. Patients should be afebrile for 48 to 72 hours before therapy is stopped
   c. Indications for longer duration of therapy
      1) Initial therapy was not active against the identified pathogen
      2) Initial therapy was complicated by extrapulmonary infection
F. Prevention
   1. Influenza vaccine
      a. Annual vaccination is recommended for all persons older than 6 months
      b. Especially important for certain groups
         1) Persons 50 years or older
         2) Persons with chronic medical conditions
         3) Household contacts of high-risk persons
         4) Health care workers
   2. Pneumococcal vaccine
      a. For persons 65 years or older
      b. For persons with selected high-risk medical conditions
   3. Smoking cessation
      a. Recommended for all patients
      b. Smoking is an important risk factor for CAP
II. Nosocomial Pneumonia
   A. Introduction
      1. *Nosocomial pneumonia*: pneumonia that develops more than 48 hours after admission to a health care facility and which was not incubating at the time of admission
      2. *Ventilator-associated pneumonia* (VAP): pneumonia developing in patients who have been intubated and mechanically ventilated in the previous 48 hours
      3. *Health care–associated pneumonia* (HCAP): a new term that describes pneumonia developing in a person who has contact with the health care system in one of several ways
         a. Received home intravenous antibiotic therapy, chemotherapy, wound care, or hemodialysis within 30 days of the onset of pneumonia
         b. Resided in a long-term care facility or nursing home within 30 days of the onset of pneumonia
         c. Was hospitalized in an acute care hospital for 2 or more days within 90 days of the onset of pneumonia
      4. HCAP is classified as nosocomial pneumonia
         a. Even though pneumonia may begin while the patient is in the community, HCAP is usually caused by antibiotic-resistant organisms like those in hospitalized patients
         b. Severity, outcome, and recommended treatments are like those of nosocomial pneumonia rather than of CAP
      5. Thus, nosocomial pneumonia includes hospital-acquired pneumonia (HAP), VAP, and HCAP
   B. Epidemiology
      1. Importance of nosocomial pneumonia
         a. Second most common nosocomial infection in the United States (after urinary tract infections)
         b. Leading cause of deaths due to nosocomial infections
         c. Increases hospital length of stay by an average of 7 to 10 days
         d. Results in an excess cost of more than $40,000 per patient
         e. Occurs at a rate of 5 to 10 cases per 1,000 hospital admissions
         f. Risks
            1) The incidence increases 6-fold to 20-fold among patients receiving mechanical ventilation
            2) Risk is higher among surgical patients than medical patients
            3) Patients undergoing cardiothoracic surgery have the highest risk
      2. Pathogens
         a. Bacteria cause the majority of cases of nosocomial pneumonia
         b. Occasionally influenza and respiratory syncytial viruses cause outbreaks of nosocomial pneumonia in high-risk patients (eg, children, the elderly, immunosuppressed patients)
         c. *Aspergillus* pneumonia can occur in severely immunosuppressed patients
         d. Overall, fungi and viruses are *not* important causes of nosocomial pneumonia
   C. Etiology
      1. The time of onset of pneumonia is an important predictor of the causative pathogen (Table 25.4)
         a. Early-onset VAP and HAP
            1) Occur within 4 days of hospitalization or intubation
            2) Usually carry a better prognosis

Table 25.4
Likely Pathogens in Early and Late Nosocomial Pneumonia

Condition	Most Likely Pathogens
Early-onset VAP or HAP	*Streptococcus pneumoniae* *Haemophilus influenzae* Methicillin-sensitive *Staphylococcus aureus* Antibiotic-sensitive gram-negative bacilli *Klebsiella pneumoniae* *Enterobacter* species
Late-onset VAP or HAP, or HCAP	*Pseudomonas aeruginosa* Resistant *Klebsiella* *Acinetobacter* Methicillin-resistant *S aureus* *Legionella pneumophila*

Abbreviations: HAP, hospital-acquired pneumonia; HCAP, health care–associated pneumonia; VAP, ventilator-associated pneumonia.

Adapted from Sampathkumar P. Nosocomial pneumonia. In: Bland KI, Buchler MW, Csendes A, Sarr MG, Garden OJ, Wong J, editors. General surgery: principles and international practice. 2nd ed. Vol 1. London: Springer; c2009. p. 287–95. Used with permission.

      3) Are more likely to be caused by antibiotic-sensitive organisms
         a) *Streptococcus pneumoniae*
         b) *Haemophilus influenzae*
         c) Antibiotic-sensitive gram-negative bacilli such as *Klebsiella* and *Enterobacter* species
   b. Late-onset HAP and VAP
      1) Occur after 5 or more days of hospitalization or intubation
      2) Generally caused by multidrug-resistant pathogens
      3) Associated with poorer outcomes
      4) Late-onset HAP and VAP pathogens are similar to those in some patients with HCAP
         a) Patients with HCAP who live in long-term care facilities
         b) Patients with HCAP who have had recent exposure to antibiotics
  2. Pneumonia due to *S aureus* is more common in certain patients
   a. Patients with diabetes mellitus
   b. Patients with head trauma
   c. Patients in ICUs
   d. Patients with a recent history of influenza
  3. Nosocomial pneumonia due to fungi such as *Aspergillus fumigatus*
   a. May occur in solid organ, bone marrow, or stem cell recipients and in otherwise severely immunocompromised patients
   b. Environmental source of fungal spores should be identified (eg, contaminated air ducts, dust from hospital renovation or construction)
  4. *Candida* and *Aspergillus* species
   a. Often colonize airway of hospitalized patients
   b. In the absence of severe immunosuppression, they do not cause pneumonia and do not require treatment
  5. Viruses
   a. Influenza A virus can be the cause of nosocomial outbreaks during influenza season (typically fall and winter)
   b. Respiratory syncytial virus outbreaks are common among pediatric patients but can also occur among adult patients, especially those with hematologic malignancies
D. Diagnosis
  1. Best diagnostic strategy is controversial
  2. For most immunocompetent patients who are not intubated, the diagnosis is made when they meet 2 clinical criteria
   a. Presence of new infiltrate on chest radiograph
   b. Clinical evidence that the infiltrate is of infectious origin
      1) New onset of fever higher than 38°C
      2) Purulent sputum
      3) Leukocytosis or leukopenia
      4) Decrease in oxygenation
  3. Confirmation of diagnosis of pneumonia is difficult, especially for intubated ICU patients, who may have many reasons for the clinical findings
   a. Drawbacks to use of clinical criteria alone to diagnose VAP
      1) May result in overdiagnosis and unnecessary use of antibiotics
      2) Does not identify the etiologic agent
   b. Lower respiratory tract culture
      1) Generally required for etiologic diagnosis
      2) Can include cultures of endotracheal aspirates, bronchoalveolar lavage (BAL) fluid, or protected specimen brush (PSB)
      3) Endotracheal aspirates
         a) Easy to obtain
         b) Usually contain the pathogens found by more invasive methods
         c) Positive culture results
            i) Colonization of the trachea is very common
            ii) Positive culture results do not distinguish a pathogen from a colonizing organism

d) Negative culture results
   i) Endotracheal aspirate cultures are most useful when culture results are negative
   ii) Pneumonia is very unlikely in a patient with negative results on endotracheal aspirate culture if the patient's antibiotics had not been changed within the previous 72 hours
4) Quantitative culture results suggestive of pneumonia
   a) BAL fluid obtained either bronchoscopically or by blind suctioning: growth of more than 10^4 colony-forming units (CFU)/mL
   b) Protected specimen brush: 10^3 CFU/mL
5) Bronchoscopic approach
   a) Disadvantages
      i) These tests are more invasive, are costly, and require specialized laboratory and clinical skills
      ii) False-negative results can occur, especially if patients had received antibiotic therapy before the sample was obtained
   b) Advantages
      i) Specificity of these tests is higher than that of sputum or endotracheal aspirate cultures
      ii) Positive culture results above the diagnostic threshold provide strong evidence that the patient has pneumonia with that organism
c. Postmortem studies of VAP have identified several characteristics pertinent to diagnostic testing
   1) Often multifocal, frequently involving both lungs, and generally in the posterior and lower segments
      a) Multifocal nature of VAP: BAL and endotracheal aspirates can provide more representative samples than PSB, which samples only 1 bronchial segment
      b) Diffuse bilateral nature of VAP and predominance in dependent lung segments: "blind" BAL and PSB may be as accurate as bronchoscopic sampling
   2) VAP is often in different phases of evolution at different sites at the same time
   3) Prior antibiotic therapy can affect the number of bacteria found in lung tissue
4. Other cultures
   a. Blood cultures
      1) Helpful when positive
      2) Overall, less than 25% of pneumonias are associated with bacteremia
   b. Pleural fluid cultures: rarely necessary to make the diagnosis of pneumonia
   c. Pleural fluid analysis
      1) May be helpful when patients do not respond to appropriate antibiotic therapy
      2) Used to identify empyema, which may need additional interventions such as a chest tube
5. Biologic markers
   a. Serum C-reactive protein and procalcitonin levels: not helpful in diagnosing pneumonia among critically ill patients, but serial procalcitonin levels may be helpful in deciding when to discontinue antibiotic therapy in patients with suspected pneumonia
   b. Triggering receptor expressed on myeloid cells (TREM-1)
      1) Appears promising
      2) A recently identified molecule involved in the inflammatory response to infection
      3) Neutrophils and monocytes expressing high levels of TREM-1 infiltrate infected tissues
      4) TREM-1 is shed by activated phagocytes and can be found in the soluble form (sTREM-1) in body fluids
         a) Presence of sTREM-1 in BAL fluid
            i) Detected rapidly with an immunoblot technique
            ii) Shown to be a strong predictor of the presence of pneumonia
         b) When it becomes commercially available, test may be helpful in distinguishing cause of pulmonary infiltrate as infectious or noninfectious
E. Treatment
   1. General principles of treatment are outlined in Box 25.1
      a. It is important to pick antibiotics that target the most likely pathogens
      b. Delayed or inappropriate antibiotic therapy is associated with poorer outcome

> **Box 25.1**
>
> **Principles of Antibiotic Therapy for Nosocomial Pneumonia**
>
> If patient is at risk for multidrug-resistant organisms, use combination antibiotic therapy
>
> Administer intravenous antibiotics initially, and then switch to oral or enteral antibiotics for selected patients with good clinical response and functioning gastrointestinal tract
>
> If patient has had recent exposure to antibiotics, choose antibiotics from different antibiotic classes for pneumonia
>
> Use local resistance patterns to guide choice of antibiotic
>
> If patient initially received an appropriate regimen, a short course of therapy (ie, 7-8 d) is adequate if the patient has a good clinical response and the targeted pathogen is not *Pseudomonas*
>
> Adapted from Sampathkumar P. Nosocomial pneumonia. In: Bland KI, Buchler MW, Csendes A, Sarr MG, Garden OJ, Wong J, editors. General surgery: principles and international practice. 2nd ed. Vol 1. London: Springer; c2009. p. 287-95. Used with permission.

> **Box 25.2**
>
> **Risk Factors for Nosocomial Pneumonia Caused by Multidrug-Resistant Pathogens**
>
> Immunosuppression
>
> Current hospitalization of ≥5 d
>
> High frequency of antibiotic resistance in the community or in the specific hospital unit
>
> Presence of risk factors for health care–associated pneumonia
>
>   Long-term hemodialysis
>
>   Residence in a long-term care facility
>
>   Receipt of home infusion therapy or wound care within 30 d of onset of pneumonia
>
>   Hospitalization in an acute care facility for ≥2 d within 90 d of onset of pneumonia
>
> Adapted from Sampathkumar P. Nosocomial pneumonia. In: Bland KI, Buchler MW, Csendes A, Sarr MG, Garden OJ, Wong J, editors. General surgery: principles and international practice. 2nd ed. Vol 1. London: Springer; c2009. p. 287-95. Used with permission.

2. Key decision in initial empirical antibiotic therapy: whether the patient has risk factors for multidrug-resistant organisms (MDROs) (Box 25.2)
   a. Patients at risk of MDROs should receive broad-spectrum coverage with antibiotics directed against those organisms
   b. Specific choice of agents
      1) Should reflect local antibiotic resistance patterns
      2) Should take into account antibiotics that the patient received within the previous 2 weeks
      3) If possible, antibiotics for empirical treatment of pneumonia should include antibiotics from drug classes that the patient has not been exposed to recently
3. Low-risk patients (ie, early-onset VAP and HAP in patients without risk factors for MDROs) (Figure 25.1)
   a. Therapy should be aimed at common community-acquired pathogens in addition to *S aureus* and *Enterobacter* species
   b. Appropriate choices
      1) Respiratory quinolone (levofloxacin or moxifloxacin)
      2) β-Lactam–β-lactamase inhibitor combination (ampicillin-sulbactam)
      3) Nonpseudomonal cephalosporin (ceftriaxone)
      4) Limited-spectrum carbapenem (ertapenem)
4. Patients with risk factors for MDROs (Figure 25.1)
   a. Combination antibiotic therapy directed against MDROs, including *Pseudomonas* and other resistant gram-negative bacteria
   b. One component of the combination should be an antipseudomonal cephalosporin (cefepime or ceftazidime), carbapenem (imipenem or meropenem), or antipseudomonal β-lactam–β-lactamase inhibitor combination (piperacillin-tazobactam)
   c. Second component of the combination should be a second antipseudomonal drug: either a quinolone (ciprofloxacin or levofloxacin) or aminoglycoside (amikacin, gentamicin, or tobramycin)
5. A quinolone is preferable to an aminoglycoside whenever possible since aminoglycosides have poor penetration into respiratory secretions and carry the risk of nephrotoxicity, especially in critically ill patients
6. Indications for adding vancomycin or linezolid to regimen
   a. Patient is known to be colonized with methicillin-resistant *S aureus* (MRSA)
   b. Patient is hospitalized in a unit that has a high prevalence of MRSA
7. Route of administration
   a. Initial therapy should be administered intravenously in all patients
   b. For selected patients who have had a good clinical response and who have a functioning gastrointestinal tract, route of administration can be switched to oral or enteral
8. Dosing: adjusted according to the patient's renal function

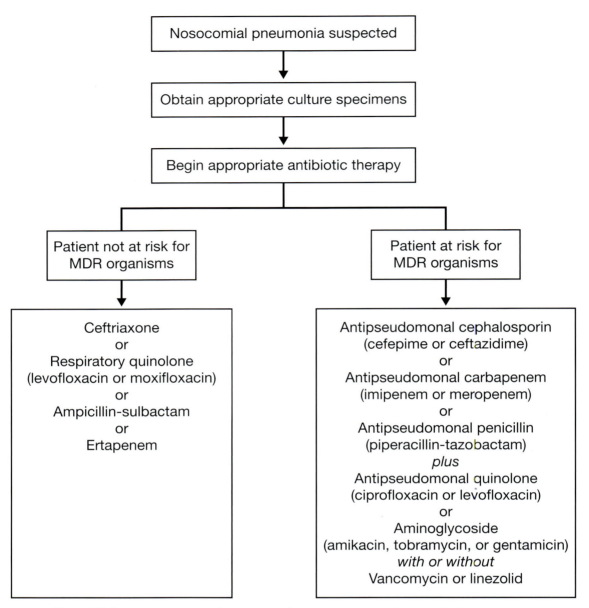

Figure 25.1. Treatment Strategy for Nosocomial Pneumonia. MDR indicates multidrug-resistant. (Adapted from Sampathkumar P. Nosocomial pneumonia. In: Bland KI, Buchler MW, Csendes A, Sarr MG, Garden OJ, Wong J, editors. General surgery: principles and international practice. 2nd ed. Vol 1. London: Springer; c2009. p. 287-95. Used with permission.)

9. Multidrug-resistant strains of *Pseudomonas* and *Acinetobacter* that are resistant to all the commonly used antipseudomonal agents are being increasingly reported worldwide
   a. Colistin: the only drug that is effective against these strains
   b. Like aminoglycosides, colistin can be administered intravenously or as an aerosol
      1) Aerosol route minimizes risks of drug toxicity
      2) Generally aerosolized antibiotics should be used in addition to—not as a substitute for—a systemic agent
10. Response to therapy
    a. Clinical improvement
       1) Usually becomes apparent after 48 to 72 hours of appropriate therapy
       2) Manifests as improvements in white blood cell count and oxygenation and resolution of fever
    b. Chest radiographs

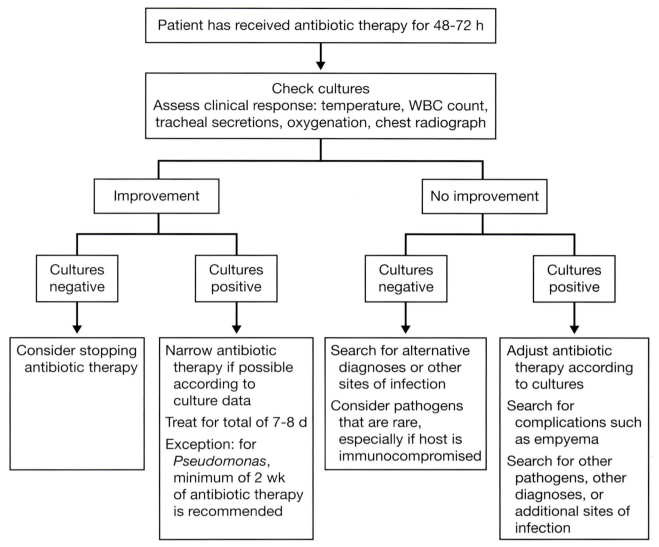

Figure 25.2. Reevaluation 48 to 72 Hours After Starting Antibiotic Therapy for Suspected Nosocomial Pneumonia. WBC indicates white blood cell. (Adapted from Sampathkumar P. Nosocomial pneumonia. In: Bland KI, Buchler MW, Csendes A, Sarr MG, Garden OJ, Wong J, editors. General surgery: principles and international practice. 2nd ed. Vol 1. London: Springer; c2009. p. 287-95. Used with permission.)

      1) Do not show improvement for several days
      2) May appear slightly worse in the first few days of treatment
   c. All patients should be reassessed at day 3 (Figure 25.2)
      1) Assess whether the initial diagnosis of nosocomial pneumonia was correct
      2) Assess whether antibiotic therapy needs to be modified according to available culture data
   d. Poor response to initial therapy

      1) Consider broadening the antibiotic coverage
      2) Simultaneously pursue further diagnostic testing
         a) Reculture lower respiratory tract specimens
         b) Look for alternative site of infection: urinary tract or bloodstream infection, surgical site infection, sinusitis, or complication of pneumonia such as empyema
         c) Search for alternative diagnosis

3) Indications for open lung biopsy
    a) To diagnose infection with an unusual pathogen or a noninfectious illness that mimics pneumonia
    b) The work-up for other sites of infection or alternative diagnoses is negative and the patient remains febrile with pulmonary infiltrates

F. Prevention
1. General measures to decrease the incidence of nosocomial pneumonia include effective infection control measures
    a. Staff education
    b. Emphasis on appropriate hand hygiene
    c. Isolation of patients with MDROs
    d. Pneumococcal and influenza vaccination
2. Intubation and mechanical ventilation
    a. Most important risk factors for pneumonia
    b. Should be avoided if possible
    c. If intubation is unavoidable, use of orotracheal intubation instead of nasotracheal intubation may decrease the risk of nosocomial sinusitis and subsequent VAP
    d. Steps to decrease the leakage of bacterial pathogens around the endotracheal cuff into the lower respiratory tract
        1) Continuously aspirating subglottic secretions
        2) Maintaining endotracheal cuff pressure at more than 20 cm water
        3) Keeping patients in the semirecumbent position (ie, elevating the head of the bed to 30°-45°)
    e. Decreased duration of mechanical ventilation may prevent VAP and can be achieved through protocols
        1) Improve the use of sedation
        2) Accelerate weaning from the ventilator
        3) Decrease the risk of pulmonary embolism by providing prophylaxis against deep vein thrombosis
3. Stress ulcer prophylaxis should be tailored to the individual patient
    a. H_2 receptor antagonists and antacids
        1) Decrease gastric acidity
        2) Associated with increased risk of nosocomial pneumonia
    b. Sucralfate
        1) Associated with lower pneumonia risk
        2) Associated with increased risk of gastrointestinal tract bleeding
4. Many institutions have adopted "bundles"
    a. Several interventions are implemented together rather than individually
    b. Example: VAP bundle promoted by the Institute for Healthcare Improvement
        1) Head of bed elevated more than 30°
        2) Daily sedation holiday and assessment of readiness for weaning
        3) Stress ulcer prophylaxis
        4) Deep vein thrombosis prophylaxis
5. Healthcare Infection Control Practices Advisory Committee (HICPAC) of the Centers for Disease Control and Prevention has published comprehensive recommendations for prevention of nosocomial pneumonia

Suggested Reading

American Thoracic Society; Infectious Diseases Society of America. Guidelines for the management of adults with hospital-acquired, ventilator-associated, and healthcare-associated pneumonia. Am J Respir Crit Care Med. 2005 Feb 15;171(4):388–416.

Mandell LA, Wunderink RG, Anzueto A, Bartlett JG, Campbell GD, Dean NC, et al; Infectious Diseases Society of America; American Thoracic Society. Infectious Diseases Society of America/American Thoracic Society consensus guidelines on the management of community-acquired pneumonia in adults. Clin Infect Dis. 2007 Mar 1;44 Suppl 2:S27–72.

Tablan OC, Anderson LJ, Besser R, Bridges C, Hajjeh R; CDC; Healthcare Infection Control Practices Advisory Committee. Guidelines for preventing health-care–associated pneumonia, 2003: recommendations of CDC and the Healthcare Infection Control Practices Advisory Committee. MMWR Recomm Rep. 2004 Mar 26;53(RR-3):1–36.

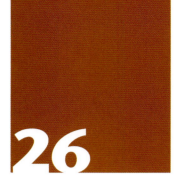

Walter C. Hellinger, MD

Urinary Tract Infections

I. Introduction
   A. Definitions Related to Presence of Bacteria
      1. *Bacteriuria:* bacteria in the urine
      2. *Significant bacteriuria:* at least 10^5 bacteria/mL of voided urine
      3. *Asymptomatic bacteriuria:* bacteria in the urine without symptoms associated with urinary tract infection
   B. Definitions Related to Infection
      1. *Urinary tract infection:* bacteriuria (or funguria) and symptoms associated with upper urinary tract infection or lower urinary tract infection (or both); urinary tract infections are sometimes characterized as asymptomatic or symptomatic, in which case *asymptomatic urinary tract infection* is synonymous with *asymptomatic significant bacteriuria*
         a. *Uncomplicated urinary tract infection:* infection of a physiologically and anatomically normal urinary tract
         b. *Complicated urinary tract infection:* infection of a physiologically or anatomically abnormal urinary tract
      2. *Cystitis:* lower urinary tract infection typically associated with urinary frequency, dysuria, or urgency
      3. *Relapse:* urinary tract infection caused by a pathogen implicated in a preceding infection
      4. *Reinfection:* second or subsequent urinary tract infection caused by a pathogen that has not caused a previous infection
      5. *Acute pyelonephritis:* upper urinary tract infection of recent onset with renal involvement; often associated with fever, chills, flank pain, or nausea
      6. *Chronic pyelonephritis:* gross or microscopic description of renal pathology (being replaced by *chronic interstitial nephritis*)
II. Pathogenesis
   A. Ascending Infection From Urethral Orifice
      1. Predisposing factors
         a. In women: intercourse, spermicidal contraceptives, and estrogen deficiency
         b. In men: condom catheters
         c. In men and women: urethral catheterization
   B. Hematogenous Seeding
      1. More frequent for gram-positive bacterial pathogens (particularly staphylococci) and *Candida*
   C. Bacterial Factors
      1. Surface adhesive characteristics of some gram-negative bacteria

a. A relatively small number of *Escherichia coli* serogroups (O1, O2, O4, O6, O7, O8, O75, and O150) account for a high proportion of all *E coli* urinary tract infections
b. Filamentous organelles, including pili and fimbriae, adhere to genitourinary mucosa
c. P fimbriae, which bind the P blood group antigen expressed on erythrocytes and uroepithelium, are frequently expressed on the surface of uropathogens
2. K capsular antigen
3. Motility
4. Endotoxin
5. Urease
6. Hemolysins
7. Aerobactin production
D. Host Factors
1. Obstruction
2. Vesicoureteral reflux
3. Stones
4. Incomplete emptying of the bladder
5. Reduced urine osmolality
6. Elevated urine or vaginal pH
7. Glycosuria
III. Epidemiology
A. Pathogens
1. Over 95% of urinary tract infections are caused by a single pathogen
2. *Escherichia coli* is the most common
3. *Staphylococcus saprophyticus* in sexually active young women
4. Other coagulase-negative staphylococci and enterococci are recovered in complicated urinary tract infections
5. Anaerobic infection is rare
6. Fungi, specifically *Candida*, are causes of catheter-associated urinary tract infection in heath care settings
7. Adenovirus is a cause of hemorrhagic cystitis in bone marrow transplant recipients
8. BK virus may cause allograft nephropathy in renal transplant recipients and, rarely, hemorraghic cystitis in recipients of renal or other solid organ transplants
9. Antibiotic resistance is associated with preceding antibiotic therapy and with infection acquired in health care settings
10. Obstruction and genital or enteric fistulization are associated with polymicrobial infections
B. Hosts
1. Significant bacteriuria occurs in preschool-aged girls (up to 4%-5%) and boys (<1%)
a. Urinary tract infection develops in many of these girls; when it does, it may cause clinically significant renal damage
b. Urinary tract infection in preschool-aged boys is frequently associated with serious congenital abnormalities
2. Bacteriuria is more common in school-aged girls than in preschool-aged girls, but it more often remains asymptomatic
3. Bacteriuria in school-aged boys is rare
4. At some time in their lives, 60% of women have a urinary tract infection
a. By age 24, 1 in 3 women have had a urinary tract infection
b. After having their first infection, 20% of women have another infection within 6 months
5. Prevalence of bacteriuria in young women is 1% to 3%
6. Prevalence of bacteriuria in young men is 0.1% or less and is associated with lack of circumcision and anal insertive intercourse
7. Prevalence of asymptomatic bacteriuria increases with age in both sexes
a. By age 65, prevalence is at least 10% among men and at least 20% among women
b. Factors associated with bacteriuria
1) Women: incomplete bladder emptying related to pelvic floor relaxation
2) Men: prostatic hypertrophy, fecal soiling, and dementia
c. High rates of spontaneous resolution and reinfection
d. Asymptomatic bacteriuria is far more common than urinary tract infection
8. Bacteriuria occurs after bladder catheterization; its prevalence increases with duration of catheterization
a. Nearly 100% of individuals with a bladder catheter in place more than 30 days have significant bacteriuria
b. Among hospitalized patients, 15% to 25% receive a bladder catheter
c. Catheter-associated urinary tract infections are the most common type of hospital-acquired infection
9. Pregnancy and renal transplant are associated with increased incidence of bacteriuria and subsequent urinary tract infection
a. The prevalence of asymptomatic bacteriuria in young women increases with

pregnancy (from 1%-3% to 4%-7%); it increases further with parity, age, diabetes mellitus, sickle cell disease, and lower socioeconomic status
      b. In 20% to 40% of women with asymptomatic bacteriuria early in pregnancy, acute pyelonephritis develops later in pregnancy
      c. An association between asymptomatic bacteriuria and premature delivery is somewhat controversial
   10. Diabetes mellitus
      a. Associated with increased incidence of bacteriuria
      b. Not clearly associated with increased risk of urinary tract infection
IV. Natural History
   A. Preschool-Aged Children
      1. For preschool-aged children who have urinary tract infection without reflux or obstruction, the prognosis is good
      2. However, 30% to 50% of these children have reflux, usually related to elevated bladder pressure from obstruction (eg, congenital anomalies in boys), delayed development of the vesicoureteral junction, a short intravesical ureter, or inflammation of the vesicoureteral junction
      3. Reflux and repeated urinary tract infection in these children may lead to renal damage, hypertension, and end-stage renal disease
      4. Reflux without infection can also lead to renal impairment in this age group
   B. Children Older Than 5 Years
      1. Reflux with or without infection rarely causes renal damage in children older than 5 years
      2. Screening for bacteriuria in school-aged children is not cost-effective
   C. Young Women
      1. The first urinary tract infection in young women usually coincides with initiation of intercourse
      2. After a woman has had 1 urinary tract infection, she is at increased risk of another
      3. Most urinary tract infections in women of childbearing age are reinfections
      4. There is no evidence that urinary tract infections in these women lead to renal damage in the absence of obstruction
      5. There is no evidence that asymptomatic bacteriuria in nonpregnant adults of any age increases the risk of infection, renal damage, or hypertension

V. Clinical Manifestations
   A. Urinary Tract Infection
      1. The clinical presentation of patients with urinary tract infection encompasses a wide spectrum of complaints and severity, with nonspecific constitutional complaints often dominating among the very young and the very old
      2. Symptoms of lower urinary tract infection: frequency, dysuria, turbid urine, suprapubic pressure or pain, and hematuria
      3. Symptoms of upper urinary tract infection: fever, flank pain, nausea with or without lower urinary tract infection, or other constitutional complaints
   B. Kidney Infection
      1. Pyelonephritis can impair renal concentration of the urine
      2. Infections of the kidney, particularly with obstruction, can lead to permanent impairment of renal function
VI. Diagnosis
   A. Direct Examination of Urine
      1. *Pyuria:* 10 leukocytes/µL or dipstick positive for leukocyte esterase
      2. Hematuria may result from cystitis
      3. Leukocyte casts may result from pyelonephritis
      4. Proteinuria (<3 g in 24 hours) may result from pyelonephritis
      5. Hematuria, leukocyte casts, and proteinuria may or may not be present with infection
      6. Presence of 1 or more bacterial organisms per field on oil-immersion examination of a Gram-stained sample of uncentrifuged urine indicates at least 10^5 bacteria/mL
      7. Absence of bacteria in several fields indicates no more than 10^4 bacteria/mL
   B. Culture
      1. Urine proximal to the bladder outlet is normally sterile
      2. Cultures of voided urine normally yield bacterial growth owing to colonization of the urethral meatus
      3. Culture of voided urine in the presence of urinary tract infection usually yields at least 10^5 colony-forming units (CFU)/mL
      4. Culture of voided urine in the absence of infection usually yields less than 10^4 CFU/mL
      5. Cultures of voided urine specimens from one-third of young women with lower urinary tract infections have less than 10^5 CFU/mL
      6. The most recent Infectious Diseases Society of America practice guideline for urinary tract

infection identifies growth of a uropathogen of at least 10^2 CFU/mL as diagnostic of cystitis in the presence of characteristic symptoms
7. Optimal voided specimens for culture are collected midstream after cleansing of the urethral meatus and, in women, the adjacent tissues
8. Cultures are performed by inoculating a specific volume of uncentrifuged urine onto the surface of an agar plate; colonies are counted after 18 to 24 hours of incubation at 37°C
9. Cultures of urine obtained by urethral catheterization with aseptic technique normally yield less than 10 to 100 CFU/mL
10. Cultures of urine obtained by suprapubic aspiration of the bladder with aseptic technique normally yield no growth
11. Colony counts in the preceding text apply to Enterobacteriacae (under similar circumstances, the colony counts of gram-positive cocci and fungi may be 1 or 2 orders of magnitude less)
12. High colony counts of mixed organisms
    a. In cultures of voided urine, high colony counts of mixed organisms usually indicate improper collection or prolonged storage at room temperature after collection
    b. In polymicrobial urinary tract infections, high colony counts may require verification with cultures of urine obtained by catheterization or bladder aspiration
13. Cultures of urine for fungus and mycobacteria should be considered if patients have pyuria and symptoms of urinary tract infection with no growth in bacterial culture
14. When symptoms and cultures do not support a diagnosis of lower urinary tract infection in women of childbearing age, exclude urethritis, vaginitis, and cervicitis

VII. Management
   A. General Considerations
      1. Urinary tract infection is symptomatic, by definition, and therefore should always be treated
      2. Antibiotic treatment without understanding and managing the predisposing risks increases the likelihood of undesirable outcomes
         a. Recurrence as relapse or reinfection
         b. Antibiotic resistance related to repeated antibiotic exposure
         c. Complications such as renal damage or urosepsis related to unrecognized anatomical or physiologic anomalies associated with obstruction
      3. Classification of responses of urinary tract infection to antibiotic treatment
         a. *Cure:* negative urine culture on treatment and negative culture 1 to 2 weeks after treatment is completed
         b. *Persistence*: urine culture yielding growth of initial pathogen after at least 48 hours of treatment
         c. *Relapse:* negative urine culture on treatment and urine culture yielding growth of initial pathogen after treatment is completed
         d. *Reinfection:* negative urine cultures on treatment and 1 to 2 weeks after treatment is completed; at subsequent urinary tract infection, urine culture yields growth of a different pathogen
   B. Acute Uncomplicated Cystitis in Women
      1. Characteristic symptoms of a first case of lower urinary tract infection are sufficient for diagnosis
         a. Subsequent infections that are suspected to be reinfections require confirmation on 1 occasion with demonstration of pyuria
         b. If relapsing infection is suspected, urine cultures should be performed
      2. Empirical treatment with trimethoprim-sulfamethoxazole for 3 days is treatment of choice if certain conditions are met
         a. No allergy to trimethoprim-sulfamethoxazole
         b. No recent antibiotic treatment (especially trimethoprim-sulfamethoxazole)
         c. No recent hospitalization
         d. Local prevalence of *E coli* resistance to trimethoprim-sulfamethoxazole is less than 20%
      3. Empirical treatment with nitrofurantoin (7 days) is recommended if trimethoprim-sulfamethoxazole cannot be given
      4. Empirical treatment with fosfomycin (single dose) is alternative to nitrofurantoin
      5. Empirical treatment with a fluoroquinolone (3 days) is alternative to nitrofurantoin and to fosfomycin
   C. Recurrent Uncomplicated Cystitis Due to Reinfection in Women
      1. Reinfections are most often related to intercourse

2. Strategies to reduce the frequency of recurrence have included postcoital voiding and enhanced perineal hygiene
3. When fewer than 3 infections occur per year, empirical therapy has been recommended (as in the management of a first case of cystitis)
4. When 3 or more infections occur per year, other interventions have been effective
    a. Long-term chemoprophylaxis (eg, one-half of a single-strength trimethoprim-sulfamethoxazole tablet or nitrofurantoin 50 mg every evening)
    b. Postcoital abortive therapy (eg, single-strength trimethoprim-sulfamethoxazole tablet or nitrofurantoin 100 mg)
D. Acute Pyelonephritis in Women
    1. High-grade bacteriuria with Gram stain of urine, pyuria, and the appropriate symptom complex are sufficient for diagnosis
    2. If there is concern about antibiotic resistance, urine culture is recommended
    3. Blood cultures are usually appropriate if the patient is hospitalized
    4. Many authorities favor fluoroquinolones for orally administered therapy in the absence of known or suspected resistance
    5. If fever, bacteriuria, or bacteremia persist after 3 days of effective therapy, further evaluation with imaging to exclude obstruction, intrarenal abscess, or perinephric infection is advisable
    6. For uncomplicated pyelonephritis, 14 days of antibiotic treatment is recommended
    7. For recurrent pyelonephritis, a second urine culture is recommended 1 to 2 weeks after treatment has ended
E. Relapsing Urinary Tract Infection in Women
    1. Diagnosis requires urine cultures of sequential infections to demonstrate persistence of a uropathogen
    2. Occasionally, relapsing infection is due to well-established infection of the renal parenchyma that resolves only after 4 to 6 weeks of antibiotic administration
    3. Alternatively, persistence may be due to obstruction, stones, foreign bodies, or urinary retention
    4. Identification and management of the predisposing anatomical or physiologic anomaly are required for antibiotic treatment to result in cure
F. Urinary Tract Infection in Men
    1. Often associated with predisposing anatomical or physiologic anomalies of the urinary tract
        a. Predisposing anomalies must be managed to achieve success with antibiotic treatment and to guide recommendations to prevent recurrence
    2. Some of these patients are also at increased risk of prostatitis, intrarenal abscess, and perinephric infection
    3. Full radiologic imaging (see the heading "L. Imaging of the Urinary Tract") and urologic evaluation of the urinary tract
        a. Measure postvoid residual volume of the bladder by ultrasonography or catheterization
        b. Computed tomographic (CT) scan of the upper and lower urinary tracts with intravenously administered radiocontrast material
        c. Cystoscopy
G. Catheter-Associated Urinary Tract Infection
    1. Diagnosis is established by identification of significant bacteriuria (or funguria) and by identification of related symptoms or invasive infection
    2. Remove the catheter whenever feasible
        a. The catheter should not be removed if obstruction or retention of urine is likely since infection can progress rapidly if drainage is inadequate
    3. Exchange the catheter when removal is not feasible
    4. Continuation of antimicrobial treatment until the catheter is removed (to maintain sterility of urine) is appropriate only if catheter removal is imminent
H. Asymptomatic Bacteriuria
    1. Indications for treatment of asymptomatic bacteriuria
        a. Young children with reflux
        b. Pregnant women
        c. Patients who are scheduled for elective, invasive urologic procedures
    2. Screening for asymptomatic bacteriuria
        a. Pregnant women: screening in first and third trimesters; treat if bacteriuria is identified
        b. Patients scheduled for elective, invasive urologic procedures: preoperative screening; treat if bacteriuria is identified
I. Prostatitis
    1. There are 2 distinct syndromes: acute and chronic
    2. Acute prostatitis
        a. Infection is associated with diffuse or segmental acute inflammation with a polymorphonuclear cellular infiltrate,

microabscess or macroabscess formation, and swelling and tenderness of the gland
   b. Symptoms include fever, chills, back or perineal pain, and often symptoms of cystitis
   c. *Escherichia coli* is most common cause
   d. Serum level of prostate-specific antigen is usually markedly increased
   e. The acutely inflamed prostate is penetrated by all antibiotics used for treatment of urinary tract infection
   f. Some recommend prolongation of treatment to 2 to 4 weeks
   g. Prostatic abscesses may require transrectal or percutaneous drainage
  3. Chronic prostatitis
   a. *Escherichia coli* or other Enterobacteriacae
    1) Less frequently, gram-positive cocci (eg, enterococci)
    2) Rarely, *Candida*, *Blastomyces dermatitidis*, *Histoplasma capsulatum*, *Cryptococcus neoformans*, and *Mycobacterium tuberculosis*
   b. Many patients are asymptomatic
   c. Symptoms: back or perineal pain, recurrent unexplained fever, relapsing urinary tract infection
   d. Diagnosis: culture of urine collected after prostatic massage
   e. Treatment: difficult owing to limited penetration of the uninflamed prostate by most antibiotics
    1) Agents that achieve satisfactory prostate levels in the absence of prostatic inflammation include trimethoprim, rifampin, and fluoroquinolones
    2) Antibiotic treatment for 6 to 12 weeks has been recommended
    3) Transurethral prostatectomy has helped some patients
 J. Chronic Pelvic Pain Syndrome
  1. Also called *prostatodynia*
  2. Attributed to nonbacterial prostatitis
  3. Has not been proved to have an infectious cause
  4. Some recommended empirical treatment for 2 to 6 weeks with a macrolide or tetracycline to exclude mycoplasma or ureaplasma infection
   a. Symptomatic improvement expected in less than 40%
   b. Refer for nonantimicrobial-based therapy
 K. Perinephric and Intrarenal Abscesses
  1. Predisposing factors: nephrourolithiasis and diabetes mellitus
  2. Pathogenesis may be obstruction with subsequent ascending infection or hematogenous seeding (intrarenal abscess) of the renal cortex with subsequent penetration of the renal capsule
  3. Most commonly recovered pathogen: gram-negative bacilli
   a. Other pathogens possible: gram-positive cocci, multiple bacterial pathogens, and fungi (particularly *Candida*)
  4. Symptoms may be nonspecific and constitutional or include signs of upper urinary tract infection with or without signs of lower urinary tract infection
  5. The time course is frequently subacute
  6. Imaging of kidney is usually necessary for diagnosis since a large proportion of intrarenal abscesses and a majority of perinephric abscesses yield nondiagnostic results in urine studies
   a. CT imaging may show inflammation of a lobe within the kidney
   b. Gas production from a facultative anaerobe leads to the appearance of emphysematous pyelonephritis
   c. Long-standing diffuse infection with obstruction, vascular insufficiency, or immune impairment may result in xanthogranulomatous pyelonephritis (in which renal parenchyma is replaced by granulomatous inflammation and lipid-laden macrophages)
  7. Antibiotic treatment alone has been effective for intrarenal abscesses less than 5 cm in diameter
  8. Larger abscesses should be assessed for diagnostic and therapeutic, radiographically directed, percutaneous drainage
  9. Surgical consultation is required when diagnostic or therapeutic drainage is necessary and not amenable to radiographically directed percutaneous interventions
 L. Imaging of the Urinary Tract
  1. Indications for imaging
   a. Severe illness
   b. Immunocompromised
   c. Pyelonephritis not responding to 72 hours of appropriate antibiotic therapy
   d. Urinary tract infection of uncertain cause
  2. CT scanning with intravenously administered radiocontrast media has replaced intravenous

pyelography as the most useful imaging method
3. Magnetic resonance imaging can be used when radiocontrast media cannot be given
4. Ultrasonography is preferred for assessments of bladder emptying, for rapid diagnosis of obstruction, and for evaluation of isolated renal anomalies
5. Voiding cystourethrograms, with or without cystoscopic retrograde pyelograms, are useful for identifying or confirming the presence of fistulae in the gastrointestinal tract or genitourinary tract

M. Prevention of Urinary Tract Infection or Related Adverse Clinical Outcomes
1. Screening and therapy for asymptomatic bacteriuria in infants and preschool-aged children
2. Contraception selection, postcoital voiding, and perineal hygiene in some women with recurrent cystitis and pyelonephritis
3. Screening and therapy for asymptomatic bacteriuria in pregnant women
4. Screening and therapy for asymptomatic bacteriuria before elective invasive urologic interventions
5. Chemoprophylaxis administered daily, or abortively after intercourse, for women with recurrent acute uncomplicated cystitis related to reinfection
6. Chemoprophylaxis for regular, intermittent straight catheterization of the bladder for management of urine retention
7. Chemoprophylaxis for the first year after kidney transplant

Suggested Reading

Gupta K, Hooton TM, Naber KG, Colgan R, Miller LG, Moran GJ, et al; Infectious Diseases Society of America; European Society for Microbiology and Infectious Diseases. International clinical practice guidelines for the treatment of acute uncomplicated cystitis and pyelonephritis in women: A 2010 update by the Infectious Diseases Society of America and the European Society for Microbiology and Infectious Diseases. Clin Infect Dis. 2011 Mar;52(5):e103-20.

Hooton TM, Besser R, Foxman B, Fritsche TR, Nicolle LE. Acute uncomplicated cystitis in an era of increasing antibiotic resistance: a proposed approach to empirical therapy. Clin Infect Dis. 2004 Jul 1;39(1):75–80. Epub 2004 Jun 14.

Hooton TM, Bradley SF, Cardenas DD, Colgan R, Geerlings SE, Rice JC, et al; Infectious Diseases Society of America. Diagnosis, prevention, and treatment of catheter-associated urinary tract infection in adults: 2009 international practice guidelines from the Infectious Diseases Society of America. Clin Infect Dis. 2010 Mar;50(5):625-63.

Johnson JR, Kuskowski MA, Wilt TJ. Systematic review: antimicrobial urinary catheters to prevent catheter-associated urinary tract infection in hospitalized patients. Ann Intern Med. 2006 Jan 17;144(2):116–26.

Nicolle LE, Bradley S, Colgan R, Rice JC, Schaeffer A, Hooton TM; Infectious Diseases Society of America; American Society of Nephrology; American Geriatric Society. Infectious Diseases Society of America guidelines for the diagnosis and treatment of asymptomatic bacteriuria in adults. Clin Infect Dis. 2005 Mar 1;40(5):643–54. Epub 2005 Feb 4. Erratum in: Clin Infect Dis. 2005 May 15;40(10):1556.

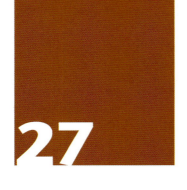

Andrew D. Badley, MD

Sepsis Syndrome

I. Introduction
   A. Definitions
      1. *Systemic inflammatory response syndrome* (SIRS): the specific host systemic response that may be elicited by various stimuli, including infection, burns, pancreatitis, ischemia, trauma, hemorrhage, immune-mediated tissue injury, and exogenous stimuli
      2. *Sepsis*: SIRS resulting from infection
      3. *Sepsis syndrome*: sepsis with altered tissue perfusion of vital organs (resulting in oliguria, hypoxemia, elevated levels of lactate, or altered mentation or any combination of these conditions)
      4. *Sepsis* and *sepsis syndrome* are distinguished from *infection* and *bacteremia*
         a. *Infection*: invasion of a normally sterile site by microorganisms
         b. *Bacteremia*: the presence of bacteria in the blood
   B. Clinical Importance
      1. Identification of cause: when a patient has SIRS, the objective is to define its cause
      2. Treatment: if SIRS is caused by infection, appropriate antibiotics must be administered and supportive care guided by the patient's history and physical examination

II. Epidemiology
   A. Increasing Incidence
      1. The incidence of sepsis has increased over the past decade
      2. In 2000, sepsis was the 10th leading cause of death overall in the United States
   B. Factors Contributing to Increasing Incidence
      1. Increased incidence and survival of persons predisposed to sepsis, such as persons infected with human immunodeficiency virus (HIV), patients with cancer, the elderly, and those who have had organ transplants
      2. Increased use of medical prostheses, such as intravascular catheters and indwelling urinary catheters
      3. Widespread (and sometimes inappropriate) use of antimicrobial agents that predispose toward the selection of multidrug-resistant pathogens

III. Pathogenesis
   A. Infectious Agents
      1. A major cause of sepsis is infection with gram-negative bacteria
         a. Lipopolysaccharide (LPS) is an integral component of the gram-negative bacterial cell wall

b. LPS initiates a cascade that results in cytokine release and the early physiologic changes associated with septic shock
c. LPS forms a complex either with bactericidal permeability-increasing protein or with LPS-binding protein
d. The complexes of LPS-binding protein and LPS bind with their receptor, CD14
 1) CD14 initiates an intracytoplasmic signaling cascade that ultimately results in the translocation of nuclear factor κB (NF-κB) into the nucleus
 2) NF-κB is a transcription factor that, while in the nucleus, initiates the transcription of numerous cytokines, including tumor necrosis factor α, interleukin (IL)-1, IL-2, IL-6, IL-8, platelet-activating factor, and interferon-γ
 3) These and other potential mediators, including nitrous oxide, intracellular adhesion molecules, prostaglandins, leukotrienes, and complement factor 5a, have been directly or indirectly implicated in the pathogenesis of septic shock
2. Sepsis syndrome may also occur after infection with gram-positive bacteria, viruses, protozoa, rickettsia, and helminths
 a. None of these agents contain LPS
 b. Alternate pathways of cytokine induction are active
3. Regardless of the organism responsible for inducing sepsis, a common final pathway characterized by the release of proinflammatory mediators is activated
 a. Proinflammatory response results in fever, hypotension, decreased organ perfusion, and other potential complications
 b. After initial proinflammatory response, an anti-inflammatory response is common and is likely a homeostatic response
4. Bacteria may be in the bloodstream only transiently; therefore, sepsis and septic shock are not always associated with bacteremia
B. Cellular Injury
1. Widespread endothelial and parenchymal cellular injury has been associated with sepsis
2. Stimuli for cellular injury are incompletely understood
 a. Ischemia or direct cellular injury by inflammatory products
 b. Ultimately, many of these cells die by apoptosis
  1) Immunosuppression results from the death of lymphocytes
  2) Anti-inflammatory cytokines are produced by macrophages, which engulf the apoptotic cells
  3) Apoptosis of gut epithelial cells causes translocation of bacteria from the gastrointestinal tract

IV. Diagnosis
A. Clinical Findings
1. Clinical findings associated with SIRS are similar regardless of the mechanism responsible for inducing the inflammatory cascade
2. Infections commonly associated with sepsis syndrome in an otherwise healthy host: pneumonia, meningitis, upper urinary tract infections, cellulitis, and intra-abdominal catastrophes (eg, perforated viscus)
B. Clinical Signs and Symptoms
1. A patient with sepsis may have few complaints or several, including fever, chills, pain, rash, or dyspnea
2. A careful physical examination should be performed to identify the source and severity of the underlying infection
 a. Vital signs: temperature, respiratory rate, and blood pressure
 b. Medical appliances (eg, intravenous lines and urinary catheters): examined for signs of infection
 c. Head and neck: examined for nuchal rigidity, conjunctival petechiae, and Roth spots
 d. Oropharynx: examined for thrush (suggesting an underlying immunosuppressive state, including chronic illness, HIV infection, malignancy, or long-term corticosteroid use), quinsy, and periodontal abscess
 e. Skin examination
  1) Rashes of disseminated meningococcemia or ecthyma gangrenosum (seen with disseminated *Pseudomonas* infection)
  2) Petechiae associated with disseminated intravascular coagulation
  3) Janeway lesions and Osler nodes
  4) Signs of cellulitis or necrotizing fasciitis are obvious clues to the cause of sepsis syndrome
 f. Pulmonary system examination
  1) Signs of pneumonitis: impaired oxygenation, pulmonary consolidation, and empyema

2) Acute respiratory distress syndrome (ARDS) often develops in patients with sepsis syndrome
3) Differentiating the pulmonary findings of pneumonia from those of ARDS may be difficult
g. Cardiac examination findings are frequently abnormal owing to the compensatory changes associated with sepsis
1) Infective endocarditis
a) Uncommon but may lead to sepsis syndrome
b) Therefore, the finding of a new or changing murmur (especially a regurgitant murmur) is important
2) Hypotension
a) Frequently, patients with sepsis syndrome are hypotensive
b) Therefore, a careful cardiac examination is needed to differentiate cardiogenic shock (with elevated jugular venous pressure, gallop rhythms, and evidence of right- or left-sided congestive failure) from noncardiogenic shock caused by sepsis (which is initially a hyperdynamic state of high cardiac output)
h. Examination of abdomen
1) Tenderness, guarding, or absence of bowel sounds, suggestive of an intra-abdominal event such as a perforated viscus
2) Presence of hepatosplenomegaly
3) Previous splenectomy and ascites, which are associated with an increased risk of certain infections
i. Examination of kidneys
1) Flank tenderness
2) Increased size (by palpation or by ballottement)
j. Thorough pelvic and rectal examinations
1) Rectal or perirectal abscess
2) Pelvic inflammatory disease
3) Prostatitis
C. Laboratory Findings
1. Laboratory findings associated with sepsis syndrome may reflect decreased organ perfusion or the underlying infection
2. Leukocytosis or leukopenia (due to lymphocyte apoptosis)
3. Anemia may be dilutional (after fluid resuscitation efforts) or associated with underlying chronic disease
4. Thrombocytopenia may signal the development of disseminated intravascular coagulation
5. Reactive thrombocythemia
6. Hypoxemia
   a. With pneumonitis or in response to the development of ARDS
   b. Hypercapnia with hypoxia signals impending respiratory failure
7. Signs of decreased organ perfusion suggestive of sepsis syndrome
   a. Increasing creatinine levels (with increasing urea levels)
   b. Increased lactate dehydrogenase levels
   c. Increasing transaminase levels
8. Microbiologic testing should be dictated by the clinical presentation
   a. At a minimum, urine, sputum, and blood should be cultured for bacteria
   b. Culture samples from vascular access lines
D. Imaging
1. No imaging procedures are specific for sepsis syndrome
2. Chest radiography should be performed for every patient
3. Computed tomography or ultrasonography of the chest or abdomen (or both) may be appropriate, depending on the presentation
V. Complications
A. Organs Involved
1. Virtually every organ system is affected in sepsis syndrome
2. Degree of involvement of each organ varies widely between patients
B. Central Nervous System
1. Toxic metabolic encephalopathy
   a. A result of cerebral hypoperfusion and hypoxia, medications, the biologically active products of the infective agent, and inflammatory mediators of sepsis
   b. May progress to coma, seizures, cerebral edema, and death
2. Critical illness polyneuropathy
   a. A distal sensory-motor polyneuropathy of unknown cause
   b. Develops in patients who are critically ill for prolonged periods
3. Cerebral hemorrhage or infarction: a result of coagulation abnormalities associated with sepsis syndrome

C. Pulmonary System
   1. Lungs may be the primary site of infection (ie, pneumonia)
   2. Lungs may be subject to the forces of increased left ventricular end-diastolic pressure characteristic of a failing left ventricle
   3. Hypoxia and hypocapnia may develop from capillary leakage
   4. Abnormalities of oxygenation and ventilation can become refractory to mechanical ventilation and lead to death
D. Cardiovascular System
   1. Cardiovascular system response may be minimal
   2. Cardiovascular system response may be increased cardiac output with low systemic vascular resistance and a loss of vascular responsiveness to sympathetic agents (such as epinephrine)
      a. Compensatory increase in heart rate maintains tissue perfusion by increasing cardiac output
      b. Failure to compensate appropriately may indicate a poor prognosis
   3. Later, myocardial dysfunction and a decrease in the ejection fraction of the left ventricle may occur as a result of a putative myocardial depressant factor
      a. If the myocardium cannot maintain adequate perfusion, cardiac ischemia may occur
      b. Cardiac ischemia may lead to arrhythmias, myocardial infarction, and death
E. Gastrointestinal System
   1. Bacterial overgrowth increases the risk of nosocomial pneumonia
   2. Impaired motility causes functional obstructions (eg, toxic megacolon)
F. Renal and Hepatic Systems
   1. Factors responsible for the dysfunction of renal and hepatic systems in sepsis syndrome
      a. Hypoperfusion
      b. Capillary leakage
      c. Concomitant medications
   2. Elevated levels of transaminases and hyperbilirubinemia are common
      a. Associated with a poor prognosis
      b. Rarely, liver injury may progress to ischemic hepatitis
   3. Prerenal azotemia secondary to hypoperfusion
      a. Most common form of renal dysfunction in sepsis syndrome
      b. Acute glomerulonephritis and interstitial nephritis may occur
G. Hematologic System
   1. Disseminated intravascular coagulation
   2. Anemia
   3. Leukopenia
   4. Thrombocytopenia
H. Musculoskeletal System
   1. Skeletal muscle dysfunction: a consequence of the effects of endotoxin and hypoperfusion
   2. Muscle injury: reflected by increasing creatine kinase levels
   3. Prolonged muscle dysfunction may lead to wasting and development of critical illness myopathy
I. Endocrine System
   1. Sepsis syndrome may unmask occult endocrine deficiency states
   2. Sepsis syndrome may induce adrenal hemorrhage, resulting in Addison disease
   3. Euthyroid sick syndrome may occur
VI. Treatment
   A. Three Aims of Treatment
      1. Eliminate infectious agents responsible for inducing sepsis
      2. Provide supportive care based in the intensive care unit to normalize oxygenation, ventilation, blood pressure, and tissue perfusion
      3. Provide therapy intended to interrupt inflammatory mediators of sepsis
   B. Elimination of Infectious Agents
      1. Principles of antibiotic use in sepsis
         a. Clinical trials comparing empirical antibiotic regimens are difficult to assess owing to the noncomparability of patient populations between studies and centers
         b. The increasing incidence of gram-positive infections as a cause of sepsis has surpassed the incidence of gram-negative infections
         c. The incidence of fungal (ie, candidal) infections as a cause of sepsis is increasing and approaching 5%
         d. Predominant sites of infections causing sepsis (in decreasing order of frequency): lungs, bloodstream, abdomen, urinary tract, skin, and soft tissue
         e. Appropriate antibiotics can reduce mortality from sepsis
         f. Choice of empirical regimens
            1) Influenced by patient history, comorbidities, and local susceptibility patterns of likely infectious agents

Table 27.1
Common Microbes That Cause Sepsis

Host Factor	Probable Pathogens
Healthy host	*Streptococcus pneumoniae, Haemophilus influenzae, Neisseria meningitidis, Staphylococcus aureus*
Interrupted integument	*Staphylococcus* species, *Streptococcus pyogenes*, Enterobacteriaceae, *Pseudomonas aeruginosa*
Abdominal urinary tract	*Escherichia coli*, Enterobacteriaceae
Alcoholism	*Klebsiella* species, *S pneumoniae*
Cirrhosis	Gram-negative rods, *Vibrio, Yersinia, Salmonella* species
Asplenia	*S pneumoniae, H influenzae, N meningitidis, Capnocytophaga canimorsus*
Diabetes mellitus	*E coli, Pseudomonas* species, fungi causing mucormycosis
Hypogammaglobulinemia	*S pneumoniae, N meningitidis, E coli, H influenzae*
Burns	*S aureus, P aeruginosa*, nosocomial gram-negative bacteria
Cystic fibrosis	Multiresistant *Pseudomonas* and *Burkholderia* species
AIDS	*Pneumocystis jiroveci, Pseudomonas* species (pneumonia), *Mycobacterium avium-intracellulare* complex, cytomegalovirus
Solid organ transplant	Gram-negative bacteria, cytomegalovirus
Intravascular devices	*S aureus*, coagulase-negative *Staphylococcus* species
Long-term use of corticosteroids	*S pneumoniae, H influenzae*
Neonate	Group B *Streptococcus, Listeria monocytogenes, S pneumoniae, H influenzae*
Postoperative patient	*S aureus*, Enterobacteriaceae, nosocomial gram-negative bacteria
Elderly patient	*S pneumoniae, H influenzae, S aureus*, Enterobacteriaceae, *L monocytogenes*

     2) Host factors that may predispose patients to certain infections are shown in Table 27.1
     3) Typical antibiotic choices: third- or fourth-generation cephalosporins, carbapenems, extended-spectrum carboxypenicillins, ureidopenicillins combined with β-lactamase inhibitors
    g. Empirical use of glycopeptides (vancomycin, teicoplanin), oxazolidinones (linezolid), streptogramins (quinupristin-dalfopristin), or daptomycin is generally not recommended but may be appropriate in select cases
    h. Empirical antifungal therapy
     1) Not necessary for most cases of sepsis
     2) Should be considered when patients may be at high risk of fungal disease (eg, organ transplant, bone marrow transplant, prolonged hospitalization with multiple prior antibiotics, etc)
    i. After microbiologic or serologic data are available, choice of antibiotics should be reevaluated
  2. Surgical drainage or débridement are critical components of treatment when indicated
 C. Supportive Care
  1. Should be based in the intensive care unit
  2. Goal: normalize oxygenation, blood pressure, and tissue perfusion
    a. Protective (low tidal volume) ventilation
    b. Aggressive fluid resuscitation
    c. Adjunctive therapy with vasopressors
 D. Activated Protein C
  1. Results of a double-blind, randomized, placebo-controlled trial with activated protein C (APC): relative reduction in mortality risk of 19.4% (absolute risk reduction, 6.1%) at 28 days
  2. Approved for treatment of patients with severe sepsis
    a. Acute Physiology and Chronic Health Evaluation (APACHE) II score: 25 or more (in the United States)
    b. Organ dysfunctions: 2 or more (in Europe)
  3. Studies involving children
    a. APC increases the incidence of intracranial hemorrhage
    b. APC has no effect on mortality
  4. Contraindications for use of APC
    a. Active internal bleeding
    b. Recent (<3 months) hemorrhagic stroke
    c. Recent (<2 months) intracranial or intraspinal surgery or head trauma
    d. Trauma with risk of life-threatening bleeding
    e. Epidural catheter
    f. Intracranial neoplasm, intracranial mass, or cerebral herniation
    g. Thrombocytopenia (platelet count ≤30,000/μL)

h. Heparin therapy at a dosage of at least 15 international units/kg per hour
5. APC has multiple biologic effects
   a. Antithrombotic anti-inflammatory effects
   b. Inhibition of NF-κB
   c. Antiapoptotic activity
   d. Which effects are responsible for the benefit seen in some patients is not clear

VII. Prognosis and Prevention and Control
   A. Prognosis
      1. Septic shock develops in 20% to 40% of patients with sepsis
      2. Crude mortality rate of septic shock: 30% to 60%
   B. Prevention and Control
      1. Early recognition of infection and appropriate therapy may help to prevent the development of the "sepsis cascade"
      2. For persons in the community, appropriate vaccinations (including pneumococcal and influenza vaccinations for patients with chronic obstructive pulmonary disease) may help to decrease the incidence of infections and sepsis syndrome
      3. For hospitalized patients, several measures may decrease the incidence of sepsis syndrome
         a. Appropriate use of prophylactic perioperative antibiotics
         b. Restriction of the use of medical appliances (such as intravenous lines) to patients who have definite indications
         c. Strict adherence to infection control procedures
            1) To decrease rate of spread of infection among other patients
            2) Includes adherence to hand-washing policies by hospital staff
      4. Patients at special risk of infections (eg, transplant recipients) who use prophylactic antibiotics (eg, trimethoprim-sulfamethoxazole) have a lower incidence of infections and therefore a lower incidence of sepsis syndrome

Suggested Reading

Bochud PY, Bonten M, Marchetti O, Calandra T. Antimicrobial therapy for patients with severe sepsis and septic shock: an evidence-based review. Crit Care Med. 2004 Nov;32 (11 Suppl):S495–512.

Hotchkiss RS, Karl IE. The pathophysiology and treatment of sepsis. N Engl J Med. 2003 Jan 9;348(2): 138–50.

Hughes M. Recombinant human activated protein C. Int J Antimicrob Agents. 2006 Aug;28(2):90–4. Epub 2006 Jul 11.

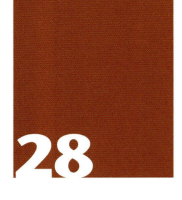

Robert Orenstein, DO

Infectious Diarrhea

I. Introduction
   A. Definition
      1. *Acute diarrhea*: usually defined as increased volume or looser consistency of stool
      2. Specifically, more than 3 loose stools daily for less than 14 days
   B. Pathophysiology
      1. Direct mucosal invasion
      2. Production of toxin that increases fluid secretion into the intestine
   C. Intervention
      1. The majority of these illnesses are self-limited
      2. The majority require no diagnostic or therapeutic interventions
II. Acute Infectious Diarrhea
   A. Etiology
      1. Noroviruses
         a. This group of caliciviruses is the most common cause of acute infectious diarrhea (two-thirds of cases)
         b. Previously known as Norwalk virus
         c. Virus is efficiently transmitted by food, water, or hands in home and institutional settings
         d. Clinical disease: rapid onset of nausea, vomiting, low-grade fever, and diarrhea lasting 3 to 5 days
      2. Diarrheogenic *Escherichia coli*: the second most frequent cause
      3. *Clostridium difficile*: a major pathogen in the health care environment, especially among the elderly
      4. When diarrhea is persistent, bloody, or associated with fever or special hosts, various epidemiologic factors should be considered to identify other causes of acute infectious diarrhea (Tables 28.1 and 28.2)
   B. Diagnosis
      1. Clinical features to be evaluated (Box 28.1)
      2. Diagnostic tests (Box 28.2)
         a. Indications for stool cultures
            1) Patient history
               a) Returning travelers
               b) Immunocompromised patients
               c) Food handlers
            2) Disease features
               a) Inflammatory diarrhea
               b) Concurrent inflammatory bowel disease
            3) Usually a single stool culture is adequate for bacterial pathogens
         b. Indications for examination for ova and parasites

Table 28.1

Epidemiologic Factors That Should Prompt Consideration of Specific Pathogens Causing Infectious Diarrhea

Epidemiologic Factor	Pathogens
Travel	*Escherichia coli, Campylobacter,* protozoa
Health care exposure	*Clostridium difficile*
Antibiotics	*C difficile*
Day care setting	Rotavirus, Norovirus, *Shigella*
Human immunodeficiency virus infection, immunosuppression	*Mycobacterium avium-intracellulare* complex, *Cryptosporidium, Giardia*
Epidemics	Norovirus
Pet exposures (reptiles)	*Salmonella*
Cruise ships	Norovirus
Poultry	*Campylobacter, Salmonella*
Shellfish	*Vibrio*, Norovirus
Soft cheeses	*Listeria, Salmonella, Campylobacter*
Raw hot dogs	*Listeria*
Camping, hiking	*Giardia, Cryptosporidium*

Box 28.1

Clinical Features to Be Evaluated for Infectious Diarrhea

Duration of symptoms: <1 wk or >2 wk
Epigastric pain
Nausea, vomiting
Watery diarrhea
Bloody diarrhea
Fever
Rectal pain, tenesmus
Fecal leukocytes

Box 28.2

Helpful Diagnostic Tests for Infectious Diarrhea

Stool test for fecal leukocytes (Gram stain or lactoferrin assay)
Stool examination for specific agents
    Enteric bacterial cultures
    Ova and parasites microscopy
    Antigen testing
        Giardia
        Cryptosporidium
        Entamoeba histolytica
Enzyme immunoassay of stool for toxins
    Shiga toxin
    Clostridium difficile toxin
Colonoscopy with biopsy for cytomegalovirus

Table 28.2

Epidemiologic Associations of Agents That Cause Diarrhea

Agent	Epidemiologic Associations
Viral	
Norovirus	Cruise ships, seafood, epidemics
Rotavirus	Winter, age <2 y, family
Astrovirus	Day care, age <1 y
Adenovirus	Transplant, age <2 y
Cytomegalovirus	AIDS, severe ulcerative colitis, transplant
Torovirus	Day care, age <2 y
Bacterial	
Clostridium difficile	Antibiotics, health care exposure
Campylobacter	Poultry, puppies
Escherichia coli	Travel, hemolytic uremic syndrome (from enterohemorrhagic *Escherichia coli*), uncooked beef, petting zoos, taco restaurants, spinach
Salmonella	Reptiles, sprouts, institutional outbreaks, peanut butter
Shigella	Day care, homosexuals
Plesiomonas	Raw oysters, Mexico, southeastern Asia, severe abdominal pain
Aeromonas	Well water and springs, brackish water, skin infection
Yersinia	Milk products, college-aged persons with pharyngitis
Tropheryma whipplei	Arthritis, middle-aged men
Vibrio	Seafood, rice
Mycobacterium avium-intracellulare complex	AIDS
Bacillus anthracis	Bioterrorism, hemorrhagic ascites, enteritis, undercooked meat
Protozoal	
Giardia	Human immunodeficiency virus infection, IgA deficiency, campers, travel in Russia
Entamoeba histolytica	Bloody diarrhea, travel, immigrants
Cryptosporidium	AIDS, transplant
Isospora belli	AIDS
Cyclospora	Imported raspberries, AIDS
Microsporidia	AIDS

    1) Patient history
        a) Immunocompromised patients
        b) Men who have sex with men
        c) Travelers and mountaineers: Nepal, southeastern Asia, Russia
    2) Disease features
        a) Persistent diarrhea (>2 weeks)
        b) Community outbreaks
        c) Bloody diarrhea
        d) Persistent diarrhea in day care settings
   3. Features reflecting pathogenesis of diarrhea (Table 28.3)
   4. Foods associated with diarrheal risks (Table 28.4)

Table 28.3
Features of Diarrhea According to Pathogenesis

Feature	Toxigenic Diarrhea	Invasive Diarrhea
Onset	Hours	Days (1-3)
Clinical signs and symptoms	Upper gastrointestinal tract symptoms; then watery diarrhea	Abdominal pain, fever, inflammatory diarrhea
Blood in stool	No fecal leukocytes	Fecal leukocytes and erythrocytes
Location	Small bowel	Colon or small bowel
Agents	Vibrio cholera	Shigella (Shigella sonnei in the United States)
	Enterotoxigenic Escherichia coli	Campylobacter jejuni
	Bacillus cereus	Salmonella
	Staphylococcus aureus	Enteroinvasive E coli
	Clostridium perfringens	Enterohemorrhagic E coli
		Yersinia enterocolitica
		Vibrio parahaemolyticus

Table 28.4
Foods Associated With Diarrheal Risks

Food	Risk (Agents, Toxins, and Diseases)
Breakfast	
Eggs	Salmonella, Campylobacter
Milk	Listeriosis
Toast and jelly (homemade)	Botulism
Homemade honey	Botulinum toxin
Lunch or dinner	
Clams, mussels, sushi, crabs	Plesiomonas, Vibrio, anisakiasis, toxins
Grouper, red snapper	Ciguatoxin
Mountain spring water	Giardia, Cryptosporidium, Cyclospora
Fruit salad	Enterotoxigenic Escherichia coli
Potato salad or mayonnaise	Staphylococcus aureus (toxigenic)
Barbecued chicken	Campylobacter, Salmonella
Fried rice, monosodium glutamate	Bacillus cereus food poisoning
Dill pickles	S aureus (toxigenic)
Chocolate mousse	Salmonella
Apple cider	Enterohemorrhagic E coli
Sprouts	Enterohemorrhagic E coli
Fried rice	B cereus

C. Clinical Disease—Special Situations
1. Intoxications from marine organisms
    a. Ciguatera
        1) Clinical signs and symptoms: nausea, vomiting, dizziness, blurred vision, and hypotension 1 to 2 hours after eating fish; reversal of hot and cold sensations
        2) Distribution: Florida, Caribbean, Hawaii
        3) Clinical course: days to months; exacerbated with caffeine or alcohol
        4) Affected fish: grouper, barracuda, snapper, mackerel; fish has normal appearance and odor
    b. Scombroid poisoning
        1) Clinical disease: histamine-like syndrome with acute onset
        2) Cause: improper refrigeration liberates histamine
        3) Clinical signs and symptoms: oral tingling, flush
        4) Affected fish: tuna, marlin, mahi-mahi, trout; dark meat of fish; fish has an amine odor and tastes peppery, salty, and bubbly
    c. Paralytic shellfish poisoning
        1) Onset: minutes to hours; toxin is preformed
        2) Clinical signs and symptoms: facial paresthesias, bulbar symptoms, paralysis
        3) Affected mollusks: mussels, clams, scallops, snails, crabs
    d. Neurotoxic shellfish poisoning
        1) Distribution: shellfish from Gulf of Mexico coast and South Atlantic Ocean
        2) Clinical signs and symptoms: ocular and respiratory changes, transient paresthesia
2. Infectious proctitis
    a. Clinical signs and symptoms: tenesmus, diarrhea, and erythrocytes and leukocytes in stool

Table 28.5

Antimicrobial Therapy for Diarrhea

Infectious Agent or Condition	Antimicrobial Agent	Alternatives
Salmonella[a]	Ciprofloxacin 500 mg twice daily for 5-7 d Azithromycin 1 g, then 500 mg daily for 6 d	Ceftriaxone 1 g daily IV for 7 d
Shigella	Ciprofloxacin 500 mg twice daily for 3 d Levofloxacin 500 mg daily for 3 d	TMP-SMX DS twice daily for 3 d Azithromycin 500 mg, then 250 mg daily for 4 d
Traveler's diarrhea	Ciprofloxacin 500 mg twice daily for 3 d Levofloxacin 500 mg daily for 3 d Azithromycin 1,000 mg for 1 dose	Rifaximin 200 mg 3 times daily
Campylobacter	Azithromycin 500 mg daily for 3 d Ciprofloxacin 500 mg twice daily for 3 d	
Escherichia coli (enterohemorrhagic E coli)	No therapy	
Yersinia	Ciprofloxacin 500 mg twice daily for 7-10 d	Doxycycline 100 mg IV twice daily *plus* gentamicin 5 mg/kg daily For severe cases: TMP-SMX
Vibrio cholerae	Ciprofloxacin 1 g for 1 d	Doxycycline 300 mg for 1 d
Aeromonas	TMP-SMX Fluoroquinolones	
Clostridium difficile	For mild to moderate disease: metronidazole 500 mg 3 times daily for 10-14 d *or* vancomycin 125 mg orally 4 times daily for 10 d For severe disease: vancomycin 125 mg orally 4 times daily for 10-14 d *with or without* metronidazole 500 mg IV 3 times daily For ileus or megacolon: consider vancomycin enemas For first relapse: repeat as in primary therapy For multiple relapses: vancomycin pulse-and-taper therapy (125 mg orally 4 times daily for 10-14 d, then 125 mg twice daily for 7 d, then 125 mg daily for 7 d, then 125 mg every 2-3 d for 2-8 wk)	
Tropheryma whipplei	Penicillin G 20 MU daily *plus* streptomycin 1 g daily for 10-14 d, then TMP-SMX DS twice daily for 1 y	Ceftriaxone 2 g daily IV
Giardia	Tinidazole 2 g for 1 d	Metronidazole 250 mg 3 times daily for 7 d Nitazoxanide 500 mg twice daily for 3 d
Entamoeba histolytica	Metronidazole 750 mg 3 times daily for 10 d *plus* iodoquinol 650 mg 3 times daily for 20 d	Tinidazole 2 g daily for 3 d *plus* iodoquinol
Cryptosporidium	Nitazoxanide 500 mg twice daily for 3 d	
Cyclospora	TMP-SMX DS twice daily for 7-10 d	Ciprofloxacin 500 mg twice daily
Isospora belli	TMP-SMX DS twice daily for 10 d	
Microsporidia	Albendazole 400 mg twice daily for 3 wk	
Cytomegalovirus	Valganciclovir 900 mg twice daily for 21 d	Ganciclovir 5 mg/kg twice daily for 21 d
Mycobacterium avium-intracellulare complex	Clarithromycin 500 mg twice daily *plus* ethambutol 15 mg/kg daily	

Abbreviations: DS, double-strength tablet; IV, intravenously; MU, million units; TMP-SMX, trimethoprim-sulfamethoxazole.

[a] No treatment for most cases.

      b. Organisms: herpes simplex virus, *Neisseria gonorrhoeae*, *Chlamydia*, *Treponema pallidum*
  D. Use of Antibiotics
    1. Indications (Table 28.5)
      a. Severe traveler's diarrhea
      b. More than 8 stools daily
      c. Duration longer than 1 week
      d. Dehydration
      e. Immunocompromised patients
      f. Fever, abdominal pain, bloody stools
  2. Complications
      a. Antibiotic-associated diarrhea
      b. *Klebsiella oxytoca*: a rare cause of hemorrhagic colitis
      c. *Clostridium difficile* infection

1) Occurs with virtually all antimicrobials (cephalosporins are a major culprit)
2) New epidemic strain: NAP1
   a) Associated with fluoroquinolone resistance
   b) May be associated with excessive toxin production
   c) More severe disease; especially in elderly
3) Diagnose from loose, unformed stools only
4) Best test: a 2-step process
   a) Enzyme immunoassay for glutamate dehydrogenase
   b) Cytotoxicity toxigenic culture assay (alternatives: *C difficile* toxin enzyme immunoassay or polymerase chain reaction)
5) Pseudomembranous colitis; occasionally ileus without diarrhea
6) Treatment (Table 28.5)
7) Do *not* perform *C difficile* toxin assay for follow-up or test of cure

Suggested Reading

Cohen SH, Gerding DN, Johnson S, Kelly CP, Loo VG, McDonald LC, et al; Society for Healthcare Epidemiology of America; Infectious Diseases Society of America. Clinical practice guidelines for *Clostridium difficile* infection in adults: 2010 update by the Society for Healthcare Epidemiology of America (SHEA) and the Infectious Diseases Society of America (IDSA). Infect Control Hospital Epidemiol. 2010 May;31(5):431–55.

Goodgame R. A Bayesian approach to acute infectious diarrhea in adults. Gastroenterol Clin North Am. 2006 Jun;35(2):249–73.

Musher DM, Musher BL. Contagious acute gastrointestinal infections. N Engl J Med. 2004 Dec 2;351(23):2417–27.

Robert Orenstein, DO

Intra-abdominal Infections

I. Introduction
   A. Role of Consultation
      1. Intra-abdominal infections are a common reason for infectious disease consultation
      2. Infectious disease consultant assists in the appropriate diagnostic evaluation and antimicrobial therapy
   B. Management of Infections
      1. These infections span the spectrum from localized organ space infections to diffuse peritonitis
      2. Management is principally by drainage (surgical, endoscopic, or image-guided needle aspiration)
II. Primary Peritonitis
   A. Clinical Importance
      1. *Primary peritonitis*: peritoneal inflammation without other apparent intra-abdominal disease
      2. Also known as spontaneous bacterial peritonitis (SBP)
      3. Risk factors
         a. Principal risk factor: cirrhotic ascites
         b. Other risk factors: recent gastrointestinal tract hemorrhage, presence of indwelling catheters (urinary or intravenous), or infection at a distant site
         c. Occasionally found in patients with congestive heart failure, malignancy, or connective tissue disorders with ascites
      4. The ascitic fluid usually has a low protein level (<1 g/dL)
   B. Clinical Disease
      1. Unexplained febrile illness (50%-80% of patients)
      2. Progressive ascites
      3. Less often: abdominal pain, nausea, and diarrhea
   C. Diagnosis
      1. Diagnosis is made through paracentesis
         a. Ascitic fluid polymorphonuclear cell count: more than 250 cells/µL (neutrocytic ascites)
         b. Gram stain: often does not show organisms (60%-80% of patients)
         c. Culture: negative in 40%
         d. Microbiology
            1) Usually aerobic gram-negative bacteria
            2) *Escherichia coli* is the most frequent isolate, followed by *Klebsiella pneumoniae*, *Streptococcus pneumoniae*, and *Enterococcus*
      2. Blood cultures positive for *E coli*, *K pneumoniae*, *S pneumoniae*, and *Enterococcus*

in the appropriate setting are highly suggestive of SBP
3. Rarely, patients with extrapulmonary tuberculosis may present with primary peritonitis
   a. Insidious onset, presence of peritoneal granulomatosis, lack of mesothelial cells, and presence of mononuclear cells in the ascitic fluid
   b. Acid-fast bacilli smears are of low yield, and adenosine deaminase levels may be elevated
   c. Polymerase chain reaction may aid with diagnosis
   d. Diagnosis usually requires a laparoscopic biopsy of peritoneal implants
D. Treatment
   1. Intravenous antibiotics
      a. Usually a third-generation cephalosporin (eg, cefotaxime or ceftriaxone)
      b. Alternatives: ureidopenicillins or fluoroquinolones
   2. Ascitic fluid white blood cell count should improve at least 25% within 48 hours
   3. Treatment should be continued for 10 to 14 days and can be switched to oral therapy when condition is stable
E. Prophylaxis
   1. Secondary prophylaxis for patients with SBP (Box 29.1)
   2. Norfloxacin 400 mg orally daily, ciprofloxacin 750 mg orally once weekly, or trimethoprim-sulfamethoxazole 1 double-strength tablet 5 days per week

III. Infection Related to Peritoneal Dialysis
   A. Etiology
      1. Peritonitis due to the presence of an indwelling peritoneal catheter for dialysis
      2. Continuous ambulatory peritoneal dialysis or automated peritoneal dialysis
   B. Diagnosis
      1. Abdominal pain
      2. Cloudy dialysate
      3. Dialysate fluid
         a. Leukocyte count is usually more than 100/μL with more than 50% polymorphonuclear cells
         b. Gram stain often does not show organisms
         c. Culture is positive in 90% of cases
            1) Coagulase-negative staphylococci, *Staphylococcus aureus*, and streptococci
            2) Occasionally gram-negative rods and fungi
   C. Treatment
      1. Intraperitoneal instillation of antibiotics (Tables 29.1 and 29.2 and Box 29.2)
         a. Empirical therapy should be directed at both gram-positive bacteria (principally staphylococci) and gram-negative bacteria
         b. Initial regimen: usually either vancomycin or cefazolin *plus* either an intraperitoneal aminoglycoside, third- or fourth-generation cephalosporin, or, rarely, a fluoroquinolone
      2. In complex cases, remove the peritoneal dialysis catheter
         a. Refractory peritonitis: no response by day 5
         b. Relapsing peritonitis: recurrence with same organism within 4 weeks
         c. Refractory exit site or tunnel infections
         d. Fungal peritonitis
      3. Duration of therapy: usually continue for 1 week after clearance
         a. For uncomplicated infections: 2 weeks
         b. For more complicated infections (*S aureus*, gram-negative bacteria, *Enterococcus*, or fungi): 3 weeks

IV. Secondary Peritonitis
   A. Clinical Features
      1. Occurs when intra-abdominal contents spill into the peritoneal cavity
      2. Risks are organ dependent
      3. Microbiologic findings reflect the flora of the disrupted viscera
         a. Flora of the stomach: principally oral bacteria (streptococci) and *Candida*

Box 29.1

Spontaneous Bacterial Peritonitis: Treatment and Prophylaxis

Treatment
    Cefotaxime 2 g IV every 8 h
        or
    Ceftriaxone 1 g IV daily
        or
    Levofloxacin 500 mg IV daily

Prophylaxis
    For patients with variceal bleeding:
        Norfloxacin 400 mg orally twice daily for 7 d
    For patients with recurrent SBP, low-protein ascites, or bilirubin >2.5 mg/dL:
        Norfloxacin 400 mg orally daily
            or
        Ciprofloxacin 750 mg weekly
            or
        Trimethoprim-sulfamethoxazole DS 5 d/wk

Abbreviations: DS, double-strength tablet; IV, intravenously; SBP, spontaneous bacterial peritonitis.

Table 29.1

Intraperitoneal Antibiotic Dosing for Peritonitis Associated With Continuous Ambulatory Peritoneal Dialysis

	Dosing		
		Continuous (All Exchanges)	
Drug	Intermittent (per Exchange, Once Daily)	Loading Dose[a]	Maintenance Dose[a]
Cephalosporins			
Cefazolin	15 mg/kg	500	125
Ceftazidime	1,000-1,500 mg	500	125
Cefepime	1,000 mg	500	125
Aminoglycosides			
Gentamicin	0.6 mg/kg	8	4
Tobramycin	0.6 mg/kg	8	4
Amikacin	2 mg/kg	25	12
Vancomycin	15-30 mg/kg every 5-7 d	1,000	25
Aztreonam	No data	1,000	250
Ciprofloxacin	No data	50	25
Penicillins			
Penicillin G	No data	50,000 units	25,000 units
Ampicillin	No data		125
Nafcillin	No data		125
Ampicillin-sulbactam	2 g every 12 h	1,000	100
Imipenem	1 g every 12 h	500	200
Quinupristin-dalfopristin	25 mg/L in alternate bags *and* 500 mg intravenously every 12 h		
Amphotericin B	No data		1.5

[a] Units are milligrams per liter unless indicated otherwise.

Table 29.2

Intermittent Dosing in Peritonitis Associated With Automated Peritoneal Dialysis

Drug	Dosing
Vancomycin	LD 30 mg/kg IP in long dwell Repeat 15 mg/kg IP in long dwell every 3-5 d Monitor trough levels and keep at approximately 15 mg/dL
Cefazolin	20 mg/kg IP daily in long dwell
Tobramycin	LD 1.5 mg/kg IP in long dwell, then 0.5 mg/kg IP daily in long dwell
Fluconazole	200 mg IP in 1 exchange daily every 24-48 h
Cefepime	1 g IP in 1 exchange daily

Abbreviations: IP, intraperitoneally; LD, loading dose.

Box 29.2

Dosing for Peritonitis Associated With Vancomycin-Resistant Enterococci and Continuous Ambulatory Peritoneal Dialysis

Ampicillin 125 mg/L with or without aminoglycoside 20 mg/L intraperitoneally if sensitive to ampicillin and gentamicin

Linezolid 600 mg intravenously twice daily if ampicillin resistant

Quinupristin-dalfopristin 25 mg/L in alternate bags *and* 500 mg intravenously every 12 h

    b. Flora of the small bowel: enteric gram-negative bacteria, *Enterococcus*, and *Bacteroides*
    c. Flora of the colon: predominantly anaerobes, *Enterococcus*, and aerobic gram-negative bacteria
  4. Patients are often very ill
    a. Fever, marked abdominal pain, and tenderness with rebound and rigidity
    b. Often have leukocytosis and may present with sepsis syndrome
 B. Diagnosis
  1. Clinical features
  2. Abdominal imaging: usually computed tomography (CT)
  3. Microbiology
    a. Polymicrobial
    b. Reflects host's flora
    c. Patients in the community typically have more susceptible organisms
    d. Patients in the hospital or other health care settings often have more resistant polymicrobial flora

Table 29.3

Treatment of Community-Acquired, Complicated Intra-abdominal Infections

Type of Therapy	Mild to Moderate Infection	Severe Infection
Single agent	Ampicillin-sulbactam	Piperacillin-tazobactam
	Ticarcillin-clavulanate	Imipenem
	Ertapenem	Meropenem
	Tigecycline	
Combination	Cefazolin + metronidazole	Third- or fourth-generation cephalosporin[b] + metronidazole
	Fluoroquinolone[a] + metronidazole	Ciprofloxacin + metronidazole
		Aztreonam + metronidazole

[a] Fluoroquinolones include levofloxacin, gatifloxacin, and ciprofloxacin.
[b] Third-generation cephalosporins include cefotaxime, ceftriaxone, and ceftazidime. Fourth-generation cephalosporins include cefepime.

C. Treatment
1. Supportive management, surgical treatment, and drainage of the affected viscera
2. Antimicrobial therapy
   a. Initially, broad-spectrum therapy directed at the suspected polymicrobial flora (Table 29.3 and Box 29.3)
   b. Duration of antimicrobial therapy depends on whether the source of the infection was completely resectable
      1) For cholecystitis or appendicitis, antibiotics are needed for only 24 hours
      2) In other cases, the duration should be limited to 5 to 7 days after surgery if the patient is improving clinically, the patient's leukocyte count is decreasing, and the patient's temperature has been less than 37.7°C for at least 24 hours
   c. The route of antibiotic administration can be switched to oral if the patient can eat
   d. For patients with persistent signs of infection after 5 to 7 days of therapy, appropriate diagnostic evaluation should be pursued along with an extended duration of antibiotic therapy
3. Two organisms often pose dilemmas for surgeons and infectious diseases consultants in the management of secondary peritonitis: *Candida* and *Enterococcus*
   a. In most instances of community-acquired infections, antimicrobial therapy for these 2 organisms is not needed and patients improve without specific therapy
   b. When these organisms are recovered in health care–acquired infections, appropriate antimicrobial therapy should be given
      1) Failure to administer antimicrobials increases morbidity and mortality
      2) If the patient is known to be colonized with vancomycin-resistant *Enterococcus faecium*, agents such as linezolid or tigecycline may be needed
   c. Indications for treating *Enterococcus* peritoneal infections
      1) Health care–associated infections
      2) Persistently positive cultures when the patient does not have clinical improvement
      3) Bacteremia with *Enterococcus*
      4) *Enterococcus* is the predominant organism on Gram stain in a life-threatening disease
   d. Treatment of *Candida* peritoneal infections
      1) *Candida* species may be isolated in 20% of patients with acute perforations of the gastrointestinal tract
      2) Antifungal therapy should not been given unless the patient is immunocompromised (eg, from chemotherapy, transplant, or

---

Box 29.3

Treatment of Health Care–Acquired, Complicated Intra-abdominal Infections

Piperacillin-tazobactam
Meropenem
Imipenem
Cefepime + metronidazole
Caspofungin or fluconazole: considered if cultures grow *Candida* species
Vancomycin: may be added if a penicillin-allergic patient has an enterococcal infection
Linezolid or tigecycline: considered with isolation of vancomycin-resistant enterococci

inflammatory disease) or has recurrent or postoperative infection
3) Caspofungin has broad activity against *Candida* and may be preferred over fluconazole until the species of *Candida* is identified

V. Tertiary Peritonitis
   A. Definition
      1. *Tertiary peritonitis*: recurrent peritonitis
      2. Usually occurs in a health care setting after surgery for an intra-abdominal infection in an ill host
   B. Clinical Features
      1. Patients have ongoing markers of inflammation despite therapy directed at the agents of secondary peritonitis
      2. Patients cannot control the infection owing to poor host defenses, inadequate source control, or inadequate antimicrobial therapy
      3. These infections are associated with health care–associated resistant organisms such as resistant gram-negative bacteria (eg, *Pseudomonas aeruginosa*, *Acinetobacter*), *Enterococcus*, and *Candida* species

VI. Intra-abdominal Abscesses
   A. Definition
      1. Collections of pus usually developing after abdominal surgery that resulted in a perforated viscus or anastomotic leak
      2. Occur in various intraperitoneal and extraperitoneal locations depending on the source
   B. Diagnosis
      1. Clinical signs and symptoms: fever and leukocytosis without specific localizing signs
      2. Best test for diagnosis: abdominopelvic CT scan
   C. Treatment
      1. CT-guided aspiration of the abscess or placement of a percutaneous drain and directed antimicrobial therapy based on aspirate findings
         a. Drain can be removed when the patient is clinically improved and the drainage is minimal
         b. A sinogram that shows collapse of the cavity usually implies that the catheter can be removed
      2. Failure to improve usually indicates inadequate drainage
      3. Antimicrobial therapy is the same as for secondary peritonitis

VII. Biliary Tract Infections
   A. Etiology
      1. Arise from obstruction of bile flow and secondary infection
      2. May result from calculous cholecystitis, acalculous cholecystitis, or ascending cholangitis
   B. Calculous Cholecystitis
      1. Occurs with intermittent obstruction of the cystic duct by a gallstone
      2. In most cases, antibiotics are not needed
   C. Acalculous Cholecystitis
      1. Occurs in critically ill patients after surgery, trauma, or sepsis
      2. Occurs in patients receiving long-term total parenteral nutrition
   D. Ascending Cholangitis
      1. Occurs with biliary obstruction
      2. Source of obstruction: usually a gallstone but may be from other causes
         a. Parasitic infection (eg, *Clonorchis sinensis*, *Opisthorchis viverrini*, *Ascaris lumbricoides*, or *Fasciola hepatica*)
         b. Stricture due to primary sclerosing cholangitis or malignancy (pancreatic, ampullary, metastatic, or cholangiocarcinoma)
         c. Human immunodeficiency virus cholangiopathy infection
         d. Manipulation of the biliary tree, an obstructed stent, or radiotherapy
   E. Diagnosis
      1. Patients typically present with fever, right upper quadrant abdominal pain, leukocytosis, and elevated levels of alkaline phosphatase and bilirubin
      2. Diagnosis is often suggested by ultrasonography or CT
   F. Treatment
      1. Most infections are from aerobic gram-negative bacilli, such as *E coli*, *Klebsiella*, and *Enterococcus*
      2. Infections are often polymicrobial
      3. Key to management: effective drainage and antibiotics (with drainage, 3 days of antibiotic therapy may be adequate)
         a. Antibiotics
            1) Broad-spectrum agents to cover aerobic gram-negative bacteria, anaerobes, and enterococci for 7 to 10 days
            2) Piperacillin-tazobactam, cefepime plus metronidazole, fluoroquinolones
         b. After there is a response to treatment, drainage can be performed in 24 to 48 hours by endoscopic retrograde cholangiopancreatography or

percutaneous transhepatic cholangiography
c. Biliary drainage can be reestablished by sphincterotomy, nasobiliary drain, stent placement, stone removal, or a combination of these

VIII. Hepatic Abscess
  A. Pathogenesis
    1. Various sources: hepatobiliary tract, portal venous circulation, or hepatic arterial circulation
    2. Pathogenesis usually determines microbiologic features
      a. Biliary tract infections often involve enteric gram-negative rods
      b. Liver abscesses resulting from a colonic infection involve anaerobic and aerobic streptococci
  B. Diagnosis
    1. CT imaging
  C. Pyogenic Liver Abscess
    1. Pathogenesis
      a. Pyogenic and amebic abscesses
        1) Most often single or multiple lesions in the right lobe
        2) Amebic abscess is best diagnosed serologically by the presence of *Entamoeba histolytica* antibodies
      b. Hydatid cysts: usually large and may contain daughter cysts (Figures 29.1-29.3)
    2. Treatment
      a. Optimal approach for pyogenic abscesses: percutaneous drainage with directed broad-spectrum antimicrobial therapy (Box 29.4)

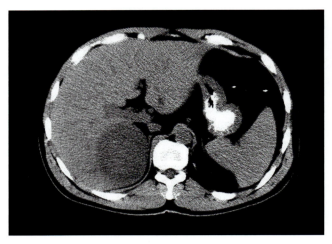

Figure 29.2. Computed Tomographic Scan Showing Liver Abscess.

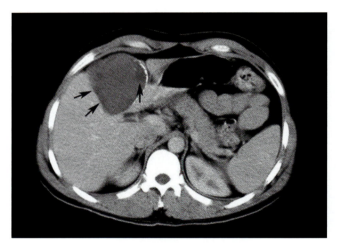

Figure 29.3. Type II Hydatid Cyst. Contrast-enhanced axial computed tomographic scan of the upper abdomen shows cystic lesion with peripheral daughter cysts and wall calcification in the left lobe of the liver. The daughter cysts have a lower attenuation value than the mother cyst (arrows). (From Yuksel M, Demirpolat G, Sever A, Bakaris S, Bulbuloglu E. Elmas N. Hydatid disease involving some rare locations in the body: a pictorial essay. Korean J Radiol. 2007 Nov-Dec;8[6]:531–40. Used with permission.)

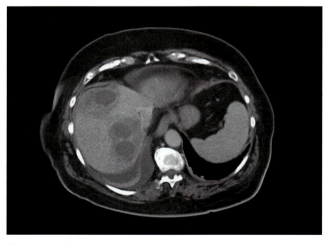

Figure 29.1. Computed Tomographic Scan Showing Hydatid Cyst.

      b. Amebic abscesses: may be treated with metronidazole 750 mg 3 times daily for 10 days
        1) Parenteral therapy for 2 to 3 weeks
        2) Then oral antibiotics for 2 to 4 weeks
      c. Follow-up CT imaging is needed to document resolution or collapse of the abscess

Box 29.4

Antimicrobial Therapy for Liver Abscesses

Pyogenic liver abscess
    Metronidazole 500 mg IV every 8 h *plus*
        Ceftriaxone 1-2 g daily IV *or*
        Cefotaxime 1-2 g every 6 h *or*
        Ciprofloxacin 400 mg IV every 12 h *or*
        Levofloxacin 500 mg IV daily
    Piperacillin-tazobactam 3.375 g IV every 6 h
    Imipenem 1 g every 6 h
    Meropenem 1 g every 8 h
    Ticarcillin-clavulanate 3.1 g IV every 4 h
    Cefoxitin 1 g IV every 4 h *or* ampicillin-sulbactam 3 g IV every 6 h
    Ertapenem 1 g IV daily
    Completion with oral therapy:
        Ciprofloxacin plus metronidazole *or*
        Amoxicillin-clavulanate
Amebic liver abscess
    Metronidazole 750 mg 3 times daily for 10 d

Abbreviation: IV, intravenously.

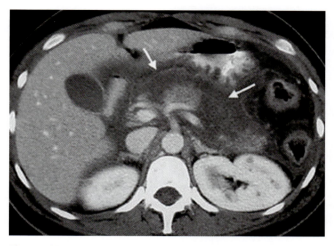

Figure 29.4. Computed tomographic scan showing necrotic lesion (arrows).

IX. Pancreatic Infections
    A. Pathogenesis
        1. Infections of the pancreas are uncommon
        2. Occur with severe necrotizing pancreatitis
        3. After several weeks, the necrotic debris may become infected by bacterial translocation across the colonic mucosa
        4. Gram-negative enteric flora (eg, *E coli*, *Klebsiella*, *S aureus*, and *Enterococcus*) may infect this necrotic debris
    B. Clinical Features
        1. Patients often present with persistent sepsis 7 to 10 days into an episode of pancreatitis
        2. They may remain febrile with abdominal pain, ileus, and leukocytosis
    C. Diagnosis
        1. Contrast CT imaging and fine-needle aspiration of the necrotic lesion (Figure 29.4)
        2. Nonspecific markers point toward infected necrosis: C-reactive protein and elevated procalcitonin levels
        3. Gram stain should direct therapy
        4. If the initial aspirate is negative and the patient's condition does not improve, follow-up aspirations should be performed every 5 to 7 days (Figure 29.5)
            a. This differs from the standard practice of many surgeons and gastroenterologists who empirically give broad-spectrum carbapenems to patients with pancreatic necrosis
            b. Recent placebo-controlled, double-blind trial results suggest that this prophylactic strategy does not improve outcomes and leads to resistant bacterial and fungal infections
    D. Treatment
        1. Best approach: look for the cause of persistent fever and leukocytosis and provide directed therapy
        2. Management of infected necrosis depends on the status of the host
            a. Early surgical débridement is optimal
            b. If patient is too ill for surgery, endoscopic or percutaneous drainage may be an option
    E. Pancreatic Abscesses
        1. Arise 5 to 6 weeks later as a complication of infected necrosis
        2. They are best managed with CT-guided drainage
X. Appendicitis
    A. Clinical Disease
        1. Acute appendicitis: one of the most common surgical emergencies
        2. Occurs when the appendiceal lumen becomes obstructed, leading to ischemia, inflammation, and perforation
    B. Diagnosis
        1. Based on clinical findings, leukocytosis, abdominal pain, anorexia, nausea and vomiting, and CT findings (Figure 29.6)
        2. Infection is typically polymicrobial: the microorganisms most often associated with appendicitis are *E coli* and *Bacteroides*
    C. Treatment
        1. Perioperatively, patients with suspected appendicitis should receive a first-, second-,

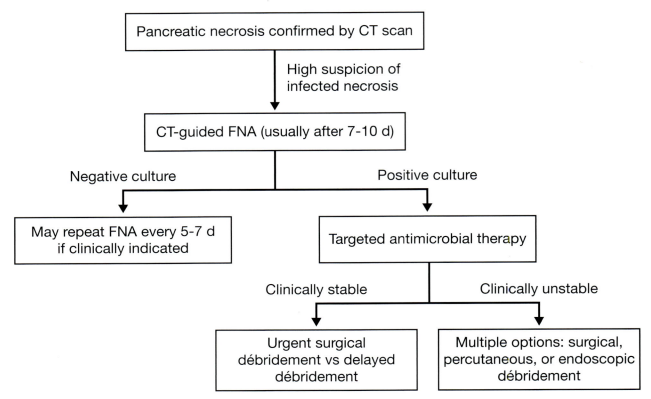

Figure 29.5. Decision Algorithm for Infected Pancreatic Necrosis. CT indicates computed tomographic; FNA, fine-needle aspiration. (From Berzin TM, Mortele KJ, Banks PA. The management of suspected pancreatic sepsis. Gastroenterol Clin North Am. 2006 Jun;35[2]: 393–407. Used with permission.)

or third-generation cephalosporin with or without anaerobic coverage (eg, cefazolin plus metronidazole)
2. Therapy is discontinued within 24 hours after surgery unless a perforation occurred
3. For perforation, antibiotic therapy (usually a fluoroquinolone or a third-generation cephalosporin plus metronidazole) is continued for 7 to 10 days
4. Oral antimicrobials can be used to complete therapy (but they may not be needed)

XI. Diverticulitis
  A. Prevalence
   1. Diverticulosis is common in the Western world: most disease involves the sigmoid colon
   2. Diverticulitis is uncommon: it occurs in only 15% to 20% of people with diverticulosis
  B. Diagnosis
   1. Patients may present with mild abdominal pain or with more severe disease that includes bleeding, abscess, peritonitis, or fistulae formation
   2. Most patients present with left lower quadrant abdominal pain, malaise, and leukocytosis
   3. CT scanning provides best imaging for diagnosis and staging of disease (Figure 29.7)
  C. Treatment
   1. Outpatient treatment of diverticulitis: clear liquid diet and a course of oral antibiotics (eg, ciprofloxacin plus metronidazole) for 7 to 10 days
   2. Most patients improve in 2 to 3 days
   3. If fever, leukocytosis, or anorexia persist, the patient should be hospitalized and receive intravenous antibiotics directed at colonic polymicrobial flora
   4. Treatment of abscesses
    a. Small localized perforation or abscess: may be managed with antibiotics alone
    b. Larger abscess: may be managed with CT-guided percutaneous drainage
    c. Patients with large abscesses should receive definitive surgical therapy within 3 to 4 weeks

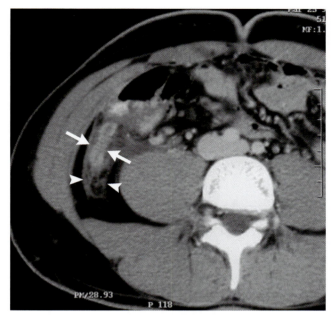

Figure 29.6. Computed Tomographic Scan of an 18-Year-Old Man With Abdominal Pain and Nausea. After the administration of intravenous and enteric contrast material, the right lower quadrant shows a dilated, fluid-filled appendix with a thickened wall (arrows). There are inflammatory changes in the adjacent fat tissue (arrowheads). Laparotomy confirmed the diagnosis of acute appendicitis, and an appendectomy was performed. The patient had an uneventful recovery. (From Paulson EK, Kalady MF, Pappas TN. Clinical practice: suspected appendicitis. N Engl J Med. 2003 Jan 16;348[3]:236–42. Used with permission.)

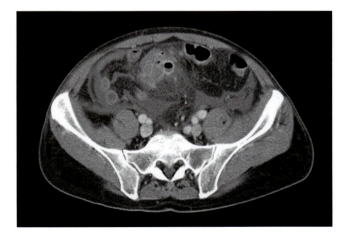

Figure 29.7. Computed Tomographic Scan Showing Diverticulitis.

XII. Typhlitis
  A. Clinical Disease
    1. Also called neutropenic enterocolitis
    2. Characterized by cecal inflammation in febrile neutropenic patients with leukemia after chemotherapy
        a. Patients may have persistent fever, right lower quadrant abdominal pain, and oral mucositis
        b. Typhlitis manifests after 10 to 14 days of neutropenia
  B. Diagnosis
    1. Any of several characteristic ultrasonographic or CT findings
        a. Fluid-filled, dilated, and distended cecum
        b. Presence of intramural edema, air, or hemorrhage
        c. Localized perforation with free air
        d. Soft tissue mass suggesting abscess formation
    2. Testing for *Clostridium difficile* toxin should be performed
  C. Treatment
    1. Parenteral nutrition
    2. Patients should not receive anything by mouth
    3. Broad-spectrum antibiotics with coverage against anaerobes (eg, imipenem, meropenem)
XIII. Hepatosplenic (Disseminated) Candidiasis
  A. Clinical Disease
    1. Disseminated candidiasis occurs after recovery from prolonged chemotherapy-induced neutropenia
    2. Fever, elevated alkaline phosphatase level, and right upper quadrant pain
  B. Diagnosis
    1. CT scan shows diffuse micronodular lesions in the liver and spleen (Figure 29.8)
  C. Treatment
    1. One of 2 options
        a. Initial course of liposomal amphotericin followed by fluconazole
        b. Prolonged course of fluconazole 400 mg daily for 4 to 12 months or until the lesions are radiographically calcified
    2. Patients requiring more chemotherapy should continue azole therapy
XIV. Peliosis Hepatis
  A. Clinical Disease
    1. Capillary dilation in the hepatic sinusoids
    2. May be associated with disseminated *Bartonella* infection in immunosuppressed patients

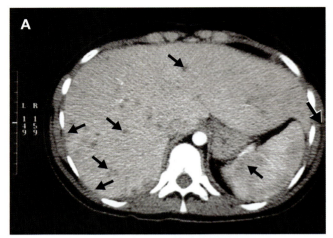

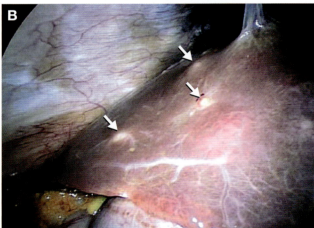

Figure 29.8. Hepatosplenic Candidiasis. A, Abdominal computed tomographic scan shows multiple hypodense lesions in the liver and spleen consistent with hepatosplenic microabscesses (arrows). B, Diagnostic laparoscopy was performed to obtain biopsy specimens of the hepatic lesions (arrows). The causative agent was identified on polymerase chain reaction assay as *Candida albicans*. (From Halkic N, Ksontini R. Images in clinical medicine: hepatosplenic candidiasis. N Engl J Med. 2007 Jan 25;356[4]:e4. Used with permission.)

B. Diagnosis
1. Patients with AIDS may present with fever, hepatomegaly, cytopenias, an elevated alkaline phosphatase level, and cutaneous bacillary angiomatosis
2. CT scan: hypodense lesions consistent with capillary dilation and hepatomegaly (Figure 29.9)

C. Treatment
1. Erythromycin 500 mg 4 times daily
2. Doxycycline 100 mg twice daily with or without rifampin 300 mg twice daily for 2 to 4 months

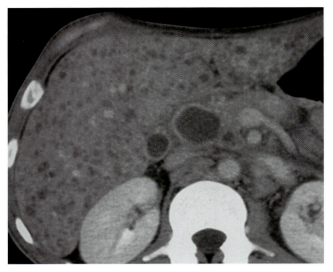

Figure 29.9. Bacillary Peliosis in a Patient With AIDS. Transverse contrast-enhanced computed tomographic image obtained after 9 months shows progression of disease with multiple hypoattenuating lesions disseminated within liver parenchyma with multiple small accumulations of contrast material in center of lesions (the so-called target sign). (From Iannaccone R, Federle MP, Brancatelli G, Matsui O, Fishman EK, Narra VR, et al. Peliosis hepatis: spectrum of imaging findings. AJR Am J Roentgenol. 2006 Jul;187[1]:W43–52. Used with permission.)

Suggested Reading

Berzin TM, Mortele KJ, Banks PA. The management of suspected pancreatic sepsis. Gastroenterol Clin North Am. 2006 Jun;35(2):393–407.

Boeschoten EW, Ter Wee PM, Divino J. Peritoneal dialysis-related infections recommendations 2005: an important tool for quality improvement. Nephrol Dial Transplant. 2006 Jul;21 Suppl 2:ii31–3.

Dominguez EP, Sweeney JF, Choi YU. Diagnosis and management of diverticulitis and appendicitis. Gastroenterol Clin North Am. 2006 Jun;35(2):367–91.

Qureshi WA. Approach to the patient who has suspected acute bacterial cholangitis. Gastroenterol Clin North Am. 2006 Jun;35(2):409–23.

Runyon BA; Practice Guidelines Committee, American Association for the Study of Liver Diseases (AASLD). Management of adult patients with ascites due to cirrhosis. Hepatology. 2004 Mar;39(3):841–56.

Solomkin JS, Mazuski JE, Bradley JS, Rodvold KA, Goldstein EJ, Baron EJ, et al. Diagnosis and management of complicated intra-abdominal infection in adults and children: guidelines by the Surgical Infection Society and the Infectious Diseases Society of America. Clin Infect Dis. 2010 Jan 15;50(2):133–64.

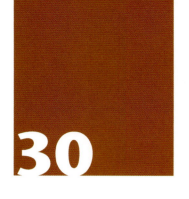

Stacey A. Rizza, MD

Viral Hepatitis

I. Introduction
   A. Viruses and Multisystem Disease
      1. Many viruses can cause multisystem disease in humans
      2. These viruses can infect the liver
   B. Hepatotropic Viruses
      1. There are 5 hepatotropic viruses that primarily infect the human liver and cause hepatitis
      2. The 5 hepatotropic viruses vary in structure
      3. Infection varies in clinical course, diagnosis, and treatment
      4. The viruses were named alphabetically in order of discovery
         a. A, B, C, D, and E
         b. In 1996 a sixth virus, hepatitis G virus, was described, but its role in human disease remains uncertain
      5. According to the Centers for Disease Control and Prevention, approximately 10 cases of viral hepatitis per 100,000 people are reported each year in the United States
      6. The disease burden is higher in many other countries throughout the world
II. Hepatitis A Virus
   A. Agent
      1. Hepatitis A virus (HAV): a member of the Picornaviridae family of viruses
      2. HAV causes about 50% of the acute hepatitis cases in the United States
      3. One-third of Americans have evidence of past infection with HAV
      4. HAV is excreted in the stool of infected persons and is spread by the fecal-oral route when an uninfected person ingests food or drink contaminated with the virus
   B. Clinical Disease
      1. People at risk of HAV infection
         a. Household or sexual contacts of infected persons
         b. Men who have sex with men
         c. Children living in an area with increased rates of hepatitis A
         d. People traveling to areas where hepatitis A is endemic
         e. Drug users (injection and noninjection)
      2. The infection is self-limited
      3. Symptoms: jaundice, nausea, fever, abdominal pain, and diarrhea
         a. Most cases of acute hepatitis are asymptomatic
         b. Symptoms generally last up to 20 days
         c. In 15% of infected people, a relapsing course lasts 6 to 9 months
      4. There are no reported cases of chronic HAV infection

5. Mortality rate is about 2 per 1,000 icteric cases
6. Immunity: lifelong immunity develops in an HAV-infected person
C. Diagnosis
1. Serologic testing for IgM and IgG antibodies from the peripheral blood
2. IgM antibody titers
   a. Become positive by the time symptoms develop
   b. Remain positive for 3 to 12 months
3. IgG antibody titers
   a. Become positive within several weeks after IgM antibody titers become positive
   b. Remain positive for life
D. Management
1. There is no treatment for HAV infection
2. Immune globulin
   a. Can provide short-term protection against hepatitis A
   b. Can be given before and within 2 weeks after exposure to HAV
3. Careful hand washing and food preparation is important
4. Hepatitis A vaccine is the best protection against infection
   a. The vaccine is administered in 2 doses 6 months apart
   b. Vaccination is recommended for certain people 1 year or older
      1) People traveling to areas with increased rates of hepatitis A
      2) Men who have sex with men
      3) Drug users (injection and noninjection)
      4) People with clotting factor disorders (ie, hemophilia)
      5) People with chronic liver disease
      6) Children living in areas with increased rates of hepatitis A
   c. Universal vaccination of American children is recommended at 1 year of age
III. Hepatitis B Virus
A. Agent
1. Hepatitis B virus (HBV): a small DNA virus in the Hepadnaviridae family
2. Approximately 400 million people are infected with HBV worldwide
B. Clinical Disease
1. Infection ranges from asymptomatic to end-stage liver disease and hepatocellular carcinoma in persons with cirrhosis
   a. Almost one-third of infected persons have no signs or symptoms
   b. Children are less likely to have symptoms than adults
2. HBV infection occurs when blood from an infected person enters a previously uninfected person
   a. Through sexual activity
   b. Through infected blood products
3. People at risk of HBV infection
   a. Also at risk of hepatitis C virus (HCV) or human immunodeficiency virus (HIV) infection
   b. People with multiple sex partners or a history of a sexually transmitted disease
   c. Men who have sex with men
   d. Sexual contacts of infected people
   e. Infants born to infected mothers
   f. Injection drug users
   g. Household contacts of chronically infected people
   h. Immigrants from areas with high rates of HBV infection
   i. Health care and public safety workers
   j. Hemodialysis patients
4. Spectrum of duration of HBV infection
   a. A self-limited acute infection
      1) Lasts up to 6 months
      2) Jaundice, fatigue, nausea, vomiting, abdominal pain, joint pain, and loss of appetite
   b. A chronic infection
      1) Develops in 90% of infants infected at birth
      2) Develops in 30% of children infected at ages 1 through 5 years
      3) Develops in 6% of people infected when older than 5 years
C. Diagnosis
1. Serology (Figure 30.1)
   a. Within weeks after exposure to HBV, hepatitis B surface antigen (HBsAg) appears in peripheral blood
   b. Hepatitis B e antigen (HBeAg) and IgM hepatitis B core antigen antibody (anti-HBc) develop shortly after
   c. If a person clears the virus, the HBsAg disappears, and IgG HBsAg antibody (anti-HBs) and anti-HBc develop
   d. If the HBsAg or HBeAg remain positive in the peripheral blood for longer than 6 months after acute infection, the patient is considered to have chronic infection
2. Molecular diagnostic techniques
   a. HBV DNA is present within days of acute infection

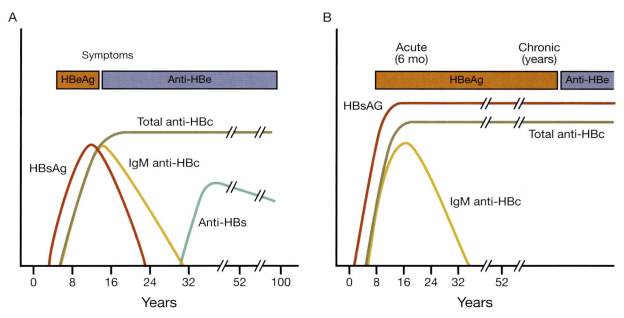

Figure 30.1. Typical Course of Hepatitis B. A, Acute hepatitis B. B, Chronic hepatitis B. Ag indicates antigen; HBc, hepatitis B core; HBe, hepatitis B e; HBs, hepatitis B surface; IgM, immunoglobulin M. (From James Koziel M, Thio CL. Hepatitis B virus and hepatitis delta virus. In: Mandell GL, Bennett JE, Dolin R, editors. Mandell, Douglas, and Bennett's principles and practice of infectious diseases. Vol 2. 7th ed. Philadelphia [PA]: Churchill Livingstone Elsevier; c2010. p. 2059-86. Used with permission.)

      b. HBV DNA levels fluctuate with disease, so they should not take the place of serologic testing for diagnosis
- D. Management
  1. Hepatitis B vaccine is the best protection against infection
     a. Efficacy is greater than 95% after 3 doses at 0, 1, and 6 months
     b. Vaccine is recommended routinely for certain groups
        1) Children up to 18 years old
        2) Adults older than 18 who are at risk of infection (see list of people at risk above)
  2. Safe sex and clean needle practices (for those who use intravenous drugs or receive tattoos)
  3. Pregnant women should undergo serologic testing for hepatitis B
  4. Infants born to HBV-infected mothers should be given hepatitis B immune globulin (HBIG) and vaccine within 12 hours after birth
- E. Treatment
  1. US Food and Drug Administration (FDA) has approved 7 drugs to treat chronic HBV infection
     a. Interferon alfa or pegylated interferon
        1) Used for 4 to 6 months to clear the infection
        2) Clears HBeAg in about 20% to 25% of the cases
        3) It is most effective in young people with high serum liver transaminase levels and low HBV viral load
        4) Cannot be used with decompensated liver disease
     b. Lamivudine
        1) Used daily to decrease viral replication and prevent liver disease during HBV infection
        2) The YMDD mutation in the polymerase gene occurs in about 70% of patients after they use lamivudine for 5 years and renders the virus resistant
        3) Lamivudine also has anti-HIV activity
     c. Adefovir
        1) A nucleotide analogue with anti-HIV activity (in higher doses)
        2) Inhibits HBV replication with a daily dosage
        3) Effective in people who have already acquired the YMDD mutation from lamivudine use

d. Entecavir
   1) A very strong inhibitor of HBV replication
   2) Also has anti-HIV activity
   3) In patients coinfected with HIV and HBV, entecavir can be used only in conjunction with effective antiretroviral therapy
e. Telbivudine
   1) A nucleoside analogue with no known HIV activity
   2) Clinical trials have shown it to be more effective than lamivudine or adefovir and less likely to cause resistance
f. Tenofovir
   1) A nucleotide analogue with strong HIV and HBV activity
   2) More effective than lamivudine or adefovir in clinical trials against HBV, with a very low incidence of resistance
2. Liver transplant
   a. Considered for people with end-stage liver disease from HBV infection
   b. HBV infection recurs in 85% to 90% of transplant recipients and can result in mild to rapidly progressive disease

IV. Hepatitis C Virus
   A. Agent
      1. HCV was first described in 1989 (previously referred to as non-A, non-B hepatitis)
      2. RNA virus in a genus of the Flaviviridae family
      3. The most common cause of viral hepatitis in the Western world
         a. More than 4 million Americans are infected with HCV
         b. The leading cause of liver failure and transplant in the United States
      4. Six genotypes of HCV have geographic distributions
         a. Genotypes 1, 2, and 3: most common in the United States and Western Europe (genotypes 2 and 3 are more common in injection drug users)
         b. Genotype 4: most common in the Middle East and North Africa
         c. Genotypes 5 and 6: most common in Asia
         d. All 6 genotypes cause identical disease and are distinguished only by their response rates to therapy
   B. Clinical Disease
      1. HCV is transmitted from an infected person through blood entering an uninfected person
         a. Risk factors are generally the same as for HBV and HIV
         b. HCV is much less likely to be transmitted sexually
         c. In addition, intranasal cocaine use with shared straws is a risk factor for HCV infection
      2. Acute infection
         a. Rarely fatal
         b. Causes symptoms such as jaundice, nausea, vomiting, abdominal pain, loss of appetite, and fatigue in about 25% of infected persons
      3. Chronic infection
         a. Approximately 15% to 40% of people who are infected with HCV clear the infection, resulting in a 60% to 85% chance of chronic infection (Figure 30.2)
            1) In 70% of those who have chronic infection, chronic liver disease develops, including cirrhosis and, in some cases, hepatocellular carcinoma
            2) Of the people with chronic infection, 1% to 5% die as a result of the HCV infection
         b. Chronic HCV infection can cause multiple extrahepatic manifestations
            1) Vasculitis: polyarteritis nodosa
            2) Cryoglobulinemia
            3) Membranous or membranoproliferative glomerulonephritis
            4) Increased risk of lymphoma

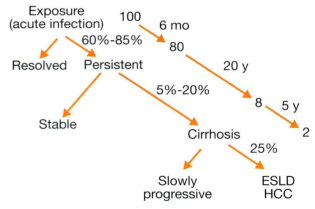

Figure 30.2. Natural History of Hepatitis C Virus Infection. Estimates of the most common outcomes of hepatitis C virus infection are provided with extrapolation to the hypothetical acute infection of 100 persons. ESLD indicates end-stage liver disease (eg, esophageal varices, ascites, hepatic encephalopathy); HCC, hepatocellular carcinoma. (From Ray SC, Thomas DL. Hepatitis C. In: Mandell GL, Bennett JE, Dolin R, editors. Mandell, Douglas, and Bennett's principles and practice of infectious diseases. Vol 2. 7th ed. Philadelphia [PA]: Churchill Livingstone Elsevier; c2010. p. 2157–94. Used with permission.)

C. Diagnosis
1. Serology
   a. Anti-HCV antibodies occur in the peripheral blood 1 to 6 months after infection
   b. These antibodies remain lifelong
2. Molecular diagnosis
   a. HCV RNA is in the peripheral blood within days of infection
   b. At 3 and 6 months after acute infection, the patient should be checked for HCV RNA
      1) If the HCV RNA level is elevated after 6 months, the patient is chronically infected
      2) If HCV RNA is undetectable at 6 months and at 12 months after infection, the patient has cleared the infection

D. Management
1. There is no vaccine to prevent HCV infection
2. Preventive behavior: avoid exposure to infected blood
   a. Use clean needles
   b. Avoid high-risk activities
3. For treatment of chronic HCV infection: pegylated interferon in combination with ribavirin
   a. Genotypes 1 and 4
      1) Require 48 weeks of therapy
      2) Response rate: approximately 50% among patients who complete therapy
   b. Genotypes 2 and 3
      1) Require 24 weeks of therapy
      2) Response rate: in nearly 85% of patients, the virus is cleared
4. HCV infection recurs almost universally after liver transplant
5. The first 2 disease-active agents for HCV infection: telaprevir and boceprevir
   a. Both are expected to be approved by the FDA in the imminent future
   b. Both are nonstructural protein 3 protease inhibitors
   c. In clinical trials, both have shown improved treatment responses compared with the traditional combination of pegylated interferon and ribavirin

V. Hepatitis D Virus
A. Agent
1. Hepatitis D virus (HDV) is a defective virus that requires HBV for support and replication
2. Can only infect people who are also infected with HBV: as a coinfection with HBV or as a superinfection

B. Clinical Disease
1. HDV is transmitted through infected blood, blood products, or bodily secretions or during child birth
2. Risk factors for HDV infection are similar to those for HBV infection
3. HDV superinfection should be considered when liver disease suddenly worsens in a patient with chronic HBV infection
4. Chronic HDV infection
   a. A person with a coinfection of HBV and HDV has only a 5% chance of a chronic HDV infection developing
   b. A person with a superinfection with HDV has a 70% chance of chronic HDV infection developing
5. HDV infection is the most likely of the chronic hepatitis virus infections to progress to cirrhosis
   a. HDV infection results in worse liver disease than HBV infection alone
   b. Mortality rate among persons with HDV infection: 2% to 20% (which is higher than with HBV infection alone)

C. Diagnosis
1. Anti-HDV antibodies in the peripheral blood (IgM and IgG anti-hepatitis D antigen)
2. Polymerase chain reaction
3. If a patient clears HBV, HDV is also cleared

D. Management
1. There is no vaccine or definitive treatment for HDV infection
2. Interferon alfa
   a. HDV infection responds to interferon alfa therapy for 9 to 12 months in doses similar to those for HBV infection
   b. Cure rate: 15% to 25%
3. Liver transplant should be considered for people with end-stage liver disease

VI. Hepatitis E Virus
A. Agent
1. Hepatitis E virus (HEV) is a small RNA calicivirus that causes acute infection
2. Found most commonly in India, Pakistan, southern and eastern Russia, China, Africa, Mexico, and South America (rare in the United States)

B. Clinical Disease
1. Infection occurs most often in people 15 to 40 years old
2. The highest mortality is among pregnant women, particularly during the third trimester
3. HEV is found in the stool of infected people and is transmitted when uninfected people ingest contaminated food or water

            a. HEV epidemics are often associated with contaminated drinking water sources
            b. Person-to-person transmission is less common than with HAV infection
        4. Acute infection frequently causes jaundice, nausea, vomiting, abdominal pain, loss of appetite, and fatigue
        5. In contrast to the other viral hepatitis viruses, HEV infection usually resembles cholestasis, resulting in dark urine and elevated serum alkaline phosphatase and bilirubin levels
        6. Chronic infection with HEV has never been reported
    C. Diagnosis
        1. HEV infection is diagnosed by finding anti-HEV antibodies in the peripheral blood
            a. Anti-HEV IgM is detectable in 96% of patients 1 to 4 weeks after the onset of disease
            b. An increasing anti-HEV IgG titer is also diagnostic
    D. Management
        1. There is no vaccine or treatment for HEV infection
        2. Careful hand washing, attention to water sources, and food preparation are recommended in areas where HEV is endemic
VII. Hepatitis G Virus
    A. Agent
        1. Described by 2 independent groups who named the virus hepatitis G virus (HGV) and hepatitis GB virus C (HGBV-C), respectively
        2. It is a single-stranded RNA virus of the Flaviviridae family and is related to HCV
        3. Approximately 1% to 2% of the general population in many countries have HGV in the peripheral blood
        4. HGV received notoriety with several studies that reported an association between improved immune status during HIV infection (and improved HIV viral load) in people who were also infected with HGV
    B. Clinical Disease
        1. HGV infection does not alter the course of infection with HAV, HBV, or HCV
        2. Thus far, no disease has been ascribed to this virus, and controversy remains as to whether it infects the liver and causes hepatitis

Suggested Reading

Centers for Disease Control and Prevention [Internet]. Viral hepatitis. [cited 2010 Jun 28]. Available from: http://www.cdc.gov/ncidod/diseases/hepatitis/.

Farrell GC, Teoh NC. Management of chronic hepatitis B virus infection: a new era of disease control. Intern Med J. 2006 Feb;36(2):100–13.

Lo Re V 3rd, Kostman JR. Management of chronic hepatitis C. Postgrad Med J. 2005 Jun;81(956):376–82.

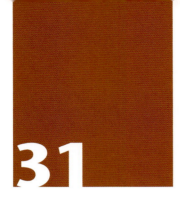

Larry M. Baddour, MD
Daniel Z. Uslan, MD

Infective Endocarditis

I. Introduction
   A. Infective Endocarditis in Clinical Practice
      1. Unlike infectious diseases that involve the respiratory tract or skin and soft tissues, infective endocarditis (IE) is uncommonly seen by primary care physicians
      2. Clinical presentation of patients with endocarditis can be nonspecific and varied
      3. IE can masquerade as other infectious syndromes, particularly at the time of clinical onset
   B. Published Treatment Guidelines
      1. Assist the clinician in managing patients with IE
      2. Guidelines specifically outline recommended antimicrobials, including dosages, route of administration, and duration
      3. Even with these guidelines, the overall care of each patient must be individualized to account for several factors
         a. Underlying comorbidities
         b. Drug interactions
         c. Infectious complications
         d. Indications for and timing of surgical interventions

II. Key Aspects of Infective Endocarditis
   A. Epidemiology
      1. Reported incidence is low: 4 to 6 cases per 100,000 person-years
         a. Increases with age
         b. Higher in males
      2. Injection drug use increases IE risk for right-sided IE or left-sided IE (or both)
      3. Majority of patients have predisposing cardiac abnormalities
         a. Highest risk groups
             1) Patients with prosthetic valves
             2) Patients who have had a previous bout of IE
         b. Mitral valve prolapse
             1) The most commonly recognized underlying predisposing cardiac condition in the United States among IE patients
             2) Valves with leaflet thickening and redundancy increase risk
      4. Health care–associated and nosocomial exposures
         a. Important in developed countries
         b. Bloodstream infection is a primary nidus for valve seeding due to infected central venous and hemodialysis catheters
   B. Pathogenesis
      1. Two modes of valve contamination
         a. Bacteremia or fungemia

b. Intraoperative contamination at the time of device placement
2. Sites of endothelial damage and subsequent platelet and fibrin deposition (so-called nonbacterial thrombotic endocarditis)
3. Staphylococci, viridans streptococci, and enterococci have unique adherence factors (adhesins) that promote valvular attachment

C. Case Definitions
1. Modified Duke Criteria
   a. Useful in clinical research and in individual patient management
   b. Blood cultures and echocardiography are pivotal
2. Transesophageal echocardiography is more sensitive than transthoracic echocardiography for detection of both vegetations and intracardiac complications (Boxes 31.1 and 31.2)

D. Etiology
1. Bacterial causes
   a. Viridans streptococci, staphylococci, and enterococci cause most cases of IE
   b. Coagulase-negative staphylococci: common causes of prosthetic valve endocarditis, particularly in the early (<60 days) postoperative period
   c. *Staphylococcus aureus*: a major cause of IE in injection drug users (other common pathogens in injection drug users: β–hemolytic streptococci, coagulase-negative staphylococci, fungi, aerobic gram-negative bacilli, and polymicrobial infection)
   d. *Staphylococcus lugdunensis*: a coagulase-negative staphylococcus that causes both native and prosthetic valve endocarditis
   e. *Streptococcus bovis*: bacteremia or IE is associated with gastrointestinal tract lesions, including colon cancer
      1) Evaluation of the gastrointestinal tract is indicated
      2) Evaluation should include colonoscopy
   f. Viridans streptococci: the most common cause of subacute IE
      1) *Streptococcus milleri* group includes *Streptococcus anginosus*, *Streptococcus intermedius*, and *Streptococcus constellatus*
      2) *Streptococcus milleri* group has a proclivity to cause abscess formation at metastatic sites of infection
   g. *Abiotrophia* and *Granulicatella* species: account for a small minority of IE cases
      1) Formerly classified as nutritionally variant streptococci
      2) *Gemella* species, like *Abiotrophia* and *Granulicatella* species, cause infections that are more difficult to treat because the bacteria have unique growth characteristics
   h. Enterococcal IE
      1) More common in elderly patients
      2) Clinical presentation is usually subacute

Box 31.1

Use of Echocardiography During Diagnosis and Treatment of Endocarditis

Early
　Echocardiography as soon as possible (<12 h after initial evaluation)
　TEE preferred, with TTE views of any abnormal findings for later comparison
　TTE if TEE is not immediately available
　TTE may be sufficient in small children
Subsequent echocardiography
　TEE after positive TTE as soon as possible in patients at high risk of complications
　TEE 7-10 d after initial TEE if suspicion exists without diagnosis of infective endocarditis or with worrisome clinical course during early treatment of infective endocarditis
Intraoperative
　Prepump: identification of vegetations, mechanism of regurgitation, abscesses, fistulae, and pseudoaneurysms
　Postpump: confirmation of successful repair of abnormal findings
　Assessment of residual valve dysfunction: elevated afterload if necessary to avoid underestimating valve insufficiency or presence of residual abnormal flow
Completion of therapy
　Establish new baseline for valve function and morphology and for ventricular size and function
　TTE usually adequate, but TEE or review of intraoperative TEE may be needed for complex anatomy to establish new baseline

Abbreviations: TEE, transesophageal echocardiography; TTE, transthoracic echocardiography.

Adapted from Baddour LM, Wilson WR, Bayer AS, Fowler VG Jr, Bolger AF, Levison ME, et al; Committee on Rheumatic Fever, Endocarditis, and Kawasaki Disease; Council on Cardiovascular Disease in the Young; Councils on Clinical Cardiology, Stroke, and Cardiovascular Surgery and Anesthesia; American Heart Association; Infectious Diseases Society of America. Infective endocarditis: diagnosis, antimicrobial therapy, and management of complications: a statement for healthcare professionals from the Committee on Rheumatic Fever, Endocarditis, and Kawasaki Disease, Council on Cardiovascular Disease in the Young, and the Councils on Clinical Cardiology, Stroke, and Cardiovascular Surgery and Anesthesia, American Heart Association: endorsed by the Infectious Diseases Society of America. Circulation. 2005 Jun 14;111(23):e394-434. Errata in: Circulation. 2007 Apr 17;115(15):e408. Circulation. 2008 Sep 16;118(12):e497. Circulation. 2007 Nov 20;116(21):e547. Circulation. 2005 Oct 11;112(15):2373. Used with permission.

> **Box 31.2**
>
> **Echocardiographic Features That Suggest Potential Need for Surgical Intervention**
>
> Vegetation
>   Persistent vegetation after systemic embolization
>   Anterior mitral leaflet vegetation, particularly with size >10 mm[a]
>   One or more embolic events during first 2 wk of antimicrobial therapy[a]
>   Increase in vegetation size despite appropriate antimicrobial therapy[a,b]
> Valvular dysfunction
>   Acute aortic or mitral insufficiency with signs of ventricular failure[b]
>   Heart failure unresponsive to medical therapy[b]
>   Valve perforation or rupture[b]
> Perivalvular extension
>   Valvular dehiscence, rupture, or fistula[b]
>   New heart block[b]
>   Large abscess or extension of abscess despite appropriate antimicrobial therapy[b]
>
> [a]Surgery may be required because of risk of embolization.
> [b]Surgery may be required because of heart failure or failure of medical therapy.
>
> Adapted from Baddour LM, Wilson WR, Bayer AS, Fowler VG Jr, Bolger AF, Levison ME, et al; Committee on Rheumatic Fever, Endocarditis, and Kawasaki Disease; Council on Cardiovascular Disease in the Young; Councils on Clinical Cardiology, Stroke, and Cardiovascular Surgery and Anesthesia; American Heart Association; Infectious Diseases Society of America. Infective endocarditis: diagnosis, antimicrobial therapy, and management of complications: a statement for healthcare professionals from the Committee on Rheumatic Fever, Endocarditis, and Kawasaki Disease, Council on Cardiovascular Disease in the Young, and the Councils on Clinical Cardiology, Stroke, and Cardiovascular Surgery and Anesthesia, American Heart Association: endorsed by the Infectious Diseases Society of America. Circulation. 2005 Jun 14;111(23):e394-434. Errata in: Circulation. 2007 Apr 17;115(15):e408. Circulation. 2008 Sep 16;118(12):e497. Circulation. 2007 Nov 20;116(21):e547. Circulation. 2005 Oct 11;112(15):2373. Used with permission.

      i. β-Hemolytic streptococci and *Streptococcus pneumoniae*
         1) Infrequent causes of IE
         2) Clinical course is acute with rapid valve destruction
      j. Organisms in the HACEK group (*Haemophilus parainfluenzae* and *Haemophilus aphrophilus*, *Actinobacillus actinomycetemcomitans*, *Cardiobacterium hominis*, *Eikenella corrodens*, and *Kingella kingae*)
         1) Subacute clinical course
         2) Prolonged incubation of specimens may be required to recover the organisms
   2. Fungal causes
      a. Fungal IE is caused by either health care–associated or nosocomial exposure in the non–injection drug use population
      b. *Candida* species are the predominant causes of fungal IE
      c. Patients usually have multiple risk factors for candidal infection
   3. Other causes
      a. Recent antibiotic use: the most common cause of IE with negative blood culture results (ie, culture-negative IE)
      b. Other more commonly recognized causes of culture-negative IE
         1) *Bartonella* species
         2) *Coxiella burnetii* (Q fever)
         3) *Brucella* species
         4) HACEK organisms
E. Treatment
   1. Antibiotic treatment regimens have been defined for the more common bacterial causes of IE (Tables 31.1-31.11)
   2. Therapy is usually administered by intravenous or intramuscular routes (exception: rifampin)
   3. Choice of antibiotic regimen for culture-negative IE may be aided by epidemiologic clues (Table 31.12)
   4. Serial laboratory screening should be performed during treatment to monitor for drug adverse events (neutropenia, renal dysfunction and nephritis, and hepatotoxicity)
F. Prophylaxis
   1. No randomized controlled studies have been conducted to evaluate the role of antibiotic prophylaxis in the prevention of IE for dental or other procedures
   2. American Heart Association 2007 guidelines have decreased the number of IE risk groups who should receive prophylaxis for certain dental or respiratory procedures
      a. In the selected groups, outcomes are more likely to be poorer if IE develops (Box 31.3)
      b. These guidelines have better clarified the dental procedures that require prophylaxis (Box 31.4)
      c. Amoxicillin, 2 g orally, approximately 1 hour before the procedure is still recommended for patients who are not allergic to penicillins (Table 31.13)
      d. Maintaining optimal dental and oral hygiene is stressed in the guidelines
      e. Antibiotic prophylaxis is no longer recommended for routine procedures involving the gastrointestinal and genitourinary tracts

Table 31.1

Therapy for Native Valve Endocarditis Caused by Highly Penicillin-Susceptible[a] Viridans Streptococci and *Streptococcus bovis*

Regimen	Dosage and Route[b,c]	Duration, wk	Strength of Recommendation[d]	Comments
Aqueous crystalline penicillin G sodium *or*	12-18 million U daily IV either continuously or in 4-6 equally divided doses	4	IA	Preferred in most patients older than 65 y and in patients with impaired function of cranial nerve VIII or impaired renal function
Ceftriaxone sodium	2 g daily IV or IM in 1 dose Pediatric: penicillin 200,000 U/kg daily IV in 4-6 equally divided doses; ceftriaxone 100 mg/kg daily IV or IM in 1 dose	4	IA	
Aqueous crystalline penicillin G sodium *or*	12-18 million U daily IV either continuously or in 6 equally divided doses	2	IB	2-wk regimen is not intended for patients with known cardiac or extracardiac abscess or for those with creatinine clearance <20 mL/min, impaired function of cranial nerve VIII, or *Abiotrophia*, *Granulicatella*, or *Gemella* species infection Gentamicin dosage should be adjusted to achieve a peak serum concentration of 3-4 μg/mL and a trough serum concentration of <1 μg/mL when 3 divided doses are used for single daily dosing
Ceftriaxone sodium *plus*	2 g daily IV or IM in 1 dose	2	IB	
Gentamicin sulfate[e]	3 mg/kg daily IV or IM in 1 dose Pediatric: penicillin 200,000 U/kg daily IV in 4-6 equally divided doses; ceftriaxone 100 mg/kg daily IV or IM in 1 dose; gentamicin 3 mg/kg daily IV or IM in 1 dose or 3 equally divided doses[f]	2		
Vancomycin hydrochloride[g]	30 mg/kg daily IV in 2 equally divided doses not to exceed 2 g daily unless concentrations in serum are inappropriately low Pediatric: 40 mg/kg daily IV in 2-3 equally divided doses	4	IB	Vancomycin therapy is recommended only for patients unable to tolerate penicillin or ceftriaxone Vancomycin dosage should be adjusted to obtain a peak (1 h after infusion completed) serum concentration of 30-45 μg/mL and a trough concentration range of 10-15 μg/mL

Abbreviations: IM, intramuscularly; IV, intravascularly; U, units.

[a] Minimum inhibitory concentration ≤0.12 μg/mL.
[b] Dosages are for patients with normal renal function.
[c] Pediatric dose should not exceed that for a healthy adult.
[d] Classification of recommendations and level of evidence are expressed in the American College of Cardiology/American Heart Association format as follows:

Classification of Recommendations

    Class I: Conditions for which there is evidence and/or general agreement that a given procedure or treatment is beneficial, useful, and effective.
    Class II: Conditions for which there is conflicting evidence and/or a divergence of opinion about the usefulness/efficacy of a procedure or treatment.
    Class IIa: Weight of evidence/opinion is in favor of usefulness/efficacy.
    Class IIb: Usefulness/efficacy is less well established by evidence/opinion.
    Class III: Conditions for which there is evidence and/or general agreement that a procedure/treatment is not useful/effective and in some cases may be harmful.

Level of Evidence

    Level of Evidence A: Data derived from multiple randomized clinical trials or meta-analyses.
    Level of Evidence B: Data derived from a single randomized trial or nonrandomized studies.
    Level of Evidence C: Only consensus opinion of experts, case studies, or standard of care.

[e] Other potentially nephrotoxic drugs (eg, nonsteroidal anti-inflammatory drugs) should be used with caution in patients receiving gentamicin therapy.
[f] Data for once-daily dosing of aminoglycosides for children exist, but there are no data for treatment of IE.

Table 31.1
(continued)

gVancomycin doses should be infused over at least 1 h to reduce risk of histamine release and red man syndrome.

Adapted from Baddour LM, Wilson WR, Bayer AS, Fowler VG Jr, Bolger AF, Levison ME, et al; Committee on Rheumatic Fever, Endocarditis, and Kawasaki Disease; Council on Cardiovascular Disease in the Young; Councils on Clinical Cardiology, Stroke, and Cardiovascular Surgery and Anesthesia; American Heart Association; Infectious Diseases Society of America. Infective endocarditis: diagnosis, antimicrobial therapy, and management of complications: a statement for healthcare professionals from the Committee on Rheumatic Fever, Endocarditis, and Kawasaki Disease, Council on Cardiovascular Disease in the Young, and the Councils on Clinical Cardiology, Stroke, and Cardiovascular Surgery and Anesthesia, American Heart Association: endorsed by the Infectious Diseases Society of America. Circulation. 2005 Jun 14;111(23):e394-434. Errata in: Circulation. 2007 Apr 17;115(15):e408. Circulation. 2008 Sep 16;118(12):e497. Circulation. 2007 Nov 20;116(21):e547. Circulation. 2005 Oct 11;112(15):2373. Used with permission.

Table 31.2
Therapy for Native Valve Endocarditis Caused by Strains of Viridans Streptococci and *Streptococcus bovis* Relatively Resistant to Penicillin[a]

Regimen	Dosage and Route[b,c]	Duration, wk	Strength of Recommendation[d]	Comments
Aqueous crystalline penicillin G sodium	24 million U daily IV either continuously or in 4-6 equally divided doses	4	IB	Patients with endocarditis caused by penicillin-resistant (MIC >5 μg/mL) strains should be treated with a regimen recommended for enterococcal endocarditis (Table 31.6)
or Ceftriaxone sodium *plus* Gentamicin sulfate[e]	2 g daily IV or IM in 1 dose	4	IB	
	3 mg/kg daily IV or IM in 1 dose	2		
	Pediatric: penicillin 300,000 U daily IV in 4-6 equally divided doses; ceftriaxone 100 mg/kg daily IV or IM in 1 dose; gentamicin 3 mg/kg daily IV or IM in 1 dose or 3 equally divided doses			
Vancomycin hydrochloride[f]	30 mg/kg daily IV in 2 equally divided doses not to exceed 2 g daily unless serum concentrations are inappropriately low	4	IB	Vancomycin therapy is recommended only for patients unable to tolerate penicillin or ceftriaxone therapy
	Pediatric: 40 mg/kg daily IV in 2 or 3 equally divided doses			

Abbreviations: IM, intramuscularly; IV, intravenously; MIC, minimum inhibitory concentration; U, units.

[a] MIC >0.12 μg/mL and ≤0.5 μg/mL.
[b] Dosages are for patients with normal renal function.
[c] Pediatric dose should not exceed that for a healthy adult.
[d] See Table 31.1 for definitions.
[e] See Table 31.1 for appropriate dosage of gentamicin.
[f] See Table 31.1 for appropriate dosage of vancomycin.

Adapted from Baddour LM, Wilson WR, Bayer AS, Fowler VG Jr, Bolger AF, Levison ME, et al; Committee on Rheumatic Fever, Endocarditis, and Kawasaki Disease; Council on Cardiovascular Disease in the Young; Councils on Clinical Cardiology, Stroke, and Cardiovascular Surgery and Anesthesia; American Heart Association; Infectious Diseases Society of America. Infective endocarditis: diagnosis, antimicrobial therapy, and management of complications: a statement for healthcare professionals from the Committee on Rheumatic Fever, Endocarditis, and Kawasaki Disease, Council on Cardiovascular Disease in the Young, and the Councils on Clinical Cardiology, Stroke, and Cardiovascular Surgery and Anesthesia, American Heart Association: endorsed by the Infectious Diseases Society of America. Circulation. 2005 Jun 14;111(23):e394-434. Errata in: Circulation. 2007 Apr 17;115(15):e408. Circulation. 2008 Sep 16;118(12):e497. Circulation. 2007 Nov 20;116(21):e547. Circulation. 2005 Oct 11;112(15):2373. Used with permission.

Table 31.3

Therapy for Endocarditis of Prosthetic Valves or Other Prosthetic Material Caused by Viridans Streptococci and *Streptococcus bovis*

Regimen	Dosage and Route[a,b]	Duration, wk	Strength of Recommendation[c]	Comments
Penicillin-Susceptible Strain (MIC ≤0.12 μg/mL)				
Aqueous crystalline penicillin G sodium	24 million U daily IV either continuously or in 4-6 equally divided doses	6	IB	Penicillin or ceftriaxone in combination with gentamicin has not demonstrated superior cure rates compared with monotherapy with penicillin or ceftriaxone for patients with a highly susceptible strain
or				
Ceftriaxone	2 g daily IV or IM in 1 dose	6	IB	
with or without				
Gentamicin sulfate[d]	3 mg/kg daily IV or IM in 1 dose Pediatric: penicillin 300,000 U/kg daily IV in 4-6 equally divided doses; ceftriaxone 100 mg/kg IV or IM once daily; gentamicin 3 mg/kg daily IV or IM in 1 dose or 3 equally divided doses	2		Gentamicin therapy should not be administered to patients who have creatinine clearance <30 mL/min
Vancomycin hydrochloride[e]	30 mg/kg daily IV in 2 equally divided doses Pediatric: 40 mg/kg daily IV or in 2 or 3 equally divided doses	6	IB	Vancomycin therapy is recommended only for patients unable to tolerate penicillin or ceftriaxone
Penicillin Relatively or Fully Resistant Strain (MIC >0.12 μg/mL)				
Aqueous crystalline penicillin sodium	24 million U daily IV either continuously or in 4-6 equally divided doses	6	IB	
or				
Ceftriaxone	2 g daily IV or IM in 1 dose	6	IB	
plus				
Gentamicin sulfate[d]	3 mg/kg daily IV or IM in 1 dose Pediatric: penicillin 300,000 U/kg daily IV in 4-6 equally divided doses	6		
Vancomycin hydrochloride[e]	30 mg/kg daily IV in 2 equally divided doses Pediatric: 40 mg/kg daily IV in 2 or 3 equally divided doses	6	IB	Vancomycin therapy is recommended only for patients unable to tolerate penicillin or ceftriaxone

Abbreviations: IM, intramuscularly; IV, intravascularly; MIC, minimum inhibitory concentration; U, units.

[a] Dosages are for patients with normal renal function.
[b] Pediatric dose should not exceed that for a healthy adult.
[c] See Table 31.1 for definitions.
[d] See Table 31.1 for appropriate dosage of gentamicin.
[e] See text and Table 31.1 for appropriate dosage of vancomycin.

Adapted from Baddour LM, Wilson WR, Bayer AS, Fowler VG Jr, Bolger AF, Levison ME, et al; Committee on Rheumatic Fever, Endocarditis, and Kawasaki Disease; Council on Cardiovascular Disease in the Young, Councils on Clinical Cardiology, Stroke, and Cardiovascular Surgery and Anesthesia; American Heart Association; Infectious Diseases Society of America. Infective endocarditis: diagnosis, antimicrobial therapy, and management of complications: a statement for healthcare professionals from the Committee on Rheumatic Fever, Endocarditis, and Kawasaki Disease, Council on Cardiovascular Disease in the Young, and the Councils on Clinical Cardiology, Stroke, and Cardiovascular Surgery and Anesthesia, American Heart Association: endorsed by the Infectious Diseases Society of America. Circulation. 2005 Jun 14;111(23):e394-434. Errata in: Circulation. 2007 Apr 17;115(15):e408. Circulation. 2008 Sep 16;118(12):e497. Circulation. 2007 Nov 20;116(21):e547. Circulation. 2005 Oct 11;112(15):2373. Used with permission.

Table 31.4

Therapy for Endocarditis Caused by Staphylococci in the Absence of Prosthetic Materials

Regimen	Dosage and Route[a,b]	Duration	Strength of Recommendation[c]	Comments
Oxacillin-Susceptible Strains				
Nafcillin[d] or Oxacillin with or without	12 g daily IV in 4-6 equally divided doses	6 wk	IA	For complicated right-sided IE and for left-sided IE; for uncomplicated right-sided IE, 2 wk
Gentamicin sulfate[e]	3 mg/kg daily IV or IM in 2 or 3 equally divided doses Pediatric: nafcillin or oxacillin 200 mg/kg daily IV in 4-6 equally divided doses; gentamicin 3 mg/kg daily IV or IM in 3 equally divided doses	3-5 d		Clinical benefit of aminoglycosides has not been established
For penicillin-allergic (nonanaphylactoid-type) patients				Consider skin testing for oxacillin-susceptible staphylococci and questionable history of immediate-type hypersensitivity to penicillin
Cefazolin with or without	6 g daily IV in 3 equally divided doses	4-6 wk	IB	Cephalosporins should be avoided in patients with anaphylactoid-type hypersensitivity to β-lactams; vancomycin should be used in these cases[f]
Gentamicin sulfate[e]	3 mg/kg daily IV or IM in 2 or 3 equally divided doses Pediatric: cefazolin 100 mg/kg daily IV in 3 equally divided doses; gentamicin 3 mg/kg daily IV or IM in 3 equally divided doses	3-5 d		Clinical benefit of aminoglycosides has not been established
Oxacillin-Resistant Strains				
Vancomycin[f]	30 mg/kg daily IV in 2 equally divided doses Pediatric: 40 mg/kg daily IV in 2 or 3 equally divided doses	6 wk	IB	Adjust vancomycin dosage to achieve 1-h serum concentration of 30-45 μg/mL and trough concentration of 10-15 μg/mL

Abbreviations: IE, infective endocarditis; IM, intramuscularly; IV, intravenously.

[a] Dosages are for patients with normal renal function.
[b] Pediatric dose should not exceed that for a healthy adult.
[c] See Table 31.1 for definitions.
[d] Penicillin G 24 million units daily may be used instead of nafcillin or oxacillin if the strain is penicillin susceptible (minimum inhibitory concentration ≤0.1 μg/mL).
[e] Gentamicin should be administered in temporal proximity to vancomycin, nafcillin, or oxacillin administration.
[f] For specific dosing adjustment and issues concerning vancomycin, see Table 31.1.

Adapted from Baddour LM, Wilson WR, Bayer AS, Fowler VG Jr, Bolger AF, Levison ME, et al; Committee on Rheumatic Fever, Endocarditis, and Kawasaki Disease; Council on Cardiovascular Disease in the Young; Councils on Clinical Cardiology, Stroke, and Cardiovascular Surgery and Anesthesia; American Heart Association; Infectious Diseases Society of America. Infective endocarditis: diagnosis, antimicrobial therapy, and management of complications: a statement for healthcare professionals from the Committee on Rheumatic Fever, Endocarditis, and Kawasaki Disease, Council on Cardiovascular Disease in the Young, and the Councils on Clinical Cardiology, Stroke, and Cardiovascular Surgery and Anesthesia, American Heart Association: endorsed by the Infectious Diseases Society of America. Circulation. 2005 Jun 14;111(23):e394-434. Errata in: Circulation. 2008 Sep 16;118(12):e497. Circulation. 2007 Apr 17;115(15):e408. Circulation. 2007 Nov 20;116(21):e547. Circulation. 2005 Oct 11;112(15):2373. Used with permission.

Table 31.5

Therapy for Prosthetic Valve Endocarditis Caused by Staphylococci

Regimen	Dosage and Route[a,b]	Duration, wk	Strength of Recommendation[c]	Comments
Oxacillin-Susceptible Strains				
Nafcillin or oxacillin	12 g daily IV in 6 equally divided doses	≥6	IB	Penicillin G 24 million U daily in 4-6 equally divided doses may be used in place of nafcillin or oxacillin if strain is penicillin susceptible (MIC ≤0.1 μg/mL) and does not produce β-lactamase
plus				
Rifampin	900 mg IV or PO in 3 equally divided doses	≤6		Vancomycin should be used in patients with immediate-type hypersensitivity reactions to β-lactam antibiotics (see Table 31.1 for dosing guidelines)
plus				
Gentamicin[d]	3 mg/kg daily IV or IM in 2 or 3 equally divided doses Pediatric: nafcillin or oxacillin 200 mg/kg daily IV in 4-6 equally divided doses; rifampin 20 mg/kg daily PO or IV in 3 equally divided doses; gentamicin 3 mg/kg daily IV or IM in 3 equally divided doses	2		Cefazolin may be substituted for nafcillin or oxacillin in patients with non-immediate hypersensitivity reactions to penicillin
Oxacillin-Resistant Strains				
Vancomycin	30 mg/kg daily in 2 equally divided doses	≥6	IB	Adjust vancomycin to achieve 1-h serum concentration of 30-45 μg/mL and trough concentration of 10-15 μg/mL
plus				
Rifampin	900 mg daily IV or PO in 3 equally divided doses	≥6		
plus				
Gentamicin[d]	3 mg/kg daily IV or IM in 2 or 3 equally divided doses Pediatric: vancomycin 40 mg/kg daily IV in 2 or 3 equally divided doses; rifampin 20 mg/kg daily IV or PO in 3 equally divided doses (up to the adult dose); gentamicin 3 mg/kg daily IV or IM in 3 equally divided doses	2		

Abbreviations: IM, intramuscularly; IV, intravenously; MIC, minimum inhibitory concentration; PO, orally; U, units.

[a] Dosages are for patients with normal renal function.
[b] Pediatric dose should not exceed that for a healthy adult.
[c] See Table 31.1 for definitions.
[d] Gentamicin should be administered in temporal proximity to vancomycin, nafcillin, or oxacillin administration.

Adapted from Baddour LM, Wilson WR, Bayer AS, Fowler VG Jr, Bolger AF, Levison ME, et al; Committee on Rheumatic Fever, Endocarditis, and Kawasaki Disease; Council on Cardiovascular Disease in the Young; Councils on Clinical Cardiology, Stroke, and Cardiovascular Surgery and Anesthesia; American Heart Association; Infectious Diseases Society of America. Infective endocarditis: diagnosis, antimicrobial therapy, and management of complications: a statement for healthcare professionals from the Committee on Rheumatic Fever, Endocarditis, and Kawasaki Disease, Council on Cardiovascular Disease in the Young, and the Councils on Clinical Cardiology, Stroke, and Cardiovascular Surgery and Anesthesia, American Heart Association: endorsed by the Infectious Diseases Society of America. Circulation. 2005 Jun 14;111(23):e394-434. Errata in: Circulation. 2007 Apr 17;115(15):e408. Circulation. 2008 Sep 16;118(12):e497. Circulation. 2007 Nov 20;116(21):e547. Circulation. 2005 Oct 11;112(15):2373. Used with permission.

Table 31.6

Therapy for Native Valve or Prosthetic Valve Enterococcal Endocarditis Caused by Strains Susceptible to Penicillin, Gentamicin, and Vancomycin

Regimen	Dosage and Route[a,b]	Duration, wk	Strength of Recommendation[c]	Comments
Ampicillin sodium *or*	12 g daily IV in 6 equally divided doses	4-6	IA	Endocarditis involving a native valve: recommended duration of therapy is 4 wk for patients with symptoms of illness ≤3 mo and 6 wk for patients with symptoms >3 mo
Aqueous crystalline penicillin G sodium *plus*	18-30 million U daily IV either continuously or in 6 equally divided doses	4-6	IA	Endocarditis involving a prosthetic valve or other prosthetic cardiac material: recommended duration of therapy is ≥6 wk
Gentamicin sulfate[d]	3 mg/kg daily IV or IM in 3 equally divided doses Pediatric: ampicillin 300 mg/kg daily IV in 4-6 equally divided doses; penicillin 300,000 U/kg daily IV in 4-6 equally divided doses; gentamicin 3 mg/kg daily IV or IM in 3 equally divided doses	4-6		
Vancomycin hydrochloride[e] *plus*	30 mg/kg daily IV in 2 equally divided doses	6	IB	Vancomycin therapy is recommended only for patients unable to tolerate penicillin or ampicillin
Gentamicin sulfate[d]	3 mg/kg daily IV or IM in 3 equally divided doses Pediatric: vancomycin 40 mg/kg daily IV in 2 or 3 equally divided doses; gentamicin 3 mg/kg daily IV or IM in 3 equally divided doses	6		Recommended duration of vancomycin therapy is 6 wk because of decreased activity against enterococci

Abbreviations: IM, intramuscularly; IV, intravenously; U, units.

[a] Dosages are for patients with normal renal function.
[b] Pediatric dose should not exceed that for a healthy adult.
[c] See Table 31.1 for definitions.
[d] The dosage of gentamicin should be adjusted to achieve a peak serum concentration of 3-4 μg/mL and a trough concentration of <1 μg/L. Patients with creatinine clearance <50 mL/min should be treated in consultation with an infectious diseases specialist.
[e] See Table 31.1 for appropriate dosing of vancomycin.

Adapted from Baddour LM, Wilson WR, Bayer AS, Fowler VG Jr, Bolger AF, Levison ME, et al; Committee on Rheumatic Fever, Endocarditis, and Kawasaki Disease; Council on Cardiovascular Disease in the Young; Councils on Clinical Cardiology, Stroke, and Cardiovascular Surgery and Anesthesia; American Heart Association; Infectious Diseases Society of America. Infective endocarditis: diagnosis, antimicrobial therapy, and management of complications: a statement for healthcare professionals from the Committee on Rheumatic Fever, Endocarditis, and Kawasaki Disease, Council on Cardiovascular Disease in the Young, and the Councils on Clinical Cardiology, Stroke, and Cardiovascular Surgery and Anesthesia, American Heart Association: endorsed by the Infectious Diseases Society of America. Circulation. 2005 Jun 14;111(23):e394-434. Errata in: Circulation. 2007 Apr 17;115(15):e408. Circulation. 2008 Sep 16;118(12):e497. Circulation. 2007 Nov 20;116(21):e547. Circulation. 2005 Oct 11;112(15):2373. Used with permission.

Table 31.7

Therapy for Native Valve or Prosthetic Valve Enterococcal Endocarditis Caused by Strains Susceptible to Penicillin, Streptomycin, and Vancomycin and Resistant to Gentamicin

Regimen	Dosage and Route[a,b]	Duration, wk	Strength of Recommendation[c]	Comments
Ampicillin sodium or	12 g daily IV in 6 equally divided doses	4-6	IA	Endocarditis involving a native valve: recommended duration of therapy is 4 wk for patients with symptoms of illness ≤3 mo and 6 wk for patients with symptoms >3 mo
Aqueous crystalline penicillin G sodium plus	24 million U daily IV continuously or in 6 equally divided doses	4-6	IA	Endocarditis involving a prosthetic valve or other prosthetic cardiac material: recommended duration of therapy is ≥6 wk
Streptomycin sulfate	15 mg/kg daily IV or IM in 2 equally divided doses Pediatric: ampicillin 300 mg/kg daily IV in 4-6 equally divided doses; penicillin 300,000 U/kg daily IV in 4-6 equally divided doses; streptomycin 20-30 mg/kg daily IV or IM in 2 equally divided doses	4-6		
Vancomycin hydrochloride[d] plus	30 mg/kg daily IV in 2 equally divided doses	6	IB	Vancomycin therapy is recommended only for patients unable to tolerate penicillin or ampicillin
Streptomycin sulfate	15 mg/kg daily IV or IM in 2 equally divided doses Pediatric: vancomycin 40 mg/kg daily IV in 2 or 3 equally divided doses; streptomycin 20-30 mg/kg daily IV or IM in 2 equally divided doses	6		

Abbreviations: IM, intramuscularly; IV, intravenously; U, units.

[a] Dosages are for patients with normal renal function. Patients with creatinine clearance <50 mL/min should be treated in consultation with an infectious diseases specialist.
[b] Pediatric dose should not exceed that for a healthy adult.
[c] See Table 31.1 for definitions.
[d] See Table 31.1 for appropriate dosing of vancomycin.

Adapted from Baddour LM, Wilson WR, Bayer AS, Fowler VG Jr, Bolger AF, Levison ME, et al; Committee on Rheumatic Fever, Endocarditis, and Kawasaki Disease; Council on Cardiovascular Disease in the Young; Councils on Clinical Cardiology, Stroke, and Cardiovascular Surgery and Anesthesia; American Heart Association; Infective endocarditis: diagnosis, antimicrobial therapy, and management of complications: a statement for healthcare professionals from the Committee on Rheumatic Fever, Endocarditis, and Kawasaki Disease, Council on Cardiovascular Disease in the Young, and the Councils on Clinical Cardiology, Stroke, and Cardiovascular Surgery and Anesthesia, American Heart Association: endorsed by the Infectious Diseases Society of America. Circulation. 2005 Jun 14;111(23):e394-434. Errata in: Circulation. 2007 Apr 17;115(15):e408. Circulation. 2008 Sep 16;118(12):e497. Circulation. 2007 Nov 20;116(21):e547. Circulation. 2005 Oct 11;112(15):2373. Used with permission.

Table 31.8

Therapy for Native Valve or Prosthetic Valve Enterococcal Endocarditis Caused by Strains Resistant to Penicillin and Susceptible to Aminoglycosides and Vancomycin

Regimen	Dosage and Route[a,b]	Duration, wk	Strength of Recommendation[c]	Comments
β-Lactamase–Producing Strain				
Ampicillin-sulbactam plus	12 g daily IV in 4 equally divided doses	6	IIaC	Unlikely that the strain will be susceptible to gentamicin
Gentamicin sulfate[d]	3 mg/kg daily IV or IM in 3 equally divided doses Pediatric: ampicillin-sulbactam 300 mg/kg daily IV in 4 equally divided doses; gentamicin 3 mg/kg daily IV or IM in 3 equally divided doses	6		If strain is gentamicin resistant, then >6 wk of ampicillin-sulbactam therapy will be needed
Vancomycin hydrochloride[e] plus	30 mg/kg daily IV in 2 equally divided doses	6	IIaC	Vancomycin therapy is recommended only for patients unable to tolerate ampicillin-sulbactam
Gentamicin sulfate[d]	3 mg/kg daily IV or IM in 3 equally divided doses Pediatric: vancomycin 40 mg/kg daily IV in 2 or 3 equally divided doses; gentamicin 3 mg/kg daily IV or IM in 3 equally divided doses	6		
Intrinsic Penicillin Resistance				
Vancomycin hydrochloride[e] plus	30 mg/kg daily IV in 2 equally divided doses	6	IIaC	Consultation with a specialist in infectious diseases is recommended
Gentamicin sulfate[d]	3 mg/kg daily IV or IM in equally divided doses Pediatric: vancomycin 40 mg/kg daily IV in 2 or 3 equally divided doses; gentamicin 3 mg/kg daily IV or IM in 3 equally divided doses	6		

Abbreviations: IM, intramuscularly; IV, intravenously.

[a] Dosages are for patients with normal renal function; see Table 31.3 for patients with creatinine clearance <30 mL/min.
[b] Pediatric dose should not exceed that for a healthy adult.
[c] See Table 31.1 for definitions.
[d] See Table 31.1 for appropriate dosing of gentamicin.
[e] See Table 31.1 for appropriate dosing of vancomycin.

Adapted from Baddour LM, Wilson WR, Bayer AS, Fowler VG Jr, Bolger AF, Levison ME, et al; Committee on Rheumatic Fever, Endocarditis, and Kawasaki Disease; Council on Cardiovascular Disease in the Young; Councils on Clinical Cardiology, Stroke, and Cardiovascular Surgery and Anesthesia; American Heart Association; Infectious Diseases Society of America. Infective endocarditis: diagnosis, antimicrobial therapy, and management of complications: a statement for healthcare professionals from the Committee on Rheumatic Fever, Endocarditis, and Kawasaki Disease, Council on Cardiovascular Disease in the Young, and the Councils on Clinical Cardiology, Stroke, and Cardiovascular Surgery and Anesthesia, American Heart Association: endorsed by the Infectious Diseases Society of America. Circulation. 2005 Jun 14;111(23):e394-434. Errata in: Circulation. 2007 Apr 17;115(15):e408. Circulation. 2008 Sep 16;118(12):e497. Circulation. 2007 Nov 20;116(21):e547. Circulation. 2005 Oct 11;112(15):2373. Used with permission.

Table 31.9

Therapy for Native Valve or Prosthetic Valve Enterococcal Endocarditis Caused by Strains Resistant to Penicillin, Aminoglycosides, and Vancomycin

Regimen[a]	Dosage and Route[b,c]	Duration, wk	Strength of Recommendation[d]	Comments
Agent: *Enterococcus faecium*				
Linezolid	1,200 mg daily IV or PO in 2 equally divided doses	≥8	IIaC	Patients with endocarditis caused by these strains should be treated in consultation with an infectious diseases specialist
or				Cardiac valve replacement may be necessary for bacteriologic cure
Quinupristin-dalfopristin	22.5 mg/kg daily IV in 3 equally divided doses	≥8	IIbC	Cure with antimicrobial therapy alone may be <50%
				Severe, usually reversible thrombocytopenia may occur with use of linezolid, especially after 2 wk of therapy
				Quinupristin-dalfopristin is effective against only *E faecium* and can cause severe myalgias, which may require discontinuation of therapy
				Only a small number of patients have reportedly been treated with imipenem-cilastatin plus ampicillin or with ceftriaxone plus ampicillin
Agent: *Enterococcus faecalis*				
Imipenem-cilastatin	2 g daily IV in 4 equally divided doses	≥8	IIbC	
plus				
Ampicillin sodium	12 g daily IV in 6 equally divided doses	≥8		
or				
Ceftriaxone sodium	2 g daily IV or IM in 1 dose	≥8	IIbC	
plus				
Ampicillin sodium	12 g daily IV in 6 equally divided doses	≥8		
	Pediatric: linezolid 30 mg/kg daily IV or PO in 3 equally divided doses; quinupristin-dalfopristin 22.5 mg/kg daily IV in 3 equally divided doses; imipenem-cilastatin 60-100 mg/kg daily IV in 4 equally divided doses; ampicillin 300 mg/kg daily IV in 4-6 equally divided doses; ceftriaxone 100 mg/kg daily IV or IM once daily			

Abbreviations: IM, intramuscularly; IV, intravenously; PO, orally.

[a] Regimens are listed in decreasing order of preference based on published data.
[b] Dosages are for patients with normal renal function.
[c] Pediatric dose should not exceed that for a healthy adult.
[d] See Table 31.1 for definitions.

Adapted from Baddour LM, Wilson WR, Bayer AS, Fowler VG Jr, Bolger AF, Levison ME, et al; Committee on Rheumatic Fever, Endocarditis, and Kawasaki Disease; Council on Cardiovascular Disease in the Young; Councils on Clinical Cardiology, Stroke, and Cardiovascular Surgery and Anesthesia; American Heart Association; Infectious Diseases Society of America. Infective endocarditis: diagnosis, antimicrobial therapy, and management of complications: a statement for healthcare professionals from the Committee on Rheumatic Fever, Endocarditis, and Kawasaki Disease, Council on Cardiovascular Disease in the Young, and the Councils on Clinical Cardiology, Stroke, and Cardiovascular Surgery and Anesthesia, American Heart Association: endorsed by the Infectious Diseases Society of America. Circulation. 2005 Jun 14;111(23):e394-434. Errata in: Circulation. 2007 Apr 17;115(15):e408. Circulation. 2008 Sep 16;118(12):e497. Circulation. 2007 Nov 20;116(21):e547. Circulation. 2005 Oct 11;112(15):2373. Used with permission.

Table 31.10
Therapy for Both Native Valve and Prosthetic Valve Endocarditis Caused by HACEK Microorganisms

Regimen	Dosage and Route[a]	Duration, wk	Strength of Recommendation[b]	Comments
Ceftriaxone sodium *or*	2 g daily IV or IM in 1 dose[c]	4	IB	Cefotaxime or another third- or fourth-generation cephalosporin may be substituted
Ampicillin-sulbactam[d] *or*	12 g daily IV in 4 equally divided doses	4	IIaB	
Ciprofloxacin[d,e]	1,000 mg daily PO or 800 mg daily IV in 2 equally divided doses Pediatric: ceftriaxone 100 mg/kg daily IV or IM once daily; ampicillin-sulbactam 300 mg/kg daily IV in 4-6 equally divided doses; ciprofloxacin 20-30 mg/kg daily IV or PO in 2 equally divided doses	4	IIbC	Fluoroquinolone therapy recommended only for patients unable to tolerate cephalosporin and ampicillin therapy Levofloxacin, gatifloxacin, or moxifloxacin may be substituted Fluoroquinolones generally not recommended for patients younger than 18 y Endocarditis involving a prosthetic valve or other prosthetic cardiac material: recommended duration of therapy is 6 wk

Abbreviations: HACEK, *Haemophilus parainfluenzae* and *Haemophilus aphrophilus, Actinobacillus actinomycetemcomitans, Cardiobacterium hominis, Eikenella corrodens,* and *Kingella kingae*; IM, intramuscularly; IV, intravenously; PO, orally.

[a] Pediatric dose should not exceed that for a healthy adult.
[b] See Table 31.1 for definitions.
[c] Patients should be informed that IM injection of ceftriaxone is painful.
[d] Dosage is for patients with normal renal function.
[e] Fluoroquinolones are highly active in vitro against HACEK microorganisms. Published data on use of fluoroquinolone therapy for endocarditis caused by HACEK are minimal.

Adapted from Baddour LM, Wilson WR, Bayer AS, Fowler VG Jr, Bolger AF, Levison ME, et al; Committee on Rheumatic Fever, Endocarditis, and Kawasaki Disease; Council on Cardiovascular Disease in the Young; Councils on Clinical Cardiology, Stroke, and Cardiovascular Surgery and Anesthesia; American Heart Association; Infectious Diseases Society of America. Infective endocarditis: diagnosis, antimicrobial therapy, and management of complications: a statement for healthcare professionals from the Committee on Rheumatic Fever, Endocarditis, and Kawasaki Disease, Council on Cardiovascular Disease in the Young, and the Councils on Clinical Cardiology, Stroke, and Cardiovascular Surgery and Anesthesia, American Heart Association: endorsed by the Infectious Diseases Society of America. Circulation. 2005 Jun 14;111(23):e394-434. Errata in: Circulation. 2008 Sep 16;118(12):e497. Circulation. 2007 Apr 17;115(15):e408. Circulation. 2007 Nov 20;116(21):e547. Circulation. 2005 Oct 11;112(15):2373. Used with permission.

Table 31.11

Therapy for Culture-Negative Endocarditis and *Bartonella* Endocarditis

Regimen	Dosage and Route[a,b]	Duration, wk	Strength of Recommendation[c]	Comments
Native Valve Endocarditis				
Ampicillin-sulbactam	12 g daily IV in 4 equally divided doses	4-6	IIbC	Patients with culture-negative endocarditis should be treated in consultation with an infectious diseases specialist
plus				
Gentamicin sulfate[d]	3 mg/kg daily IV or IM in 3 equally divided doses	4-6		
Vancomycin[e]	30 mg/kg daily IV in 2 equally divided doses	4-6	IIbC	Vancomycin is recommended only for patients who are unable to tolerate penicillins
plus				
Gentamicin sulfate	3 mg/kg daily IV or IM in 3 equally divided doses	4-6		
plus				
Ciprofloxacin	1,000 mg daily PO or 800 mg daily IV in 2 equally divided doses Pediatric: ampicillin-sulbactam 300 mg/kg daily IV in 4-6 equally divided doses; gentamicin 3 mg/kg daily IV or IM in 3 equally divided doses; vancomycin 40 mg/kg daily in 2 or 3 equally divided doses; ciprofloxacin 20-30 mg/kg daily IV or PO in 2 equally divided doses	4-6		
Early (≤1 y) Prosthetic Valve Endocarditis				
Vancomycin	30 mg/kg daily IV in 2 equally divided doses	6	IIbC	
plus				
Gentamicin sulfate	3 mg/kg daily IV or IM in 3 equally divided doses	2		
plus				
Cefepime	6 g daily IV in 3 equally divided doses	6		
plus				
Rifampin	900 mg daily PO or IV in 3 equally divided doses Pediatric: vancomycin 40 mg/kg daily IV in 2 or 3 equally divided doses; gentamicin 3 mg/kg daily IV or IM in 3 equally divided doses; cefepime 150 mg/kg daily IV in 3 equally divided doses; rifampin 20 mg/kg daily PO or IV in 3 equally divided doses	6		
Late (>1 y) Prosthetic Valve Endocarditis				
Same regimens as listed above for native valve endocarditis		6	IIbC	
Suspected *Bartonella* Endocarditis (Culture Negative)				
Ceftriaxone sodium	2 g daily IV or IM in 1 dose	6	IIaB	Patients with *Bartonella* endocarditis should be treated in consultation with an infectious diseases specialist
plus				
Gentamicin sulfate	3 mg/kg daily IV or IM in 3 equally divided doses	2		
with or without				
Doxycycline	200 mg/kg daily IV or PO in 2 equally divided doses	6		

Documented *Bartonella* Endocarditis (Culture Positive)

Doxycycline	200 mg daily IV or PO in 2 equally divided doses	6	
plus			
Gentamicin sulfate	3 mg/kg daily IV or IM in 3 equally divided doses	2	IIaB	If gentamicin cannot be given, replace it with rifampin, 600 mg daily PO or IV in 2 equally divided doses
	Pediatric: ceftriaxone 100 mg/kg daily IV or IM once daily; gentamicin 3 mg/kg daily IV or IM in 3 equally divided doses; doxycycline 2-4 mg/kg daily IV or PO in 2 equally divided doses; rifampin 20 mg/kg daily PO or IV in 2 equally divided doses		

Abbreviations: IM, intramuscularly; IV, intravenously; PO, orally.

[a] Dosages are for patients with normal renal function; see Table 31.3 for patients with creatinine clearance <30 mL/min.
[b] Pediatric dose should not exceed that for a healthy adult.
[c] See Table 31.1 for definitions.
[d] See Table 31.1 for appropriate dosing of gentamicin.
[e] See Table 31.1 for appropriate dosing of vancomycin.

Adapted from Baddour LM, Wilson WR, Bayer AS, Fowler VG Jr, Bolger AF, Levison ME, et al; Committee on Rheumatic Fever, Endocarditis, and Kawasaki Disease; Council on Cardiovascular Disease in the Young; Councils on Clinical Cardiology, Stroke, and Cardiovascular Surgery and Anesthesia; American Heart Association; Infectious Diseases Society of America. Infective endocarditis: diagnosis, antimicrobial therapy, and management of complications: a statement for healthcare professionals from the Committee on Rheumatic Fever, Endocarditis, and Kawasaki Disease, Council on Cardiovascular Disease in the Young, and the Councils on Clinical Cardiology, Stroke, and Cardiovascular Surgery and Anesthesia, American Heart Association: endorsed by the Infectious Diseases Society of America. Circulation. 2005 Jun 14;111(23):e394–434. Errata in: Circulation. 2007 Apr 17;115(15):e408. Circulation. 2008 Sep 16;118(12):e497. Circulation. 2007 Nov 20;116(21):e547. Circulation. 2005 Oct 11;112(15):2373. Used with permission.

Table 31.12

Epidemiologic Clues in Etiologic Diagnosis of Culture-Negative Endocarditis

Epidemiologic Feature	Common Microorganisms
Injection drug use	*Staphylococcus aureus*, including community-acquired oxacillin-resistant strains Coagulase-negative staphylococci β-Hemolytic streptococci Fungi Aerobic gram-negative bacilli, including *Pseudomonas aeruginosa* Polymicrobial populations
Indwelling cardiovascular medical devices	*S aureus* Coagulase-negative staphylococci Fungi Aerobic gram-negative bacilli *Corynebacterium* species
Genitourinary tract disorders, infection, or manipulation, including pregnancy, delivery, and abortion	*Enterococcus* species Group B streptococci (*Streptococcus agalactiae*) *Listeria monocytogenes* Aerobic gram-negative bacilli *Neisseria gonorrhoeae*
Chronic skin disorders, including recurrent infections	*S aureus* β-Hemolytic streptococci
Poor dental health or dental procedures	Viridans streptococci "Nutritionally variant streptococci" *Abiotrophia defectiva* *Granulicatella* species *Gemella* species HACEK organisms
Alcoholism or cirrhosis	*Bartonella* species *Aeromonas* species *Listeria* species *Streptococcus pneumoniae* β-Hemolytic streptococci
Burn patients	*S aureus* Aerobic gram-negative bacilli, including *Pseudomonas aeruginosa* Fungi
Diabetes mellitus	*S aureus* β-Hemolytic streptococci *S pneumoniae*
Early (≤1 y) prosthetic valve placement	Coagulase-negative staphylococci *S aureus* Aerobic gram-negative bacilli Fungi *Corynebacterium* species *Legionella* species
Late (>1 y) prosthetic valve placement	Coagulase-negative staphylococci *S aureus* Viridans streptococci *Enterococcus* species Fungi *Corynebacterium* species
Dog or cat exposure	*Bartonella* species *Pasteurella* species *Capnocytophaga* species
Contact with contaminated milk or infected farm animals	*Brucella* species *Coxiella burnetii* *Erysipelothrix* species
Homelessness or body lice	*Bartonella* species
AIDS	*Salmonella* species *S pneumoniae* *S aureus*
Pneumonia or meningitis	*S pneumoniae*

Table 31.12
(continued)

Epidemiologic Feature	Common Microorganisms
Solid organ transplant	S aureus
	Aspergillus fumigatus
	Enterococcus species
	Candida species
Gastrointestinal tract lesions	Streptococcus bovis
	Enterococcus species
	Clostridium septicum

Abbreviation: HACEK, *Haemophilus parainfluenzae* and *Haemophilus aphrophilus*, *Actinobacillus actinomycetemcomitans*, *Cardiobacterium hominis*, *Eikenella corrodens*, and *Kingella kingae*.

Adapted from Baddour LM, Wilson WR, Bayer AS, Fowler VG Jr, Bolger AF, Levison ME, et al; Committee on Rheumatic Fever, Endocarditis, and Kawasaki Disease; Council on Cardiovascular Disease in the Young; Councils on Clinical Cardiology, Stroke, and Cardiovascular Surgery and Anesthesia; American Heart Association; Infectious Diseases Society of America. Infective endocarditis: diagnosis, antimicrobial therapy, and management of complications: a statement for healthcare professionals from the Committee on Rheumatic Fever, Endocarditis, and Kawasaki Disease, Council on Cardiovascular Disease in the Young, and the Councils on Clinical Cardiology, Stroke, and Cardiovascular Surgery and Anesthesia, American Heart Association: endorsed by the Infectious Diseases Society of America. Circulation. 2005 Jun 14;111(23):e394-434. Errata in: Circulation. 2007 Apr 17;115(15):e408. Circulation. 2008 Sep 16;118(12):e497. Circulation. 2007 Nov 20;116(21):e547. Circulation. 2005 Oct 11;112(15):2373. Used with permission.

Table 31.13
Regimens for a Dental Procedure

		Regimen: Single Dose 30-60 min Before Procedure	
Situation	Agent	Adults	Children
Oral administration	Amoxicillin	2 g	50 mg/kg
Unable to take oral medication	Ampicillin	2 g IM or IV	50 mg/kg IM or IV
	or		
	Cefazolin or ceftriaxone	1 g IM or IV	50 mg/kg IM or IV
Allergic to penicillins or ampicillin: oral administration	Cephalexin[a,b]	2 g	50 mg/kg
	or		
	Clindamycin	600 mg	20 mg/kg
	or		
	Azithromycin or clarithromycin	500 mg	15 mg/kg
Allergic to penicillins or ampicillin and unable to take oral medication	Cefazolin or ceftriaxone[b]	1 g IM or IV	50 mg/kg IM or IV
	or		
	Clindamycin	600 mg IM or IV	20 mg/kg IM or IV

Abbreviations: IM, intramuscularly; IV, intravenously.

[a] Or other first- or second-generation oral cephalosporin in an equivalent adult or pediatric dosage.

[b] Cephalosporins should not be used in a patient who has a history of anaphylaxis, angioedema, or urticaria with penicillins or ampicillin.

Adapted from Wilson W, Taubert KA, Gewitz M, Lockhart PB, Baddour LM, Levison M, et al; American Heart Association Rheumatic Fever, Endocarditis, and Kawasaki Disease Committee; American Heart Association Council on Cardiovascular Disease in the Young; American Heart Association Council on Clinical Cardiology; American Heart Association Council on Cardiovascular Surgery and Anesthesia; Quality of Care and Outcomes Research Interdisciplinary Working Group. Prevention of infective endocarditis: guidelines from the American Heart Association: a guideline from the American Heart Association Rheumatic Fever, Endocarditis, and Kawasaki Disease Committee, Council on Cardiovascular Disease in the Young, and the Council on Clinical Cardiology, Council on Cardiovascular Surgery and Anesthesia, and the Quality of Care and Outcomes Research Interdisciplinary Working Group. Circulation. 2007 Oct 9;116(15):1736-54. Epub 2007 Apr 19. Erratum in: Circulation. 2007 Oct 9;116(15):e376-7. Used with permission.

Box 31.3

Cardiac Conditions Associated With the Highest Risk of Adverse Outcomes From Endocarditis for Which Prophylaxis With Dental Procedures Is Reasonable

Prosthetic cardiac valve or prosthetic material used for cardiac valve repair
Previous infective endocarditis
Congenital heart disease (CHD)[a]
- Unrepaired cyanotic CHD, including palliative shunts and conduits
- Completely repaired congenital heart defect with prosthetic material or device, whether placed by surgery or by catheter intervention, during the first 6 mo after the procedure[b]
- Repaired CHD with residual defects at the site or adjacent to the site of a prosthetic patch or prosthetic device (which inhibit endothelialization)

Cardiac valvulopathy that develops in cardiac transplant recipients

[a] Antibiotic prophylaxis is no longer recommended for CHD except for the conditions listed.
[b] Prophylaxis is reasonable because endothelialization of prosthetic material occurs within 6 months after the procedure.

Adapted from Wilson W, Taubert KA, Gewitz M, Lockhart PB, Baddour LM, Levison M, et al; American Heart Association Rheumatic Fever, Endocarditis, and Kawasaki Disease Committee; American Heart Association Council on Cardiovascular Disease in the Young; American Heart Association Council on Clinical Cardiology; American Heart Association Council on Cardiovascular Surgery and Anesthesia; Quality of Care and Outcomes Research Interdisciplinary Working Group. Prevention of infective endocarditis: guidelines from the American Heart Association: a guideline from the American Heart Association Rheumatic Fever, Endocarditis, and Kawasaki Disease Committee, Council on Cardiovascular Disease in the Young, and the Council on Clinical Cardiology, Council on Cardiovascular Surgery and Anesthesia, and the Quality of Care and Outcomes Research Interdisciplinary Working Group. Circulation. 2007 Oct 9;116(15):1736-54. Epub 2007 Apr 19. Erratum in: Circulation. 2007 Oct 9;116(15):e376-7. Used with permission.

Box 31.4

Dental Procedures for Which Endocarditis Prophylaxis Is Reasonable for Patients in Box 31.3

All dental procedures that involve manipulation of gingival tissue or the periapical region of teeth or perforation of the oral mucosa[a]

[a] Prophylaxis is not needed for the following procedures and events: routine anesthetic injections through noninfected tissue, dental radiographs, placement of removable prosthodontic or orthodontic appliances, adjustment of orthodontic appliances, placement of orthodontic brackets, shedding of deciduous teeth, and bleeding from trauma to the lips or oral mucosa.

Adapted from Wilson W, Taubert KA, Gewitz M, Lockhart PB, Baddour LM, Levison M, et al; American Heart Association Rheumatic Fever, Endocarditis, and Kawasaki Disease Committee; American Heart Association Council on Cardiovascular Disease in the Young; American Heart Association Council on Clinical Cardiology; American Heart Association Council on Cardiovascular Surgery and Anesthesia; Quality of Care and Outcomes Research Interdisciplinary Working Group. Prevention of infective endocarditis: guidelines from the American Heart Association: a guideline from the American Heart Association Rheumatic Fever, Endocarditis, and Kawasaki Disease Committee, Council on Cardiovascular Disease in the Young, and the Council on Clinical Cardiology, Council on Cardiovascular Surgery and Anesthesia, and the Quality of Care and Outcomes Research Interdisciplinary Working Group. Circulation. 2007 Oct 9;116(15):1736-54. Epub 2007 Apr 19. Erratum in: Circulation. 2007 Oct 9;116(15):e376-7. Used with permission.

Suggested Reading

Baddour LM, Bettmann MA, Bolger AF, Epstein AE, Ferrieri P, Gerber MA, et al; AHA. Nonvalvular cardiovascular device-related infections. Circulation. 2003 Oct 21;108(16):2015–31.

Baddour LM, Wilson WR, Bayer AS, Fowler VG Jr, Bolger AF, Levison ME, et al; Committee on Rheumatic Fever, Endocarditis, and Kawasaki Disease; Council on Cardiovascular Disease in the Young; Councils on Clinical Cardiology, Stroke, and Cardiovascular Surgery and Anesthesia; American Heart Association; Infectious Diseases Society of America. Infective endocarditis: diagnosis, antimicrobial therapy, and management of complications: a statement for healthcare professionals from the Committee on Rheumatic Fever, Endocarditis, and Kawasaki Disease, Council on Cardiovascular Disease in the Young, and the Councils on Clinical Cardiology, Stroke, and Cardiovascular Surgery and Anesthesia, American Heart Association: endorsed by the Infectious Diseases Society of America. Circulation. 2005 Jun 14;111(23):e394–434. Errata in: Circulation. 2007 Apr 17;115(15):e408. Circulation. 2008 Sep 16;118(12):e497. Circulation. 2007 Nov 20;116(21):e547. Circulation. 2005 Oct 11;112(15):2373.

Wilson W, Taubert KA, Gewitz M, Lockhart PB, Baddour LM, Levison M, et al; American Heart Association Rheumatic Fever, Endocarditis, and Kawasaki Disease Committee; American Heart Association Council on Cardiovascular Disease in the Young; American Heart Association Council on Clinical Cardiology; American Heart Association Council on Cardiovascular Surgery and Anesthesia; Quality of Care and Outcomes Research Interdisciplinary Working Group. Prevention of infective endocarditis: guidelines from the American Heart Association: a guideline from the American Heart Association Rheumatic Fever, Endocarditis, and Kawasaki Disease Committee, Council on Cardiovascular Disease in the Young, and the Council on Clinical Cardiology, Council on Cardiovascular Surgery and Anesthesia, and the Quality of Care and Outcomes Research Interdisciplinary Working Group. Circulation. 2007 Oct 9;116(15):1736–54. Epub 2007 Apr 19. Erratum in: Circulation. 2007 Oct 9;116(15):e376-7.

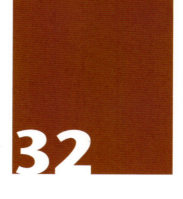

Michael R. Keating, MD

Infections of the Central Nervous System

I. Acute Meningitis
   A. Introduction
      1. Meningitis is diagnosed by the presence of white blood cells in the cerebrospinal fluid (CSF)
      2. Duration of acute infection before presentation: a few hours to a few days
      3. Acute meningitis may be infectious or noninfectious
      4. Clinical signs and symptoms
         a. Key features: fever, headache, neck stiffness, and altered mental status
         b. If stupor or coma is prominent, distinguishing encephalitis from meningitis can be difficult
      5. Aseptic meningitis
         a. Usually associated with lymphocytic pleocytosis
         b. Has no apparent cause after initial evaluation of CSF
            1) Viruses account for most cases of aseptic meningitis
            2) Nonviral causes can be infectious or noninfectious
         c. Aseptic meningitis cannot be reliably distinguished from bacterial meningitis without an examination of spinal fluid
   B. Epidemiology
      1. Annual incidence
         a. Acute bacterial meningitis
            1) Overall: 3 per 100,000 population
            2) Males: 3.3 per 100,000 population
            3) Females: 2.6 per 100,000 population
            4) Increased incidence among neonates and the elderly
         b. Viral meningitis: 10.5 per 100,000 population
      2. Mortality
         a. Bacterial meningitis: greater than 20%
         b. Viral meningitis: less than 1%, with the greatest mortality among the elderly and neonates
         c. Mortality by bacterial pathogen
            1) *Streptococcus pneumoniae*: 18% to 30%
            2) *Listeria monocytogenes*: 15%
            3) *Neisseria meningitidis*: 4% to 7%
   C. Etiology
      1. The cause of acute bacterial meningitis varies according to age (Table 32.1) and risk factors (Table 32.2)
      2. The cause of viral meningitis varies according to season
         a. Summer and fall: enteroviral meningitis and insect-borne meningitis are more common

Table 32.1

Incidence of Bacterial Meningitis in the United States According to Causative Organism and Patient Age, 1995

Organism	Percentage of Total Cases by Patient Age				
	<1 mo	1-23 mo	2-18 y	19-59 y	>60 y
Streptococcus pneumoniae	10	45	28	60	68
Neisseria meningitidis	0	30	59	18	3
Haemophilus influenzae	0	5	8	12	4
Listeria monocytogenes	20	0	2	7	22
Streptococcus agalactiae	70	20	3	3	3

Adapted from Schuchat A, Robinson K, Wenger JD, Harrison LH, Farley M, Reingold AL, et al. Bacterial meningitis in the United States in 1995. N Engl J Med. 1997;337:970–6. Used with permission.

   b. Spring and winter: mumps and lymphocytic choriomeningitis viral infections are more common
D. Diagnosis
   1. Clinical signs and symptoms
      a. Classic triad
         1) Fever, nuchal rigidity, and altered sensorium
         2) May not be present in up to one-third of patients
      b. A fourth common symptom: headache (Table 32.3)
      c. Rash (uncommon) suggests infection with N meningitidis
      d. Concomitant pneumonia, sinusitis, or otitis media suggests pneumococcus as the causative agent
      e. Bacterial meningitis is more likely to rapidly progress to lethargy and coma than aseptic meningitis
      f. Elderly or immunocompromised patients may have only fever and altered sensorium as the presenting signs and symptoms
   2. Laboratory testing
      a. All patients with suspected meningitis should undergo lumbar puncture and CSF examination
      b. Key CSF findings for aseptic and bacterial meningitis are summarized in Table 32.4
      c. CSF examination and prompt initiation of appropriate antibiotic therapy should not be delayed while waiting for the results of imaging studies
   3. Imaging
      a. In the following conditions, imaging should be completed before lumbar puncture is performed
         1) Immunocompromised state (eg, human immunodeficiency virus [HIV] infection, immunosuppressive therapy, after solid organ or bone marrow transplant)
         2) History of central nervous system disease (mass lesion, stroke, or focal infection)

Table 33.2

Association Between Risk Factors and Cause of Bacterial Meningitis

Risk Factor	Bacterial Agent
Age	
<1 mo	Streptococcus pneumoniae, Escherichia coli, Listeria monocytogenes, Klebsiella pneumoniae
1-23 mo	Streptococcus agalactiae, E coli, Haemophilus influenzae, S pneumoniae, Neisseria meningitidis
2-50 y	S pneumoniae, N meningitidis
>50 y	S pneumoniae, L monocytogenes, N meningitidis, aerobic gram-negative bacilli
Immunocompromised state	S pneumoniae, L monocytogenes, N meningitidis, aerobic gram-negative bacilli (including Pseudomonas aeruginosa)
Basilar skull fracture	S pneumoniae, H influenzae, group A β-hemolytic streptococci
Head trauma; postneurosurgery	Staphylococcus aureus, coagulase-negative staphylococci, aerobic gram-negative bacilli (including P aeruginosa)

Adapted from Tunkel AR, van de Beek D, Scheld WM. Acute meningitis. In: Mandell GL, Bennett JE, Dolin R, editors. Mandell, Douglas, and Bennett's principles and practice of infectious diseases. Vol 1. 7th ed. Philadelphia (PA): Churchill Livingstone/Elsevier; c2010. p. 1189–230. Used with permission.

Table 32.3

Signs and Symptoms of Meningitis

Sign or Symptom	Relative Frequency, %
Headache	≥85
Fever	≥80
Meningismus	≥80
Altered sensorium	≥75
Kernig or Brudzinski sign	50
Vomiting	35
Seizure	30
Focal neurologic findings	10-35
Papilledema	<5

Adapted from Tunkel AR, van de Beek D, Scheld WM. Acute meningitis. In: Mandell GL, Bennett JE, Dolin R, editors. Mandell, Douglas, and Bennett's principles and practice of infectious diseases. Vol 1. 7th ed. Philadelphia (PA): Churchill Livingstone/Elsevier; c2010. p. 1189–230 as originally adapted from Gnann JW Jr. Meningitis and encephalitis caused by mumps virus. In: Scheld WM, Whitley RJ, Marra CM, editors. Infections of the Central Nervous System. 3rd ed. Philadelphia: Lippincott Williams & Wilkins; 2004:231–41. Used with permission.

   3) New-onset seizure (within 1 week of presentation)
   4) Papilledema
   5) Abnormal level of consciousness
   6) Focal neurologic deficit
  b. If imaging will delay the initiation of therapy, blood should be cultured and age-appropriate antibiotics administered empirically before imaging is done
 E. Treatment
  1. Antibacterial therapy for acute bacterial meningitis
   a. May be empirically based on the presence of neutrophils if Gram stain does not show organisms (Table 32.5)
   b. May be based on the CSF Gram stain (Table 32.6)
   c. May be definitively based on culture results and susceptibility data (Table 32.7)
  2. Corticosteroid therapy with dexamethasone
   a. Given to all patients with suspected pneumococcal meningitis
   b. Continued in patients who have confirmed pneumococcal infection
   c. Discontinued if cultures yield a microorganism other than pneumococcus
   d. Corticosteroid therapy has no role after antibiotic therapy has been started
   e. Consider discontinuing corticosteroid therapy if a penicillin-resistant organism is recovered from cultures
  3. Duration of therapy
   a. For meningococcal meningitis: 7 days
   b. For pneumococcal meningitis: 10 to 14 days of antibiotic therapy and 4 days of dexamethasone therapy
   c. For *Streptococcus agalactiae* meningitis: 21 days
   d. For *Listeria* meningitis: 21 days
  4. Antiviral therapy
   a. For most causes of aseptic viral meningitis, there is no specific antiviral therapy
   b. Acyclovir
    1) Should be administered when primary herpes simplex virus 1 infection is complicated by meningitis
    2) Herpes simplex virus 2 meningitis is a self-limited infection, and treatment with acyclovir is optional
 F. Specific Pathogens
  1. Bacteria
   a. *Streptococcus pneumoniae*

Table 32.4

Cerebrospinal Fluid Findings in Aseptic and Bacterial Meningitis

Feature	Reference Values	Bacterial Meningitis	Aseptic Meningitis
Opening pressure, mm water	90-180	>180	90-200
White blood cell count, cells/μL	0-5 lymphocytes	1,000-5,000 polymorphonuclear cells	10-300 lymphocytes[a]
Glucose, mg/dL	50-75	≤40	Normal[b]
Protein, mg/dL	15-40	100-500	50-100
Gram stain	Negative	60%-90%	Negative
Culture	Negative	70%-85%	Occasionally positive
Polymerase chain reaction	Negative	Promising	Enterovirus, herpes simplex virus 2

[a]Neutrophils may predominate in early aseptic meningitis.
[b]Glucose concentration may be low with mumps and lymphocytic choriomeningitis.

Adapted from Razonable RR, Keating MR. Meningitis: treatment & medication. Updated 2009 Aug 26 [cited 2010 Dec 14]. Available from: http://emedicine.medscape.com/article/232915-treatment.

Table 32.5

Empirical Therapy for Bacterial Meningitis When Gram Stain Results Are Negative

Predisposing Factor	Preferred Therapy	Alternative Therapy
Age		
<1 mo	Ampicillin plus cefotaxime	Ampicillin plus an aminoglycoside
1-23 mo	Vancomycin plus a third-generation cephalosporin[a]	Vancomycin plus ampicillin plus chloramphenicol
2-50 y	Vancomycin plus a third-generation cephalosporin[a]	
>50 y	Vancomycin plus ampicillin plus a third-generation cephalosporin[a]	
Immunocompromised state	Vancomycin plus ampicillin plus an antipseudomonal cephalosporin[b]	
Basilar skull fracture	Vancomycin plus a third-generation cephalosporin[a]	
Head trauma; postneurosurgery	Vancomycin plus an antipseudomonal cephalosporin[b]	

[a] Cefotaxime or ceftriaxone; cefepime may also be used.
[b] Cefepime or ceftazidime.

Adapted from Tunkel AR, van de Beek D, Scheld WM. Acute meningitis. In: Mandell GL, Bennett JE, Dolin R, editors. Mandell, Douglas, and Bennett's principles and practice of infectious diseases. Vol 1. 7th ed. Philadelphia (PA): Churchill Livingstone/Elsevier; c2010. p. 1189–230. Used with permission.

1) Most common cause of bacterial meningitis in the United States
2) Infection results in the highest mortality rate (up to 30%)
3) Often accompanies another focus of infection, including pneumonia, sinusitis, otitis media, mastoiditis, and endocarditis
4) Incidence is higher among patients with predisposing conditions, including alcoholism, diabetes mellitus, chronic kidney disease, chronic liver disease, hypogammaglobulinemia, splenectomy or asplenic states, and multiple myeloma

b. *Neisseria meningitidis*
1) Most common in children and young adults
2) Nasopharyngeal colonization usually precedes invasive disease
3) Occurs in outbreaks where crowding occurs, such as military barracks and college dormitories
4) Increased risk of infection in persons with terminal complement deficiencies (C5, C6, C7, and C8)
5) Serogroups B, C, and Y account for most cases in the United States
6) Epidemics are now unusual in the developed world but occur throughout the developing world, particularly in sub-Saharan Africa, which is often referred to as the meningitis belt

c. *Listeria monocytogenes*
1) Most common in infants younger than 1 month and adults older than 60 years
2) Also occurs in transplant recipients, other immunosuppressed patients, alcoholics, cancer patients, and patients with diabetes mellitus, chronic kidney disease, collagen-vascular diseases, or conditions associated with iron overload

Table 32.6

Empirical Therapy for Bacterial Meningitis When Cerebrospinal Fluid Gram Stain Results Are Known

Gram Stain Morphology	Antibiotic Therapy
Gram-positive cocci	Vancomycin plus ceftriaxone
Gram-negative cocci	Penicillin G
Gram-positive bacilli	Ampicillin plus aminoglycoside
Gram-negative bacilli	Cephalosporin plus aminoglycoside[a]

[a] Use an antipseudomonal agent if the patient is immunocompromised or postneurosurgical or if the patient had head trauma.

Adapted from Razonable RR, Keating MR. Meningitis: treatment & medication. Updated 2009 Aug 26 [cited 2010 Dec 14]. Available from: http://emedicine.medscape.com/article/232915-treatment.

Table 32.7

Definitive Therapy for Bacterial Meningitis

Microorganism	Preferred Therapy	Alternative Therapy
Streptococcus pneumoniae		
Penicillin MIC <0.1 µg/mL	Penicillin G or ampicillin	Third-generation cephalosporin Vancomycin
Penicillin MIC 0.1-1.0 µg/mL	Third-generation cephalosporin[a]	Meropenem Vancomycin
Penicillin MIC >1.0 µg/mL	Vancomycin plus a third-generation cephalosporin	Third-generation cephalosporin plus moxifloxacin
Neisseria meningitidis	Penicillin G or ampicillin[b]	Third-generation cephalosporin Chloramphenicol Meropenem Moxifloxacin
Listeria monocytogenes	Ampicillin[c]	Trimethoprim-sulfamethoxazole Meropenem
Streptococcus agalactiae	Penicillin G or ampicillin	Third-generation cephalosporin Vancomycin
Haemophilus influenzae	Third-generation cephalosporin[d]	Third-generation cephalosporin Cefepime Aztreonam
Enterobacteriaceae	Third-generation cephalosporin[c]	Aztreonam Trimethoprim-sulfamethoxazole Meropenem[c]
Pseudomonas aeruginosa	Cefepime or ceftazidime[c]	Meropenem Aztreonam Moxifloxacin[c]
Staphylococcus aureus		
Methicillin sensitive	Nafcillin	Vancomycin
Methicillin resistant	Vancomycin	
Coagulase-negative staphylococci	Vancomycin	

Abbreviation: MIC, minimum inhibitory concentration.

[a] Cefotaxime or ceftriaxone; cefepime can also be used.
[b] Penicillin G or ampicillin for rare penicillin-resistant strains.
[c] Consider adding an aminoglycoside.
[d] Ampicillin may be used for β-lactamase–negative strains.

Adapted from Tunkel AR, van de Beek D, Scheld WM. Acute meningitis. In: Mandell GL, Bennett JE, Dolin R, editors. Mandell, Douglas, and Bennett's principles and practice of infectious diseases. Vol 1. 7th ed. Philadelphia (PA): Churchill Livingstone/Elsevier; c2010. p. 1189–230. Used with permission.

    3) Portal of entry is gastrointestinal tract
    4) Both sporadic cases and outbreaks occur
  d. *Haemophilus influenzae*
    1) Dramatic decrease in the rate of invasive diseases after the introduction of the conjugate vaccine for *H influenzae* type B in 1987
    2) Associated with underlying conditions, including diabetes mellitus, alcoholism, splenectomy and asplenic states, hypogammaglobulinemia, head trauma, and respiratory tract infection (eg, pneumonia, sinusitis)
    3) Mortality rate: usually less than 6%
  e. *Streptococcus agalactiae*
    1) Major cause of meningitis among newborns and children younger than 2 years
    2) Both vertical and horizontal transmission contribute to disease in the newborn
    3) Increasing incidence of invasive disease, including meningitis in adults
    4) Risk factors for invasive disease in adults include pregnancy, postpartum state, diabetes mellitus, age older than 60 years, chronic renal disease, cirrhosis, decubitus ulcers, and corticosteroid therapy

f. Aerobic gram-negative bacilli
   1) Most cases are accounted for by *Escherichia coli*, *Serratia marcescens*, *Klebsiella* species, *Salmonella* species, and *Pseudomonas aeruginosa*
   2) Usually associated with head trauma or postneurosurgical infection
   3) Other occurrences
      a) Newborns (especially *E coli*): vertical and horizontal transmission are important
      b) Immunocompromised patients: may be a marker for *Strongyloides* hyperinfection syndrome
      c) Elderly patients
      d) Patients with overwhelming gram-negative bacillary sepsis
g. *Staphylococcus* species
   1) *Staphylococcus aureus* meningitis
      a) Mortality: from less than 15% to more than 75%
      b) Usually associated with head trauma or postneurosurgical infection
      c) Also occurs with various other predisposing conditions, including stage 5 kidney disease, alcoholism, diabetes mellitus, injection drug use, endocarditis, *S aureus* sepsis, and other *S aureus* infection
   2) Both *S aureus* and coagulase-negative staphylococci can cause meningitis related to a neurosurgical device (eg, ventriculoperitoneal shunt, external ventricular drain)
h. Spirochetes
   1) *Borrelia burgdorferi*
      a) Clinical syndrome of aseptic meningitis but with frequent cranial neuropathies and variable, often fluctuating levels of cerebral symptoms (eg, memory loss, somnolence, depression)
      b) Infection is more likely to manifest as a subacute or chronic syndrome
      c) Clues to the diagnosis: exposure to *Ixodes* tick, tick bite, or recent erythema migrans
   2) *Treponema pallidum*
      a) Incidence of syphilitic aseptic meningitis is greatest in the first 2 years after infection
      b) Increased incidence among patients coinfected with HIV
      c) Clinical syndrome is aseptic meningitis but more commonly as a subacute or chronic condition
      d) Cranial nerve palsies are common, especially involving cranial nerves VII and VIII and the ocular cranial nerves
2. Viruses
   a. Enteroviruses
      1) Nonpolio enteroviruses account for more than 85% of all cases of aseptic meningitis
      2) Predominate during summer and fall, especially in temperate climates
      3) Echoviruses and coxsackieviruses constitute the majority of isolates recovered when cultures are done
      4) Clues to the diagnosis include other manifestations of enterovirus infection, such as conjunctivitis, maculopapular rash, herpangina, and pleurodynia
      5) In patients with hypogammaglobulinemia, chronic meningitis or meningoencephalitis can develop
   b. Arboviruses
      1) More likely to cause encephalitis than meningitis but the distinction can be difficult
      2) St Louis encephalitis virus
         a) Aseptic meningitis in 15% of cases
         b) Sporadic cases and occasional summertime epidemics
      3) California encephalitis virus group
         a) La Crosse virus, Jamestown Canyon virus, snowshoe hare virus
         b) Mainly in northern United States
         c) Asymptomatic in most patients
      4) Eastern equine encephalomyelitis virus
         a) Rare but lethal mosquito-borne virus of the eastern coastal United States
         b) Mortality: 50% to 70%
      5) Western equine encephalomyelitis virus
         a) Rare mosquito-borne virus west of the Mississippi River
         b) Mortality less than 4%
      6) Venezuelan equine encephalomyelitis virus
         a) Common mosquito-borne virus in tropical area of South and Central America
         b) Mild infection (mortality <1%)

7) West Nile virus
   a) Usually causes an encephalitis, less frequently an asymmetric paralysis similar to poliomyelitis
   b) Occasional cause of aseptic meningitis
   c) Recent report of transmission by solid organ transplant
8) Mumps virus
   a) Aseptic meningitis is a common, self-limited manifestation of mumps infection and can occur in the absence of parotiditis
   b) More likely to induce a low CSF glucose level than other forms of aseptic meningitis
   c) Other extraglandular infections are rare but manifest as encephalitis, neuritis, and seizures
9) Lymphocytic choriomeningitis virus
   a) Transmitted to humans after exposure to rodents—no human-to-human transmission
   b) Occurs more frequently in winter and spring
   c) Recent report of transmission by solid organ transplant
10) Human immunodeficiency virus
    a) Aseptic meningitis is a frequent manifestation of primary HIV infection, often as part of a mononucleosis syndrome
    b) Cranial nerve palsies may occur
    c) Aseptic meningitis or a mononucleosis-like syndrome in a patient with high-risk behavior is an indication for HIV screening
11) Herpesviruses
    a) Primary genital herpes simplex virus 2 (HSV2) infection is complicated by aseptic meningitis in more than 30% of women and more than 10% of men
    b) Primary herpes simplex virus 1 (HSV1) infection is rarely associated with meningitis
    c) Varicella-zoster virus (VZV), cytomegalovirus (CMV), and Epstein-Barr virus (EBV) rarely cause meningitis
       i) VZV: with or without the presence of skin lesions
       ii) CMV and EBV: usually with a mononucleosis syndrome
    d) Human herpes virus 6–associated meningitis can occur as a complication of exanthema subitum
3. Protozoa and helminths
   a. *Angiostrongylus cantonensis*
      1) Acute meningitis syndrome
         a) After ingestion of raw or undercooked snails or crabs
         b) Characterized by a predominance of eosinophils in the CSF
      2) Epidemic and sporadic disease occurs in Southeast Asia and the South Pacific
      3) Usually a self-limited illness, although frequently the course is prolonged (up to 2 months)
   b. Amebas: *Naegleria fowleri* and *Acanthamoeba* species
      1) Cause meningoencephalitis in persons exposed to warm freshwater lakes and ponds
      2) Very rare, rapidly progressive illness that is nearly uniformly fatal within 1 week of symptom onset
      3) Examination of CSF shows motile trophozoites
4. Rare agents of acute meningitis are listed in Box 32.1
G. Noninfectious Causes
   1. Noninfectious causes of acute meningitis are listed in Box 32.2
H. Special Situations
   1. Recurrent meningitis
      a. Recurrent community-acquired meningitis
         1) Pneumococcus and meningococcus most commonly, but often cultures are negative
         2) Patients usually have CSF leak or remote history of head trauma or neurosurgery
         3) Leak can usually be detected with high-resolution computed tomography (CT), but occasionally fluorescein instillation or radionuclide scanning is necessary
      b. Recurrent nosocomial meningitis
         1) Gram-negative bacilli and staphylococci cause most cases
         2) Occurs after neurosurgical procedures and often is associated with indwelling devices (eg, Ommaya reservoir, ventricular shunt)
      c. Benign recurrent aseptic meningitis (Mollaret meningitis)

> **Box 32.1**
> **Rare Infectious Causes of Acute Meningitis**
> Bacteria
>   *Acinetobacter* species
>   *Bacillus anthracis*
>   *Capnocytophaga canimorsus*
>   *Enterococcus* species
>   *Fusobacterium necrophorum*
>   *Mycobacterium tuberculosis*
>   *Nocardia* species
>   *Pasteurella multocida*
>   *Streptococcus bovis*
>   *Streptococcus pyogenes*
>   Viridans streptococci
> Fungi
>   *Coccidioides immitis*
>   *Cryptococcus neoformans*
> Helminths
>   *Baylisascaris procyonis*
>   *Strongyloides stercoralis*
> Rickettsiae
>   *Anaplasma* species
>   *Ehrlichia* species
>   *Orientia tsutsugamushi*
>   *Rickettsia conorii*
>   *Rickettsia prowazekii*
>   *Rickettsia rickettsii*
>   *Rickettsia typhi*
> Spirochetes
>   *Leptospira* species
> Viruses
>   Adenovirus
>   Human parainfluenza virus 3
>   Human parvovirus B19
>   Influenza A virus
>   Influenza B virus
>   Measles virus
>   Poliovirus

> **Box 32.2**
> **Noninfectious Causes of Acute Meningitis**
> Antimicrobial agents
>   Ciprofloxacin
>   Cotrimoxazole
>   Isoniazid
>   Metronidazole
>   Penicillin
>   Pyrazinamide
>   Sulfamethoxazole
>   Sulfasoxazole
>   Trimethoprim
> Biologics
>   Immune globulins
>   Muromonab-CD3 (OKT3)
> Intracranial tumors and cysts
>   Craniopharyngioma
>   Dermoid or epidermoid cyst
>   Teratoma
> Miscellaneous
>   Migraine headache
>   Seizures
> Nonsteroidal anti-inflammatory drugs
>   Diclofenac
>   Ibuprofen
>   Ketoprofen
>   Naproxen
>   Rofecoxib
>   Sulindac
>   Tolmentin
> Other medications
>   Azathioprine
>   Carbamazepine
>   Cytosine arabinoside
>   Phenazopyridine
>   Ranitidine
> Procedure-related causes
>   After intrathecal injection of air, isotopes, antimicrobics, antineoplastic agents, corticosteroids, or contrast media
>   Chymopapain injection
>   Postneurosurgical state
>   Spinal anesthesia
> Systemic illnesses
>   Behçet disease
>   Cerebral vasculitis
>   Kawasaki disease
>   Multiple sclerosis
>   Polyarteritis nodosa
>   Rheumatoid arthritis
>   Sarcoidosis
>   Sjögren syndrome
>   Systemic lupus erythematosus
>   Vogt-Koyanagi-Harada syndrome

       1) HSV2 causes more than 85% of cases; recurrences are suppressed with antiviral therapy
       2) Genital lesions rarely appear during recurrence
       3) Cause of non-HSV2–associated cases is uncertain: possibly from HSV1, EBV, or hypersensitivity reaction
    2. Parameningeal focus of infection
       a. Infection adjacent to the meninges induces a neutrophilic CSF pleocytosis and is usually associated with negative cultures
       b. Examples include sinusitis, otitis, brain abscess, pituitary abscess, cranial osteomyelitis, intracranial epidural abscess, and venous sinus thrombosis
I. Prevention and Chemoprophylaxis
    1. Immunoprophylaxis
       a. *Haemophilus influenzae*
       1) The *H influenzae* type b vaccine has been highly effective in reducing the incidence of invasive disease among children
       2) There is no standard recommendation for its use in adults

b. *Neisseria meningitidis*
  1) New tetravalent conjugated *N meningitidis* vaccine (serogroups A, C, Y, and W-135)
    a) Recommended for routine use in children aged 11 to 12 years and for adolescents not previously vaccinated when they enter high school
    b) Recommended for patients at high risk of meningococcal meningitis
      i) Patients with terminal complement deficiency
      ii) Patients with anatomical or functional asplenia
      iii) Travelers to areas where meningococcal meningitis is hyperendemic or epidemic
      iv) Military recruits
      v) College students living in dormitories
      vi) Close contacts of cases of meningococcal disease
  2) The older unconjugated tetravalent vaccine may be substituted if the conjugated vaccine is not available
 c. *Streptococcus pneumoniae*
  1) The role of the 23-valent pneumococcal vaccine in preventing meningitis has not been determined
 2. Chemoprophylaxis
  a. *Neisseria meningitidis*
   1) Postexposure chemoprophylaxis is recommended for close contacts of a person with meningococcal meningitis
     a) Household contacts
     b) Day care center attendees
     c) Anyone having direct contact with the patient's oral secretions (eg, through kissing, mouth-to-mouth resuscitation, endotracheal intubation, or endotracheal tube management)
   2) Recommended options
     a) Rifampin 600 mg orally twice daily for 2 days (4 doses)
     b) Ciprofloxacin 500 mg once
     c) Ceftriaxone 250 mg intramuscularly once
II. Chronic Meningitis
 A. Introduction
  1. *Chronic meningitis*: meningitis lasting for 4 or more weeks
  2. Diverse infectious and noninfectious causes
  3. Symptoms include fever, headache, altered mental status, meningismus, nausea, and vomiting; hence, it can be challenging to distinguish this rare condition from acute meningitis and encephalitis early in its clinical evolution
  4. Given that this condition has diverse causes, it is critical to establish a precise diagnosis and avoid empirical therapy until a meticulous evaluation has been completed
 B. Etiology
  1. Identified causes of chronic meningitis: infectious, malignant, inflammatory, and noninfectious (Box 32.3)
  2. Most common causes: tuberculosis, carcinoma, and *Cryptococcus neoformans*
  3. At least one-third of cases are idiopathic

Box 32.3

Infectious and Noninfectious Causes of Chronic Meningitis

Bacterial
 Actinomyces
 Borrelia burgdorferi
 Brucella species
 Ehrlichia chaffeensis
 Francisella tularensis
 Leptospira
 Listeria monocytogenes
 Nocardia
 Treponema pallidum
Fungal
 Blastomyces dermatitidis
 Coccidioides immitis
 Cryptococcus neoformans
 Histoplasma capsulatum
Noninfectious conditions
 Behçet disease
 Central nervous system vasculitis
 Chemical- or drug-induced meningitis
 Fabry disease
 Neoplasm
 Sarcoidosis
 Systemic lupus erythematosus
 Vogt-Koyanagi-Harada syndrome
 Wegener granulomatosis
Parasitic
 Acanthamoeba
 Angiostrongylus cantonensis
 Schistosoma species
 Taenia solium
 Toxoplasma
Viral
 Cytomegalovirus
 Enterovirus
 Epstein-Barr virus
 Herpes simplex virus
 Human immunodeficiency virus
 Varicella-zoster virus

C. Diagnosis
   1. Evaluation of the patient with chronic meningitis is a formidable diagnostic challenge
   2. Requires a careful, systematic approach
      a. Epidemiologic clues from the history will help guide the evaluation (Table 32.8)
      b. Physical examination findings may suggest the diagnosis (Table 32.9)
      c. Laboratory evaluation must be comprehensive and include tests that can identify unusual causes of this condition (Box 32.4)
      d. Evaluation may be streamlined by following an algorithm that combines predisposing conditions, exposure history, and physical findings (Figures 32.1 and 32.2)
      e. Characteristics of the CSF provide important clues to the diagnosis (Box 32.5)
      f. Brain or meningeal biopsy
         1) Should be considered when less invasive diagnostic studies have not yielded a diagnosis and the patient's condition is worsening despite empirical therapy
         2) Yield on biopsy is quite low but is enhanced when biopsy is directed toward a focal brain lesion seen on imaging or an area of meningeal enhancement on magnetic resonance imaging (MRI)
D. Treatment
   1. Directed therapy based on results of diagnostic tests is always preferred over empirical therapy, but therapeutic trials are often required for the patient with progressive disease before a diagnosis has been clearly established
      a. One-third of patients do not have a definitive diagnosis
      b. Frequently, results of serological tests are delayed
      c. While receiving empirical therapy, the patient should be carefully monitored for response to therapy, and diagnostic efforts should continue
   2. Antitubercular therapy should always be considered
      a. Tuberculous meningitis is a common cause of chronic meningitis, especially where tuberculosis is endemic

Table 32.8
Epidemiologic or Historical Clues to the Diagnosis of Chronic Meningitis

Clue	Diagnosis
Travel or residence in semiarid regions of southwestern United States, Mexico, or Central or South America	Coccidioidomycosis
Travel or residence in the developing world	Tuberculosis
Prior residence in Mexico, Central America, India, the Caribbean, or sub-Saharan Africa	Cysticercosis
New sex partner or high-risk activity for acquiring HIV	HIV
Consumption of unpasteurized milk	Brucellosis
Work in a meatpacking house or other exposure to cows, goats, sheep, or swine	Brucellosis
History of tick exposure or rash resembling erythema migrans	Lyme disease
Travel or residence in the Mississippi, Ohio, or St Lawrence river valleys or the southeastern United States	Blastomycosis
Exposure to bat or avian habitats (guano)	Histoplasmosis
Contact with birds	Cryptococcosis
History of cancer	Neoplastic meningitis
Immunocompromised state	Cryptococcosis, toxoplasmosis, tuberculosis, endemic mycoses

Abbreviation: HIV, human immunodeficiency virus.

Table 32.9
Physical Examination Findings That Suggest the Cause of Chronic Meningitis

Physical Finding	Possible Diagnosis
Cranial nerve deficits	Neurosyphilis, Lyme disease, sarcoidosis, brucellosis, tuberculosis
Oral and genital ulcerations	Behçet disease, Sjögren syndrome, SLE, sarcoidosis
Uveitis or iritis	Sarcoidosis, Behçet disease, Vogt-Koyanagi-Harada syndrome
Poliosis (whitening of hair and eyelashes)	Vogt-Koyanagi-Harada syndrome
Skin rash or lesions	Cryptococcosis, sarcoidosis, coccidioidomycosis, blastomycosis, *Acanthamoeba* infection, syphilis
Subcutaneous nodules	Cysticercosis, metastatic cancer

Abbreviation: SLE, systemic lupus erythematosus.

> **Box 32.4**
>
> **Diagnostic Laboratory Evaluation of the Patient With Chronic Meningitis**
>
> General blood testing
>   Complete blood cell count and differential blood count
>   Liver function
>   Renal function
>   Serum angiotensin-converting enzyme
>   Erythrocyte sedimentation rate
> Serologies and molecular diagnostics
>   Serology for human immunodeficiency virus, syphilis, cryptococcal antigen, toxoplasma, Lyme disease, antinuclear antibody
>   CSF PCR for tuberculosis, *Borrelia burgdorferi*
>   CSF cryptococcal antigen
>   PPD (repeat in 2-4 wk if negative and evaluation is nondiagnostic)
> Cultures
>   Blood for mycobacteria and fungi by lysis centrifugation
>   Blood for aerobic and anaerobic bacteria
>   Urine for fungi and mycobacteria
>   CSF (large volume) for fungi and mycobacteria
> CSF examination
>   Opening pressure
>   Cell count with differential
>   Glucose level
>   Protein level
>   Gram stain
>   Stain for eosinophils
>   VDRL test
>   Cytology
> Imaging
>   Chest radiograph
>   MRI of brain with and without gadolinium
> Exposure-directed studies
>   Serum serology for histoplasmosis, blastomycosis, coccidioidomycosis, sporotrichosis, brucellosis
>   CSF serology for histoplasmosis, coccidioidomycosis, blastomycosis, brucellosis, cysticercosis (*Taenia solium*), sporotrichosis, histoplasma antigen
> Extended studies for a patient without a diagnosis
>   Serum immunoglobulins and enterovirus CSF PCR if low
>   Bone marrow biopsy
>   Other extraneural biopsies according to findings
>   Brain or meningeal biopsy
>
> Abbreviations: CSF, cerebrospinal fluid; MRI, magnetic resonance imaging; PCR, polymerase chain reaction; PPD, purified protein derivative (tuberculin).

  b. If epidemiologic clues or clinical data suggest tuberculosis but a definitive diagnosis has not been made, empirical therapy should be started after adequate cultures have been obtained
  c. Unless the patient has severe symptoms, concurrent corticosteroid therapy should be avoided
  d. If there is no response to antitubercular therapy after 4 to 6 weeks, therapy should be discontinued

 3. Empirical antifungal therapy with fluconazole or a newer azole
    a. Can be considered if clinical features strongly suggest an undiagnosed fungal infection
    b. Published data supporting this approach are scant
 4. Corticosteroids
    a. May be considered in selected patients with chronic meningitis if an infectious cause has been reasonably excluded
    b. Success as high as nearly 50% has been reported with this approach
E. Differential Diagnosis
 1. Tuberculous meningitis
    a. Most common cause of chronic meningitis
    b. Tuberculin purified protein derivative (PPD) test is negative in 50% to 65% of patients
    c. Typical CSF profile (but not specific)
       1) Lymphocytic pleocytosis (100-500 cells/μL)
       2) Elevated protein level
       3) Low glucose level
    d. CSF glucose levels that decrease on serial lumbar punctures without treatment also suggest tuberculous meningitis
    e. Other features of cases
       1) CSF acid-fast bacilli (AFB) smear is positive in 10% to 20%
       2) CSF culture is positive in 40% to 90%
       3) Concurrent sputum AFB culture is positive in 14% to 50%
    f. CSF polymerase chain reaction (PCR) is now considered a standard
       1) Sensitivity: as high as 85%
       2) Specificity: 95% to 100%
 2. Cryptococcal meningitis
    a. Most frequently occurs in patients with a clinically significant defect in cellular immunity (eg, AIDS, high-dose corticosteroid use), but it can occur in previously healthy persons
    b. Course is most often subacute and slowly progressive, but it can be rapidly progressive, especially in persons with AIDS
    c. Typical CSF profile
       1) Lymphocytic pleocytosis (40-400 cells/μL)
       2) Decreased glucose level
       3) India ink staining is positive in about 50% of cases
       4) CSF cryptococcal antigen is positive in more than 85%

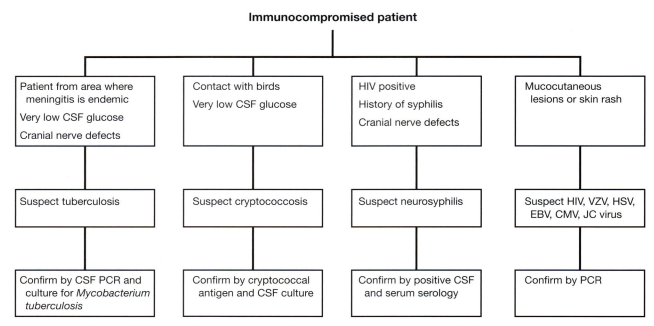

Figure 32.1. Algorithm for Evaluation of Immunocompromised Patient With Chronic Meningitis. Causes of the immunocompromised state include human immunodeficiency virus (HIV) infection, corticosteroid or other immunosuppressive therapy, bone marrow or solid organ transplant, and lymphoma. CMV indicates cytomegalovirus; CSF, cerebrospinal fluid; EBV, Epstein-Barr virus; HSV, herpes simplex virus; PCR, polymerase chain reaction; VZV, varicella-zoster virus. (Adapted from Hildebrand J, Aoun M. Chronic meningitis: still a diagnostic challenge. J Neurol. 2003 Jun;250[6]:653–60. Used with permission.)

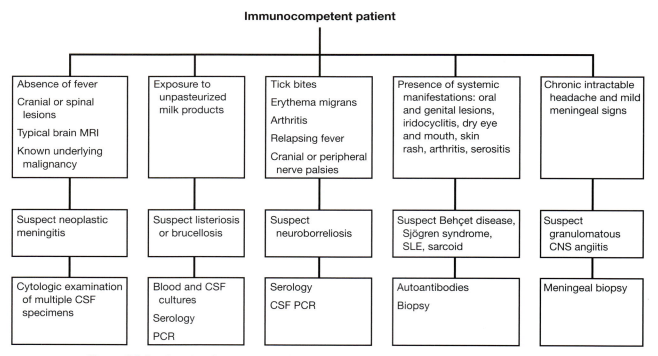

Figure 32.2. Algorithm for Evaluation of Immunocompetent Patient With Chronic Meningitis. CNS indicates central nervous system; CSF, cerebrospinal fluid; MRI, magnetic resonance imaging; PCR, polymerase chain reaction; SLE, systemic lupus erythematosus. (Adapted from Hildebrand J, Aoun M. Chronic meningitis: still a diagnostic challenge. J Neurol. 2003 Jun;250[6]:653–60. Used with permission.)

Box 32.5

Diagnostic Clues From Characteristics of Cerebrospinal Fluid Profile in Chronic Meningitis

Pleocytosis <50 cells/μL
    Behçet disease
    Benign lymphocytic meningitis
    Carcinoma
    Cryptococcus in HIV-infected patient
    Sarcoidosis
    Vasculitis
Neutrophilic pleocytosis
    Actinomyces
    Aspergillus
    Candida
    Chemical
    Nocardia
    SLE
Eosinophilic pleocytosis
    Angiostrongylus
    Chemical
    Coccidioides
    Cysticercus
    Lymphoma
    Schistosoma
Low glucose level
    Actinomyces
    Carcinoma
    Chronic enterovirus infection
    CMV in HIV-infected patient
    Cysticercus
    Fungi
    Mycobacterium tuberculosis
    Nocardia
    Postsubarachnoid hemorrhage
    Sarcoidosis
    Syphilis
    Toxoplasma

Abbreviations: CMV, cytomegalovirus; HIV, human immunodeficiency virus; SLE, systemic lupus erythematosus.

Adapted from Behlau I, Ellner JJ. Chronic meningitis. In: Mandell GL, Bennett JE, Dolin R, editors. Mandell, Douglas, and Bennett's principles and practice of infectious diseases. Vol 1. 6th ed. Philadelphia (PA): Elsevier/Churchill Livingstone; c2005. p. 1132–43. Used with permission.

       5) Culture is positive in more than 75% (percentage increases with serial cultures of CSF)
  3. Neoplastic meningitis
    a. Frequency is increasing owing to longer survival of cancer patients
    b. Most common primary lesions or sites: melanoma, lung, breast, stomach, pancreas, and hematologic malignancies
    c. Symptom complex is identical to that of meningitis from infectious and other noninfectious causes
       1) Usually occurs with a known malignancy
       2) The challenge is to distinguish infectious chronic meningitis that is emerging after treatment of malignancy from failure of antineoplastic therapy and disease progression or paraneoplastic syndrome
    d. There is no characteristic CSF profile, but a very low glucose level with only mild pleocytosis is most suggestive
  4. Sarcoid meningitis
    a. Occurs in less than 5% of sarcoid patients
    b. Basilar meningitis is most common
       1) Results in cranial nerve palsies
       2) Can progress to involve the hypothalamus
          a) Leads to diabetes insipidus
          b) Seems to be unique to sarcoid meningitis (in contrast to other causes of chronic meningitis)
    c. CSF profile: usually mild lymphocytic pleocytosis and decreased glucose level
    d. Diagnosis is supported by evidence of sarcoid at other sites (>65% have evidence of thoracic sarcoidosis)
  5. Coccidioidal meningitis
    a. Exposure history
       1) Important epidemiologic clue to this geographically restricted mycosis
       2) Disease can occur years after initial exposure
    b. Manifestations: may be only neurologic or may occur with involvement at other sites (eg, pulmonary, cutaneous)
    c. Causes an eosinophilic pleocytosis
    d. Diagnosis
       1) Positive CSF complement fixation antibody, positive CSF culture, or presence of eosinophilic meningitis
       2) Positive serum complement fixation antibody titer
  6. *Histoplasma* meningitis
    a. Unusual manifestation of *Histoplasma* infection
    b. Occurs without extraneural infection in 25% of cases
    c. Diagnosis
       1) CSF cultures: often negative
       2) CSF and blood should be checked for *Histoplasma* antibodies and blood
       3) CSF and urine should be checked for *Histoplasma* antigen
       4) Blood cultures may be positive by the lysis centrifugation technique
  7. Neuroborreliosis
    a. Cranial and peripheral neuropathies
       1) Common
       2) Important diagnostic clues

b. Detection of intrathecal antibody production
1) A specific diagnostic test
2) PCR is most specific but lacks sensitivity (<40%)
8. Cysticercosis
a. Manifests as chronic meningitis in 25% of patients owing to cysts in the subarachnoid space in contrast to the more common brain parenchymal disease, which manifests with seizure
b. Symptoms can occur decades after exposure to the eggs of the tapeworm *Taenia solium*
c. CSF and serum antibody detection is diagnostic, but serum results are negative in 50% of cases and CSF results are negative in 15%

III. Encephalitis
A. Introduction
1. *Encephalitis*: inflammation of the brain caused by infection
a. Most cases are caused by viruses
b. Other cases are caused by bacteria, fungi, and protozoa
2. Pathologically, infectious agent directly invades brain parenchyma
3. Hallmark of encephalitis: altered brain function and an impaired level of mental status
4. Distinguishing meningitis from encephalitis during the acute phase can be difficult
a. Distinction is important
b. Cause of each—and hence management of each—is different
B. Epidemiology and Etiology
1. Many viral and nonviral infectious causes of encephalitis are recognized (Boxes 32.6 and 32.7)
2. Noninfectious causes can create an encephalitis syndrome that is difficult to distinguish from infectious causes (Box 32.8)
3. Seasonal variation
a. Diseases from mosquito-borne agents (eg, arboviruses, West Nile virus) and tick–borne infections (eg, Lyme disease, Rocky Mountain spotted fever) occur from late spring into fall
b. Enterovirus infections peak during the summer and are rare during the winter
c. Measles and mumps tend to occur during late winter to early spring
d. Herpes simplex virus (HSV) encephalitis is sporadic and can occur at any time during the year

---

Box 32.6
Viral Causes of Encephalitis[a]

Bunyaviridae
 California encephalitis virus
 La Crosse virus
 Rift Valley fever virus
Flaviviridae
 Japanese encephalitis virus
 Murray Valley encephalitis virus
 St Louis encephalitis virus
 West Nile virus
Herpesviridae
 Cytomegalovirus
 Epstein-Barr virus
 Herpes simplex virus 1 and 2
 Herpesvirus B
 Human herpesvirus 6
 Varicella-zoster virus
Togaviridae
 Eastern equine encephalomyelitis virus
 Venezuelan equine encephalomyelitis virus
 Western equine encephalomyelitis virus
Other viruses
 Adenovirus
 Colorado tick fever virus
 Ebola virus
 Enteroviruses
 Human immunodeficiency virus
 Marburg virus
 Rabies virus

[a]Boldface type indicates causes that are more commonly encountered.

Box 32.7
Nonviral Infectious Causes of Encephalitis[a]

Acanthamoeba
Brucella species
Cat-scratch disease
Cerebral malaria
Chlamydia
Cryptococcosis
Cysticercosis
Ehrlichiosis
Legionella
Leptospirosis
Listeria monocytogenes
Lyme disease
Mycoplasma
Naegleria
Q fever
Rocky Mountain spotted fever
Schistosomiasis
Tertiary syphilis
Toxoplasmosis
Trypanosomiasis
Tuberculosis
Typhus
Whipple disease

[a]Boldface type indicates causes that are more commonly encountered.

Box 32.8

Noninfectious Causes of an Encephalitis Syndrome

Acute electrolyte imbalance
Behçet disease
Carcinoma
Cerebral vasculitis
Drug reactions
Heavy metal poisoning
Lupus cerebritis
Reye syndrome

Table 32.10

Signs and Symptoms Suggesting the Cause of Encephalitis

Sign or Symptom	Possible Cause of Encephalitis
Personality change, bizarre behavior, hallucinations, aphasia	Herpes simplex virus
Parkinsonian-like movement	Japanese encephalitis virus
Tongue, eyelid, lip, or extremity tremors	St Louis virus, WEE virus, West Nile virus
Ataxia	Measles, tertiary syphilis, St Louis virus, EBV, varicella-zoster virus, echovirus
Herpes zoster ophthalmicus and contralateral hemiparesis	Varicella-zoster virus
Cranial nerve palsies	Lyme neuroborreliosis
Asymmetrical flaccid paralysis and muscular pain	Poliovirus, enterovirus, Japanese encephalitis virus, West Nile virus, Colorado tick fever virus
Vesicular rash	Herpes simplex virus, varicella-zoster virus
Petechial rash	Rocky Mountain spotted fever, arboviruses, Colorado tick fever virus
Erythema multiforme	Mycoplasma, herpes simplex virus
Maculopapular rash	Measles, rubella, HIV, EBV, WEE virus, lupus cerebritis, West Nile virus
Paresthesia at site of a bite, hydrophobia, aerophobia, hyperactivity, pharyngeal spasms	Rabies
Seizures	California encephalitis virus, EEE virus, herpes simplex virus 1, VEE virus, rabies
Coma	Herpes simplex virus 1, EEE virus, WEE virus, rabies, VEE virus, Colorado tick fever virus, California virus
Rapid onset of disease	Arboviruses
Pneumonia	Adenovirus, influenza virus, mycoplasma, legionella
Diarrhea	Enterovirus, legionella, Whipple disease, mycoplasma, VEE virus
Parotitis, orchitis	Mumps

Abbreviations: EBV, Epstein-Barr virus; EEE, eastern equine encephalomyelitis; HIV, human immunodeficiency virus; VEE, Venezuelan equine encephalomyelitis; WEE, western equine encephalomyelitis.

4. Arbovirus-associated encephalitis may occur sporadically or in epidemics

C. Diagnosis
   1. Clinical signs and symptoms
      a. Mental status or cognitive capabilities are usually altered, although sometimes to a very mild degree, especially in subacute cases
      b. Meningeal irritation often coexists, resulting in headache and meningismus
      c. Focal neurologic deficits
      d. Seizures are common
      e. Abnormal movements and paralysis may be present
      f. Progression of disease
         1) Progression of infection may be rapid and result in coma and death (eg, eastern equine encephalomyelitis infection)
         2) Progression may be slow, with mild symptoms and prompt recovery (eg, Venezuelan equine encephalomyelitis infection)
      g. Asymptomatic seroconversion is common with some viruses (eg, West Nile virus)
      h. Findings on physical examination often provide important clues to the diagnosis (Table 32.10)
   2. Laboratory testing
      a. CSF examination usually shows a lymphocytic pleocytosis with 10 to 2,000 cells/μL
         1) Neutrophils may predominate early in acute infection
         2) Presence of red blood cells is common with HSV encephalitis and *Naegleria* infection
         3) Eosinophils are present with *Coccidioides* and helminth infections
      b. CSF glucose level: usually normal in viral and rickettsial infections and decreased to various degrees in other infections
      c. CSF protein level: usually elevated
      d. Serum and CSF antibody levels should be checked for specific pathogens
         1) If level of CSF antibody against a specific pathogen is equivalent to or higher than the serum antibody level,

the specific pathogen probably caused the infection
            2) Acute and convalescent serum antibody levels may also be used to establish a diagnosis
        e. PCR of the CSF is available for many pathogens known to cause encephalitis
        f. Electroencephalography can be helpful in establishing the diagnosis of HSV encephalitis by showing early temporal lobe localization
    3. Imaging
        a. MRI: optimal imaging for encephalitis and meningoencephalitis
        b. MRI can show enhancement at the focus of infection (eg, temporal lobe in HSV encephalitis), edema, demyelination, or mass-occupying lesions
    4. A definitive diagnosis is made for less than 50% of cases
D. Treatment
    1. High-dose acyclovir
        a. Administered empirically for encephalitis until HSV has been excluded as the cause
        b. Therapy should be continued for 3 weeks if the diagnostic evaluation confirms HSV encephalitis
    2. VZV encephalitis: treated with acyclovir
    3. CMV encephalitis: treated with ganciclovir
    4. All other forms of viral encephalitis: managed with supportive care
E. Selected Specific Pathogens
    1. Herpes simplex virus
        a. Most common cause of viral encephalitis
        b. Annual incidence rate: 1 in 300,000 persons
        c. HSV1 accounts for more than 95% of the cases
        d. Temporal lobe localization leads to behavioral symptoms, which may aid in the diagnosis
        e. CSF PCR: the standard for establishing the diagnosis
    2. Arboviruses
        a. Eastern equine encephalomyelitis virus
            1) Most lethal of the arboviruses: mortality rate in adults is up to 70%
            2) Geographic distribution
                a) Occurs in North and South America
                b) North American cases are restricted to the eastern seaboard: Florida, Georgia, Massachusetts, and New Jersey
            3) On average, fewer than 15 cases per year nationally
            4) High fevers are characteristic
            5) Rapidly progressive
        b. Western equine encephalomyelitis virus
            1) Usually a mild encephalitis, although fatalities occur
            2) Frequently subacute
            3) Geographic distribution
                a) Reported in all states in the upper Midwest west of Ohio
                b) Reported in all states west of the Mississippi River except Idaho, Nevada, and Utah
                c) Most cases occur in Colorado, Texas, California, and North Dakota
        c. Venezuelan equine encephalomyelitis virus
            1) Geographic distribution
                a) Occurs throughout North America, Central America, and South America
                b) Most cases in the United States occur in southern Texas and southern Florida
            2) May occur sporadically or in epidemics
            3) Pharyngitis and conjunctivitis
                a) Usually present
                b) Virus can be recovered from throat cultures in 40% of cases
            4) Disease is usually very mild or subclinical
        d. California encephalitis virus group
            1) Approximately 70 cases per year in the United States: Great Lakes states and mid-Atlantic states
            2) Disease is usually mild, but seizures and coma occasionally occur
            3) Case fatality rate: less than 1%
        e. St Louis virus
            1) Geographic distribution
                a) North America, Central America, and northern South America
                b) In the United States it is most prevalent along the Mississippi River
            2) Occasional seasonal epidemics
            3) Infection occurs most commonly in persons older than 60 years
        f. West Nile virus
            1) First case in North America occurred in 1999
                a) Has since spread rapidly across the continent
                b) Occurs in seasonal epidemics and sporadic cases throughout North America during late summer and early fall
                c) Most common mosquito-borne infection in the United States

2) Also endemic in Europe, Asia, Africa, and Australia
3) Clinical disease
   a) In 80% of persons infected, asymptomatic infection and seroconversion occur
   b) In less than 20%, a flulike illness develops
      i) Fever, headache, arthralgias, and myalgias
      ii) Some have lymphadenopathy and a maculopapular rash
      iii) Symptoms last from a few days to a few weeks
   c) In less than 1%, severe symptoms of encephalitis develop or, less frequently, meningitis or polio-like paralysis
   d) Persons older than 50 years are more likely to have serious symptoms
g. Japanese encephalitis virus
   1) Endemic in Japan, eastern and southern China, India, Southeast Asia, Malaysia, Indonesia, and the Philippines
      a) Leading cause of encephalitis in Asia: mortality rate 30% to 40%
      b) Causes seasonal epidemics most frequently in rural areas
   2) Rare North American cases occur in travelers and military personnel who have been where virus is endemic
   3) Extrapyramidal symptoms are characteristic
   4) Vaccine
      a) Prevents disease
      b) Can be offered to persons spending 1 month or more where virus is endemic during the transmission season, especially if travel will include rural areas
h. Colorado tick fever
   1) Tick-borne virus endemic at elevations above 1,200 meters in western United States and Canada
   2) Flulike illness, with neuroinvasive disease occurring occasionally in children
      a) Fever and symptoms commonly recur 2 to 3 days after apparent recovery
      b) Petechial or maculopapular rash in 15% of cases
i. Rocky Mountain spotted fever
   1) Occurs in southeastern United States west to Texas and Oklahoma and in South Dakota and Montana

2) Neurologic symptoms
   a) Altered mental status, meningismus, seizures, and coma
   b) Headache in more than 90% of patients
3) CSF abnormalities
   a) More than 30% of patients: increased white blood cell count and protein level
   b) Glucose level is usually normal
4) Mortality rate
   a) Untreated: 30%
   b) With appropriate therapy: 3% to 5%

IV. Myelitis
   A. Definitions
      1. *Myelitis*: infection or inflammation of the spinal cord
      2. *Encephalomyelitis* is the term frequently used because most causes of encephalitis can cause myelitis with or without encephalitis
   B. Notable Myelitis Syndromes
      1. Transverse myelitis
         a. Acute infection or inflammation of the spinal cord, causing rostral motor and sensory deficits and bowel and bladder dysfunction
         b. Onset usually evolves over 2 to 24 hours
         c. Infectious causes: syphilis, schistosomiasis, human T-lymphotropic virus 1 (HTLV-1), CMV, VZV, Lyme disease, and *Toxoplasma*
         d. Clinical features suggest an apparent transection at a discrete level (usually thoracic), but MRI shows evidence of inflammation extending along several levels
         e. Must be distinguished from multiple sclerosis, anterior spinal artery thrombosis, dissecting aneurysm, cord compression, and arteriovenous malformation
      2. Flaccid paralysis caused by involvement of anterior horn cells of the spinal cord
         a. Usually with evidence of encephalitis but can be isolated myelitis
         b. Common causes: poliovirus, other enteroviruses, rabies virus, and arboviruses

V. Postinfectious Encephalitis
   A. Clinical Features
      1. Acute encephalitis syndrome occurring several days after an infection and characterized by recrudescent fever with neurologic signs and symptoms
      2. Invasion of the brain parenchyma by the infectious agent is not apparent, but perivascular inflammation and demyelination are present

3. Annual incidence rate: 1 per 100,000 population
4. Postvaccinal encephalitis causes a similar syndrome with an incidence rate ranging from 1 per 100,000 vaccine recipients (varicella) to less than 1 per 1,000,000 (mumps)

B. Etiology
1. Delayed onset and histologic features suggest an immune-mediated cause
2. Causes of postinfectious and postvaccinal encephalitis are summarized in Box 32.9

VI. Suppurative Infections of the Central Nervous System
A. Brain Abscess
1. Introduction
a. Focal or multifocal intracerebral collection of pus usually surrounded by an abscess wall
b. Frequently preceded by cerebritis characterized by an infectious inflammatory process without a well-defined capsule
c. Previously a lethal infection, but with modern imaging and neuroinvasive procedures, mortality has dramatically decreased
2. Epidemiology
a. Overall incidence rate
   1) Approximately 1.3 per 100,000 person-years
   2) Slightly bimodal distribution with increased rates among children aged 5 to 9 years and adults older than 60
b. Although cryptogenic infection can occur, most brain abscesses develop with a recognized predisposing condition (Table 32.11)
c. The microbiologic features of a brain abscess are also influenced by the predisposing condition (Table 32.11)
3. Diagnosis
a. Clinical manifestations of brain abscess are summarized in Table 32.12
b. Laboratory findings are not specific
   1) White blood cell count: may be elevated but is normal in 40%
   2) Erythrocyte sedimentation rate: usually elevated
   3) C-reactive protein level: usually elevated
c. Imaging
   1) CT or MRI should be performed on all patients with suspected brain abscess
   2) MRI is more sensitive and will detect cerebritis, edema, and early satellite lesions better than CT
4. Initial management and empirical therapy
a. Lesions smaller than 2.5 cm or lesions in the cerebritis stage
   1) Treated without drainage with empirical antibiotic therapy (Table 32.13) and monitored for response
   2) For multiple lesions, consider stereotactic aspiration for microbiologic diagnosis
b. All lesions larger than 2.5 cm should be drained emergently either stereotactically or by craniotomy, preferably before antibiotic therapy is initiated
c. Evaluate patient for focus of infection predisposing to brain abscess formation
d. Consider adding corticosteroid therapy if there is significant edema or a mass effect
e. Consider adding prophylactic anticonvulsant therapy
5. Definitive therapy
a. Empirical therapy can be modified according to the results of cultures and susceptibility data
b. Monitor response to therapy with serial CT or MRI

Box 32.9
Causes of Postinfectious and Postvaccinal Encephalitis

Postinfectious
  Campylobacter jejuni
  Epstein-Barr virus
  Influenza
  Measles
  Mumps
  Mycoplasma pneumoniae
  Nonspecific gastrointestinal tract infection
  Nonspecific upper respiratory infection
  Rubella
  Smallpox
  Streptococcus pyogenes
  Varicella-zoster virus
Postvaccinal
  Diphtheria and tetanus toxoids
  Haemophilus influenzae type b vaccine
  Inactivated *Vibrio cholerae* vaccine
  Japanese encephalitis virus vaccine
  Measles vaccine
  Oral poliovirus vaccine
  Pertussis vaccine
  Rubella virus vaccine
  Tetanus toxoid
  Varicella virus vaccine

Table 32.11

Predisposing Conditions, Locations, and Microbiologic Features of Brain Abscesses

Predisposing Condition	Location	Usual Microbiologic Features
Otitis media or mastoiditis	Temporal lobe, cerebellum	Streptococci (aerobic and anaerobic), *Bacteroides* species, *Prevotella* species, Enterobacteriaceae
Paranasal sinusitis	Frontal lobe, temporal lobe	Streptococci, *Bacteroides* species, Enterobacteriaceae, *Staphylococcus aureus*
Dental infection or dental procedure	Frontal lobe	Streptococci, *Bacteroides* species, *Prevotella* species, *Fusobacterium*
Trauma or postneurosurgery	According to surgical or penetrating trauma site	*S aureus*, coagulase-negative staphylococci, streptococci, Enterobacteriaceae, *Pseudomonas aeruginosa*
Cyanotic heart disease	Middle cerebral artery distribution	Streptococci, *Haemophilus* species
Pyogenic lung disease[a]	Middle cerebral artery distribution	Streptococci, *Bacteroides* species, *Prevotella* species, *Fusobacterium*, *Actinomyces* species, *Nocardia* species
Meningitis	Frontal lobe, cerebellum	Enterobacteriaceae, *Listeria*
Bacterial endocarditis	Middle cerebral artery distribution	*S aureus*, viridans streptococci, enterococci
Neutropenia	Middle cerebral artery distribution	Enterobacteriaceae, *P aeruginosa*, *Aspergillus* species, Mucorales, *Candida* species
AIDS	Middle cerebral artery distribution	*Toxoplasma gondii*, *Nocardia* species, *Listeria*, *Cryptococcus*, *Mycobacterium* species
Transplant	Middle cerebral artery distribution	*Aspergillus* species, Mucorales, *Candida* species, *Nocardia* species, *Toxoplasma*, Enterobacteriaceae

[a] Lung abscess, bronchiectasis, or empyema.

Adapted from Tunkel AR. Brain abscess. In: Mandell GL, Bennett JE, Dolin R, editors. Mandell, Douglas, and Bennett's principles and practice of infectious diseases. Vol 1. 7th ed. Philadelphia (PA): Churchill Livingstone/Elsevier; c2010. p. 1265–78. Used with permission.

    c. Continue parenteral antimicrobial therapy for 4 to 6 weeks if lesions were drained
    d. Patients treated empirically should receive therapy for at least 2 months
 6. Selected specific pathogens
    a. Streptococci
       1) Organisms in the *Streptococcus anginosus* group (*S anginosus*, *Streptococcus constellatus*, and *Streptococcus intermedius*) account for up to 70% of brain abscesses
       2) Overt or occult focus of primary infection is usually present
    b. *Nocardia* species
       1) Usually in patients with impaired T-cell immunity (from transplant, AIDS, corticosteroid therapy, etc) but also in patients who do not have underlying conditions
       2) Isolated brain abscess or in association with pulmonary or cutaneous nocardiosis
    c. Fungal pathogens
       1) *Candida* species
          a) Most common cause of fungal brain abscess
          b) Risk factors: corticosteroid use, long-term central venous catheter use, broad-spectrum antibiotics, malignancy, diabetes mellitus, and other chronic conditions
          c) Diagnosis is often made at autopsy
       2) *Aspergillus* species
          a) Usually in association with neutropenia and hematologic malignancies

Table 32.12

Clinical Manifestations of Brain Abscess

Clinical Manifestation	Frequency, %
Headache	70[a]
Somnolence, altered mental status	≤70
Focal neurologic findings	>60
Triad of headache, fever, and focal deficit	<50
Fever	45-50
Nausea and vomiting	25-50
Seizures	25-35
Meningismus	25[a]
Papilledema	25[a]

[a] Approximately.

Adapted from Tunkel AR. Brain abscess. In: Mandell GL, Bennett JE, Dolin R, editors. Mandell, Douglas, and Bennett's principles and practice of infectious diseases. Vol 1. 7th ed. Philadelphia (PA): Churchill Livingstone/Elsevier; c2010. p. 1265–78. Used with permission.

Table 32.13

Empirical Therapy for Brain Abscess by Predisposing Condition

Predisposing Condition	Empirical Therapy
Otitis media or mastoiditis	Third-generation cephalosporin[a] plus metronidazole
Paranasal sinusitis	Third-generation cephalosporin[a] plus metronidazole
Dental infection or dental procedure	Penicillin plus metronidazole
Trauma or postneurosurgery	Vancomycin plus antipseudomonal cephalosporin[b]
Cyanotic heart disease	Third-generation cephalosporin[a]
Pyogenic lung disease[c]	Third-generation cephalosporin[a] plus metronidazole[d]
Bacterial endocarditis	Ampicillin plus gentamicin plus antistaphylococcal penicillin[e]
Neutropenia	Antipseudomonal cephalosporin[b]
AIDS	Trimethoprim-sulfamethoxazole
Transplant	Variable
Cryptogenic	Vancomycin plus a third-generation cephalosporin[a] plus metronidazole

[a] Cefotaxime or ceftriaxone.
[b] Therapy with ceftazidime or cefepime should continue until *Pseudomonas* infection is excluded.
[c] Lung abscess, bronchiectasis, or empyema.
[d] Consider adding sulfonamide if *Nocardia* is a consideration.
[e] Vancomycin plus gentamicin as an alternative.

Adapted from Tunkel AR. Brain abscess. In: Mandell GL, Bennett JE, Dolin R, editors. Mandell, Douglas, and Bennett's principles and practice of infectious diseases. Vol 1. 7th ed. Philadelphia (PA): Churchill Livingstone/Elsevier; c2010. p. 1265–78. Used with permission.

b) Also in patients with advanced liver disease, transplant recipients, and other patients with impaired immune function
c) Hematogenous dissemination from a pulmonary infection is most common, but direct invasion from the sinuses also occurs
3) Mucorales
a) Rhinocerebral form of disease follows direct extension from the sinuses and occurs most frequently in patients with diabetes mellitus and acidosis
b) Other risk factors: malignancies, organ transplant, injection drug use, and deferoxamine use
4) *Scedosporium apiospermum*
a) Disseminated infection, including brain abscess, has been reported in survivors of near drowning

b) Also occurs in immunocompromised hosts
c) Rarely occurs in healthy hosts
d. *Toxoplasma gondii*
1) Intracranial infection usually results from reactivation of latent disease in persons with impaired cellular immunity
2) Most common in persons with AIDS but also occurs in others
a) Transplant recipients
b) Persons with malignancies receiving cytotoxic therapy
c) Other persons receiving immunosuppressive therapy
B. Epidural Abscess
1. Introduction
a. Focal collection of pus in the epidural space
b. May occur intracranially or, more commonly, in the spinal canal
2. Epidemiology
a. Cranial epidural abscess: occurs after direct extension from adjacent infected sinus, mastoid air cells, or middle ear
b. Spinal epidural abscess: occurs most frequently by hematogenous dissemination from a remote infection or by extension from an adjacent disk space infection
c. Cranial or spinal epidural abscess may occur after blunt trauma
d. Pathogens
1) *Staphylococcus aureus* accounts for more than half of the cases
2) Streptococci and gram-negative bacilli account for most others
3) Various other organisms from case reports: *Nocardia*, fungi, and *Mycobacteria*
3. Clinical and imaging features
a. Cranial infection
1) Usually insidious
2) Headache is usually present
3) May manifest with focal neurologic symptoms
b. Spinal infection
1) Acute or chronic
2) Chronic evolution of symptoms is more common
a) Localized spinal pain is the initial symptom
b) Neurologic deficits emerge as the abscess enlarges
c) Often associated with disk space infection and adjacent vertebral osteomyelitis

c. Fever is frequently absent
d. MRI is the diagnostic procedure of choice for cranial or spinal epidural abscess
4. Management
   a. Cranial epidural abscess: surgical drainage and directed antibiotic therapy based on culture results
   b. Spinal epidural abscess: may be treated with antibiotic therapy alone if there are no neurologic deficits
   c. Antibiotic therapy
      1) Therapy based on results of CT-guided aspiration is preferred to empirical therapy
      2) Serial neurologic examination and imaging should be performed to assess response to therapy
      3) Antibiotic therapy should be continued for at least 8 weeks
   d. Emergency decompressive laminectomy should be performed when there is neurologic dysfunction

C. Subdural Empyema
1. Collection of pus spreading through the space between the dura and arachnoid
2. Epidemiology and etiology
   a. Occurrence
      1) Direct extension from adjacent infection (in descending order of frequency: sinusitis, otitis or mastoiditis, cranial osteomyelitis)
      2) After neurosurgery or after trauma
      3) Occasionally from hematogenous source
   b. Most cases spreading from adjacent infection involve streptococci, *S aureus*, aerobic gram-negative bacilli, and anaerobes
   c. Staphylococci predominate after neurosurgery and after trauma
   d. Polymicrobial infection is common
3. Clinical and imaging features
   a. Usually a rapidly progressive infection with signs and symptoms similar to those of acute bacterial meningitis but with prominent focal neurologic deficits and altered mental status
   b. MRI or CT is diagnostic, but MRI provides greater detail
   c. Lumbar puncture is contraindicated owing to the risk of herniation
4. Management
   a. Medical emergency
      1) Requires combined medical and surgical intervention
      2) Emergent decompression and culture of purulent material by burr hole or craniotomy should be done as soon as possible after the diagnosis is suspected
   b. Empirical therapy
      1) Vancomycin and an antipseudomonal carbapenem *or* vancomycin, an antipseudomonal cephalosporin, and metronidazole
      2) Empirical therapy should be continued until culture results, including anaerobic culture results, and susceptibility data are available

D. Suppurative Intracranial Venous Sinus Thrombosis
1. Combination of thrombosis and purulent infection in any of the intracranial venous sinuses or veins
2. Epidemiology
   a. Can occur as a complication of infection involving the sinuses, ears, mastoid air cells, or oropharynx by direct extension
   b. Can occur as a complication of subdural empyema, epidural abscess, or bacterial meningitis
   c. Microbiologic features are similar to those of subdural empyema
      1) *Staphylococcus aureus* predominates
      2) Streptococci and gram-negative bacilli account for most other cases
3. Clinical and imaging features
   a. Signs and symptoms depend on the site of suppurative thrombosis
      1) Cavernous sinus thrombosis
         a) Periorbital swelling, proptosis, diplopia, headache, and altered mental status
         b) Initially unilateral
         c) Becomes bilateral as contralateral cavernous sinus is involved
      2) Lateral sinus thrombosis
         a) Headache, photophobia, nausea, vomiting, facial pain
         b) Otitis media is usually present
      3) Superior sagittal sinus thrombosis
         a) Meningismus, altered mental status, focal neurologic deficits
         b) Papilledema
   b. MRI or magnetic resonance angiography is diagnostic
   c. High-resolution CT is acceptable but less sensitive
   d. CSF examination: slow, slight pleocytosis with elevated protein level
   e. CSF culture may be positive
4. Management
   a. Empirical antibiotic therapy should be initiated with the same regimen outlined above for subdural empyema

b. Surgical therapy
1) May be required if therapy with parenteral antibiotics fails
2) Most often required in cavernous sinus suppurative thrombophlebitis

VII. Cerebrospinal Fluid Shunt Infections
A. Introduction
1. Shunts are used to divert excess CSF in patients with hydrocephalus
a. Ventriculoperitoneal (VP)
b. Ventriculoatrial (VA)
c. Occasionally, lumboperitoneal (LP)
2. Use of externalized intraventricular catheters
a. Temporary CSF drainage
b. Monitoring of CSF pressure in the intensive care unit
c. Management of shunt infections
B. Epidemiology and Etiology
1. Incidence rate for shunt infections
a. With current devices and surgical technique: less than 4%
b. With external devices: 5% to 10%
2. Pathogens
a. Staphylococci account for more than 75% of infections (coagulase-negative staphylococci predominate)
b. Other skin flora organisms: *Corynebacteria* and *Propionibacterium* in up to 15% of infections
c. Enterobacteriaceae and other gram-negative bacilli are occasionally involved
3. Mechanisms of infection
a. Usually colonization of the shunt at the time of implantation
b. Retrograde spread from contamination of the distal end (eg, enteric perforation of the peritoneal catheter, with spread to the CSF)
c. Hematogenous seeding
d. Breakdown of skin over the tunneled catheter allows contamination of the shunt
C. Diagnosis
1. Signs and symptoms of infection depend on several factors
a. Type of shunt
b. Whether the proximal (ie, intraventricular) end, the distal end, or the entire shunt is infected
c. Virulence of the infecting organism
d. Proximal infections: symptoms of meningitis or ventriculitis
e. Distal shunt infections: evidence of peritonitis or increased symptoms of hydrocephalus owing to shunt obstruction and failure
2. Clinical features may be indolent and insidious, so that establishing the diagnosis is challenging
3. CSF evaluation
a. CSF cultures should be obtained from the device reservoir if possible
b. CSF should be analyzed for cell count and differential count, protein, and glucose
4. Blood cultures
a. Positive in more than 90% of VA shunts
b. Usually negative in VP or LP shunts
D. Management
1. Shunt removal is necessary
a. Treatment of shunt infection with retention of the device is rarely successful
b. A temporary, external CSF drain is usually required until the shunt can be replaced
2. Antibiotic therapy
a. Empirical antibiotic therapy with vancomycin and an antipseudomonal cephalosporin or carbapenem is appropriate until definitive culture and susceptibility results are available
b. Intraventricular vancomycin combined with oral rifampin is advocated by some experts to overcome the low CSF levels of vancomycin when given systemically
c. For *S aureus* and gram-negative bacillary infection, 14 to 21 days of therapy is recommended
3. With coagulase-negative staphylococcal infection, the shunt can be replaced after 7 to 10 days of antibiotic therapy if subsequent CSF cultures are negative

Suggested Reading

Coyle PK. Overview of acute and chronic meningitis. Neurol Clin. 1999 Nov;17(4):691–710.

Cunha BA. Differential diagnosis of West Nile encephalitis. Curr Opin Infect Dis. 2004 Oct;17(5):413–20.

Hildebrand J, Aoun M. Chronic meningitis: still a diagnostic challenge. J Neurol. 2003 Jun;250(6):653–60.

Solomon T. Flavivirus encephalitis. N Engl J Med. 2004 Jul 22;351(4):370–8.

Tunkel AR, Glaser CA, Bloch KC, Sejvar RR, Marra CM, Roos KL, et al. The management of encephalitis: clinical practice guidelines by the Infectious Diseases Society of America. Clin Infect Dis. 2008 Aug 1;47(3):303–27.

Tunkel AR, Hartman BJ, Kaplan SL, Kaufman BA, Roos KL, Scheld WM, et al. Practice guidelines for the management of bacterial meningitis. Clin Infect Dis. 2004 Nov 1;39(9):1267–84. Epub 2004 Oct 6.

van de Beek D, de Gans J, Tunkel AR, Wijdicks EF. Community-acquired bacterial meningitis in adults. N Engl J Med. 2006 Jan 5;354(1):44–53.

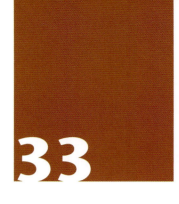

Imad M. Tleyjeh, MD, MSc
Larry M. Baddour, MD

33

Skin and Soft Tissue Infections

I. Common Skin and Soft Tissue Infections
  A. Impetigo
    1. *Impetigo*: a superficial pustular skin infection
    2. Multiple lesions occur on exposed skin of the face and extremities
    3. Associated with little or no systemic toxicity
    4. Usually occurs in warm, humid conditions
    5. Risk factors
       a. Poverty
       b. Crowding
       c. Poor personal hygiene
       d. Carriage of group A streptococcus or *Staphylococcus aureus*
    6. Etiology
       a. Minor skin trauma (eg, from insect bites or abrasions) often predisposes to the development of impetigo
       b. *Staphylococcus aureus* causes most cases
       c. In the remainder, group A streptococcus is the pathogen, either alone or with *S aureus*
    7. Three types of lesions (in order of decreasing frequency)
       a. Nonbullous vesicular impetigo
       b. Bullous impetigo due to *S aureus* exfoliative toxin A
       c. Ulcerated impetigo, known as ecthyma
    8. Treatment
       a. For localized disease: topical antibiotic with either fusidic acid or mupirocin
       b. For extensive disease: oral antibiotic with cephalexin
  B. Folliculitis
    1. *Folliculitis*: a superficial skin infection of hair follicles
    2. Erythematous lesions
       a. Diameter of 5 mm or less
       b. Central pustule may be present
       c. Usually cluster in groups
       d. Often pruritic
    3. Most common pathogens responsible for folliculitis (with corresponding risk factors)
       a. *Staphylococcus aureus* (nasal carriage of *S aureus*)
       b. *Pseudomonas aeruginosa* (contaminated water or hot tub use)
       c. *Candida* species (antibiotic administration and corticosteroid therapy)
    4. Treatment
       a. Warm saline compresses
       b. Topical antibacterial or antifungal agents (depending on epidemiologic clues) are usually sufficient

C. Furunculosis and Carbunculosis
 1. *Furuncle*: a purulent, painful nodular skin infection involving the hair follicle that is usually a complication of folliculitis
 2. *Carbuncle*: a cluster of abscesses in subcutaneous tissue that drain through hair follicles
 3. Prevailing pathogen for both furuncles and carbuncles: S aureus
 4. The back of the neck, face, axillae, and buttocks are commonly involved
 5. Treatment
    a. For most patients with furuncles and carbuncles: warm compresses to promote spontaneous drainage
    b. Surgical drainage may be required in cases in which spontaneous drainage does not occur
D. Skin Abscess
 1. Skin abscesses involve the dermis and deeper skin tissues
    a. Painful and fluctuant
    b. Often a pustule is present on the skin
 2. Pathogens
    a. For most cases: S aureus
    b. Other pathogens, either alone or with additional organisms, also can cause skin abscess
 3. Treatment
    a. Incision and drainage are required
    b. Antibiotics are not needed except in the presence of multiple lesions, cutaneous gangrene, immunosuppression, surrounding cellulitis, or systemic symptoms
E. Cellulitis
 1. Cellulitis involves skin and subcutaneous tissues
    a. Clinical manifestations: swelling, erythema, tenderness, and warmth
    b. Systemic manifestations: usually mild
 2. Pathogens
    a. The most common causative organism varies, depending on the location of cellulitis, associated venous and lymphatic compromise, immune status of the host, and exposure history
    b. Non–group A β-hemolytic streptococci (groups B, C, G, and F streptococci)
       1) Common causes of cellulitis
       2) Tend to cause cellulitis when venous or lymphatic compromise is present
    c. Group A streptococci can also cause cellulitis as can various other organisms
    d. *Staphylococcus aureus*: usually associated with skin breakdown from trauma or a wound
 3. Diagnosis
    a. Cellulitis is a clinical diagnosis
    b. Many noninfectious maladies mimic cellulitis (Table 33.1)
 4. Treatment
    a. Initial choice of antimicrobial therapy is usually empirical because identifying a specific microbial causative agent is uncommon
    b. Culturing of blood or skin can be helpful for patients in several circumstances
       1) Immunosuppression
       2) Systemic toxicity
       3) No response to therapy
       4) Unusual exposures (eg, water, animals)
       5) Recurrent infection
    c. Cultures are also helpful when there is a risk of community-acquired methicillin-resistant S aureus (CA-MRSA) cellulitis
    d. Treatment options are detailed in Table 33.2 for specific cellulitis syndromes
F. Erysipelas
 1. *Erysipelas*: a superficial cellulitis of skin with prominent lymphatic involvement
 2. Clinical features
    a. Painful lesion
    b. Bright red, edematous, indurated appearance
    c. Raised border that is sharply demarcated from adjacent normal skin
 3. Almost always caused by group A streptococci
II. Necrotizing Skin and Soft Tissue Infections
 A. Introduction
  1. Necrotizing infections of the skin and fascia
     a. Necrotizing forms of cellulitis
     b. Necrotizing fasciitis types I and II
  2. Clinical features: fulminant destruction of tissue and systemic toxicity
     a. Extensive tissue destruction
     b. Thrombosis of blood vessels, leading to necrosis
     c. Bacteria spreading along fascial planes are seen on histopathologic examination
  3. Signs of necrotizing deep tissue infection
     a. Pain disproportionate to the physical findings
     b. Violaceous bullae
     c. Cutaneous hemorrhage
     d. Skin sloughing
     e. Skin anesthesia
     f. Rapid progression of signs and symptoms
     g. Gas in the tissue

Table 33.1
Syndromes That Mimic Cellulitis

Syndrome	Mechanism	Distinctive Features
Stasis dermatitis	Chronic venous insufficiency Chronic edema and inflammation	No fever
Cutaneous expansion syndrome	Rapid expansion of edema with stretching of the skin	No fever Extremities are affected bilaterally
Superficial thrombophlebitis	Intravenous needle or catheter	Tender cord
Deep vein thrombosis	Vein thrombosis with edema, warmth, and erythema	No fever, palpable clot, or engorgement of veins Duplex ultrasonographic findings Risk factors
Contact dermatitis	Inflammation related to toxin or irritant	Sharply demarcated and confined to area of exposure
Insect bites	Local inflammatory reaction	Pruritus History
Sweet syndrome	Neutrophilic dermatosis	Associated with malignancies (eg, acute myelogenous leukemia)
Gouty arthritis	Arthritis with cutaneous erythema	Location History Joint examination findings
Lymphedema without cellulitis	Lymphedema	No fever No response to antibiotics

      h. Severe systemic manifestations such as severe sepsis and shock
 4. Accurate diagnosis is required along with early surgical intervention
 B. Necrotizing Cellulitis
  1. Types of necrotizing cellulitis
   a. Clostridial and nonclostridial anaerobic infections
   b. Meleney synergistic gangrene
   c. Synergistic necrotizing cellulitis
  2. There is significant overlap between these cellulitis syndromes and deeper necrotizing soft tissue infections
   a. They must be distinguished from myonecrosis and necrotizing fasciitis
   b. Diagnosis requires prompt surgical exploration or imaging studies (or both)
  3. Cellulitis caused by *Clostridium perfringens*
   a. Usually related to local trauma or surgical procedure
   b. Gas is present in skin but not in deeper structures
  4. Nonclostridial anaerobic cellulitis
   a. Caused by both anaerobic and aerobic organisms
   b. Gas is produced in tissues
   c. Foul odor is often present
   d. Persons usually have diabetes mellitus
  5. Meleney synergistic gangrene
   a. A rare infection
   b. Occurs in postoperative patients
   c. Characterized by a slowly expanding ulceration that is confined to the superficial fascia
   d. Results from a synergistic interaction between *S aureus* and microaerophilic streptococci
  6. Synergistic necrotizing cellulitis
   a. Confined to the skin
   b. A variant of necrotizing fasciitis type I, which involves the skin, muscle, fat, and fascia
   c. Usually found on the legs or perineum
   d. Diabetes mellitus is a known risk factor
 C. Necrotizing Fasciitis
  1. Necrotizing fasciitis involves the subcutaneous tissue
   a. With or without skin involvement
   b. Fascia and fat are progressively destroyed
  2. Early recognition of necrotizing fasciitis is important
   a. Fulminant clinical course
   b. Extensive tissue destruction
   c. Systemic toxicity
   d. Risk of need for limb amputation
   e. Risk of death

Table 33.2
Specific Cellulitis Syndromes: Organisms and Empirical Therapy

Syndrome	Location	Likely Organisms	Source	Empirical Parenteral Therapy	Oral Regimens
Extremity cellulitis	Lower extremity	Group A β-hemolytic streptococci *Staphylococcus aureus*	Macerated or fissured interdigital toe spaces	Cefazolin 1–2 g IV every 8 h or nafcillin 2 g IV every 6 h In penicillin-allergic patients (immediate-type hypersensitivity reaction) or in patients with possible community-acquired or health care–related ORSA or MRSA: vancomycin 15 mg/kg IV every 12 h (dose based on actual body weight and used for patients with calculated creatinine clearance >50 mL/min) If patient is intolerant of vancomycin: linezolid 600 mg IV every 12 h or daptomycin 4 mg/kg IV every 24 h	Dicloxacillin 500 mg orally every 6 h or cephalexin 500 mg orally every 6 h In penicillin-allergic patients (immediate-type hypersensitivity reaction): clindamycin 300 mg orally every 6 h (unless clindamycin resistance among strains of β-hemolytic streptococci is prevalent) or linezolid 600 mg orally every 12 h
Preseptal cellulitis	Periorbital	*Streptococcus pneumoniae* *Staphylococcus aureus* Coagulase-negative staphylococci Anaerobes *Haemophilus influenzae* type b (unvaccinated children)	Contiguous infection of the soft tissues of the face and eyelids caused by local trauma, insect bites, or foreign bodies	Ampicillin-sulbactam 3 g IV every 6 h *or* Levofloxacin 750 mg IV every 24 h plus metronidazole 500 mg IV every 8 h	Amoxicillin-clavulanate 875 mg orally every 12 h *or* Levofloxacin 750 mg orally every 24 h plus metronidazole 500 mg orally every 8 h
Orbital cellulitis	Orbital	Streptococci *Staphylococcus aureus* Non–spore-forming anaerobes	Sinusitis Orbital trauma with fracture or foreign body Dacryocystitis Infection of the teeth, middle ear, or face	Same as for preseptal cellulitis	Same as for preseptal cellulitis
Erysipelas	Face and lower extremity	Group A streptococci	Antecedent streptococcal respiratory tract infection, skin ulcers, local trauma or abrasions, or psoriatic or eczematous lesions	Same as for extremity cellulitis If organism is confirmed: penicillin G (2 million to 4 million units every 4 h)	Same as for extremity cellulitis If organism is confirmed: penicillin V (500 mg every 6 h)
Postmastectomy cellulitis	Ipsilateral arm	Non–group A β-hemolytic streptococci	Complication of operations that involve lymph node dissection	Same as for extremity cellulitis	Same as for extremity cellulitis

Postlumpectomy cellulitis	Ipsilateral breast (can extend to the remainder of the breast, anterior shoulder, back, and ipsilateral upper extremity)	Non–group A β-hemolytic streptococci	Complication of operations that involve limited lymph node dissection and breast conservation and radiotherapy	Same as for extremity cellulitis
Post-saphenous venectomy cellulitis	Lower extremity	Non–group A β-hemolytic streptococci	Occur months to years after saphenous venectomy Disruption of the cutaneous barrier Lymphedema Venous insufficiency	Same as for extremity cellulitis
Perineal or postgynecologic surgery cellulitis	Abdominal wall Inguinal area Proximal thigh	Non–group A β-hemolytic streptococci *Staphylococcus aureus* Enterococci *Escherichia coli* *Peptostreptococcus* species *Prevotella* species *Porphyromonas* species *Bacteroides fragilis* group *Clostridium* species	Surgical procedures with local lymph node dissection and radiotherapy for several types of gynecologic cancer	Same as for preseptal cellulitis
Abdominal wall cellulitis	Abdominal wall May extend to thighs	β-Hemolytic streptococci	Morbid obesity Abdominal wall lymphedema	Same as for extremity cellulitis

(continued)

Table 33.2
(continued)

Syndrome	Location	Likely Organisms	Source	Empirical Parenteral Therapy	Oral Regimens
Clostridial cellulitis	Varies	*Clostridium perfringens* and other *Clostridium* species	Local trauma or recent surgery	Penicillin (3 million to 4 million units every 4 h IV) plus clindamycin (600-900 mg every 8 h IV) *or* Tetracycline (500 mg every 6 h IV)	Not recommended initially
Nonclostridial anaerobic cellulitis	Varies	Both anaerobic and aerobic organisms (*Bacteroides*, peptostreptococci, *Klebsiella*, *E coli*)	Diabetes mellitus	Same as for preseptal cellulitis	Not recommended initially
Gangrenous cellulitis (immunosuppressed host)	Varies	*Pseudomonas* *Aspergillus* Agents of mucormycosis	Immunosuppression	Requires biopsy and microbial confirmation	Not recommended initially
Bacterial cellulitis in immunosuppressed patients	Varies	Group A β-hemolytic streptococci *Staphylococcus aureus* *Pseudomonas aeruginosa* *Serratia* *Proteus* Enterobacteriaciae	Immunosuppression Bacteremia	Cefepime 2 g IV every 12 h *or* Imipenem 500 mg IV every 6 h *or* Piperacillin-tazobactam 3.375 g IV every 4-6 h In the penicillin-allergic (immediate-type hypersensitivity reaction) patient: moxifloxacin 400 mg IV every 24 h If fluoroquinolone resistance is prevalent among local strains of *P aeruginosa*: add tobramycin 5-7 mg/kg IV every 24 h (dosing per Hartford Hospital nomogram) In patients with possible community-acquired or health care-related ORSA or MRSA: same as for extremity cellulitis	Not recommended initially
Dog and cat bite cellulitis	Varies	*Pasteurella* Staphylococci Streptococci *Capnocytophaga* *Bacteroides* species Fusobacteria *Porphyromonas* species *Prevotella heparinolytica* Propionibacteria Peptostreptococcus	Oral and skin flora	Same as for preseptal cellulitis	Same as for preseptal cellulitis

Human bite cellulitis	Varies	Normal oral flora of the biter Streptococci (especially viridans streptococci), staphylococci, Haemophilus species, and Eikenella Anaerobes, including Fusobacterium nucleatum and other Fusobacterium species, Peptostreptococcus, Prevotella species, and Porphyromonas species	Same as for preseptal cellulitis	Same as for preseptal cellulitis
Freshwater exposure cellulitis	Varies	Aeromonas hydrophila	Freshwater	Levofloxacin 750 mg IV every 24 h or Cefepime 1-2 g IV every 24 h or Meropenem 1 g IV every 8 h or Other carbapenems: imipenem-cilastatin and ertapenem	Levofloxacin 750 mg IV every 24 h
Saltwater exposure cellulitis	Varies	Vibrio species, particularly Vibrio vulnificus	Saltwater Ingestion of raw or undercooked seafood	Minocycline 200 mg IV as loading dose; then 100 mg IV every 12 h plus cefotaxime 2 g IV every 8 h or Levofloxacin 750 mg IV daily	Minocycline 200 mg orally as loading dose; then 100 mg orally every 12 h or Levofloxacin 750 mg orally daily
Aquaculture cellulitis	Varies	Streptococcus iniae	Fish	Penicillin G (2 million to 4 million units every 4 h) Empirical coverage is same as for extremity cellulitis	Penicillin V (500 mg every 6 h) Empirical coverage is same as for extremity cellulitis
Meat handling cellulitis	Hands	Erysipelothrix rhusiopathiae	Meat Poultry Hides Saltwater fish Shellfish	Penicillin G (2 million to 4 million units every 4 h) Alternative therapies include ceftriaxone (2 g once daily), imipenem (500 mg every 6 h), or fluoroquinolones (ciprofloxacin 400 mg every 12 h or levofloxacin 500 mg once daily)	Penicillin V (500 mg every 6 h) If the patient is penicillin allergic: ciprofloxacin (250 mg every 12 h), clindamycin (200 mg every 8 h), or erythromycin (500 mg every 6 h)

Abbreviations: IV, intravenously; MRSA, methicillin-resistant *Staphylococcus aureus*; ORSA, oxacillin-resistant *S aureus*.

3. Two clinical types
   a. Type I necrotizing fasciitis
      1) Infection with both aerobic and anaerobic bacteria (eg, *S aureus*, streptococci, enterococci, *Escherichia coli*, *Peptostreptococcus* species, *Prevotella* species, *Porphyromonas* species, *Bacteroides fragilis* group, *Clostridium* species)
      2) Typical occurrence
         a) After surgical procedures
         b) In patients with diabetes mellitus and peripheral vascular disease
         c) In head and neck region (cervical necrotizing fascitiis) or perineum (Fournier gangrene)
            i) Cervical necrotizing fasciitis results from disruption of the mucous membranes
               (a) After surgical procedure
               (b) After use of instruments
               (c) With an odontogenic infection
            ii) Fournier gangrene results from enteric organisms penetrating the gastrointestinal or urethral mucosa
   b. Type II necrotizing fasciitis
      1) Caused by group A streptococci
      2) Can be associated with toxic shock syndrome
      3) Predisposing factors
         a) Blunt trauma, laceration, or surgical procedure
         b) Varicella
         c) Injection drug use
         d) Childbirth
         e) Exposure to a case
         f) Burns
      4) Methicillin-resistant *S aureus* (MRSA) has been reported to cause type II necrotizing fasciitis
4. Clinical features
   a. Fever and signs of toxicity
   b. Skin involvement
   c. Pain greater than suggested by clinical findings
   d. Elevated levels of creatine kinase
5. Diagnosis
   a. Magnetic resonance imaging can help to delineate the extent of soft tissue involvement
   b. Surgical exploration is the only definite way to ascertain the diagnosis
6. Treatment
   a. Early surgical intervention is key in reducing mortality
      1) Surgically resected tissue should be sent for microbiologic analysis
      2) Determine pathogens involved and susceptibility for selection of antibiotic therapy
   b. Repeated surgical débridement to define the extent of disease and resect necrotic tissue
   c. Hemodynamic support
   d. Empirical antibiotic therapy initially
   e. Antibiotic therapy should later be based on operative culture results and susceptibility patterns
   f. Type I necrotizing fasciitis
      1) Empirical antibiotic therapy should cover aerobic and anaerobic organisms
      2) For patients who have been hospitalized previously, gram-negative coverage should be improved to protect against resistant organisms
   g. Type II necrotizing fasciitis
      1) Combination therapy with clindamycin and penicillin may be more effective than penicillin monotherapy
         a) Clindamycin is not affected by inoculum size or stage of growth
         b) Clindamycin suppresses toxin production
         c) Clindamycin facilitates phagocytosis of *Streptococcus pyogenes* by inhibiting M-protein synthesis
         d) Clindamycin has a long postantibiotic effect
      2) Empirical coverage for MRSA may be indicated in selected cases while awaiting microbiologic confirmation
      3) Limited evidence supports routine use of intravenous immunoglobulin
III. Specific Situations Involving Skin and Soft Tissue Infections
   A. Water Exposure
      1. Five microorganisms most commonly cause skin and soft tissue infections after water exposure
         a. With 4 of them, cellulitis is a well-recognized manifestation that often occurs as a complication of a traumatic wound and can range from trivial to severe
            1) *Aeromonas* species
            2) *Vibrio vulnificus*
            3) *Erysipelothrix rhusiopathiae*
            4) *Edwardsiella tarda*

b. With the fifth agent, *Mycobacterium marinum*, a subacute lymphadenitis syndrome is more characteristic
2. Typical associations
   a. *Aeromonas* species: freshwater exposure
   b. *Vibrio vulnificus*: saltwater exposure
   c. *Erysipelothrix rhusiopathiae*: handling fish or other marine life for meal preparation
   d. *Edwardsiella tarda*: various marine exposures
   e. *Mycobacterium marinum*: fish tank cleaning
3. Treatment
   a. Treatment choices are outlined in Table 33.2
   b. Regardless of the type of water exposure, empirical therapy should include antibiotics that have activity against the most common causes of cellulitis: β-hemolytic streptococci and *S aureus*

B. Animal and Human Bites
1. Cellulitis and deeper soft tissue infections can occur after animal or human bites
   a. Usually polymicrobial infection
   b. Usually caused by normal flora of the oral cavity
2. Causes of infections related to animal bites: *Pasteurella* species, staphylococci and streptococci, *Capnocytophaga*, *Bacteroides* species, fusobacteria, *Porphyromonas* species, *Prevotella heparinolytica*, propionibacteria, and *Peptostreptococcus*
3. Causes of infections related to human bites
   a. Normal oral flora of the biter, including streptococci (especially viridans streptococci), staphylococci, *Haemophilus* species, *Eikenella*
   b. Anaerobes, including *Fusobacterium nucleatum* and other *Fusobacterium* species, *Peptostreptococcus*, *Prevotella* species, and *Porphyromonas* species
4. Treatment choices are outlined in Table 33.2

C. Immunocompromised Hosts
1. Reasons for immunocompromised status
   a. Neutropenia
   b. Cellular immune deficiency, such as in lymphoma
   c. Blood, bone marrow, or solid organ transplant
   d. AIDS
   e. Treatment with corticosteroids or other immune suppressants
2. Opportunistic pathogens should be considered in every immunosuppressed host
3. Every effort should be made to establish a pathologic and microbiologic diagnosis, particularly for patients who have no response to empirical therapy or who have signs of systemic toxicity or deep tissue infection
4. Immunocompromised patients are predisposed to a different spectrum of etiologic agents that cause skin and soft tissue infections
   a. β-Hemolytic streptococci and *S aureus*
   b. Various unusual pathogens may invade the skin of immunocompromised patients spontaneously or after local trauma
      1) Fungi: *Aspergillus*, *Rhizopus*, *Apophysomyces elegans*, *Paecilomyces*, *Penicillium*, *Trichosporon*, *Fusarium*, *Alternaria*
      2) Nontuberculous mycobacteria: *Mycobacterium marinum* and rapidly growing mycobacteria
5. Skin lesions
   a. Localized or disseminated nodules, papules, or necrotizing infections
   b. Gangrenous cellulitis
6. Specific syndromes
   a. Gangrenous cellulitis and ecthyma gangrenosum
      1) Caused by various organisms
      2) *Pseudomonas* bacteremia, for example, can produce gangrenous cellulitis in immunocompromised hosts
      3) Gangrenous skin lesions may also occur with infection caused by other gram-negative bacilli and with disseminated aspergillosis
   b. Mucormycotic necrotizing angioinvasive cellulitis
      1) Caused by *Apophysomyces elegans* (class Zygomycetes) after a traumatic injury that involved contamination with soil or by *Rhizopus* species from contaminated tape
      2) Course of infection varies
         a) Indolent course: minimal fever and a slowly enlarging black ulcer
         b) Rapidly progressive, febrile course
      3) Clinical features
         a) Characteristic lesion consists of a central black, necrotic area with a surrounding raised zone of violaceous cellulitis and edema
         b) Superficial vesicles and blistering may occur in the gangrenous area
      4) Diagnosis: identification of the cause is best obtained from biopsy specimens

c. Cryptococcal cellulitis
   1) Occurs in severely immunocompromised hosts
   2) Extremely rare
   3) If cryptococcal infection is considered, every effort (skin biopsy and serum cryptococcal antigen) should be made to secure a diagnosis
   4) Empirical antifungal therapy should be avoided
7. Treatment
   a. Immunocompromised hosts with cellulitis should receive broad-spectrum antimicrobial therapy
   b. Causative organisms can be multidrug resistant and may be identified in blood cultures
   c. Drug resistance
      1) More likely in patients who have received prior antibiotic therapy
      2) Empirical antibiotic regimens that provide coverage for both aerobic gram-negative bacilli and gram-positive cocci (β-hemolytic streptococci and *S aureus*) should be used (Table 33.2)

Suggested Reading

Bjornsdottir S, Gottfredsson M, Thorisdottir AS, Gunnarsson GB, Rikardsdottir H, Kristjansson M, et al. Risk factors for acute cellulitis of the lower limb: a prospective case-control study. Clin Infect Dis. 2005 Nov 15;41(10):1416–22. Epub 2005 Oct 13.

McNamara DR, Tleyjeh IM, Berbari EF, Lahr BD, Martinez J, Mirzoyev SA, et al. A predictive model of recurrent lower extremity cellulitis in a population-based cohort. Arch Intern Med. 2007 Apr 9;167(7):709–15.

Stevens DL, Bisno AL, Chambers HF, Everett ED, Dellinger P, Goldstein EJ, et al; Infectious Diseases Society of America. Practice guidelines for the diagnosis and management of skin and soft-tissue infections. Clin Infect Dis. 2005 Nov 15;41(10):1373–406. Epub 2005 Oct 14. Erratum in: Clin Infect Dis. 2006 Apr 15;42(8):1219. Dosage error in article text. Clin Infect Dis. 2005 Dec 15;41(12):1830.

Elie F. Berbari, MD
Douglas R. Osmon, MD

34

Osteomyelitis, Infectious Arthritis, and Orthopedic Device Infection

I. Osteomyelitis
   A. Pathogenesis
      1. Despite recent advances in its medical and surgical management, osteomyelitis is a challenge for clinicians
      2. Two major mechanisms by which osteomyelitis occurs
         a. Contiguous inoculation
            1) Occurs when microorganisms contaminate the bone directly through an ulcer adjacent to the bone, trauma, or surgery on the bone
            2) Integrity of the cortex is breached
            3) Over time, microbial contamination causes progressive destruction of the bone and formation of sequestra
            4) This mechanism of infection is a common consequence of diabetic foot ulcers, open fractures, or surgical procedures
         b. Hematogenous seeding of bone
            1) Site of infection is elsewhere in the body
            2) This route of infection is common in acute long bone osteomyelitis in children and vertebral osteomyelitis in adults
   B. Classification Schemes
      1. Cierny-Mader classification: based on the infected portion of the bone, the physiologic status of the host, and the local environment of the infected bone (Box 34.1)
      2. Waldvogel classification: based on the duration of illness (ie, acute or chronic), the mechanism of infection (ie, hematogenous or contiguous), and the presence of vascular insufficiency
   C. Microbiology
      1. Many microorganisms can cause osteomyelitis
         a. Most common: *Staphylococcus aureus*
         b. In certain situations: coagulase-negative staphylococci and other organisms such as streptococci, enterococci, *Pseudomonas aeruginosa*, *Enterobacter* species, *Escherichia coli*, *Serratia* species, and others (Box 34.2)
         c. Occasionally: fungi and mycobacteria
      2. Contiguous-focus osteomyelitis
         a. Very common in adults
         b. Usually associated with vascular insufficiency or peripheral neuropathy and the appearance of skin ulcers
         c. Commonly seen in patients with advanced diabetes mellitus or in patients with paraplegia and decubitus pressure ulcers
         d. Often polymicrobial

> **Box 34.1**
>
> **Cierny-Mader Staging System for Osteomyelitis**
>
> Anatomical type
>   Stage 1: medullary osteomyelitis
>   Stage 2: superficial osteomyelitis
>   Stage 3: localized osteomyelitis
>   Stage 4: diffuse osteomyelitis
> Physiologic class
>   A host: normal host
>   B host
>   Systemic compromise (Bs)
>   Local compromise (Bl)
>   Systemic and local compromise (Bls)
>   C host: treatment worse than the disease
> Systemic or local factors that affect immune surveillance, metabolism, and local vascularity
>   Systemic (Bs)
>   Malnutrition
>   Renal, hepatic failure
>   Diabetes mellitus
>   Chronic hypoxia
>   Immune disease
>   Malignancy
>   Extremes of age
>   Immunosuppression
>   Local (Bl)
>   Chronic lymphedema
>   Major vessel compromise
>   Small vessel disease
>   Vasculitis
>   Venous stasis
>   Extensive scarring
>   Radiation fibrosis
>   Neuropathy
>   Tobacco abuse
>
> Adapted from Mader JT, Shirtliff M, Calhoun JH. Staging and staging application in osteomyelitis. Clin Infect Dis. 1997 Dec;25(6):1303–9. Used with permission.

> **Box 34.2**
>
> **Microbiology of Osteomyelitis**
>
> Common (>50% of cases)
>   *Staphylococcus aureus*
>   Coagulase-negative staphylococci
> Occasional (25%-50% of cases)
>   Streptococci
>   Enterococci
>   *Pseudomonas* species
>   *Enterobacter* species
>   *Proteus* species
>   *Escherichia coli*
>   *Serratia* species
>   Anaerobes (*Peptostreptococcus* species, *Clostridium* species, *Bacteroides fragilis* group)
> Rare (<5% of cases)
>   *Mycobacterium tuberculosis*
>   *Mycobacterium avium-intracellulare* complex
>   Rapidly growing mycobacteria
>   Dimorphic fungi
>   *Candida* species
>   *Aspergillus* species
>   *Mycoplasma* species
>   *Tropheryma whipplei*
>   *Brucella* species
>   *Salmonella* species
>   *Actinomyces*
>
> Adapted from Berbari EF, Steckelberg JM, Osmon DR. Osteomyelitis. In: Mandell GL, Bennett JE, Dolin R, editors. Mandell, Douglas, and Bennett's principles and practice of infectious diseases. Vol 1. 7th ed. Philadelphia (PA): Churchill Livingstone/Elsevier; c2010. p. 1457–68. Used with permission.

3. Osteomyelitis occurring as a consequence of an open fracture
   a. Multiple possible sources of pathogens
      1) Normal skin flora
      2) Organisms in the soil, debris, or vegetation that contaminate the wound at the time of the injury
      3) Nosocomial pathogens acquired at the time of fracture fixation
   b. Most common pathogens: *S aureus*, coagulase-negative staphylococci, aerobic gram-negative bacilli
4. Hematogenous osteomyelitis in adults
   a. Most common pathogen: *S aureus*
   b. Less frequent: β-hemolytic streptococci and aerobic gram-negative bacilli
   c. β-Hemolytic streptococcal infection commonly occurs in patients with diabetes mellitus or cancer or in elderly patients
5. Vertebral osteomyelitis
   a. Most common causes: hematogenous spread from skin or soft tissue infection, genitourinary tract infection, infective endocarditis, infected intravenous sites, intravenous drug abuse, or respiratory tract infection
   b. Common pathogen: *S aureus*
   c. Microorganisms in patients who abuse injection drugs: *P aeruginosa* and *Candida* species
   d. Spinal infections due to *Mycobacterium tuberculosis* and *Brucella* spondylodiskitis are common in patients who live where these pathogens are endemic
D. Diagnosis
   1. Clinical features
      a. Often nonspecific pain centered on the involved bone
      b. Typically, systemic symptoms are absent
      c. Fever and chills can occur with certain conditions
         1) Vertebral osteomyelitis complicated by bacteremia or abscess

2) Contiguous osteomyelitis complicated by concomitant soft tissue infection
  d. Draining sinus tract that extends to the involved bone may be present
  e. Neurologic dysfunction may be present in certain patients
    1) When bone infection or concomitant soft tissue infection or abscess impinges on neurologic structures
    2) Most common in cases of vertebral osteomyelitis and epidural abscess
  f. SAPHO syndrome
    1) Acronym for *s*ynovitis, *a*cne, *p*ustulosis, *h*yperostosis, and *o*steitis
    2) A consideration when patient has multifocal osteomyelitis and negative bone culture results
    3) Etiology is unknown
2. Diagnostic testing
  a. Detection of osteomyelitis depends on several factors
    1) Type of osteomyelitis
    2) Duration of symptoms
    3) Presence of underlying fracture fixation devices, joint prostheses, or spinal stabilization devices
  b. White blood cell count, sedimentation rate, or C-reactive protein level
    1) Often increased but can be normal
    2) Can be helpful in monitoring the progress of the disease with treatment
  c. Probe-to-bone test
    1) For patients suspected of having contiguous osteomyelitis involving an ulcer over the bone
    2) Clinician uses a metal probe to determine whether there is exposed bone at the depth of a wound
    3) Sensitive, specific, and inexpensive test
    4) Reported positive predictive value: 89%
  d. Plain radiographs
    1) Abnormalities may not be apparent for up to 2 weeks in most types of osteomyelitis, including contiguous osteomyelitis
    2) Thus, normal findings on plain film should not dissuade the clinician from the diagnosis of contiguous osteomyelitis
  e. Technetium Tc 99m methylene diphosphonate bone scan
    1) With or without indium In 111–labeled white blood cell scan
    2) Low specificity, particularly with other bone disease such as neuropathic bone disease or radiation necrosis
  f. Magnetic resonance imaging (MRI)
    1) Very sensitive and usually very specific for the diagnosis of osteomyelitis
    2) Exception: with neuropathic bone disease, MRI can lack specificity
  g. Computed tomography (CT)
    1) Less sensitive and specific than MRI
  h. Presence of orthopedic hardware
    1) CT or MRI images may be degraded and thus have less sensitivity and specificity
    2) In this situation, radionuclide imaging may be the most helpful
      a) Gallium Ga 67 citrate scanning seems to be very sensitive and specific for the diagnosis of diskitis
      b) Gallium Ga 67 citrate scanning is very sensitive and specific for spinal infection and is often used when MRI cannot be used
  i. All imaging techniques may be less sensitive and specific after recent surgery in the area of interest
  j. Gold standard for the diagnosis of osteomyelitis: deep bone culture that yields an organism or bone biopsy that yields pathologic evidence of infection
    1) Bone culture
      a) Administration of all antimicrobials should be withheld until a bone biopsy culture has been prepared
      b) Exception: presence of soft tissue infection or sepsis syndrome
      c) Culture results allow medical management to be directed to the microorganisms grown in culture and to avoid prolonged empirical therapy
    2) Bone biopsy
      a) Closed needle biopsy or open surgical procedure
      b) Several closed biopsies may be required to make a diagnosis of vertebral osteomyelitis
      c) Surgeons often describe soft or necrotic bone at the depth of a contiguous ulcer, which is helpful in determining whether disease is osteomyelitis
E. Therapy
  1. Surgical therapy
    a. In most cases of chronic osteomyelitis, surgical débridement is required

b. Principles of surgical therapy
   1) Adequate drainage and débridement of all infected tissue
   2) Removal of all infected orthopedic hardware (may need to be delayed to allow adequate fracture healing or surgical stabilization to occur)
   3) Management of dead space and adequate soft tissue coverage
      a) May require the use of muscle flaps and skin grafts
      b) Surgeons place temporary, antibiotic-impregnated polymethylmethacrylate beads in and around infected bone to manage dead space and to provide local antimicrobial therapy
   4) Vascular supply to an area of osteomyelitis should always be assessed and revascularization performed
      a) Improves the outcome of osteomyelitis surgery
      b) Minimizes the extent of any amputation that may be required if surgical débridement is not possible
2. Antimicrobial therapy (Table 34.1)

Table 34.1
Antimicrobial Therapy for Chronic Osteomyelitis in Adults for Selected Microorganisms

Microorganism	First Choice[a]	Alternative Choice[a]
Staphylococci		
Oxacillin sensitive	Nafcillin sodium or oxacillin sodium 1.5-2.0 g IV every 4 h for 4-6 wk *or* Cefazolin 1-2 g IV every 8 h for 4-6 wk	Vancomycin 15 mg/kg IV every 12 h for 4-6 wk
Oxacillin resistant	Vancomycin[b] 15 mg/kg IV every 12 h for 4-6 wk	Linezolid 600 mg orally or IV every 12 h for 6 wk *or* Levofloxacin[b] 500-750 mg orally or IV daily plus rifampin 600 mg orally daily for 6 wk
Penicillin-sensitive streptococci	Aqueous crystalline penicillin G 20×10^6 units daily IV continuously or in 6 equally divided daily doses for 4-6 wk *or* Ceftriaxone 1-2 g IV or IM every 24 h for 4-6 wk *or* Cefazolin 1-2 g IV every 8 h for 4-6 wk	Vancomycin 15 mg/kg IV every 12 h for 4-6 wk
Enterococci or streptococci with an MIC ≥0.5 μg/mL or nutritionally variant streptococci	Aqueous crystalline penicillin G 20×10^6 units daily IV continuously or in 6 equally divided daily doses for 4-6 wk *or* Ampicillin sodium 12 g daily IV continuously or in 6 equally divided daily doses *Optional:* addition of gentamicin sulfate 1 mg/kg IV or IM every 8 h for 1-2 wk	Vancomycin[b] 15 mg/kg IV every 12 h for 4-6 wk *Optional:* addition of gentamicin sulfate 1 mg/kg IV or IM every 8 h for 1-2 wk
Enterobacteriaciae	Ceftriaxone 2 g IV daily for 4-6 wk	Ciprofloxacin[b] 500-750 mg orally every 24 h for 4-6 wk
Pseudomonas aeruginosa or *Enterobacter* species	Cefepime 2 g IV every 12 h for 4-6 wk *or* Meropenem 1 g IV every 8 h for 4-6 wk	Ciprofloxacin[b] 750 mg orally every 12 h for 4-6 wk *or* Ceftazidime 2 g IV every 8 h

Abbreviations: IM, intramuscularly; IV, intravenously; MIC, minimum inhibitory concentration.

[a] Antimicrobial selection should be based on in vitro sensitivity data.
[b] Should be avoided if possible in pediatric patients and in osteomyelitis associated with fractures.

Adapted from Berbari EF, Steckelberg JM, Osmon DR. Osteomyelitis. In: Mandell GL, Bennett JE, Dolin R, editors. Mandell, Douglas, and Bennett's principles and practice of infectious diseases. Vol 1. 7th ed. Philadelphia (PA): Churchill Livingstone/Elsevier; c2010. p. 1457–68. Used with permission.

a. Osteomyelitis surgery typically precedes antimicrobial therapy
b. In some situations, broad-spectrum empirical therapy may need to precede surgical therapy
    1) Concomitant soft tissue infection
    2) Sepsis syndrome with osteomyelitis
    3) This approach is common when patients with diabetes mellitus have osteomyelitis in a foot
c. Conclusions from experimental model evidence and results of multiple cohort studies concerning treatment of chronic osteomyelitis after adequate débridement and removal of orthopedic hardware
    1) Intravenous antimicrobial therapy or highly bioavailable oral antimicrobial therapy is required for 4 to 6 weeks
    2) Success rates: typically 80% with the first attempt at therapy for chronic osteomyelitis
d. Randomized clinical trial data are insufficient to guide clinicians on the optimal type and duration of antimicrobial therapy
e. Selected acute hematogenous cases with vertebral osteomyelitis
    1) Antimicrobial therapy alone can be sufficient
    2) Duration of therapy: typically 4 to 6 weeks
    3) Duration of therapy may be prolonged if coexisting abscesses are managed with medical therapy alone
f. Options when orthopedic hardware cannot be removed at the time of surgical débridement owing to the need to stabilize a fracture
    1) Treatment initially with intravenous antimicrobial therapy followed by long-term oral antimicrobial suppression until fracture is healed
    2) Quinolone in combination with rifampin after initial intravenous antimicrobial therapy without the long-term use of oral antimicrobial suppression
        a) Studied with staphylococcal infection of fracture fixation device when the hardware must be retained
        b) Successful outcomes have been reported with this strategy
        c) Concerns of the effect of quinolones on fracture healing have been raised on the basis of in vitro and experimental models, but human data are lacking
g. Relapse of infection with retained hardware
    1) Remove the orthopedic hardware
    2) Administer intravenous or highly bioavailable oral antimicrobial therapy based on deep intraoperative cultures for 4 to 6 weeks
3. Hyperbaric oxygen therapy
    a. Has been used as an adjunctive measure for patients with chronic or refractory osteomyelitis
    b. A detailed discussion of the pros and cons is beyond the scope of this chapter

II. Infectious Arthritis Due to Bacteria
  A. Epidemiology and Pathogenesis
    1. Mechanisms
      a. Most cases of infectious arthritis due to bacteria are the consequence of hematogenous seeding from an infection elsewhere in the body
      b. Direct inoculation of the joint through surgical procedures, such as arthroscopy or therapeutic injections, also occurs
      c. Infections of the small joints of the hands and feet are often the result of contiguous trauma, animal or human bites, or surgery
    2. Infectious arthritis can cause irreversible cartilage damage and irreversible dysfunction of the joint from recruitment of leukocytes that release enzymes that destroy cartilage
    3. Patients at increased risk of infection
      a. Patients with systemic immune dysfunction, such as rheumatoid arthritis or malignancy
      b. Patients with joint abnormalities, such as severe degenerative arthritis
      c. Patients at increased risk of bacteremia, such as those with long-term intravenous catheters
    4. Microorganisms
      a. *Staphylococcus aureus*: most common cause of infectious arthritis in adults, in part because it binds to sialoprotein, a glycoprotein found in joints
      b. Coagulase-negative staphylococci: can be pathogens after manipulation of the joint at surgery
      c. *Neisseria gonorrhoeae*: a common pathogen in young adults
      d. Infections due to gram-negative bacteria: more common in the elderly

e. Infections due to fungi, mycobacteria, *Borrelia burgdorferi*, and viruses occur but are discussed in other chapters
B. Diagnosis
 1. Clinical features
    a. Acute onset of joint pain in combination with systemic symptoms is common
    b. A longer duration for symptoms is more common with mycobacterial and fungal infection
    c. Affected joints
       1) Septic arthritis is most frequently diagnosed in the knee, followed by the hip, ankle, elbow, wrist, and shoulder
       2) Polyarticular disease
          a) Common in patients with rheumatoid arthritis and in patients with *S aureus* bacteremia
          b) Other bacterial pathogens that cause polyarticular sepsis: gonococci, pneumococci, group B streptococci, and gram-negative bacilli
 2. Diagnostic testing
    a. Leukocyte count, sedimentation rate, and C-reactive protein level are often elevated
    b. Plain films typically show only soft tissue swelling
    c. CT or MRI is helpful in diagnosing coexisting periarticular osteomyelitis
    d. Diagnostic arthrocentesis results are required for the diagnosis of infectious arthritis
       1) Synovial fluid analysis showing more than 50,000 cells/μL is commonly used as a threshold for diagnosis and initiation of therapy
       2) Other conditions that can cause an elevated synovial fluid cell count include crystalline arthritis and other inflammatory arthritides
       3) Cultures
          a) Synovial fluid cultures are often needed to confirm the diagnosis
          b) Blood culture results are often positive
          c) When disseminated gonococcal disease is suspected, cultures from the urethra, cervix, rectum, and pharynx may yield the diagnosis since synovial fluid cultures are often negative for bacteria
C. Management
 1. Goals in management of septic arthritis: prevent cartilage damage and eradicate the infection
 2. Antimicrobial therapy and drainage should be implemented as soon as possible
    a. Antimicrobial therapy
       1) Should start immediately after obtaining samples for blood and synovial fluid cultures in most circumstances
       2) Initial antimicrobial choice
          a) Should be based on results of Gram stain
          b) Should be active in vitro against staphylococci or other organisms that might be present on the basis of the typical organisms that have been reported to cause bacterial arthritis in specific hosts
          c) Should be active against gonococci in young adults
       3) After culture results are available, antimicrobial therapy can be modified on the basis of those results
          a) Duration and type of antimicrobial therapy depend on the type of microorganism and in vitro susceptibility
          b) Most cases of infectious arthritis are treated with parenteral antimicrobial therapy for 2 to 4 weeks
          c) Duration of therapy may be longer if concomitant osteomyelitis, bacteremia, or infective endocarditis is present
    b. Surgical drainage
       1) Drainage can be done through repeated aspiration, open arthrotomy, or arthroscopic débridement
       2) Controversy still exists about the optimal type of drainage procedure in patients with bacterial septic arthritis
       3) Arthrotomy
          a) Recommended when the condition has not improved with conservative therapy
          b) Recommended when it is difficult or impossible to drain the joint with repeated aspiration or arthroscopy
 3. Gonococcal arthritis
    a. Often treated with antimicrobial therapy alone
       1) In patients who do not have β-lactam allergies, ceftriaxone should be administered intravenously
       2) After 48 to 72 hours, intravenous antimicrobial therapy can be switched to an oral agent such as cefixime or a quinolone

b. Recommended antimicrobial therapy for gonococcal arthritis is updated frequently by the Centers for Disease Control and Prevention (CDC)
   1) Recommendations are based on emerging data on antimicrobial resistance among gonococci
   2) CDC should be consulted for current recommendations

III. Prosthetic Joint Infection
   A. Epidemiology and Pathogenesis
      1. Prosthetic joints
         a. A major advancement in orthopedic management
         b. Used to treat painful arthritides, to relieve pain in patients with spinal stenosis, and to fix fractures in patients with long bone fractures
         c. Results are often excellent, but infection is a major complication of the procedures
      2. Etiology
         a. Infection may start with intraoperative contamination despite systemic antimicrobial prophylaxis, modern surgical technique, and clean operating rooms
         b. Infection may start with wound healing difficulties in the early postoperative period
         c. Only a small percentage of the patients have infections that result from occult bacteremia
         d. Pathogens
            1) *Staphylococcus aureus* and coagulase-negative staphylococci are the pathogens in more than 60% of patients with orthopedic hardware infections
            2) Aerobic gram-negative bacilli, anaerobes, enterococci, and *Candida* species account for most of the other infections
      3. Risk of infection
         a. Estimated rate of infection among patients undergoing total joint arthroplasty: 1% to 5%
         b. Patient risk factors for prosthetic joint infection
            1) Rheumatoid arthritis
            2) Medical comorbidities
            3) Prior arthroplasty
            4) History of malignancy
         c. It is also believed that in a small percentage of patients, prosthetic joint infection develops from an occult bacteremia after an invasive procedure such as dental surgery or an infection at a distant site
      4. Biofilm formation: a hallmark of prosthetic joint infection
         a. Bacteria adhere to implanted biomaterial and produce extracapsular glycocalyx
         b. Glycocalyx provides a mechanical barrier that allows bacteria to evade host defense mechanisms and antimicrobial therapy
         c. Microorganisms embedded in the biofilm are more resistant to antimicrobials
   B. Diagnosis
      1. Clinical features
         a. Various manifestations
            1) Acute arthritis syndrome
            2) Early postoperative wound healing complications
            3) Chronic pain syndrome without systemic symptoms owing to prosthesis dysfunction and loosening
         b. Sinus tract that communicates with the joint
            1) Present in a minority of cases
            2) If present, it is pathognomonic of infection
      2. Diagnostic testing
         a. Leukocyte count, sedimentation rate, and C-reactive protein level
            1) May be elevated in patients with a septic arthritis syndrome
            2) May be only mildly abnormal or normal in patients with pain due to prosthesis dysfunction
         b. Plain films and arthrograms
            1) Can show loosening of the prosthesis
            2) Loosening may or may not result from infection
         c. Radionuclide imaging
            1) Reasonably sensitive and specific for infection if done soon after joint implantation
            2) Expensive
            3) Not available at all centers
         d. Arthrocentesis for culture and leukocyte count
            1) Reasonably sensitive and specific
            2) Cost-effective
         e. Diagnostic requirements if all preoperative testing results are normal and chronic prosthetic joint infection is present
            1) Pathologic examination of the tissue surrounding the prosthesis for acute inflammatory cells
            2) Multiple cultures with positive results

C. Therapy
1. Surgical management (Table 34.2)
    a. Depends on several factors
        1) Whether the prosthesis is well fixed
        2) Stage of infection
        3) Duration of infection
    b. For patients with an early or acute infection, a well-fixed prosthesis, and no sinus tract: débridement with component retention is the surgical procedure of choice
    c. For patients with a chronic infection or a prosthesis that is not well fixed: resection arthroplasty followed by a delayed reimplantation is the typical surgical strategy
        1) Delay between resection arthroplasty and reimplantation
            a) For a total knee arthroplasty infection: 6 to 8 weeks
            b) For a total hip arthroplasty infection: 3 months
        2) One-stage replacement can be successful in selected patients, such as patients with a good tissue envelope when the infection is caused by a pathogen with low virulence
2. The use of other surgical procedures, such as arthrodesis or amputation, or the use of antimicrobial therapy alone is much less common
    a. Amputation is used when there is uncontrolled infection
    b. Antimicrobial therapy alone is used when reconstructive surgery is not an option owing to medical comorbidities or technical issues
3. Antimicrobial therapy: essential to treatment of prosthetic joint infection (Table 34.2)
    a. Duration of therapy and type of antimicrobial depend on the surgical strategy used to treat the infection
        1) Patients who undergo removal of the prosthesis: typically 4 to 6 weeks of intravenous antimicrobial therapy
        2) Patients with a susceptible staphylococcal prosthetic joint infection that is treated with débridement and retention of the prosthesis
            a) Often managed with parenteral antistaphylococcal antimicrobial therapy plus rifampin for 2 to 6 weeks followed by rifampin in combination with a quinolone for 3 to 6 months
                i) Strategy has been reported to be successful in 1 small clinical trial
                ii) With increasing resistance to quinolones among staphylococci, other agents, such as co-trimoxazole, are being used in combination with rifampin

Table 34.2

Medical and Surgical Management of Prosthetic Joint Infection

Type of Infection	Time of Onset	Surgical Treatment	Medical Management
Positive intraoperative cultures after revision surgery	Intraoperative	One-stage exchange arthroplasty	4-6 wk of IV antimicrobial therapy with or without long-term oral antimicrobial suppression
Early postoperative infection	First month	Débridement with retention of the prosthesis	2-6 wk of IV antimicrobial therapy plus long-term oral antimicrobial suppression Combination rifampin if susceptible staphylococcal PJI (see text)
Acute infection	Late acute onset	Débridement with retention of the prosthesis	2-6 wk of IV antimicrobial therapy plus long-term oral antimicrobial suppression Combination rifampin if susceptible staphylococcal PJI (see text)
Late chronic infection	Late (chronic) infection	Resection arthroplasty	4-6 wk of IV antimicrobial therapy

Abbreviations: IV, intravenous; PJI, prosthetic joint infection.

Data from Segawa H, Tsukayama DT, Kyle RF, Becker DA, Gustilo RB. Infection after total knee arthroplasty: a retrospective study of the treatment of eighty-one infections. J Bone Joint Surg Am. 1999 Oct;81(10):1434-45 and Tsukayama DT, Estrada R, Gustilo RB. Infection after total hip arthroplasty: a study of the treatment of one hundred and six infections. J Bone Joint Surg Am. 1996 Apr;78(4):512–23.

b) Combination therapy with rifampin is required owing to the high level of resistance emerging among staphylococci if rifampin is used alone
c) Long-term antimicrobial suppression when the prosthesis is retained
   i) Recommended by many clinicians unless rifampin is used
   ii) Recommended by some investigators even if rifampin is used but eradication of infection is not possible
   iii) The goal with this treatment is to preserve a functional prosthesis, not to eradicate the infection
b. For patients undergoing 1-stage exchange, 4 to 6 weeks of treatment with appropriate antimicrobial therapy is often sufficient, although long-term oral antimicrobial suppression is also used in some cases

Suggested Reading

Berbari EF, Osmon DR, Steckelberg JM. Infective and reactive arthritis. In: Cohen J, Powderly WG, Berkley SF, Calandra T, Clumeck N, Finch RG, et al, editors. Infectious diseases. Vol 1. 2nd ed. Edinburgh: Mosby; c2004. p. 563–9.

Berbari EF, Steckelberg JM, Osmon DR. Osteomyelitis. In: Mandell GL, Bennett JE, Dolin R, editors. Mandell, Douglas, and Bennett's principles and practice of infectious diseases. Vol 1. 7th ed. Philadelphia (PA): Churchill Livingstone/Elsevier; c2010. p. 1457–68.

Tsukayama DT, Estrada R, Gustilo RB. Infection after total hip arthroplasty: a study of the treatment of one hundred and six infections. J Bone Joint Surg Am. 1996 Apr;78(4): 512–23.

Zimmerli W, Trampuz A, Ochsner PE. Prosthetic-joint infections. N Engl J Med. 2004 Oct 14;351(16):1645–54.

Zimmerli W, Widmer AF, Blatter M, Frei R, Ochsner PE; Foreign-Body Infection (FBI) Study Group. Role of rifampin for treatment of orthopedic implant-related staphylococcal infections: a randomized controlled trial. JAMA. 1998 May 20;279(19):1537–41.

Randall S. Edson, MD

35

Sexually Transmitted Diseases

I. Introduction
   A. Significant Public Health Problem
   B. Estimates From the Centers for Disease Control and Prevention
      1. Approximately 19 million new cases of sexually transmitted diseases (STDs) annually
      2. Estimated cost of $15.5 billion each year
      3. Approximately half of all STDs occur in persons aged 15 to 24 years
      4. Figures are clearly an underestimate of the true burden of STDs
         a. Many cases are not diagnosed
         b. Infections due to herpes simplex virus (HSV) and human papillomavirus are not reportable
   C. Suggested Reading
      1. All treatment recommendations in this chapter have been adapted from the references in "Suggested Reading" at the end of this chapter
      2. Those references provide a more comprehensive review of this vast topic
II. Genital Ulcer Diseases
   A. Etiology
      1. Syphilis
      2. Herpes simplex virus
      3. Chancroid
      4. Lymphogranuloma venereum
      5. Granuloma inguinale (donovanosis)
   B. Evaluation
      1. Serologic evaluation for syphilis
      2. Dark-field examination
      3. Culture and antigen test for HSV
      4. If chancroid is suspected, culture for *Haemophilus ducreyi*
   C. Associations
      1. Increased risk of human immunodeficiency virus (HIV) acquisition
      2. Increased risk of HIV transmission
III. Syphilis
   A. Epidemiology
      1. Causative agent: *Treponema pallidum*
      2. Incidence of syphilis among men who have sex with men (MSM) is increasing significantly
   B. Clinical Manifestations
      1. Primary chancre (Figure 35.1)
         a. Single or multiple at site of "inoculation"
         b. Serology may be negative, so need dark-field examination (Figure 35.2)
      2. Secondary syphilis (a "systemic" disease): 6 to 8 weeks after chancre resolves
         a. Generalized rash (palms and soles) (Figure 35.3)

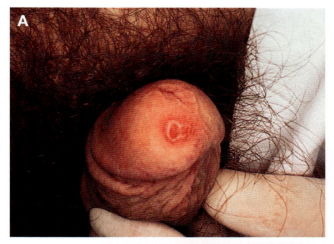
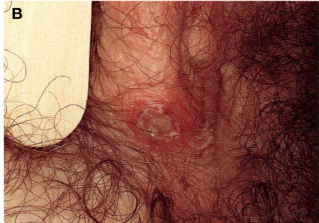
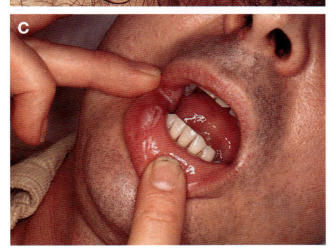

Figure 35.1. Chancres in Primary Syphilis. A, Penile chancre. B, Female genital chancre. C, Oral chancre.

  b. Mucous patches (Figure 35.4)
  c. Condylomata lata (Figure 35.5)
  d. Alopecia and lymphadenopathy
  e. Nontreponemal and treponemal serologic results are strongly positive

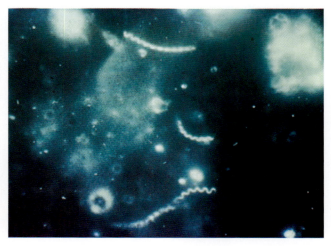

Figure 35.2. *Treponema pallidum* on Dark-field Examination.

  f. Untreated secondary syphilis may "relapse" after resolution
 3. Late (tertiary) syphilis
  a. Occurs in approximately one-third of untreated patients
  b. Neurologic features
   1) Lymphocytic meningitis
   2) Stroke
   3) Charcot joint
   4) Posterior column disease (tabes dorsalis)
  c. Cardiac features
   1) Aneurysm of proximal aorta (Figure 35.6)
   2) Aortic regurgitation
  d. *Gummas*: destructive granulomatous lesions
 C. Diagnosis
  1. Nontreponemal tests (often used in screening)
   a. VDRL test
   b. Cerebrospinal fluid VDRL test: highly specific but insensitive in diagnosis of neurosyphilis
   c. Rapid plasma reagin (RPR) test for detection of reagin antibodies
   d. Inexpensive
   e. Antibodies disappear with treatment
    1) Primary syphilis: seronegative in 1 year
    2) Secondary syphilis: seronegative in 2 years
    3) Later stages of syphilis: may take years to become seronegative or may not revert to negative

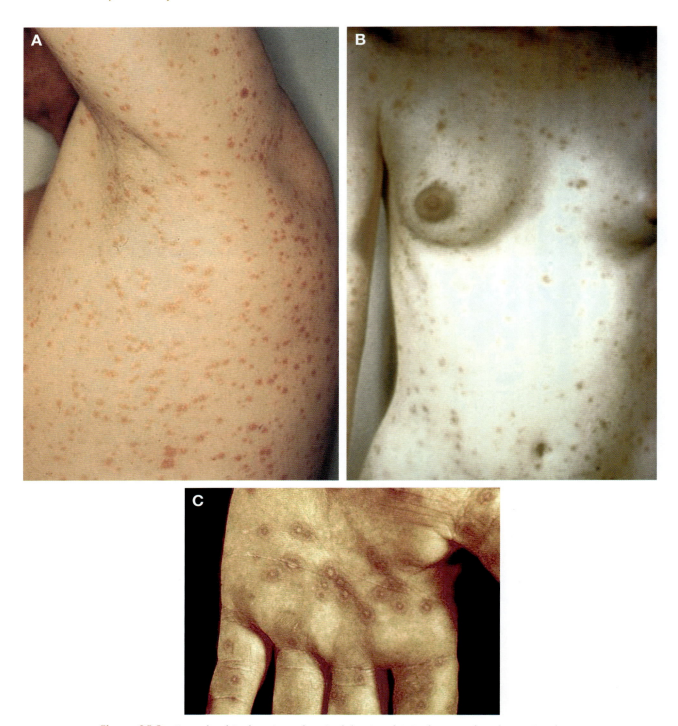

Figure 35.3. Generalized Rash in Secondary Syphilis. A and B, Rash on trunk and arm. C, Palmar rash.

    f. Decreased sensitivity in later disease even without treatment (up to 25%)
    g. False-positive results occur in acute viral illness, connective tissue disease, and pregnancy
2. Treponemal tests

    a. Fluorescent treponemal antibody absorption (FTA-ABS) test
    b. Microhemagglutination assay for *T pallidum* (MHA-TP)
    c. CAPTIA Syphilis-G enzyme immunoassay (Figure 35.7)

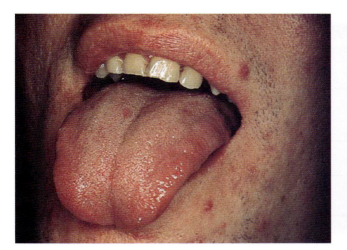

Figure 35.4. Mucous Patches in Secondary Syphilis.

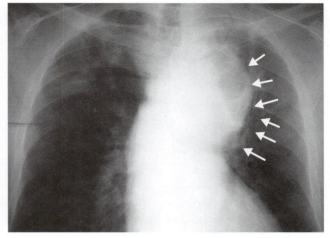

Figure 35.6. Aortic Aneurysm in Tertiary Syphilis. Arrows point to aneurysm of proximal aorta.

        d. More specific and more sensitive
        e. Results are usually positive after treatment
   D. Treatment
     1. Treatment of choice: penicillin G benzathine
        a. Bicillin L-A
          1) Preparation of penicillin G benzathine
          2) Acceptable to use
        b. Bicillin C-R
          1) Combination preparation of penicillin G benzathine and penicillin G procaine
          2) Should *not* be used
          3) Has been associated with treatment failures
     2. Treatment guidelines for syphilis are presented in Box 35.1

IV. Herpes Simplex Virus Genital Infection
   A. Epidemiology
     1. Causative agent: HSV-1 or HSV-2
     2. Most common genital ulcer disease in the United States (prevalence about 20%)
     3. Asymptomatic transmission due to viral shedding is common
     4. Risk of transmission to neonate
        a. High (30%-50%) with near-term acquisition of HSV
        b. Decreased in recurrent disease
     5. Acyclovir may be used in pregnancy to treat primary or recurrent disease
   B. Clinical Manifestations
     1. Primary infection may be asymptomatic or symptomatic
     2. Symptomatic primary infection: genital ulcers or anal ulcers (or both) with fever, lymphadenopathy, malaise, and urinary retention (Figure 35.8)
     3. Grouped vesicles on erythematous base: heals with crusting
        a. May have extensive, erosive disease in HIV infection (Figure 35.9)
        b. May cause mucopurulent cervicitis
     4. Recurrent infection
        a. Rate of recurrence
          1) Varies significantly
          2) Genital herpes is less frequently recurrent with HSV-1 than with HSV-2
        b. Recurrent lymphocytic meningitis may occur
        c. HSV-1 and HSV-2 can cause urethritis in men
   C. Diagnosis
     1. Tzanck smear: insensitive

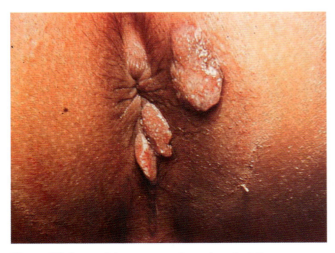

Figure 35.5. Condyloma Lata in Secondary Syphilis.

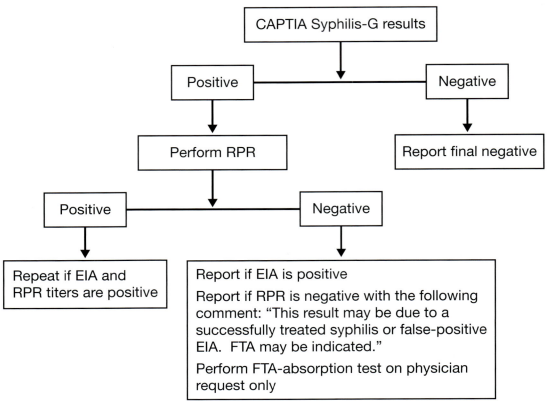

Figure 35.7. Interpretation of CAPTIA Syphilis-G Enzyme Immunoassay Results. EIA indicates enzyme immunoassay; FTA, fluorescent treponemal antibody; RPR, rapid plasma reagin.

Box 35.1

Treatment Guidelines for Syphilis

Primary and secondary syphilis
   Recommended regimen
      Penicillin G benzathine, 2.4 million units IM
   For patients with penicillin allergy[a]
      Doxycycline 100 mg twice daily for 14 d
      Ceftriaxone 1 g IM or IV daily for 8-10 d (limited studies)
      Azithromycin 2 g orally for 1 dose (preliminary data)
   Response to treatment
      No definitive criteria for cure or failure are established
      Reexamine clinically and serologically at 6 and 12 mo
      Consider treatment failure if signs or symptoms persist or if nontreponemal test shows a sustained 4-fold increase in titer
      Treatment failure: HIV test, CSF analysis, and administration of penicillin G benzathine weekly for 3 wk
      Additional therapy is not warranted if titers do not decrease despite normal CSF findings and repeated therapy
   Response to treatment in patients with HIV infection
      Most respond appropriately to penicillin G benzathine 2.4 million units IM
      Some experts recommend CSF examination before therapy and additional therapy (ie, weekly penicillin G benzathine for 3 wk)
      Clinical/serologic evaluation at 3, 6, 9, 12, and 24 mo; some perform CSF examination at 6 mo
      For treatment of serologic failure (6-12 mo after treatment): CSF examination, re-treatment with penicillin G benzathine 2.4 million units weekly for 3 wk
Latent syphilis
   Recommended regimen
      Penicillin G benzathine 2.4 million units IM for 1-wk intervals for 3 doses
   For patients with penicillin allergy

Box 35.1

(continued)

    Duration of therapy, 28 days
    Close clinical and serologic follow-up
    Data to support alternatives to penicillin are limited
        Doxycycline 100 mg orally twice daily
            or
    Tetracycline 500 mg orally 4 times daily
    Management considerations
        Clinical evaluation of tertiary disease (aortitis, gumma, iritis)
        CSF analysis, neurologic or ophthalmic signs/symptoms, active tertiary disease, treatment failure, HIV infection
        Some experts recommend CSF examination in those with nontreponemal titer ≥1:32
        Pharmacologic considerations suggest that an interval of 10-14 d between penicillin G benzathine doses may be acceptable before restarting treatment course in nonpregnant patients
    Response to treatment
        Limited data available to guide evaluation
        Repeat quantitative nontreponemal tests at 6, 12, and 24 mo
        Perform CSF examination and re-treat for latent syphilis if there is a 4-fold increase in titer, initial nontreponemal titer ≥1:32 does not decrease 12-24 mo after treatment, or signs or symptoms develop
    Response to treatment in patients with HIV infection
        CSF examination before treatment
        Normal findings on CSF examination: penicillin G benzathine 2.4 million units IM weekly for 3 wk
        Clinical and serologic evaluation at 6, 12, 18, and 24 mo
        Development of symptoms or 4-fold titer increase: repeat CSF examination and treat
        Repeat CSF examination and treatment if nontreponemal titer does not decrease in 12-24 mo
    Management of sexual partners
        Identification of at-risk sexual partners: duration of symptoms >3 mo for primary syphilis, >6 mo for secondary syphilis, and 1 y for early latent syphilis
        For exposure to primary, secondary, or early latent syphilis within 90 d, treat presumptively
        For patients with exposure to latent syphilis and high nontreponemal titers (≥1:32), consider presumptive treatment for early syphilis

Neurosyphilis and uveitis or ocular disease
    Recommended regimen
        Aqueous crystalline penicillin G, 18-24 million units administered as 3-4 million units IV every 4 h for 10-14 d
    Alternative regimen
        Penicillin G procaine 2.4 million units IM daily
            plus
        Probenecid 500 mg orally 4 times daily for 10-14 d
    Some experts administer penicillin G benzathine 2.4 million units IM weekly for 3 wk after completion of these regimens to provide duration of treatment comparable with that of latent syphilis
    For patients with penicillin allergy
        Ceftriaxone 2 g daily IM or IV for 10-14 d
        Consideration of cross reactivity
        Pregnant patients should undergo skin testing and penicillin desensitization if skin test is positive
        Other regimens have not been evaluated
    Response to treatment
        Initial CSF pleocytosis: repeat CSF examination every 6 mo until cell count is normal
        CSF VDRL test results and protein level decrease slowly
        Consider re-treatment if cell count has not decreased by 6 mo or if CSF is not normal by 2 y
    Treatment in pregnancy
        Screen for syphilis at first prenatal visit; repeat rapid plasma reagin test in the third trimester and at delivery for those at high risk or in high-prevalence areas
        Treat for appropriate stage of syphilis
        Some experts recommend additional penicillin G benzathine (2.4 million units IM) after the initial dose for primary, secondary, or early latent syphilis
        Management and counseling may be facilitated by sonographic fetal evaluation for congenital syphilis in the second half of pregnancy

Abbreviations: CSF, cerebrospinal fluid; HIV, human immunodeficiency virus; IM, intramuscularly; IV, intravenously.

[a] Use of the following regimens in HIV infection has not been studied.

Adapted from Centers for Disease Control and Prevention; Workowski KA, Berman SM. Sexually transmitted diseases treatment guidelines, 2006. MMWR Recomm Rep. 2006 Aug 4;55(RR-11):1-94. Erratum in: MMWR Recomm Rep. 2006 Sep 15;55(36):997.

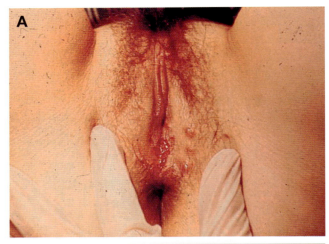

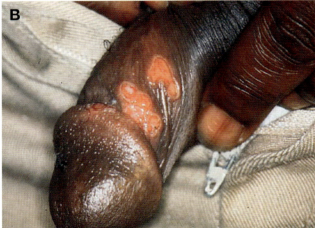

Figure 35.8. Herpes Simplex Virus Genital Infection. A, Female genital infection. B, Male genital infection.

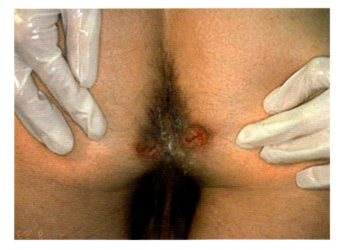

Figure 35.9. Erosive Perirectal Herpes Simplex Virus Infection in Patient With Human Immunodeficiency Virus Infection.

2. Culture: slow and expensive
3. Direct antigen and DNA amplification: rapid, sensitive, and specific
4. Type-specific HSV serology: uncertain role but may be helpful in pregnancy if seronegative woman has partner with known HSV infection

D. Treatment
1. Treatment is outlined in Table 35.1

V. Chancroid
A. Epidemiology
1. Causative agent: *H ducreyi*
2. Increased incidence in the United States
3. Worldwide problem in developing countries
4. Associated with HIV transmission and acquisition
5. Incubation: 4 to 7 days

B. Clinical Manifestations
1. Multiple, painful ulcers (Figure 35.10)
2. Regional lymphadenopathy

C. Diagnosis
1. Culture: 80% sensitivity
2. Polymerase chain reaction (PCR) testing: greater than 90% sensitivity but not widely available

D. Treatment
1. Azithromycin 1 g orally
2. Ceftriaxone 250 mg intramuscularly
3. Ciprofloxacin 500 mg orally twice daily for 3 days
4. Erythromycin 500 mg 3 times daily for 7 days

VI. Lymphogranuloma Venereum
A. Epidemiology
1. Causative agent: *Chlamydia trachomatis*, serovars L1, L2, and L3

B. Clinical Manifestations
1. Painless genital ulcer, followed by significant inguinal lymphadenopathy ("groove" sign) (Figure 35.11)
2. Recent reports of hemorrhagic proctitis in MSM (often HIV infected)

C. Diagnosis
1. Serology
2. Direct identification (by Centers for Disease Control and Prevention [CDC]) from lesion aspirate

D. Treatment
1. Doxycycline 100 mg twice daily for 21 days
2. Erythromycin 500 mg 4 times daily for 21 days

VII. Granuloma Inguinale (Donovanosis)
A. Epidemiology
1. Causative agent: *Calymmatobacterium granulomatis*
2. Rare in the United States; seen in India and Latin America

Table 35.1
Treatment of Genital Herpes Infection

Drug	Dosage		
	First Episode (7-10 d)	Recurrent Episodes (5 d)	Long-term Suppression
Acyclovir	400 mg 3 times daily[a]	400 mg twice daily	400 mg twice daily
Valacyclovir	1,000 mg twice daily	500 mg twice daily	500 mg or 1 g daily[b]
Famciclovir	250 mg 3 times daily	125 mg twice daily[c]	250 mg twice daily

[a] Daily treatment with valacyclovir decreases herpes simplex virus transmission in discordant (ie, source partner has a history of genital herpes) heterosexual couples.
[b] Also acyclovir 800 mg twice daily for 5 days or 800 mg 3 times daily for 2 days.
[c] New recommendation: famciclovir 1,000 mg twice daily for 1 day.

   B. Clinical Manifestations
      1. Painless anogenital ulcers
      2. Ulcers heal with fibrosis and scarring in the inguinal areas
   C. Diagnosis
      1. Donovan bodies (Figure 35.12)
         a. Intracellular rod-shaped chromatin condensations
         b. Seen on biopsy
   D. Treatment
      1. Doxycycline 100 mg twice daily for 21 days
      2. Double-strength trimethoprim-sulfamethoxazole twice daily for 21 days
      3. Ciprofloxacin 750 mg twice daily for 21 days
      4. Erythromycin base 500 mg 4 times daily for 21 days
      5. Azithromycin 1 g weekly for 21 days
VIII. Urethritis
   A. Definition (Includes 3 Criteria)
      1. Mucopurulent or purulent discharge
      2. Five white blood cells (WBCs) per oil-immersion field
      3. Leukocyte esterase in first voided urine or 10 or more WBCs per high-power field
   B. Epidemiology
      1. Gonococcal urethritis
         a. *Neisseria gonorrhoeae*
      2. Nongonococcal urethritis
         a. *Chlamydia trachomatis*
         b. *Mycoplasma genitalium*: may be associated with up to 30% of nongonococcal urethritis
         c. *Ureaplasma urealyticum*: some organisms may be resistant to tetracyclines, requiring azalide or fluoroquinolone therapy
         d. *Trichomonas vaginalis*: men are usually asymptomatic but may be symptomatic and not responsive to usual treatment of urethritis
         e. HSV: HSV-1 may be associated with urethritis in men
         f. Unknown cause

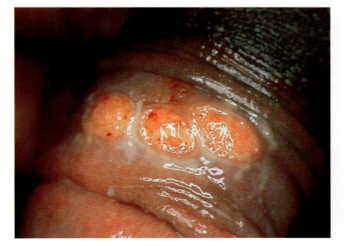

Figure 35.10. Chancroid Ulcers.

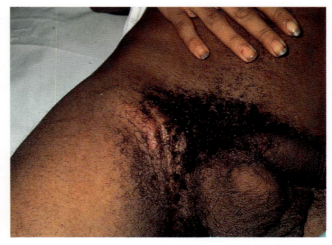

Figure 35.11. "Groove" Sign in Lymphogranuloma Venereum.

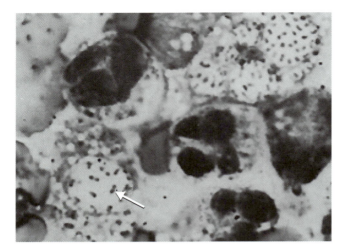

Figure 35.12. Granuloma Inguinale. Donovan body (arrow).

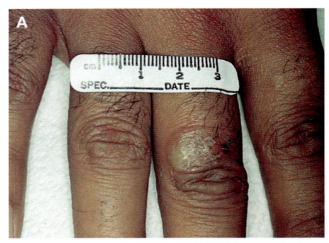
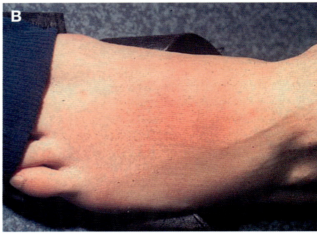

Figure 35.13. Disseminated Gonococcal Infection. A, Rash. B, Tenosynovitis.

IX. Gonorrhea
   A. Epidemiology
      1. Causative agent: *N gonorrhoeae*, a gram-negative diplococcus
   B. Clinical Manifestations
      1. May be asymptomatic
      2. Pharyngeal infection
      3. Disseminated disease (Figure 35.13)
         a. May complicate genital or pharyngeal infection
         b. Rash, tenosynovitis, and arthritis (also occurs in terminal complement deficiency)
      4. Men
         a. Urethritis
         b. Epididymitis
      5. Women
         a. Mucopurulent cervicitis (other causes include *Chlamydia* and HSV)
         b. Pelvic inflammatory disease (PID)
         c. Bartholin gland abscess and skin abscess
   C. Diagnosis
      1. Gram stain
         a. Symptomatic men: urethral Gram staining sensitivity is 95% (Figure 35.14)
         b. Cervical Gram staining is insensitive but specific
      2. Nonculture, molecular diagnostic testing
         a. Ligase chain reaction and PCR testing
         b. Have supplanted culture in both men and women
         c. Highly sensitive and specific
         d. Similar tests are used to detect *Chlamydia*
         e. Allows for urine-based testing, which is far more acceptable to patients
   D. Treatment
      1. Therapeutic considerations
         a. Antimicrobial resistance: penicillin and tetracyclines
         b. Emerging fluoroquinolone resistance
            1) MSM and persons in Asia, Pacific Islands, Hawaii, and California
            2) Fluoroquinolones are no longer recommended for treatment of gonorrhea because of increasing resistance
         c. Spectinomycin and cefixime are no longer reliably available
      2. Coexisting *Chlamydia*
         a. In 15% to 25% of men
         b. In 25% to 50% of women
      3. Specific treatment regimens (must include anti-*Chlamydia* treatment): cephalosporins
         a. Ceftriaxone 125 mg intramuscularly (IM) for 1 dose

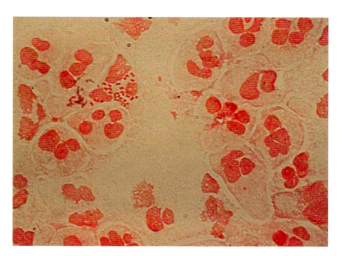

Figure 35.14. *Neisseria gonorrhoeae* (Gram stain).

Box 35.2

Treatment Regimens for *Chlamydia trachomatis* Infection

Recommended regimens
    Azithromycin 1 g for 1 dose
        or
    Doxycycline 100 mg twice daily for 7 d
Alternative regimens
    Erythromycin base 500 mg 4 times daily for 7 d
        or
    Erythromycin ethylsuccinate 800 mg 4 times daily for 7 d
        or
    Ofloxacin 300 mg twice daily for 7 d
        or
    Levofloxacin 500 mg for 7 d
Treatment in pregnancy
    Recommended regimens
        Erythromycin base 500 mg 4 times daily for 7 d
            or
        Amoxicillin 500 mg 3 times daily for 7 d
    Alternative regimens
        Erythromycin base 250 mg 4 times daily for 14 d
            or
        Erythromycin ethylsuccinate 800 mg 4 times daily for 14 d
            or
        Erythromycin ethylsuccinate 400 mg 4 times daily for 14 d
            or
    Azithromycin 1 g for 1 dose
Treatment of urethritis of unknown cause
    Metronidazole 2 g or tinidazole 2 g
        plus
    Azithromycin 1 mg for 1 dose

Adapted from Centers for Disease Control and Prevention; Workowski KA, Berman SM. Sexually transmitted diseases treatment guidelines, 2006. MMWR Recomm Rep. 2006 Aug 4;55(RR-11): 1-94. Erratum in: MMWR Recomm Rep. 2006 Sep 15;55(36):997.

---

        b. Cefpodoxime 400 mg orally for 1 dose
        c. Cefuroxime 1 g orally for 1 dose
    4. Disseminated infection
        a. Ceftriaxone 1 g IM or intravenously (IV) every 24 hours
        b. Cefotaxime or ceftizoxime 1 g IV every 8 hours
        c. Levofloxacin 250 mg IV every 24 hours
X. *Chlamydia trachomatis* Infection
    A. Clinical Manifestations
        1. Same as for *N gonorrhoeae*
    B. Screening
        1. Annual screening is suggested for sexually active women 25 years or younger
        2. Rescreening should occur 3 to 4 months after treatment owing to the high prevalence of recurrent infection
    C. Diagnosis
        1. Same as for gonorrhea
        2. Urine, urethral, or cervical specimens for detection with ligase chain reaction or PCR testing (highly sensitive and specific)
    D. Treatment
        1. Treatment regimens are summarized in Box 35.2
XI. Pelvic Inflammatory Disease
    A. Epidemiology
        1. Causative agents
            a. Sexually transmitted organisms: *N gonorrhoeae* and *C trachomatis*
            b. Bacterial vaginosis organisms: anaerobes, *Gardnerella vaginalis*, mycoplasmas, and ureaplasmas
            c. Vaginal flora microorganisms: gram-negative rods and *Streptococcus agalactiae*
        2. Screening for *Chlamydia*: associated with decreased incidence of pelvic inflammatory disease
    B. Clinical Manifestations
        1. Symptoms
            a. Lower abdominal pain
            b. Dyspareunia
            c. Discharge may be present
        2. Signs
            a. Adnexal tenderness
            b. Pain with cervical motion
    C. Diagnosis
        1. Minimum diagnostic criterion: uterine, adnexal, or cervical motion tenderness
        2. Additional diagnostic criteria
            a. Oral temperature higher than 38.3°C
            b. Cervical *C trachomatis* or *N gonorrhoeae*
            c. WBCs on saline microscopy

d. Elevated erythrocyte sedimentation rate
e. Elevated C-reactive protein
f. Cervical discharge
D. Treatment
1. Indications for hospitalization
a. Pregnancy
b. Systemic toxicity
c. Tubo-ovarian abscess
2. Treatment regimens are listed in Box 35.3
E. Complications
1. Ectopic pregnancy
2. Tubal infertility
3. Chronic pelvic pain
XII. Epididymitis
A. Epidemiology
1. In men younger than 35 years: *N gonorrhoeae* and *C trachomatis*
2. In MSM: *N gonorrhoeae*, *C trachomatis*, and enteric pathogens from rectal intercourse
3. In men older than 35 years: organisms causing urinary tract infection (identify with urine culture)
B. Clinical Manifestations
1. Unilateral testicular pain, tenderness, and swelling
C. Treatment
1. Treatment regimens are listed in Box 35.4
XIII. Vaginal Discharge Syndromes
A. Clinical Manifestations
1. Vulvovaginal candidiasis, bacterial vaginosis, and trichomoniasis
2. Distinguishing features are summarized in Table 35.2
B. Treatment and Other Clinical Considerations
1. Vulvovaginal candidiasis (Figure 35.15)
a. Treatment
1) Intravaginal topical antifungals (therapy of choice in pregnancy)
2) Fluconazole 150 mg (1 dose)
b. For frequent recurrences: consider HIV infection and diabetes mellitus
2. Bacterial vaginosis
a. Shift of vaginal microbial flora from predominance of lactobacilli to polymicrobial anaerobic population (Figure 35.16)
b. Considerations for pregnant women
1) Symptomatic pregnant women should be treated because of risk of adverse pregnancy outcomes (eg, preterm

---

Box 35.3

Treatment Regimens for Pelvic Inflammatory Disease

Parenteral regimen A
  Cefotetan 2 g IV every 12 h or cefoxitin 2 g IV every 6 h
      plus
  Doxycycline 100 mg orally or IV every 12 h
Parenteral regimen B
  Clindamycin 900 mg IV every 8 h
      plus
  Gentamicin loading dose (2 mg/kg) IV or IM followed by maintenance dose (1.5 mg/kg) every 8 h (single daily dosing may be substituted)
Alternative parenteral regimens
  Ofloxacin 400 mg IV every 12 h or levofloxacin 500 mg IV once daily
      with or without
  Metronidazole 500 mg IV every 8 h
  Ampicillin-sulbactam 3 g IV every 6 h
      plus
  Doxycycline 100 mg orally or IV every 12 h
Oral regimen A
  Ofloxacin 400 mg twice daily for 14 d or levofloxacin 500 mg once daily for 14 d
      with or without
  Metronidazole 500 mg twice daily for 14 d
Oral regimen B
  Ceftriaxone 250 mg IM for 1 dose or cefoxitin 2 g IM for 1 dose with probenecid 1 g administered concurrently
      plus
  Doxycycline 100 mg twice daily for 14 d
      with or without
  Metronidazole 500 mg twice daily for 14 d

Abbreviations: IM, intramuscularly; IV, intravenously.

Adapted from Crossman SH. The challenge of pelvic inflammatory disease. Am Fam Physician. 2006 Mar 1;73(5):859-64. Erratum in: Am Fam Physician. 2006 Dec 15;74(12):2024. Used with permission.

Box 35.4

Treatment Regimens for Epididymitis

For infection most likely caused by gonococci or chlamydiae
  Ceftriaxone 250 mg IM for 1 dose
      plus
  Doxycycline 100 mg twice daily for 10 d
For infection most likely caused by enteric organisms or for patients who are older than 35 y
  Ofloxacin 300 mg twice daily for 10 d
      or
  Levofloxacin 500 mg once daily for 10 d

Abbreviation: IM, intramuscularly.

Adapted from Centers for Disease Control and Prevention; Workowski KA, Berman SM. Sexually transmitted diseases treatment guidelines, 2006. MMWR Recomm Rep. 2006 Aug 4;55(RR-11):1-94. Erratum in: MMWR Recomm Rep. 2006 Sep 15;55(36):997.

Table 35.2

Distinguishing Features of Diseases Characterized by Vaginal Discharge

Feature	Vulvovaginal Candidiasis	Bacterial Vaginosis	Trichomoniasis
Symptoms	Pruritus Discharge	Malodorous discharge	Malodorous discharge
Findings	Erythema Thick discharge	Adherent, thin discharge	Vulvovaginal erythema Discharge
pH of vaginal fluid	4-4.5	>4.5	>4.5
Amine test	Negative	Positive	Negative
KOH smear	Pseudohyphae	Negative	Negative
Diagnosis	KOH microscopy	Several criteria[a]	Motile trichomonads or wet preparation culture (very sensitive)[b]
Treatment of partner	No	No	Yes

Abbreviation: KOH, potassium hydroxide.

[a] Homogeneous gray discharge, pH >4.5, "whiff" test with KOH, and "clue" cells on microscopy.
[b] The OSOM Trichomonas Rapid Test and the Affirm are rapid tests with increased sensitivity and specificity.

      labor, low birth weight, postpartum endometritis)
- 2) Existing data do not support use of topical agents in pregnancy
- 3) Asymptomatic women at high risk of preterm delivery (ie, they have had a preterm birth)
    - a) Some experts recommend screening and treating at the first prenatal visit
    - b) Optimal regimen has not been established
- c. Treatment regimens are listed in Box 35.5
3. Trichomoniasis (Figure 35.17)
    - a. Treatment regimens are listed in Box 35.6
    - b. If treatment fails
        - 1) Treat again: metronidazole 500 mg twice daily for 7 days
        - 2) If treatment fails again
            - a) Change regimen: metronidazole 2 g once daily for 3 to 5 days
            - b) Metronidazole susceptibility testing is available through the CDC

XIV. Human Papillomavirus
  A. Epidemiology
    1. Causative agent: double-stranded DNA virus

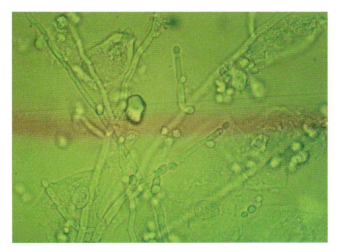

Figure 35.15. Vulvovaginal Candidiasis. Wet preparation.

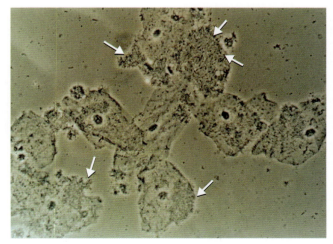

Figure 35.16. Bacterial Vaginosis. "Clue" cells (arrows).

> **Box 35.5**
> **Treatment Regimens for Bacterial Vaginosis**
> Recommended regimens
>   Metronidazole 500 mg twice daily for 7 d
>   *or*
>   Metronidazole gel 0.75%, 5 g intravaginally once daily for 5 d
>   *or*
>   Clindamycin cream 2%, 5 g intravaginally at bedtime for 7 d
> Alternative regimens
>   Clindamycin 300 mg twice daily for 7 d
>   *or*
>   Clindamycin ovules 100 g intravaginally at bedtime for 3 d
> No longer recommended: single-dose therapy with metronidazole 2 g
> Pregnant women: recommended regimens
>   Metronidazole 250 mg 3 times daily for 7 d
>   *or*
>   Metronidazole 500 mg twice daily for 7 d
>   *or*
>   Clindamycin 300 mg twice daily for 7 d
>
> Adapted from Centers for Disease Control and Prevention; Workowski KA, Berman SM. Sexually transmitted diseases treatment guidelines, 2006. MMWR Recomm Rep. 2006 Aug 4;55(RR-11):1-94. Erratum in: MMWR Recomm Rep. 2006 Sep 15;55(36):997.

> **Box 35.6**
> **Treatment Regimens for Trichomoniasis**
> Recommended regimen
>   Tinidazole 2 g orally for 1 dose
> Alternative regimen
>   Metronidazole 500 mg twice daily for 7 d
> Pregnancy
>   Metronidazole 2 g orally for 1 dose
>
> Adapted from Centers for Disease Control and Prevention; Workowski KA, Berman SM. Sexually transmitted diseases treatment guidelines, 2006. MMWR Recomm Rep. 2006 Aug 4;55(RR-11):1-94. Erratum in: MMWR Recomm Rep. 2006 Sep 15;55(36):997.

2. Ubiquitous among sexually experienced adults
3. Mostly asymptomatic
4. May become extensive in the presence of immunosuppression (HIV infection or transplant)

B. Clinical Manifestations
  1. External genital or anal warts: human papillomavirus (HPV) types 6, 11, 42, 43, 44, and 58
  2. Cervical or rectal cancer: HPV types 16, 18, 31, 33, 39, and 45

C. Diagnosis
  1. Inspection (Figure 35.18)
  2. Cytology (cervical or anal Papanicolaou smear)
  3. Biopsy and histology

D. Treatment
  1. Treatment regimens are listed in Box 35.7
  2. Treatment in pregnancy
    a. Contraindicated: imiquimod, podophyllum resin, and podofilox
    b. Wart removal may be beneficial because warts can proliferate and become friable
    c. Respiratory papillomatosis may develop in infants and children from HPV types 6 and 11
    d. Cesarean delivery
      1) Possible indication: pelvic outlet obstruction
      2) Preventive value is unknown

E. Additional Considerations
  1. Management of sexual partners of patient with HPV
    a. Colposcopic examination of male and female asymptomatic partners
    b. Cervical cytology
  2. Vaccine has been approved by the US Food and Drug Administration
    a. Directed against types 16 and 18 (responsible for 70% of cervical cancer)
    b. Highly efficacious

XV. Men Who Have Sex With Men
  A. Routine Annual Screening for Sexually Active MSM
    1. HIV serology if it was negative but was not tested within previous year

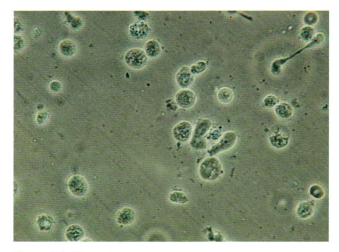

Figure 35.17. *Trichomonas*. Wet preparation.

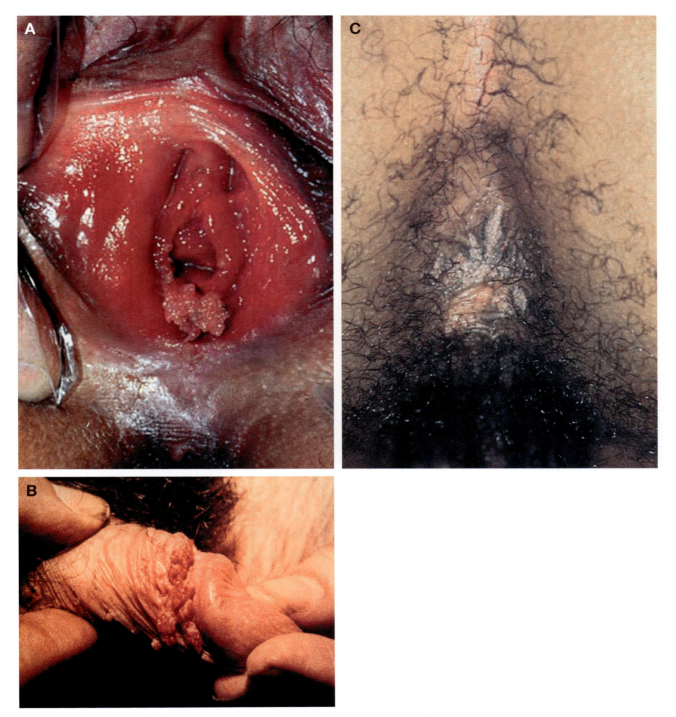

Figure 35.18. Human Papillomavirus. A, Female genital warts. B, Penile warts. C, Anal warts.

2. Syphilis serology
3. Men practicing insertive intercourse during previous year
   a. Test for urethral infection with *N gonorrhoeae* and *C trachomatis*
4. Men practicing receptive anal intercourse during previous year
   a. Test for rectal infection (*C trachomatis, N gonorrhoeae*)
   b. Consider testing for rectal lymphogranuloma venereum in patients with symptomatic proctitis
5. Men practicing receptive oral intercourse during previous year

Box 35.7

Treatment Regimens for Human Papillomavirus Warts

Provider-administered treatment
    Cryotherapy
        Liquid nitrogen or cryoprobe
        Repeat every 1-2 wk
    Podophyllum resin
        10%-25% in a compound tincture of benzoin
        Repeat weekly as needed
    Trichloroacetic acid 80%-90%
        Repeat weekly as needed
    Surgical removal
Patient-applied treatment
    Podofilox (Condylox) 0.5% solution or gel
        Apply twice daily for 3 d, followed by 4 d of no therapy
        Repeat 3 cycles if needed
    Imiquimod (Aldara) 5% cream
        Apply at bedtime 3 times weekly for as long as 16 wk

Adapted from Centers for Disease Control and Prevention; Workowski KA, Berman SM. Sexually transmitted diseases treatment guidelines, 2006. MMWR Recomm Rep. 2006 Aug 4;55(RR-11):1-94. Erratum in: MMWR Recomm Rep. 2006 Sep 15;55(36):997.

      a. Test for pharyngeal infection with *N gonorrhoeae*
  B. Vaccinations Recommended in Absence of Documented Prior Infection or Immunization
    1. Hepatitis A and hepatitis B
    2. Vaccine-associated adverse effects are not increased if patient was previously immune

Suggested Reading

Centers for Disease Control and Prevention. Sexually transmitted diseases treatment guidelines, 2010. MMWR 2010;59(No. RR-12):1–108.

Mandell GL, Bennett JE, Dolin R, editors. Mandell, Douglas, and Bennett's principles and practice of infectious diseases. Vol 1. 7th ed. Philadelphia (PA): Churchill Livingstone/Elsevier; c2010.

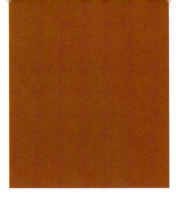

Select Major Clinical Syndromes
Questions and Answers

Questions

Multiple Choice (choose the best answer)

1. Which of the following statements is true about the pathogenesis of sepsis?
   a. Lipopolysaccharide (LPS) binding to CD14 may initiate nuclear factor-κB–driven proinflammatory responses.
   b. Toll-like receptor (TLR) ligation may initiate NF-κB–driven proinflammatory responses.
   c. In sepsis, exaggerated lymphoid and epithelial apoptosis may exacerbate sepsis.
   d. After the initial proinflammatory response, an anti-inflammatory response occurs.
   e. All of the above are true.

2. Which of the following should be included in the empirical antimicrobial treatment of patients with sepsis?
   a. A single broad-spectrum agent, vancomycin, and an antifungal for all patients
   b. A single broad-spectrum agent and vancomycin for all patients, with an antifungal for some patients
   c. A single broad-spectrum agent for all patients, with vancomycin and an antifungal for some patients
   d. Empirical coverage against *Pseudomonas* for all patients
   e. Double gram-negative coverage for all patients

3. Which of the following is *not* a contraindication for use of activated protein C?
   a. Recent heparin treatment
   b. Platelet count of 23,000/μL
   c. Splenic contusion
   d. Hemorrhagic stroke 6 weeks ago
   e. Epidural catheter

4. Concerning the epidemiology of infectious risks in selected populations, which of the following is *false*?
   a. *Listeria monocytogenes* is a special consideration for elderly or neonatal patients.
   b. Splenectomized patients have a higher risk of infection with pneumococcus or *Haemophilus influenzae*.
   c. Organ transplant recipients have a high risk of cytomegalovirus disease.
   d. Patients with a history of abnormal urinary tract anatomy have a high incidence of infection with Enterobacteriaciae.
   e. *Pneumocystis jiroveci* is the most common cause of pneumonia in patients infected with human immunodeficiency virus (HIV).

5. Which patients meet the classic criteria for fever of unknown origin (FUO)?
   a. A 28-year-old man who has a human immunodeficiency virus (HIV) infection has had an intermittent fever up to 38.5°C for the past month.

There are no clues to a diagnosis after his first 2 clinic visits and routine laboratory testing.
b. A previously healthy 74-year-old man reports muscle pain, headache, and fever up to 38.5°C off and on for the past month. Physical examination findings are normal. He has seen his primary care physician on 2 occasions. Laboratory evaluation shows only an elevated white blood cell count and an elevated erythrocyte sedimentation rate.
c. A 26-year-old woman with complaints of sore throat, fatigue, and fever up to 37.8°C over the past 4 months has had an extensive but unrevealing evaluation by her primary physician.
d. A 44-year-old man is referred to you by his physician assistant because he has lost 9 kg and has had a fever up to 39°C over the past 6 weeks. No testing has been done.
e. A 20-year-old man has had a fever up to 39°C and a headache for the past week. On physical examination, he has cervical and axillary lymphadenopathy. Initial laboratory tests reveal only mild leukopenia.
  a. Only *b*
  b. Only *b* and *e*
  c. Only *b*, *d*, and *e*
  d. All 5 patients
  e. None of the 5 patients

6. Which statement about evaluating a patient with fever of unknown origin (FUO) is true?
   a. Bone marrow cultures have a high yield when the fever is greater than 39°C and other testing has been unrevealing.
   b. A temporal artery biopsy is a reasonable test to perform next for a 75-year-old man who has FUO and no localizing complaints, an erythrocyte sedimentation rate greater than 100 mm/h, mild anemia, normal blood chemistry results, and negative blood cultures at 3 days and who has not had any other evaluation.
   c. Lumbar puncture should be done on every patient with FUO.
   d. When there are no clues to the underlying diagnosis, extensive serologic testing for unusual infections is often helpful.
   e. Liver biopsy is unlikely to be helpful in a patient with FUO and miliary tuberculosis.

7. Which statement is true about fever of unknown origin (FUO)?
   a. Empirical treatment with tetracycline is indicated whenever infection is suspected but the specific diagnosis for a patient with classic FUO is not forthcoming.
   b. Empirical antitubercular treatment would be reasonable in a 42-year-old immigrant from India who has granulomas but no organisms in her liver, a positive tuberculin skin test, and an otherwise extensive evaluation that is negative for the cause of FUO.
   c. An empirical trial of corticosteroids is almost always indicated when the erythrocyte sedimentation rate is high and an extensive FUO evaluation has been negative.
   d. Few cases of FUO (<10%) remain undiagnosed after careful evaluation in current case series.
   e. Patients with undiagnosed FUO generally have a poor prognosis.

8. Eosinophilia is frequently seen with fever of unknown origin from all but 1 of the following illnesses. Which illness is *not* frequently associated with eosinophilia?
   a. Systemic lupus erythematosus (SLE)
   b. Drug fever
   c. Tuberculosis
   d. Myeloproliferative disease
   e. Polyarteritis nodosa (PAN)

9. Which of the following patients is a candidate for screening and therapy for asymptomatic bacteriuria?
   a. A 70-year-old man who is hospitalized for congestive heart failure and has a bladder catheter in place
   b. A 45-year-old woman who has type 1 diabetes mellitus and a serum creatinine level of 2.5 mg/dL
   c. A 28-year-old woman (gravida 2, para 1 with 1 living child) in her 10th week of an uncomplicated pregnancy
   d. A 75-year-old woman who has had a total hip arthroplasty and is hospitalized with acute coronary syndrome
   e. A 50-year-old man who is undergoing a general medical examination and who had an aortic valve replacement 2 years earlier

10. Which of the following agents is recommended for treatment of the first case of uncomplicated cystitis in a 22-year-old woman who is allergic to sulfa?
    a. Cefixime
    b. Nitrofurantoin
    c. Azithromycin
    d. Levofloxacin
    e. Clindamycin

11. Which of the following is *not* a candidate for antibiotic prophylaxis of urinary tract infection?
    a. A 65-year-old man with asymptomatic bacteriuria who is scheduled for cystoscopic evaluation of a bladder mass
    b. A 35-year-old man 2 weeks after cadaveric renal transplant for end-stage renal disease from diabetes mellitus
    c. A 70-year-old woman with relapsing asymptomatic bacteriuria after hysterectomy

d. A 25-year-old woman with the third episode of uncomplicated cystitis in 9 months
   e. A 52-year-old paraplegic woman who is catheterized with a urinary straight catheter in an intermittent catheterization program for managing continence and voiding

12. Which agent would *not* be expected to reach therapeutic levels in an uninflamed prostate?
    a. Norfloxacin
    b. Trimethoprim
    c. Sulfamethoxazole
    d. Rifampin
    e. Ciprofloxacin

13. What would be the single best study for radiologic examination of a 74-year-old man with a serum creatinine level of 1.2 mg/dL and a relapsing urinary tract infection?
    a. Intravenous pyelography
    b. Magnetic resonance imaging of the abdomen and pelvis
    c. Computed tomographic (CT) scan of the abdomen and pelvis
    d. Ultrasonography
    e. Renal scan with radioisotope

14. After falling out of a tree stand, a healthy 52-year-old hunter is found by his brother and complains of severe abdominal pain, nausea, and low back ache. He is taken to the local emergency department, where a computed tomographic scan of the abdomen shows a small liver laceration and perihepatic hemorrhage. He is admitted for observation. Two days later, a fever develops (40°C), and his abdominal pain worsens. While the patient undergoes a laparotomy, the surgeon identifies several enterotomies in the small bowel and purulent material adherent to the peritoneum. A Gram stain is not performed, but cultures are begun and the patient is given meropenem 1 g every 8 hours. His condition is improving 72 hours postoperatively, but the cultures of the peritoneal fluid are growing extended-spectrum β-lactamase (ESBL)–producing *Escherichia coli*, *Bacteroides fragilis*, viridans group streptococci, *Enterococcus faecalis*, and *Candida albicans*. An infectious diseases consultation is requested for further antibiotic recommendations. Which of the following recommendations would you suggest?
    a. Discontinue use of meropenem and begin use of cefepime and metronidazole.
    b. Continue use of meropenem and add vancomycin.
    c. Continue use of meropenem and add fluconazole.
    d. Continue use of meropenem and add fluconazole and vancomycin.
    e. Continue use of meropenem.

15. A 52-year-old diabetic woman receiving long-term continuous ambulatory peritoneal dialysis works 2 jobs to support her family and complains of 2 days of cloudy fluid during her exchanges. This is similar to 3 previous episodes she has had in the past 3 months. Her last episode was 4 weeks ago and her cultures grew coagulase-negative *Staphylococcus*. When she received a 2-week course of intravenous vancomycin, her condition rapidly improved. Cultures from the first 2 episodes were negative, but she had a good response to cefepime and vancomycin. Now the peritoneal fluid cell count is 180/µL with 53% polymorphonuclear cells. No organisms are seen with Gram stain, and her culture is growing a gram-positive coccus in clusters. Her nephrologist calls to tell you that the patient declined hemodialysis and to ask for your best advice for managing this situation. Which of the following would you recommend?
    a. Give her another 2-week course of intravenous (IV) vancomycin.
    b. Give her IV vancomycin, immediately remove the catheter, and tell her that she must begin hemodialysis since she cannot properly care for the peritoneal dialysis catheter.
    c. Leave the catheter in and begin intraperitoneal (IP) vancomycin and treat for 6 weeks.
    d. Leave the catheter in and treat with IP vancomycin until the fluid clears, and then replace the catheter and give IV vancomycin for 2 more weeks.
    e. There is no need to treat because coagulase-negative *Staphylococcus* is a contaminant.

16. You are asked to see a 19-year-old day care worker with nausea, vomiting, and diarrhea who requests a prescription for ciprofloxacin. She says that 14 other persons from the same day care center were seen at a local emergency department earlier today and given antibiotics. All became ill 2 hours after they ate catered Chinese food at a party to celebrate the Chinese New Year. Which of the following would you recommend?
    a. Begin treatment with ciprofloxacin 500 mg twice daily for 5 days.
    b. Check for hepatitis A IgM and give an injection of immune globulin.
    c. Give her prochlorperazine 10 mg for nausea.
    d. Immediately contact the local health department about a possible bioterrorism event.
    e. Begin treatment with azithromycin 250 mg orally once daily for 5 days.

17. A 47-year-old lumberjack from northern Minnesota is admitted with 1-day onset of dizziness, blurred vision, slurred speech, difficulty swallowing, and nausea. In the emergency department, he had right eye ptosis, paralysis of cranial nerves V and VII, palatal weakness, and impaired gag reflex. When respiratory distress developed, his trachea was intubated and he was transported to the intensive care unit, where he required mechanical ventilation. He had no history of hypertension, diabetes

mellitus, or heart disease. He recalled no tick exposure, and he had already received the Lyme vaccine. His wife, who had been out of town, said that he was well previously, he worked hard outdoors yesterday, and then ate a hearty meal of stew containing roast beef and potatoes, which she had made for him 3 days earlier and which had been sitting on the stove. Which of the following diagnostic tests or test results would best help explain his symptoms?
   a. Western blot positive for Lyme disease
   b. Stool culture showing a large gram-positive rod
   c. Stool culture showing a curved gram-negative rod
   d. Cerebrospinal fluid analysis positive for cryptococcal antigen
   e. Toxin assay on the stew

18. A 46-year-old female marathon runner presented to her local physician in January, 1 week before a big race in Miami, Florida. She complained of persistent watery diarrhea for 2 weeks, anorexia, and dehydration, which had affected her ability to train. She is surprised that she has diarrhea because she eats a healthful diet with plenty of fiber and grains. For the past month she has been eating lots of yogurt, granola, and fresh raspberries, which she purchased at a local health food store in Iowa. Her local physician could not find anything remarkable on routine stool cultures and referred the patient to you. You obtain more stool samples for bacterial culture and an examination for ova and parasites. The laboratory report states that a large, round acid-fast organism was found. Which of the following antimicrobial agents would you recommend?
   a. Ciprofloxacin 500 mg twice daily for 5 days
   b. Trimethoprim-sulfamethoxazole double-strength tablet (DS) twice daily for 7 to 10 days
   c. Nitazoxanide 500 mg twice daily for 3 days
   d. Tinidazole 2 g for 1 dose
   e. Azithromycin 1 g orally every day for 3 days

19. A 22-year-old man presents to the emergency department after having abdominal pain, diarrhea, and tooth pain for 2 days. He and his bride have returned from a honeymoon on a Caribbean island, where they stayed at an all-inclusive resort. They walked the sandy beaches barefoot, received several insect bites, and drank the local water. All their meals were served at the resort. On the final day, they had a beach banquet of lobster, shrimp, grouper, red snapper, steamed clams, mussels, corn, and potatoes. His wife does not have diarrhea, but she began to complain that her cigarettes felt like icicles in her mouth. The man took 1 dose of ciprofloxacin, but it did not help his symptoms. An abdominal computed tomographic scan appears normal. He is referred to the Travel Clinic for further evaluation and recommendations. Which of the following would you recommend?
   a. Continue use of ciprofloxacin for 4 more days.
   b. Check a blood smear for malaria, and examine a stool sample for ova and parasites.
   c. Inform the patient that his symptoms may get worse with alcohol or caffeine.
   d. Administer albendazole 400 mg twice daily for 3 weeks.
   e. Administer hepatitis immune serum globulin.

20. An 82-year-old man with a permanent pacemaker is scheduled for an elective dental visit for routine cleaning. He has no known antibiotic allergies and has no acute dental complaints. Which of the following is correct?
   a. Amoxicillin should be prescribed before the procedure.
   b. Ampicillin should be administered intravenously before and after the procedure.
   c. Erythromycin should be given before the procedure.
   d. No antibiotic prophylaxis is required before the procedure.
   e. Antibiotic prophylaxis is required owing to the patient's age.

21. A 21-year-old injection drug user is being evaluated for infective endocarditis. He presents with fever and pleuritic chest pain, but no murmur is heard. Which of the following is correct?
   a. The most likely organism causing infective endocarditis is *Staphylococcus aureus*.
   b. Transthoracic echocardiography should be sufficient to evaluate for evidence of endocarditis.
   c. The pulmonic valve is the most likely site of infection.
   d. *Streptococcus bovis* is a frequent cause of endocarditis in injection drug users.
   e. Methicillin-resistant *S aureus* (MRSA) is usually not a cause of endocarditis in injection drug users.

22. Which of the following is the most common cause of endocarditis with negative cultures?
   a. *Bartonella* species
   b. *Coxiella burnetii* (Q fever)
   c. HACEK organisms (*Haemophilus parainfluenzae* and *Haemophilus aphrophilus*, *Actinobacillus actinomycetemcomitans*, *Cardiobacterium hominis*, *Eikenella corrodens*, and *Kingella kingae*)
   d. Prior antibiotic administration
   e. *Tropheryma whipplei*

23. Which of the following conditions do *not* predispose a patient to endocarditis?
   a. Mitral valve prolapse
   b. Coronary artery disease

c. Injection drug abuse
d. Prosthetic cardiac valve
e. Prior episode of endocarditis

24. A 75-year-old man with diabetes mellitus presents with a fever and a 3-week-old foot ulcer over the head of his fifth metatarsal. There is surrounding cellulitis and purulent drainage from the wound. The leukocyte count is 15×10⁹/L, and the erythrocyte sedimentation rate is 55 mm/h. Which of the following tests would *not* have reasonable sensitivity and specificity in diagnosing osteomyelitis in this patient?
    a. Probe-to-bone test
    b. Magnetic resonance imaging scan
    c. Technetium Tc 99m bone scan
    d. Plain radiograph
    e. Technetium Tc 99m bone scan plus indium In 111–labeled white blood cell scan

25. A 75-year-old healthy patient who had a total hip arthroplasty 12 years ago presents with a painful, loose prosthesis. The pain has been present for 18 months and is progressive. The erythrocyte sedimentation rate is 75 mm/h, and the C-reactive protein level is 1.5 mg/L. Culture of arthrocentesis fluid shows growth of *Staphylococcus aureus*. What would be the most appropriate management strategy to treat this infection at this time?
    a. Débridement with retention of the prosthesis and 6 weeks of intravenous antimicrobial therapy
    b. Prosthesis removal and 6 weeks of intravenous antibiotic therapy followed by reimplantation arthroplasty
    c. Intravenous antimicrobial therapy for 6 weeks
    d. Oral linezolid and rifampin for 6 weeks
    e. Long-term antimicrobial suppression with oral trimethoprim-sulfamethoxazole

26. A 48-year-old man presents with lumbar spine pain of 6 weeks' duration that started 2 weeks after treatment of a finger felon. The only abnormalities on a plain film of the spine are degenerative changes. The erythrocyte sedimentation rate is 45 mm/h, and the C-reactive protein level is 1.5 mg/L. Which of the following would be the next appropriate diagnostic test?
    a. Intravenous cefazolin for 6 weeks
    b. Magnetic resonance imaging (MRI) of the spine
    c. Another plain film in 1 month to see whether osteomyelitis is present
    d. Technetium Tc 99m bone scan
    e. Gallium Ga 67 citrate scan

27. A 60-year-old man undergoes débridement with retention of components for a methicillin-sensitive *Staphylococcus aureus* total hip arthroplasty infection. If he has no antimicrobial allergies, what would be the appropriate antimicrobial regimen?
    a. Nafcillin 2 g intravenously (IV) every 4 hours for 6 weeks
    b. Ceftriaxone 2 g IV every 24 hours for 6 weeks
    c. Daptomycin 6 mg/kg IV every 24 hours
    d. Cefazolin 2 g IV every 8 hours for 4 weeks plus rifampin, then levofloxacin plus rifampin for 2 months, and then long-term antimicrobial suppression with cefadroxil
    e. Vancomycin 15 mg/kg IV every 12 hours for 6 weeks

28. A 57-year-old man has a painful, loose prosthesis from a total hip arthroplasty. His sedimentation rate and C-reactive protein level are abnormal without obvious explanation. What would be the best diagnostic test to perform next?
    a. Aspiration for cell count and aerobic and anaerobic cultures
    b. Magnetic resonance imaging (MRI)
    c. Technetium Tc 99m bone scan
    d. Gallium Ga 67 citrate scan
    e. All of the above

29. Which viral hepatitis is rare in the United States, is characterized by water-borne epidemics in underdeveloped countries, and is associated with a high mortality rate among pregnant women?
    a. Hepatitis A
    b. Hepatitis B
    c. Hepatitis C
    d. Hepatitis D
    e. Hepatitis E

30. A patient with serologic results that are positive for hepatitis B surface antigen and negative for IgM hepatitis B core antigen antibody has signs and symptoms of acute hepatitis. Which of the following would *not* be consistent with these findings?
    a. Hepatitis D virus (HDV) superinfection with chronic hepatitis B virus (HBV) infection
    b. HDV-HBV coinfection
    c. Hepatitis C virus superinfection with chronic HBV infection
    d. Ischemic liver injury with chronic HBV infection
    e. Medication-related liver injury with chronic HBV infection

31. A 25-year-old male injection drug user presents to your office with 3 days of nausea, vomiting, anorexia, and abdominal pain. On evaluation, you note icterus and right upper quadrant abdominal pain. Which of the following blood tests would *not* help you?
    a. Anti–hepatitis A virus (HAV) antibody

b. Anti–hepatitis C virus (HCV) antibody and HCV RNA
c. Hepatitis B surface antigen, hepatitis B e antigen, and hepatitis B core antigen antibody
d. Anti–hepatitis D virus (HDV) antibody
e. Hepatitis B virus (HBV) DNA

32. Which of the following statements about hepatitis G virus (HGV)/hepatitis GB virus C (HGBV-C) is *false*?
    a. HGV/HGBV-C is an RNA virus belonging to the Flaviviridae family.
    b. Less than 2% of the adult population have HGV/HGBV-C in the peripheral blood.
    c. Patients coinfected with human immunodeficiency virus (HIV) and HGV have improved survival compared with patients infected with HIV alone.
    d. Patients coinfected with hepatitis C virus (HCV) and HGV have a more clinically severe course of illness than those infected with HCV alone.
    e. No disease has been ascribed to HGV

33. Which of the following is often required immediately for management of deep facial space infections?
    a. Suspicion of a neoplastic growth requiring an oncology consultation
    b. Use of an initial oral antibiotic regimen that covers aerobic pathogens
    c. Thoracic radiographic studies to identify the likely source of infection
    d. Use of an initial parenteral antibiotic regimen that includes anaerobic coverage and surgical drainage
    e. Careful search for the presence of an infected embryonic cyst

34. What is the source of most deeper face, neck, and head infections?
    a. Nearby lymphatic infections
    b. Upper respiratory tract infections
    c. Infections of the teeth or periodontal tissues
    d. Trauma or other penetrating wounds
    e. Perforations of the pharynx or upper esophagus

35. A 42-year-old man attending a football game was punched in the mouth after he irritated a fan of the opposing team. The punch loosened a left maxillary molar. Although he felt some discomfort, he did not seek dental help for his injury. Nine days later, he awoke with left cheek swelling that extended to his left lower eyelid. In the emergency department, he reported little pain or difficulty chewing from the swelling, but the affected molar was sensitive to touch and heat. A computed tomographic scan showed periapical molar inflammation and an abscess in the deep temporal space. A syringe aspirate showed gram-negative bacilli. Surgical drainage was scheduled. You are consulted for antibiotic recommendations. Which of the following would you recommend?
    a. Linezolid 600 mg intravenously (IV) every 12 hours
    b. Cefazolin 1 g IV every 8 hours
    c. Tetracycline 250 mg orally every 6 hours
    d. Nafcillin 2 g IV every 4 hours
    e. Ampicillin-sulbactam 3 g IV every 6 hours

36. A 30-year-old-man presents to the emergency department complaining of difficulty swallowing and regurgitation, occasionally through his nose. He also reports fever, chills, and some difficulty breathing over the past 24 to 48 hours. He mentions that he had a molar removed 2 weeks ago, and he still has some lower jaw pain. A computed tomographic (CT) scan shows bulging of the posterior pharyngeal wall and marked widening of the retropharyngeal space surrounding the esophagus and trachea. What course of action should the physician recommend?
    a. Review latest dental records to ascertain history of tooth or periodontal disorders.
    b. Proceed with syringe aspirate culture of abscess material and surgical drainage.
    c. Allow 2 to 4 days for culture results before administering intravenous antibiotics.
    d. Administer analgesics and topical antiseptics for the mouth and throat.
    e. Arrange a consultation with a gastroenterologist for endoscopic follow-up to confirm the CT scan findings.

37. A 25-year-old woman in her second trimester of pregnancy has a positive rapid plasma reagin test (1:32) with a moderately reactive fluorescent treponema test; she is asymptomatic. She has an unremarkable past medical history and takes only prenatal vitamins. She recalls "hives" developing when she was treated for a prolonged sore throat and adenopathy as a teenager. What should be the next step in the management of this patient?
    a. Begin treatment with penicillin G benzathine.
    b. Begin treatment with penicillin G procaine and probenecid.
    c. Begin treatment with doxycycline.
    d. Perform a penicillin skin test.
    e. Begin treatment with ceftriaxone.

38. If the patient in the previous question has a positive penicillin skin test, what should you do next?
    a. Begin treatment with ceftriaxone administered intramuscularly.
    b. Begin treatment with doxycycline.
    c. Begin treatment with azithromycin.
    d. Desensitize and begin treatment with penicillin G benzathine.
    e. Request a cerebrospinal fluid examination.

39. A 40-year-old man infected with human immunodeficiency virus (HIV) returns from a trip to the Netherlands with a 3-month history of tenesmus, rectal pain, and blood-streaked diarrhea. Physical examination findings are normal except for prominent inguinal adenopathy. Proctoscopic examination discloses proctitis. Results are negative for both the Gram stain and the polymerase chain reaction test for herpes simplex virus. What would be the most appropriate therapy?
    a. Ceftriaxone 1 g intramuscularly
    b. Levofloxacin 500 mg orally daily for 1 week
    c. Doxycycline 100 mg orally for 1 week
    d. Azithromycin 1 g now
    e. Doxycycline 100 mg orally twice daily for 21 days

40. You are asked to give a presentation to the local medical society about sexually transmitted disease screening, with specific attention to *Chlamydia*. Which of the following statements about chlamydial screening is correct?
    a. Annual screening is recommended for asymptomatic sexually active men younger than 25 years.
    b. Annual screening is recommended for asymptomatic sexually active women younger than 25 years.
    c. Urine-based DNA-amplification tests are less sensitive than testing of cervical specimens.
    d. Most women with chlamydial cervicitis are symptomatic.
    e. Pharyngitis is a common clinical manifestation.

41. A 35-year-old Hispanic woman presents to the outpatient clinic with a 3-day history of malodorous vaginal discharge. Pelvic examination findings are negative. The vaginal discharge has a pH of 6, and large epithelial cells are noted with adherent, small coccobacillary organisms. Which of the following statements about this disease is *false*?
    a. It facilitates acquisition of other sexually transmitted diseases, including infection with human immunodeficiency virus.
    b. It may be responsible for preterm labor and delivery.
    c. Screening and treatment in pregnancy may prevent postpartum complications.
    d. It may be seen in women who are not sexually active.
    e. Sexual partners should be treated.

42. A 48-year-old woman is admitted from the emergency department with a 4-week history of severe headache, night sweats, and neck pain. She reports temperatures as high as 39°C. She is lethargic but arousable. Her temperature is 38.5°C. She cannot adduct either eye. The other physical examination findings are normal. Computed tomography of the head findings are normal. Cerebrospinal fluid (CSF) examination results are as follows:

Component	Finding
Cell count, cells/µL	20 erythrocytes
	125 leukocytes (85% lymphocytes)
Protein, mg/dL	300
Glucose, mg/dL	20 (plasma glucose 100)
Gram stain	Negative
Acid-fast stain	Negative
Cryptococcal antigen	Negative

CSF was submitted to the microbiology laboratory for bacterial, mycobacterial, and fungal cultures. Empirical therapy with ampicillin and ceftriaxone was begun. Two days later, the patient's condition is unchanged and she continues to have a severe headache. Cultures of the CSF remain negative. The lumbar puncture is repeated, and there is no change in the results. What is the most likely diagnosis?
    a. *Listeria monocytogenes* meningitis
    b. Brain abscess
    c. *Mycobacterium tuberculosis* meningitis
    d. Pneumococcal meningitis
    e. Cryptococcal meningitis

43. A previously healthy 28-year-old medical intern who just started his residency is evaluated in the emergency department for a 5-day history of a progressively severe headache with intermittent fevers. He describes a mostly frontal headache with radiation into the neck. There is no history of recent travel and he is not aware of any sick contacts. He can recall childhood varicella but no other childhood illnesses. He has no risk factors for human immunodeficiency virus and has never had a blood transfusion. On physical examination he is pale and diaphoretic. He requests that the lights be left off. His temperature is 37.7°C. His vital signs are stable. A fine erythematous papular rash is present on the neck and forearms. Ophthalmologic examination findings are negative, and the remainder of the physical examination findings are unremarkable. Cerebrospinal fluid (CSF) examination results are as follows:

Component	Finding
Opening pressure, mm water	150
Cell count, cells/µL	0 erythrocytes
	72 leukocytes (10% neutrophils, 87% lymphocytes, 3% monocytes)
Protein, mg/dL	40
Glucose, mg/dL	58 (plasma glucose 95)

What is the most likely diagnosis?
a. Mumps meningitis
b. Herpes simplex virus 2 infection
c. Leptospirosis
d. Enterovirus infection
e. Ehrlichiosis

44. A 35-year-old woman who recently returned home from Christmas vacation in North Dakota presents to the emergency department with a 2-day history of fever, headaches, stiff neck, and photophobia. This is the third episode that she has had in the past 2 years. Both prior episodes resolved without therapy after about 5 days of symptoms, but she is concerned about the cause. She is otherwise in good health. On physical examination she is pleasant and cooperative but prefers to have the lights dimly lit. Her temperature is 38.5°C and her blood pressure, heart rate, and respiratory rate are normal. There is mild nuchal rigidity, and the remainder of the physical examination findings are normal. Cerebrospinal fluid (CSF) examination results are as follows:

Component	Finding
Cell count, cells/µL	175 leukocytes (95% lymphocytes, 5% neutrophils)
Protein, mg/dL	110
Glucose, mg/dL	70
Gram stain	No organisms seen

CSF was submitted for bacterial, fungal, and mycobacterial cultures and for cryptococcal antigen testing. Which of following is most likely to be positive?
a. Herpes simplex virus 2 polymerase chain reaction (PCR) on CSF
b. Enterovirus PCR on CSF
c. Mumps virus culture
d. Serum cryptococcal antigen
e. Serum antinuclear antibody

45. A 48-year-old man with end-stage renal disease who receives outpatient hemodialysis 3 times per week is admitted with fever, productive cough, and pleuritic chest pain. Chest radiography shows a left lower lobe infiltrate. He is hemodynamically stable, and his oxygen saturation is 90% on room air. He does not have any antibiotic allergies. What would be the most appropriate choice of empirical antibiotics for this patient?
a. Ceftriaxone in combination with azithromycin
b. Ceftriaxone in combination with levofloxacin
c. Cefepime in combination with levofloxacin
d. Cefepime
e. Piperacillin-tazobactam

46. Which of the following statements is true?
a. Blood cultures are positive for less than 25% of patients with pneumonia.
b. All patients with ventilator-associated pneumonia must have a bronchoscopic examination.
c. Pneumonia cannot be prevented by vaccination.
d. All pneumonia should be treated with antibiotics for a minimum of 2 weeks.
e. Treatment of pneumonia with oral antibiotics is never appropriate.

47. In a 55-year-old man who has polytrauma and who is receiving mechanical ventilation, a new left lower lobe infiltrate develops on day 8 of his hospitalization. Bronchial washings grow methicillin-resistant *Staphylococcus aureus* (3+) and *Candida albicans*. Which of the following regimens is *least* appropriate?
a. Vancomycin intravenously (IV)
b. Linezolid IV
c. Daptomycin IV in combination with fluconazole IV
d. Vancomycin IV in combination with trimethoprim-sulfamethoxazole (TMP-SMX) by feeding tube
e. Vancomycin IV in combination with TMP-SMX IV

48. For which patient listed below would an 8-day course of antibiotics *not* be appropriate?
a. A 75-year-old trauma patient with early ventilator-associated pneumonia (VAP) and tracheal cultures that have grown penicillin-resistant pneumococci
b. A 75-year-old man with respiratory failure after cardiac surgery and VAP with *Pseudomonas*
c. A 75-year-old woman receiving long-term hemodialysis who is admitted to the hospital with *Klebsiella* pneumonia
d. A 75-year-old man with recent influenza and methicillin-sensitive *Staphylococcus aureus* in tracheal secretions
e. A 75-year-old man with community-acquired aspiration pneumonia

49. A 35-year-old woman with lower extremity lymphedema presents with her first episode of cellulitis. She has no acute skin injuries but has chronic tinea pedis. Which of the following is correct?
a. Blood cultures will probably define the pathogen.
b. She is at low risk of another bout of lower extremity cellulitis.
c. Swab cultures of the toe web spaces should be used to identify the likely cause of cellulitis, a β-hemolytic streptococcus.
d. Cellulitis is the most frequent skin infection syndrome caused by community-acquired methicillin-resistant *Staphylococcus aureus* (CA-MRSA).
e. Macrolides are an appropriate choice of therapy.

50. A 52-year-old diabetic woman presents with sudden onset of severe pain in her right calf and high fever. On physical examination, there are necrotic-appearing skin lesions over the calf, which is indurated, painful on palpation, and diffusely erythematous. Which of the following is correct?
    a. Gentamicin should be included in the empirical treatment regimen.
    b. Magnetic resonance imaging should be scheduled for the next day to evaluate for a Baker cyst.
    c. This definitely is a polymicrobial infection.
    d. Emergent surgical evaluation should be obtained.
    e. Disseminated infection with *Histoplasma capsulatum* should be considered in the differential diagnosis for this diabetic patient.

51. A 21-year-old male college football player presents with a skin abscess on his posterior right shoulder. He indicated that he had a similar infection 6 months earlier and that 3 other team members had been treated for the same condition. He has noted no fever or chills and otherwise feels well. What would be the optimal choice of antibiotic therapy?
    a. Cephalexin
    b. Amoxicillin
    c. Cefadroxil
    d. Ciprofloxacin
    e. In addition to incision and drainage, there is controversy as to whether antibiotic therapy is needed. Because *Staphylococcus aureus*, including community-acquired methicillin-resistant *S aureus* (CA-MRSA) strains, is the most likely pathogen, trimethoprim-sulfamethoxazole is a preferred choice.

52. A 42-year-old diabetic woman presents with a subacute presentation of nodular lymphadenitis advancing up the arm from the dorsal hand to the proximal forearm. She has noted no systemic toxicity. The only pet exposure has been to fish in 3 different fish tanks that she manages. What is the most likely pathogen?
    a. *Streptococcus pyogenes*
    b. *Pseudomonas aeruginosa*
    c. *Mycobacterium marinum*
    d. *Vibrio vulnificus*
    e. Varicella-zoster virus

Answers

1. Answer e.
Multiple signals may contribute to the proinflammatory response of sepsis, including but not limited to LPS binding to CD14 and activation of TLR. This activation promotes apoptosis of epithelial cells and lymphoid cells contributing to more bacterial translocation from the gut and to decreased immunocompetence, which in turn exacerbates the septic response. Several days after the onset of sepsis, an anti-inflammatory phase ensues.

2. Answer c.
The cornerstone of empirical antimicrobial treatment for sepsis is broad-spectrum agents such as third- or fourth-generation cephalosporins, carbapenems, extended-spectrum carboxypenicillins, and ureidopenicillins combined with β-lactamase inhibitors. The empirical use of glycopeptides, antifungals, or agents against *Pseudomonas* is generally not recommended but may be appropriate in select cases.

3. Answer a.
Unlike ongoing treatment with heparin at more than 15 international units/kg per hour, a history of recent heparin treatment per se, without thrombocytopenia or active bleeding, is not a contraindication to administering activated protein C.

4. Answer e.
Although HIV-infected patients with CD4 cell counts less than 200 μL or 14% have a higher risk of *Pneumocystis jiroveci* infection than the general population, the most common cause of pneumonia in HIV-infected patients is bacterial pneumonia. According to the World Health Organization, the most common bacterial cause is pneumococcus.

5. Answer a.
The patient in *b* meets the classic criteria for FUO (presumably the initial laboratory evaluation included a complete blood cell count with differential, blood chemistry tests that included liver function testing, urinalysis and culture, blood cultures, and chest radiography). He is reportedly not immunosuppressed, he has been ill for more than 3 weeks, and his fever has been higher than 38.3°C on several occasions.

The patient in *a* does not meet the classic criteria for FUO since he has an HIV infection. Patients who have HIV infection or other illnesses that compromise the immune system frequently have FUO from causes that are different from those in otherwise healthy adults.

The patient in *c* does not meet the classic criteria for FUO since her fever has been low grade. If a patient with a low-grade fever appears healthy, extensive testing is highly unlikely to be beneficial.

The patient in *d* does not meet the classic criteria for FUO because he has not had any evaluation. If his illness remains uncertain after a comprehensive history, physical examination, and initial laboratory testing, he would meet the classic criteria for FUO.

The patient in *e* has not been ill long enough to meet the classic criteria for FUO. To assume that this patient has FUO would mean considering unlikely possibilities and subjecting him to an intensive evaluation when his illness may well spontaneously resolve.

6. Answer b.
Statement *a* is false. Bone marrow cultures from an immunocompetent patient are unlikely to be positive when there are no hematologic abnormalities, particularly if pathologic examination of the bone marrow does not suggest infection.

Statement *b* is true. Patients with temporal arteritis may present with no symptoms other than fever. Temporal arteritis should be strongly considered when trying to diagnose FUO in an elderly patient. In some series, temporal arteritis has been the most common cause of FUO in the elderly. Although invasive, temporal artery biopsy is usually safe and well tolerated.

Statement *c* is false. Cerebrospinal fluid evaluation is unlikely to be helpful unless there has been confusion, memory difficulty, or other symptoms or signs of meningitis or encephalitis, and it is not routinely recommended in evaluation of FUO.

Statement *d* is false. Although it is often tempting to order a battery of serologic tests, the results are as likely to be misleading as diagnostic. Since each test can have a false-positive result, testing should be ordered only if there is a reasonable chance that a test will yield a true-positive result.

Statement *e* is false. Liver biopsy findings are often positive with staining and in culture when patients have miliary tuberculosis even when other biopsy results are nondiagnostic.

7. Answer b.
Statement *a* is false. Most patients with suspected infection and FUO remain clinically stable and do not require empirical antibiotic treatment. This should be considered when the likelihood of an unusual infection seems probable and the patient's clinical condition is poor.

Statement *b* is true. *Mycobacterium tuberculosis* can be difficult to culture even from patients who are later documented to have tuberculosis. Granulomas, particularly caseating or necrotizing granulomas, greatly increase the likelihood of tuberculosis; when granulomas are found in a patient with known exposure to tuberculosis, empirical treatment is often reasonable.

Statement *c* is false. Administering an empirical trial of corticosteroids is often tempting; however, a response is not helpful in arriving at a diagnosis since corticosteroids can suppress fever from inflammatory illnesses of any cause as well as fever from infection and malignancy. Corticosteroids may be detrimental when infection is present and not yet identified.

Statement *d* is false. In most current case series from the United States or Europe, a diagnosis was not confirmed in 15% to 25% of cases. This may partially reflect the fact that most series are from tertiary care centers and most patients who are referred have already undergone a fairly extensive evaluation. A 1992 US series of 86 patients seen in a community hospital reported an inability to arrive at a diagnosis in only 9%.

Statement *e* is false. Most patients who did not receive a diagnosis in FUO case series had a favorable prognosis and many had spontaneous resolution of their illness. This may be misleading since clinicians aggressively pursue a diagnosis in patients who appear severely ill. When patients die and the diagnosis remains unknown at death, autopsy findings usually secure a diagnosis.

8. Answer c.
Drug fever is often associated with significant eosinophilia. SLE, myeloproliferative diseases, and PAN are frequently associated with eosinophilia. Tuberculosis and other bacterial illnesses are rarely associated with eosinophilia.

9. Answer c.
Screening and therapy for asymptomatic bacteriuria is indicated only for young children with vesicoureteral reflux, pregnant women, and patients scheduled for elective, invasive urologic procedures.

10. Answer b.
Of the 5 agents listed, only nitrofurantoin is endorsed by the Infectious Diseases Society of America guidelines. The other agents are unnecessarily broad in their spectrum of antimicrobial activity, incapable of achieving reliably active levels in the urinary space, or more expensive.

11. Answer c.
A woman with asymptomatic bacteriuria after hysterectomy does not have an indication for treatment or prophylaxis of bacteriuria. The other patients listed for this question have conditions for which prophylaxis is indicated.

12. Answer c.
Fluoroquinolones and trimethoprim—and to a less degree, rifampin—diffuse into prostatic fluid in the absence of inflammation. Sulfonamides, including sulfamethoxazole, do not diffuse readily into prostatic fluid.

13. Answer c.
Anatomical and physiologic anomalies that would increase the risk of relapsing urinary tract infection in this patient could reside in the prostate or the kidneys or anywhere between. Unlike the other options for diagnostic evaluation, a CT scan with intravenous radiocontrast material would identify many of these. There is no indication that the patient is at significantly increased risk of contrast-induced nephrotoxicity. It may be prudent to discuss imaging selection and ordering with a local radiologist before the study is performed, since some centers use specialized protocols to optimize administration of contrast material.

14. Answer e.
In this patient, acute secondary peritonitis developed after small-bowel perforation from blunt abdominal trauma. Patients with community-onset peritonitis are infected with bowel flora that is usually susceptible to most combination regimens. This patient had no previous health care or antimicrobial exposure and would not be expected to be at high risk of multiresistant pathogens. Use of meropenem should be continued because it is effective for most enteric gram-negative bacteria, *E faecalis*, anaerobes, and the ESBL-producer that was identified. *Candida* and *Enterococcus* do not need to be considered in the treatment at this time. Studies have specifically looked at whether coverage against these organisms in community-onset peritonitis is necessary. Results did not show improvement in outcome when compared with regimens without that coverage.

15. Answer d.
This woman has had relapsing infections with coagulase-negative *Staphylococcus*. They result from either poor preparation of the skin surface or the presence of biofilm on the peritoneal dialysis catheter. Because she declined hemodialysis and needs to work, she must continue peritoneal dialysis. The best approach is to treat the infection until the effluent clears and then remove the catheter because biofilm may be causing relapses. She can then complete her therapy with intravenous antibiotics and a new peritoneal dialysis catheter.

16. Answer c.
The Chinese food syndrome is most often associated with *Bacillus cereus* food poisoning due to contamination of fried rice. Gastroenteritis and a history of eating fried rice should prompt one to consider *B cereus*, which causes 2 forms of gastroenteritis: 1) an emetic syndrome that resembles one caused by *Staphylococcus aureus* and is characterized by an incubation period of 1 to 6 hours and 2) a diarrheal illness characterized by an incubation period of 6 to 24 hours. Fever is uncommon in either syndrome. *Bacillus cereus* is frequently present in uncooked rice, and heat-resistant spores may survive cooking. If cooked rice is held at room temperature, vegetative forms multiply, and heat-stable toxin is produced that can survive brief heating, such as stir-frying. This does not reflect a bioterrorism event; however, foodborne outbreaks should be reported to the local public health authorities. This patient should be treated symptomatically with prochlorperazine for nausea and provided adequate hydration. The syndrome is self-limited.

17. Answer e.
Botulism is a paralytic illness resulting from a toxin produced under anaerobic conditions by *Clostridium botulinum*. The diagnosis is suggested by clinical manifestations that begin with cranial nerve palsies (ptosis and extraocular palsies) and progress to descending paralysis involving the extremities. A good mnemonic is the 4 *Ds*—dry mouth,

*d*ysphagia, *d*iplopia, and *d*ysarthria—which occur in almost 90% of cases. The incubation period is 18 to 36 hours. Patients presenting with clinical signs and symptoms of botulism should have serum analysis for toxin by bioassay in mice, which can be obtained from the health department. Analysis of stool, vomitus, and suspected food items may also show toxin, which is diagnostic when coupled with the appropriate clinical and neurologic findings. A botulinum toxin assay should be performed on the contaminated stew. In the present case, the heat-resistant *C botulinum* spores either survived the initial cooking or were introduced afterward; the spores subsequently germinated and produced toxin. The lid on the pot of stew most likely produced the anaerobic environment necessary for toxin production. Most outbreaks of foodborne botulism result from eating improperly preserved home-canned vegetables (especially asparagus, green beans, and peppers). Treatment is administration of antitoxin.

18. Answer b.

Cyclospora cayetanensis is a coccidian protozoan that causes diarrheal illness in persons in the United States, in travelers, and in patients with AIDS. It has been associated with outbreaks of foodborne illness in the United States, especially related to imported raspberries. It is transmitted by the fecal-oral route. Most cases occur in spring and summer; however, cases associated with imported fruits may occur in the winter. The average incubation period is 1 week. Illness may be protracted (from days to weeks) with frequent, watery stools and other gastrointestinal tract symptoms that may remit and relapse. Diagnosis is made by microscopy. The organisms are acid-fast and resemble large *Cryptosporidium* ("Crypto Grande"). Treatment is with trimethoprim-sulfamethoxazole DS twice daily for 7 days.

19. Answer c.

Ciguatoxin is a neurotoxin from dinoflagellates that are ingested by carnivorous fish found in the warm waters of the Caribbean Sea. Grouper, barracuda, red snapper, and mackerel are often the culprits. These fish look and taste fine, and the toxins are heat stable. Although some patients present 1 to 2 days after ingestion with gastroenteritis, many complain of bizarre dysesthesias, such as tooth pain, reversal of hot and cold sensations, and blurry vision. The symptoms are exacerbated by caffeinated beverages and alcohol and may persist for weeks. Although mannitol has been used, there is no specific antidote for this illness.

20. Answer d.

The American Heart Association does not recommend the administration of antibiotic prophylaxis before dental procedures to patients with permanent pacemakers or implantable cardioverter-defibrillators.

21. Answer a.

Transthoracic echocardiography is less sensitive than transesophageal echocardiography (TEE) in evaluating cardiac valves and associated infection complications; thus, TEE should be used. Pulmonic valve infection is rare, even among injection drug users who are at increased risk of right-sided endocarditis. *Streptococcus bovis* is infrequently identified among pathogens causing endocarditis in injection drug users. MRSA, in contrast, has been identified as a cause of endocarditis in this population.

22. Answer d.

Although several of the listed organisms can cause endocarditis with negative blood cultures, by far the most common cause of "culture-negative" endocarditis is recent antibiotic administration. If endocarditis is clinically suspected, blood cultures should be obtained before administration of antibiotics. The other organisms may be considered in the proper epidemiologic context.

23. Answer b.

Coronary artery disease is not an established risk factor for endocarditis. All the other conditions listed may either cause endothelial damage or otherwise predispose to bacterial adherence, ultimately leading to vegetation formation.

24. Answer d.

Plain radiography is associated with low sensitivity and specificity in the diagnosis of contiguous osteomyelitis. Bone infection may be present for 2 weeks before changes appear on a plain radiograph. Furthermore, bone remodeling or Charcot arthropathy can have findings similar to those of osteomyelitis.

25. Answer b.

A high success rate has been associated with prosthesis removal followed by a course of antimicrobial therapy before final reimplantation. The presence of a chronic infection precludes the use of débridement and retention as a first choice. Antimicrobial therapy alone is associated with a high failure rate.

26. Answer b.

MRI of the spine is the most sensitive and specific diagnostic test for a patient who may have a disk space infection. Plain films and technetium Tc 99m bone scans have low specificity and sensitivity and are not typically useful. Empirical therapy with prolonged antimicrobial therapy is not justified according to the information provided from the preliminary assessment.

27. Answer d.

When components are retained, an antimicrobial regimen that has activity against biofilm organisms is appropriate and has been shown to be effective in randomized trials and cohort studies. Rifampin has activity against biofilm organisms but must be given with a companion drug to avoid emergence of resistance.

28. Answer a.

The most cost-effective test is aspiration for cell count and cultures. It will provide microbiologic and susceptibility data to guide empirical therapy after surgery. MRI is associated with significant image distortion. Technetium Tc 99m and gallium Ga 67 citrate scans are sensitive but not specific tests.

29. Answer e.
Hepatitis E is a serious liver disease that usually results in an acute infection. Although rare in the United States, hepatitis E is common in many parts of the world, especially in countries with contaminated water supplies and poor sanitation. Hepatitis E can cause severe liver disease in pregnant women.

30. Answer b.
The serologic results suggest a chronic HBV infection. Therefore, a new HBV infection (choice b) is the exception. All the other choices would result in acute hepatitis in a patient with chronic HBV infection.

31. Answer d.
The symptoms suggest that acute hepatitis developed from a bloodborne hepatitis virus; however, 3 days is too soon for an antibody response to develop. Antigens to HBV (choice c) would be present, and genomic material for HCV and HBV (choices b and e) would be present, but antibody to HDV would not have time to develop. HAV is generally not transmitted through blood.

32. Answer d.
HGV is a single-stranded RNA virus and is a new genus within the Flaviviridae family. Studies have repeatedly shown that HGV has no effect on the clinical, biochemical, histologic, or virologic course of HCV infection. Several studies have shown that HIV-infected patients who are coinfected with HGV have better overall survival and a longer interval to development of AIDS than people who are infected with HIV alone.

33. Answer d.
It is important to begin use of antibiotics with anaerobic coverage and to provide surgical intervention as soon as possible to prevent potential life-threatening complications from these infections. The regimen in response b does not provide anaerobic coverage. The other 3 responses describe diagnostic procedures not relevant to the problem.

34. Answer c.
Most deep head, face, and neck infections spread from teeth or periodontal tissues. Unless the patient has had notable trauma, the clinician should assume that the source was an odontogenic infection, manage the acute problem, and focus the patient on preventive oral hygiene. The other responses describe unlikely sources for these infections.

35. Answer e.
Only the ampicillin-sulbactam combination provides good anaerobic and gram-negative coverage. Other good antibiotic choices include 1) clindamycin, 2) moxifloxacin, or 3) metronidazole with either penicillin or levofloxacin. Linezolid and nafcillin provide only gram-positive coverage, and cefazolin has poor anaerobic coverage. Tetracycline is less effective than its more recent analogues such as doxycycline.

36. Answer b.
The syringe aspirate should be protected from ambient oxygen and cultured for anaerobes. Blood cultures too often provide false-negative results. Reviewing dental records and requesting a consultation with endoscopic follow-up would waste critical time and diagnostic resources. Intentionally waiting to begin antibiotic therapy is wrong because appropriate antibiotic coverage should begin immediately, before confirmative culture results are available. After culture results are available, the antibiotic regimen can be adjusted. Topical antiseptics are useless against deeper serious infections. Although analgesics may provide relief, they can mask a serious, perhaps life-threatening infection.

37. Answer d.
Penicillin is always the treatment of choice in pregnant women with syphilis. A negative result from a penicillin skin test has a high negative predictive value for anaphylaxis, even though a rash may develop with treatment. A positive result from a skin test predicts anaphylaxis. Desensitization and penicillin therapy are mandated.

38. Answer d.
A positive result from a skin test predicts anaphylaxis. Desensitization and penicillin therapy are mandated.

39. Answer e.
This patient most likely has a newly described manifestation of lymphogranuloma venereum with hemorrhagic proctocolitis, seen exclusively in HIV-infected patients.

40. Answer b.
This is an official recommendation of the US Preventive Services Task Force. None of the other statements are true.

41. Answer e.
There is no indication to treat the sexual partners of women with bacterial vaginosis.

42. Answer c.
The duration of symptoms and the cranial nerve deficits are key factors in this case. Pneumococcal meningitis can be excluded as a likely cause owing to the duration of symptoms. The remaining options could produce a clinical picture similar to this, but the cranial nerve palsies are most likely caused by M tuberculosis, which commonly causes a basilar meningitis. It is also the most likely organism to produce such a low glucose level in the CSF.

43. Answer d.
This clinical scenario is compatible with aseptic meningitis, which could involve each of the answer choices. Mumps meningitis can occur without parotiditis but is very rare and commonly produces a low glucose level in the CSF. Herpes simplex virus 2 meningitis would produce this CSF profile, but the presence of a rash and no history of recurrences suggest an alternative diagnosis. There is no history to suggest exposure to Leptospira, and there is no mention of either conjunctival suffusion on physical examination or myalgias by history, both of which are common manifestations of

leptospirosis. Ehrlichiosis is a rare cause of aseptic meningitis, but the history contains no supporting epidemiologic clues such as exposure to ticks. Finally, enterovirus infection is the most common cause of aseptic meningitis and occurs most frequently during the summer and fall. A maculopapular rash is frequently present. Other common features include conjunctivitis, herpangina, and pleurodynia.

44. Answer a.
The key feature is the recurrent nature of the patient's symptoms. Of the options presented, only herpes simplex virus 2 is commonly associated with recurrences. The time of year (December or January) would be unusual for enteroviral infection. Mumps meningitis is rare, and the patient has no associated symptoms to suggest it. Most cases of cryptococcal meningitis occur in patients who are immunosuppressed, either from AIDS or from immunosuppressive therapy for malignancies or inflammatory disorders. The CSF in cryptococcal meningitis usually has a decreased glucose level, and lymphocytes usually predominate. Systemic lupus erythematosus (SLE) can cause aseptic meningitis, but the patient has no other features to suggest SLE.

45. Answer c.
Long-term hemodialysis is a risk factor for colonization with multidrug-resistant (MDR) organisms. Therefore, this patient has health care–associated pneumonia with possible MDR pathogens. The recommended antibiotic regimen is a cephalosporin, carbapenem, or β-lactam–β-lactamase inhibitor combination with antipseudomonal activity and either a quinolone with antipseudomonal activity or a macrolide. Ceftriaxone would not be adequate against *Pseudomonas*. The other 2 choices, cefepime alone and piperacillin-tazobactam alone, would also not be adequate according to the 2004 American Thoracic Society and the Infectious Diseases Society of America guideline.

46. Answer a.
Although blood cultures are helpful when positive, they are positive for less than 25% of patients with pneumonia. Pneumococcal pneumonia can be prevented by vaccination. Influenza vaccination can prevent both primary viral pneumonia and postviral bacterial pneumonia. An 8-day course of therapy is adequate for most pneumonia. The exception is *Pseudomonas* pneumonia. Respiratory fluoroquinolones and macrolides have good bioavailability and are good choices for oral antibiotic regimens for pneumonia.

47. Answer c.
Daptomycin is inactivated by pulmonary surfactant. Hence, it is not an appropriate choice for treatment of a pulmonary infection, even if the organisms targeted are susceptible to daptomycin. *Candida* is frequently isolated from respiratory specimens, but it is a very infrequent cause of pneumonia and a cause only in immunocompromised patients. It does not need to be treated in the majority of patients.

48. Answer b.
A 7- to 8-day course of antibiotics is adequate for the treatment of most uncomplicated pneumonias, including health care–associated pneumonia. The exception is patients with *Pseudomonas* pneumonia, for which a minimum of 2 weeks of antibiotic therapy is recommended. Shorter durations of therapy have been associated with treatment failure.

49. Answer c.
The yield of blood cultures from patients with cellulitis is low (2%-4%). The risk of recurrent cellulitis is at least 20%. Abscess is the most common skin syndrome caused by CA-MRSA. Owing to development of resistance to macrolides by some β-hemolytic streptococci, macrolides are no longer an appropriate choice of empirical therapy for cellulitis.

50. Answer d.
Gentamicin is not considered first-line therapy for necrotizing infections. A Baker cyst is not likely to manifest with necrotizing skin lesions. Monomicrobial infection due to β-hemolytic streptococci could account for this presentation. Disseminated histoplasmosis is not likely to cause an acute necrotizing presentation.

51. Answer e.
Because CA-MRSA is a common cause of skin abscess and this pathogen is resistant to cephalexin, amoxicillin, and cefadroxil, these drugs would not be appropriate treatment options. Ciprofloxacin does not have reliable activity against gram-positive cocci, including CA-MRSA. If an antibiotic is chosen for use, then trimethoprim-sulfamethoxazole would be desired.

52. Answer c.
The subacute presentation of lymphadenitis would not be characteristically due to *S pyogenes, P aeruginosa, V vulnificus*, or varicella-zoster virus. *Mycobacterium marinum* is the most likely cause from the presentation and epidemiology.

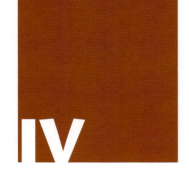

Special Hosts and Situations

36

Zelalem Temesgen, MD

Human Immunodeficiency Virus Infection[a]

I. Human Immunodeficiency Virus
   A. Classification
      1. Human immunodeficiency virus (HIV) is a lentivirus, a member of the Retroviridae family (retroviruses)
         a. The Retroviridae family is a large group of ubiquitous viruses that infect all classes of vertebrates
         b. Retroviruses share several characteristics
            1) A unique viral-encoded enzyme: reverse transcriptase
            2) Reverse flow of genetic information from RNA to DNA
            3) Integration of the reverse-transcribed viral complementary DNA (cDNA) into the genome of the host cell
            4) The integrated viral cDNA (the proviral DNA) serves as the template for viral replication
         c. Retroviruses are classified into 7 genera on the basis of similarities in amino acid sequences in the reverse transcriptase proteins
            1) Alpha (eg, avian leukosis virus)
            2) Beta (eg, mouse mammary tumor virus)
            3) Gamma (eg, feline leukemia virus)
            4) Delta (eg, human T-lymphotropic virus [HTLV]-1 and HTLV-2)
            5) Epsilon (eg, reticuloendotheliosis virus)
            6) *Lentivirus* (eg, HIV-1 and HIV-2)
            7) *Spumavirus* (eg, human foamy virus)
         d. Retroviruses are also classified as simple and complex
            1) Complex retroviruses (including HIV, *Spumavirus*, and HTLV) contain several regulatory genes in addition to 3 main structural genes (*gag*, *pol*, and *env*)
      2. There are 2 genetically distinct types of HIV: HIV-1 and HIV-2
         a. HIV-1
            1) Further classified into subtypes, also known as clades
               a) Group M (main): clades A through K
               b) Group O (outlier): primarily present in Cameroon

---

[a] Portions of the text have been adapted from Warnke D, Barreto J, Temesgen Z. Antiretroviral drugs. J Clin Pharmacol. 2007 Dec;47(12):1570-9. Used with permission.

c) Group N (non-M, non-O): very rare
2) In the United States, 98% of HIV is HIV-1 clade B
3) HIV-1 is the predominant HIV type globally
4) Donated blood has been screened for HIV-1 since 1985 in the United States

b. HIV-2
1) Amino acid homology with HIV-1: 40% to 60%
2) Epidemic subtypes (A and B) and nonepidemic subtypes (C through G)
3) Mode of transmission: same as for HIV-1
4) Clinical picture: same as for HIV-1
5) Transmission: less efficient than for HIV-1
6) Viral load: lower than for HIV-1
7) Rate of progression: slower than for HIV-1
8) Prevalent in West Africa but has been identified elsewhere (eg, India)
9) Donated blood has been screened for HIV-2 since 1992 in the United States

B. Origin
1. HIV is believed to have originated in the first half of the 20th century as a result of independent cross-species transmission events
2. HIV-1 is closely related to simian immunodeficiency virus (SIV) strains that infect central African chimpanzees (*Pan troglodytes troglodytes*) (SIVcpzPTT strains)
3. HIV-2 is closely related to SIV from sooty mangabeys (SIVsm strains)

C. Structure
1. HIV envelope is a lipid bilayer that is acquired from the host cell plasma membrane as the virus buds through the cell membrane (Figure 36.1)

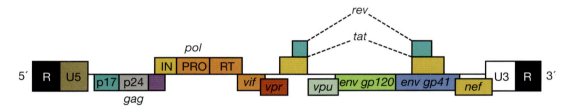

Virion-associated components

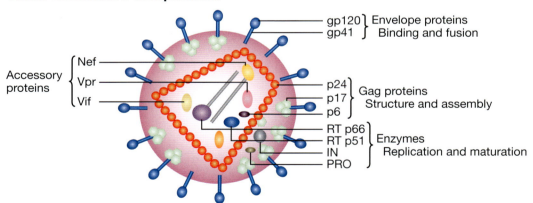

Cell-associated components
Rev Posttranscriptional processing
Tat Transcriptional activation
Vpu CD4 degradation, virion production

Figure 36.1. Genetic Organization of Human Immunodeficiency Virus Type 1. The virus is an enveloped retrovirus with a plus-stranded RNA genome that contains genes for proteins with structural, enzymatic, and regulatory functions. (From Maldarelli F. Diagnosis of human immunodeficiency virus infection. In: Mandell, Douglas, and Bennett's principles and practice of infectious diseases. Vol 1. 6th ed. Philadelphia [PA]: Elsevier/Churchill Livingstone; c2005. p. 1506-27. Used with permission.)

a. Two major proteins are associated with the HIV envelope: gp120 and gp41
b. In each envelope structure, the cap or knob is formed by gp120 molecules and the stalk is formed by the transmembrane gp41 anchored in the viral lipid bilayer
2. HIV genomic material is in the form of 2 identical single-strand RNA molecules that are contained within a nucleocapsid core
3. Core contains viral enzymes: reverse transcriptase, integrase, and protease
4. Core contains other proteins with structural and regulatory functions
D. Genome
1. Two functionally active single-stranded RNA molecules, each approximately 9 kilobases in length (Figure 36.2)
2. Three major retroviral genes: *gag*, *pol*, and *env*
3. Six auxiliary genes: *tat*, *rev*, *nef*, *vif*, *vpr*, and *vpu*
E. Life Cycle
1. HIV cell entry occurs in 3 stages (Figure 36.3)
a. Attachment
1) First step in HIV replication cycle: interaction between the envelope proteins of the virus and specific host-cell surface receptors (eg, CD4 receptor) of the host cell
2) However, binding to the CD4 receptor by itself is not sufficient for entry of the virus into the cell, and a coreceptor for entry into target cells is required

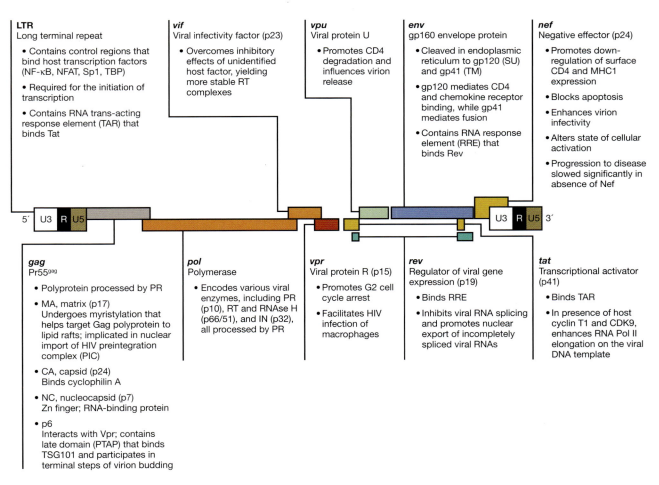

Figure 36.2. Human Immunodeficiency Virus (HIV) Proviral Genome and Gene Product Functions. An overview of the organization of the (approximately) 9-kilobase genome of the HIV provirus and a summary of the functions of its 9 genes encoding 15 proteins. MHC indicates major histocompatibility complex; PR, protease; RT, reverse transcriptase. (From Greene WC, Peterlin BM. Molecular insights into HIV biology. U.S. Department of Veterans Affairs. February 2003. [cited 2010 Nov 30]. Available from: http://hivinsite.ucsf.edu/InSite?page=kb-02091-01. Used with permission.)

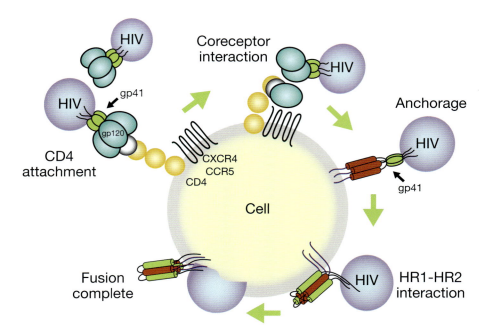

Figure 36.3. The 3 stages of human immunodeficiency virus (HIV) cell entry are attachment, coreceptor binding, and fusion. HR indicates heptad repeat. (From the World Wide Web [cited 2010 Nov 30]. Available from: http://www.roche.com/pages/facets/16/hiv_3_e.jpg.)

b. Coreceptor binding
  1) The chemokine receptors CXCR4 and CCR5 are the principal coreceptors for entry of HIV into its target cells
     a) *Chemokines* (short for *chemo*attractant cyto*kines*): a group of structurally related glycoproteins involved in activating the immune system's response to infection
     b) Chemokine receptors: a family of structurally related receptors that mediate the actions of chemokines
  2) Different HIV-1 isolates have distinct tropisms for various CD4+ human target cell types in vitro
     a) Some replicate only in transformed T-cell lines and in activated primary T cells (designated T-tropic)
     b) Other HIV-1 strains (designated M-tropic) replicate only in cells from the macrophage or monocyte lineage and in activated primary T cells
  3) Viral isolates from persons in the early stages of HIV infection are predominantly M-tropic
     a) Chemokine receptor CCR5 is the major coreceptor for M-tropic HIV-1 isolates
  4) T-tropic virus is more common at lower CD4 cell counts and higher viral loads
     a) Chemokine receptor CXCR4 is the major coreceptor for T-tropic strains
c. Fusion
  1) Binding of HIV to coreceptors causes conformational changes in the envelope proteins, ultimately resulting in the "fusion" of the viral envelope and the host cytoplasmic membrane
     a) Fusion creates a pore through which the viral capsid enters the cell
2. After cell entry, other steps occur (Figure 36.4)
  a. Reverse transcription: the viral reverse transcriptase enzyme catalyzes the conversion of viral RNA into DNA
  b. Integration
    1) The enzyme integrase catalyzes the process of entry of the viral DNA into the host cell nucleus and its integration into the host genome
    2) The integration of the viral DNA into the host chromosome occurs through a 3-step series of DNA cutting and joining reactions

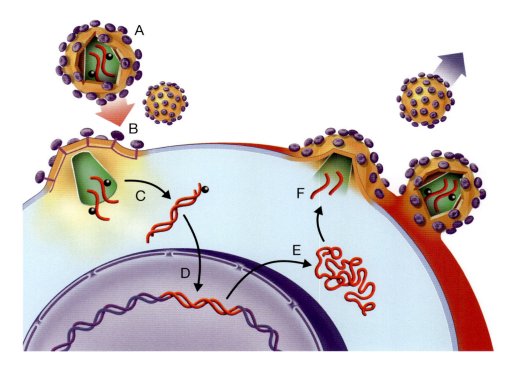

Figure 36.4. Life Cycle of Human Immunodeficiency Virus. A, The virus is an enveloped virus that contains viral genomic RNA and various Gag and Pol protein products. B, The interaction between the envelope proteins of the virus and CD4 receptor and other receptors of the host cell leads to the binding of the viral envelope and the host cytoplasmic membrane. C, The viral reverse transcriptase enzyme catalyzes the conversion of viral RNA into DNA. D, The viral DNA enters the nucleus and becomes inserted into the chromosomal DNA of the host cell. E, Expression of the viral genes leads to production of viral RNA and proteins. F, These viral proteins, as well as viral RNA, are assembled at the cell surface into new viral particles and leave the host cell by a process called budding. During the process of budding, they acquire the outer layer and envelope. At this stage, the protease enzyme cleaves the precursor Gag and Gag-Pol proteins into their mature products. (From Temesgen Z, Kasten MJ. HIV infection. In: Ghosh AK, editor. Mayo Clinic Internal Medicine Board Review. 9th ed. New York: Oxford University Press; c2010. p. 429-50. Used with permission of Mayo Foundation for Medical Education and Research.)

- a) First step: removal of 2 nucleotides from each 3′ end of the viral DNA (catalyzed by HIV-1 integrase)
- b) Second step (called DNA strand transfer): the processed viral DNA ends are inserted or joined into the host DNA (catalyzed by HIV-1 integrase)
- c) Third step: cellular enzymes repair the single gaps in the DNA chain by removing the 2 unpaired nucleotides at the 5′ ends of the viral DNA
- c. Assembly and budding
  1) Expression of the viral genes leads to production of precursor viral proteins
  2) The protease enzyme cleaves the precursor viral proteins into their mature products
  3) These proteins and viral RNA are assembled at the cell surface into new viral particles
  4) New viral particles leave the host cell by a process called budding, during which the virion acquires the outer layer and envelope
- F. Transmission
  1. Involved in HIV transmission
    a. Sexual contact: the most common mode of transmission
      1) Traumatic intercourse (eg, receptive anal intercourse) increases the risk of HIV transmission

2) Ulcerative genital infections increase the risk of HIV transmission
3) The proper use of condoms greatly reduces the risk of HIV transmission
  b. Perinatal infection
  c. Parenteral inoculation (intravenous drug injection, occupational exposure)
  d. Receipt of blood products
  e. Receipt of donated organs or semen
 2. Not involved in HIV transmission
  a. Kissing or hugging
  b. Having contact with saliva, tears, or sweat
  c. Receiving insect bites
  d. Sharing utensils
G. Immunopathogenesis
 1. Dendritic cells (bone marrow–derived progenitor cells)
  a. Migrate to regions of inflammation in mucous membranes
  b. Function as antigen-presenting cells
  c. Transport and present HIV to regional lymphoid tissue
 2. Systemic dissemination and viremia typically develop a few days after initial infection
 3. After viremia develops, HIV extensively seeds lymphoid organs and the central nervous system
H. Immune Deficiency Due to HIV
 1. Progressive depletion in the numbers of circulating $CD4^+$ T cells is the hallmark of HIV infection
 2. HIV-induced immune deficiency is broad and includes several features
  a. Diminished T-cell repertoire
  b. Reduced lymphocyte function
  c. Reduced delayed hypersensitivity response to recall antigens
  d. Reduced phagocytosis
  e. Reduced chemotaxis
  f. Reduced intracellular killing
  g. Reduced natural killer cell–mediated killing
  h. Loss of specific antibody responses
  i. Increased immune activation
  j. Disruption of immunoregulatory cytokine expression and production
   1) Decreased interleukin (IL)-2, interferon-γ, and IL-12
   2) Increased IL-1, IL-6, and tumor necrosis factor α (proinflammatory cytokines)
I. Natural History
 1. Typical course of HIV infection is shown in Figure 36.5

II. Acute and Chronic HIV Infection
 A. Acute HIV Infection
  1. Two to 4 weeks after acquiring HIV infection, at least half of infected persons present with a recognizable illness known as acute or primary HIV infection
  2. Most common presentation is mononucleosis-like syndrome
   a. Fever, sore throat, headache, swollen lymph nodes in the neck, liver or spleen enlargement, muscle and joint pain, and rash
   b. Onset is usually abrupt, and course is usually self-limiting with resolution over a period of weeks
  3. Other conditions that have been associated with acute HIV infection
   a. Ulcers involving the mouth and genitals
   b. Aseptic meningitis
   c. Guillain-Barré syndrome
   d. Encephalopathy
  4. Laboratory abnormalities are variable and nonspecific
   a. CD4 cell counts are reduced
   b. Atypical lymphocytes may be present (similar to what is observed with Epstein-Barr virus infection–associated mononucleosis)
   c. Total white blood cell count may be reduced
   d. Liver enzymes may be elevated
   e. Viral loads are typically very high (usually >100,000 copies/mL): acute HIV infection represents a period of high infectivity
  5. Diagnosis of acute HIV infection
   a. HIV antibody tests are often negative during HIV infection
    1) This is the "window period" after infection has occurred but before enough specific antibodies have developed to be detected by current tests (seroconversion)
    2) Therefore, diagnosis of acute HIV infection requires either antibody testing a few weeks later (allowing time for seroconversion) or the use of other methods, if available, for detecting HIV infection
     a) These methods include tests for detecting HIV RNA and tests for detecting the p24 antigen (an HIV protein that is detectable about 1-3 weeks after acquiring infection)

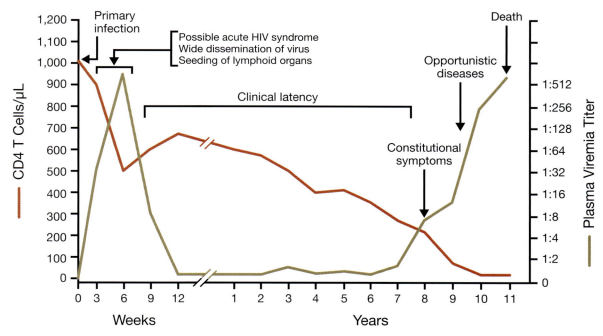

Figure 36.5. Typical Course of Human Immunodeficiency Virus (HIV) Infection. During the early period after primary infection, there is widespread dissemination of virus and a sharp decrease in the number of CD4 T cells in peripheral blood. An immune response to HIV ensues, with a decrease in detectable viremia followed by a prolonged period of clinical latency. The CD4 T-cell count continues to decrease during the following years, until it reaches a critical level below which there is a substantial risk of opportunistic diseases. (From Pantaleo G, Graziosi C, Fauci AS. New concepts in the immunopathogenesis of human immunodeficiency virus infection. N Engl J Med. 1993 Feb 4;328[5]:327-35. Used with permission.)

B. Chronic HIV Infection
1. Persons with HIV infection mount an immune response that consists of a humoral response (production of antibodies against HIV) and a cell-mediated response (CD4 and CD8)
2. However, this response cannot eliminate the virus from the body and resolve the infection
    a. Over a period of 6 to 12 months, the immune response reaches a steady state (also known as a set point) at which the HIV RNA level stabilizes and fluctuates around a certain value
    b. In most patients, the viral load increases and the CD4 cell count decreases over the subsequent years, with progression of immune deficiency and eventual development of opportunistic infections and conditions
        1) This progression of HIV disease is variable and may take 8 to 11 years for advanced immune deficiency to manifest clinically
    2) However, there are 2 small groups of HIV-infected persons in whom the disease progression is considerably slower in the absence of treatment
        a) *Long-term nonprogressors* have detectable viral loads but maintain adequate CD4 cell counts and remain asymptomatic
        b) *Elite controllers* have normal CD4 cell counts and undetectable viral loads and are asymptomatic
III. Diagnostic Testing for HIV Infection
    A. Antibody Detection
        1. Screening test: enzyme-linked immunosorbent assay (ELISA) is most commonly used
            a. Steps
                1) HIV antigen is attached to a well and reacts with HIV antibody, if present in the patient sample
                2) An antihuman immunoglobulin with a bound enzyme is added and binds the HIV antigen-antibody complex

3) Addition of more substrate leads to color development that is detected by a spectrophotometer
  b. Positive results require verification or confirmation with an additional test
    1) Screening test should be repeated in duplicate
    2) If repeatedly reactive, a confirmatory test should be performed
    3) ELISA has high sensitivity and specificity (>99.97%) but low predictive value in populations with low prevalence of HIV
  c. Causes of false-negative results
    1) Preseroconversion (window) period
    2) Replacement transfusions
    3) Bone marrow transplant
    4) Agammaglobulinemia
    5) Seroreversion in late-stage disease
    6) Unusual HIV subtypes (HIV-2, clade O or N)
    7) Atypical immune response
    8) Technical or laboratory error
  d. Causes of false-positive results
    1) Cross-reacting antibodies
      a) Multiparous women
      b) Multiple transfusions
    2) HIV vaccine recipients
    3) Technical or laboratory error
2. Confirmatory test: Western blot is most commonly used
  a. Steps
    1) Electrophoresis separates purified HIV antigens onto a polyacrylamide gel slab according to their molecular weights
    2) Proteins on the gel are transferred to nitrocellulose paper, which is cut into a test strip
    3) Test strip is incubated with a patient's test sample
    4) If HIV antibody is present in the patient's sample, a reaction (antigen-antibody complex) occurs, which manifests itself as a colored band (Figure 36.6)
  b. Positive result requires reactivity to 2 of the following major HIV antigens: p24, gp41, and gp120/160
  c. Negative result: absence of all bands
  d. Indeterminate result: reactivity to 1 or more antigens but not fulfilling the criterion for positivity
    1) If indeterminate, repeat in 4 to 6 weeks and at 6 months
    2) If still indeterminate, patient is considered HIV negative
    3) Molecular tests are not approved by the US Food and Drug Administration (FDA) for diagnostic purposes and are not generally recommended for resolving indeterminate Western blot results
  B. Rapid HIV Testing
    1. Sensitivities and specificities are comparable to those of ELISA
    2. No need for sophisticated laboratory equipment and highly trained technicians
    3. Clinical Laboratory Improvement Amendments (CLIA) are waived
    4. Point-of-care HIV testing is feasible (in emergency departments, sexually transmitted disease clinics, physician offices, etc)
    5. Sample used: oral fluid, finger stick, or whole blood
    6. Results available in minutes
    7. Still need confirmatory testing
IV. Treatment
  A. Antiretroviral Drugs
    1. There are 22 FDA-approved antiretroviral drugs
    2. Classified into 6 categories on the basis of their mechanism of action (Box 36.1)
      a. Nucleoside/nucleotide analogue reverse transcriptase inhibitor (NRTI)
      b. Nonnucleoside reverse transcriptase inhibitor (NNRTI)
      c. Protease inhibitor (PI)
      d. Fusion inhibitor
      e. Chemokine receptor CCR5 antagonist
      f. Integrase inhibitor
    3. Nucleoside/nucleotide analogue reverse transcriptase inhibitors
      a. The word *analogue* is used because NRTIs are structurally similar to the building blocks of nucleic acids (RNA, DNA)
      b. NRTIs block reverse transcriptase activity by competing with the natural substrates and incorporating into viral DNA to act as chain terminators in the synthesis of proviral DNA
      c. To exert their antiviral activity, NRTIs must first be intracellularly phosphorylated to their active 5′-triphosphate forms by cellular kinases
      d. Tenofovir
        1) The only currently available nucleotide analogue
        2) Already contains a phosphate molecule in its structure

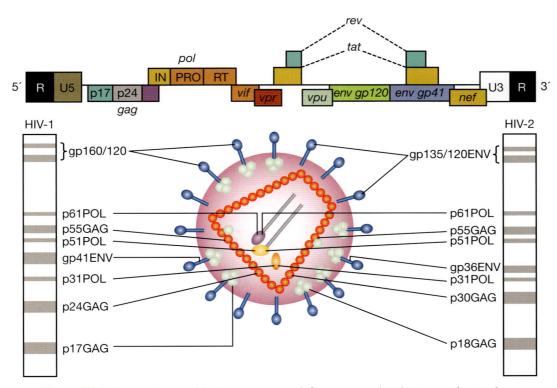

Figure 36.6. Proteins Detected by Human Immunodeficiency Virus (HIV) Western Blot. Viral lysates are disrupted and subjected to sodium dodecyl sulfate–polyacrylamide gel electrophoresis (SDS-PAGE), and proteins are separated according to molecular size. Positions of viral proteins in typical Western blot strips for HIV-1 and HIV-2 are indicated. The location of each protein in the virion is indicated and the position of the genes encoding relevant proteins is color-coded in the HIV-genome map. (From Maldarelli F. Diagnosis of human immunodeficiency virus infection. In: Mandell, Douglas, and Bennett's principles and practice of infectious diseases. Vol 1. 6th ed. Philadelphia [PA]: Elsevier/Churchill Livingstone; c2005. p. 1506-27. Used with permission.)

3) Thus, it requires phosphorylation by cellular enzymes only to its diphosphate form to exert antiviral activity
e. General characteristics of currently available nucleoside analogue reverse transcriptase inhibitors are shown in Table 36.1
f. Two important NRTI-associated adverse events
1) Hyperlactatemia
a) Hyperlactatemia results from abnormal mitochondrial toxicity caused by NRTIs that inhibit the enzyme mitochondrial DNA polymerase γ
b) This inhibition results in decreased energy production and increased levels of lactic acid
i) Incidence of asymptomatic or mildly symptomatic lactic acidemia is 8% to 21% of patients receiving at least 1 NRTI
ii) Lactic acidemia with significant symptoms occurs less frequently, with an estimated incidence of 1.5% to 2.5% among persons taking NRTIs
c) Onset of hyperlactatemia is typically months to years after starting antiretroviral therapy (ART) that includes NRTI
d) Most common symptoms: nausea, vomiting, abdominal pain, weight loss, fatigue, myalgias, tender hepatomegaly, peripheral edema, ascites, and encephalopathy
i) Later symptoms may include dyspnea and cardiac dysrhythmias
ii) Some patients may also have signs or symptoms of other mitochondrial toxicities, such

> **Box 36.1**
> **FDA-Approved Antiretroviral Drugs**
> NRTIs
>   Zidovudine
>   Didanosine
>   Stavudine
>   Lamivudine
>   Abacavir
>   Tenofovir
>   Emtricitabine
> NNRTIs
>   Nevirapine
>   Delavirdine
>   Efavirenz
>   Etravirine
> Protease inhibitors
>   Saquinavir
>   Indinavir
>   Ritonavir
>   Nelfinavir
>   Lopinavir-ritonavir
>   Fosamprenavir
>   Atazanavir
>   Tipranavir
>   Darunavir
> Fusion inhibitor
>   Enfuvirtide
> Chemokine receptor CCR5 antagonist
>   Maraviroc
> Integrase inhibitor
>   Raltegravir
>
> Abbreviations: FDA, US Food and Drug Administration; NNRTI, nonnucleoside reverse transcriptase inhibitor; NRTI, nucleoside/nucleotide analogue reverse transcriptase inhibitor.

        as peripheral neuropathy and lipoatrophy
- e) Risks associated with agents
  - i) Stavudine and didanosine are the most likely NRTIs to cause this complication, especially if used together
  - ii) Zidovudine poses some risk but significantly less than either stavudine or didanosine
  - iii) Tenofovir, abacavir, emtricitabine, and lamivudine appear to pose the least risk
- f) In addition to the use of NRTIs, there are other risk factors for hyperlactatemia
  - i) Pregnancy
  - ii) Female gender
  - iii) Obesity
  - iv) Decreased creatinine clearance
  - v) Concurrent treatment with ribavirin, hydroxyurea, or metformin
- g) Other causes of elevated lactate levels besides NRTIs
  - i) Inappropriate sample collection or processing
  - ii) Dehydration
  - iii) Vigorous exercise
  - iv) Alcohol intoxication
  - v) Sepsis
  - vi) Renal failure
  - vii) Pancreatitis
  - viii) Hyperthyroidism
  - ix) Toxicity from medications other than antiretrovirals
- h) Treatment of hyperlactatemia
  - i) Treatment is primarily supportive: hydration, replacement of electrolytes as needed, and discontinued use of the causative drug
  - ii) Indications for discontinuing use of the entire antiretroviral regimen immediately
    - (a) Serum lactate level greater than 10 mmol/L (90 mg/dL), regardless of clinical symptoms
    - (b) Serum lactate level 5 to 10 mmol/L (45-90 mg/dL) in conjunction with significant clinical symptoms
  - iii) Otherwise, another antiretroviral agent should be substituted for the causative drug
    - (a) Clinical signs, symptoms, and serum lactate levels should be monitored
    - (b) It may take more than 3 months for lactate levels to return to normal
2) Abacavir hypersensitivity
  - a) Abacavir hypersensitivity reaction is a systemic illness that occurs in approximately 5% to 8% of HIV-infected patients receiving treatment with abacavir
  - b) It is manifested by signs or symptoms from at least 2 of these groups
    - i) Fever
    - ii) Rash
    - iii) Constitutional: fatigue, myalgias, and generalized malaise
    - iv) Gastrointestinal tract
    - v) Respiratory: dyspnea, cough, and sore throat

Table 36.1
General Characteristics of Nucleoside Analogue Reverse Transcriptase Inhibitors

Drug Name (Alias)	Dosing and Adjustments	Metabolism	Toxic or Adverse Effects
Abacavir (ABC)	300 mg twice daily or 600 mg once daily No food effect No adjustment needed for renal insufficiency Dose adjustment for hepatic impairment required	Hepatic by alcohol dehydrogenase and glucuronyl transferase	Diarrhea, anorexia, nausea, vomiting, headache, fatigue, hypersensitivity reaction
Didanosine (ddI)	Body weight ≥60 kg: 400 mg once daily Body weight <60 kg: 250 mg once daily Take 0.5 h before or 2 h after a meal Dose adjustment for renal insufficiency required	Unknown	Rash, abdominal pain, diarrhea, nausea, vomiting, asthenia, headache, fever, pancreatitis, peripheral neuropathy
Emtricitabine (FTC)	200-mg capsule once daily or 240 mg (24 mL) oral solution once daily Take without regard to meals Dose adjustment for renal insufficiency required	Limited: oxidation and conjugation	Hyperpigmentation of skin, rash, diarrhea, nausea, vomiting, headache
Lamivudine (3TC)	150 mg twice daily or 300 mg once daily Take without regard to meals Dose adjustment for renal insufficiency required	5.6% to transsulfoxide metabolite	Decrease in appetite, nausea, vomiting, headache, fatigue, pancreatitis in children
Stavudine (d4T)	Body weight ≥60 kg: 40 mg twice daily Body weight <60 kg: 30 mg twice daily Take without regard to meals Dose adjustment for renal insufficiency required	Intracellular phosphorylation to active metabolite	Rash, diarrhea, nausea, vomiting, headache, lipoatrophy, hyperlipidemia, peripheral neuropathy, muscle weakness
Tenofovir (TDF)	300 mg once daily Take without regard to meals Dose adjustment for renal insufficiency required	Intracellular hydrolysis	Diarrhea, flatulence, nausea, vomiting, osteopenia, renal impairment
Zidovudine (ZDV)	300 mg twice daily or 200 mg 3 times daily Take without regard to meals Dose adjustment for renal insufficiency required	Hepatic glucuronidation	Headache, nausea, anorexia, vomiting, anemia, leukopenia, myopathy, lipoatrophy, hyperlipidemia

Adapted from Panel on Antiretroviral Guidelines for Adults and Adolescents. Guidelines for the use of antiretroviral agents in HIV-1-infected adults and adolescents. Department of Health and Human Services. December 1, 2009; 1-161. [cited 2010 Nov 29]. Available from: http://www.aidsinfo.nih.gov/ContentFiles/AdultandAdolescentGL.pdf.

    c) Symptoms become evident within hours of taking abacavir and progressively worsen with each subsequent dose

    d) If present, laboratory abnormalities are nonspecific and may include leukopenia, anemia, thrombocytopenia, and elevations in transaminases, creatinine, and lactate dehydrogenase

    e) Symptoms usually resolve promptly with discontinued use of abacavir

    f) However, immediate, severe, life-threatening reactions (including hypotension, renal failure, and bronchoconstriction) have been noted when patients with prior abacavir hypersensitivity were rechallenged

    g) Abacavir hypersensitivity has been associated with the genetic marker HLA-B*5701: screening for HLBA-B*5701 should be performed before any patient begins receiving an abacavir-containing regimen

g. NRTIs and drug interactions
    1) Because NRTIs are neither substrates nor inducers or inhibitors of the cytochrome p450 (CYP450) system, interactions with other drugs do not pose significant problems
    2) Among NRTIs, the buffered formulation of didanosine has the most significant drug interactions
    3) Notable NRTI-related drug interactions
        a) Magnesium and calcium contained in the buffered tablet formulation of didanosine may bind quinolones and tetracyclines, thereby reducing their absorption
        b) The buffered tablet formulation of didanosine also affects the absorption of atazanovir, which

requires an acidic environment for optimal absorption
- c) Plasma levels of didanosine are significantly reduced when administered with tenofovir
  - i) The mechanism of this interaction is thought to be through tenofovir's inhibition of purine nucleoside phosphorylase (PNP), an enzyme that normally metabolizes cellular inosine monophosphate (IMP)
  - ii) Increased rates of pancreatitis and peripheral neuropathy have been observed with the coadministration of tenofovir and didanosine
  - iii) Coadministration should be avoided or the dose of didanosine reduced
- d) Ribavirin increases the intracellular concentration of didanosine
  - i) Fatal liver failure and other didanosine-related side effects have been reported with coadministration of ribavirin and didanosine
  - ii) Therefore, the concomitant use of ribavirin and didanosine is contraindicated
- e) Ribavirin inhibits phosphorylation of zidovudine, potentially increasing the likelihood of zidovudine-related side effects: avoid coadministration or closely monitor for side effects

4. Nonnucleoside reverse transcriptase inhibitors
   a. Bind directly and noncompetitively to a site on the enzyme reverse transcriptase that is distinct from the substrate (deoxynucleoside triphosphate) binding site
   b. Block DNA polymerase activity by causing a conformational change and disrupting the catalytic site of the enzyme
   c. Do not require phosphorylation to become active
   d. Have no activity against HIV-2
   e. Important drug interaction issues
      1) Nevirapine and efavirenz are inducers of the hepatic CYP450 system
      2) Delavirdine inhibits CYP450
   f. General characteristics of currently available NNRTIs are shown in Table 36.2
   g. Important adverse events associated with the use of NNRTIs
      1) Nevirapine-related hepatotoxicity
         a) An asymptomatic increase in hepatic transaminase levels develops in about 5% to 15% of patients taking nevirapine

Table 36.2

General Characteristics of Nonnucleoside Reverse Transcriptase Inhibitors

Drug Name (Alias)	Dosing and Adjustments	Metabolism	Toxic or Adverse Effects
Delavirdine (DLV)	400 mg 3 times daily Take without regard to meals No adjustment for renal insufficiency	CYP substrate CYP3A4 inhibitor	Rash, hepatotoxicity, headache
Efavirenz (EFV)	600 mg once daily at or before bedtime Take on an empty stomach to reduce side effects No adjustment for renal insufficiency	CYP, CYP3A4, and CYP2B6 substrate Mixed CYP3A4 inducer or inhibitor	Rash, central nervous system symptoms (dizziness, light-headedness, abnormal dreams, difficulty with concentration), hepatotoxicity
Etravirine (ETR)	200 mg twice daily Take after a meal No adjustment for renal insufficiency	CYP3A4, CYP2C9, and CYP2C19 substrate CYP3A4 inducer CYP2C9 and CYP2C19 inhibitor	Rash, hypersensitivity reaction
Nevirapine (NVP)	200 mg once daily for 14 d (lead-in period); thereafter, 200 mg twice daily Take without regard to meals No adjustment for renal insufficiency	CYP3A4 substrate CYP3A4 inducer	Rash, hepatotoxicity, including symptomatic hepatitis and fatal hepatic necrosis

Abbreviation: CYP, cytochrome P450.

Adapted from Panel on Antiretroviral Guidelines for Adults and Adolescents. Guidelines for the use of antiretroviral agents in HIV-1-infected adults and adolescents. Department of Health and Human Services. December 1, 2009; 1-161. [cited 2010 Nov 29]. Available from: http://www.aidsinfo.nih.gov/ContentFiles/AdultandAdolescentGL.pdf.

b) Symptomatic hepatitis is noted in approximately 4%
c) Risk factors for hepatotoxicity while receiving nevirapine
   i) Female gender: particularly pregnant women
   ii) CD4 cell count greater than 250/μL in females before use of nevirapine
   iii) CD4 cell count greater than 400/μL in males before use of nevirapine
   iv) Abnormal baseline hepatic transaminase levels
   v) Concomitant liver disease
      (a) Chronic hepatitis B
      (b) Chronic hepatitis C
      (c) Alcoholic liver disease
d) Generally, symptoms develop within 18 weeks after starting the use of nevirapine
e) Symptoms include fever, myalgia, fatigue, malaise, nausea and vomiting, and skin rash
f) Management considerations
   i) Do not use nevirapine in patients with severe liver disease
   ii) Use nevirapine with caution in patients with mild to moderate hepatic impairment
   iii) Nevirapine treatment should be initiated with a dosage of 200 mg once daily for 14 days (lead-in period), followed by an increase to the full dosage of 200 mg twice daily
   iv) If rash develops during the lead-in period, the dosage should not be increased until the rash has resolved
   v) Monitor transaminase levels closely during the first 18 weeks and every 3 months thereafter
   vi) If treatment is interrupted for more than 7 days, resumption of nevirapine therapy should include a 14-day lead-in period
   vii) If nevirapine-associated hepatotoxicity develops, the patient should not receive nevirapine in the future

2) Nevirapine-associated rash
   a) Rash is the most frequent nevirapine-associated adverse event
   b) Reported in up to 35% of people receiving nevirapine
   c) Rash most commonly occurs in the first 6 weeks of exposure to nevirapine
   d) Rash is generally mild and self-limited, but grade 3 or 4 rash, including Stevens-Johnson syndrome, can occur in a significant minority of patients
   e) Predisposing factors or the mechanism of nevirapine-related rash remains to be determined
   f) Management of nevirapine-related rash depends on the extent and severity of the rash
      i) If the rash is mild to moderate, nevirapine therapy can be continued without interruption
      ii) If the toxicity occurred during the lead-in period, the full dosage should not be administered until the rash has resolved
      iii) If the rash is associated with systemic or constitutional signs and symptoms (eg, fever, malaise, myalgia, arthralgia, blistering, facial swelling, oral lesions), nevirapine therapy should be immediately discontinued and nevirapine should never be reintroduced
      iv) If the rash is severe, including Stevens-Johnson syndrome, nevirapine therapy should be immediately discontinued and nevirapine should never be reintroduced

3) Efavirenz-associated neuropsychiatric adverse events
   a) Efavirenz use is commonly associated with central nervous system adverse events, which have been reported in approximately half of patients receiving efavirenz in clinical trials
      i) These adverse events include dizziness, abnormal dreams, insomnia, somnolence, and impaired concentration

ii) Symptoms usually begin soon after the first dose of efavirenz and usually resolve after the first 2 to 4 weeks of therapy
b) Psychiatric adverse events (eg, depression, suicidal ideation, paranoia, manic reactions) have also been reported with the use of efavirenz
i) Factors that have been associated with these psychiatric adverse events include history of injection drug use and history of psychiatric illness or treatment
4) Efavirenz and teratogenicity
a) Use of efavirenz has been associated with teratogenic effects
i) Significant abnormalities, such as anencephaly, microphthalmos, and anophthalmia, were observed in monkeys exposed to efavirenz during pregnancy
ii) Cases of central nervous system neural tube defects have been reported in human infants with first-trimester exposure to efavirenz
iii) Retrospective studies and review of the antiretroviral pregnancy registry do not indicate that there is a substantially increased risk of teratogenicity with the use of efavirenz
b) Until there is more conclusive evidence, current guidelines designate efavirenz as contraindicated during the first trimester of pregnancy
5) NNRTIs and drug interactions
a) Nevirapine, efavirenz, and etravirine are inducers of CYP450, but their interactions are not entirely identical
b) Select drug interactions of currently available NNRTIs are listed in Table 36.3
5. Protease inhibitors
a. PIs exert their antiviral effect by inhibiting the enzyme HIV-1 protease, an enzyme responsible for cleaving the large viral

Table 36.3
Select Drug Interactions of Currently Available Nonnucleoside Reverse Transcriptase Inhibitors

Drug	Contraindications	Interactions Requiring Dosage Modification
Efavirenz	Antihistamines (astemizole and terfenadine) Benzodiazepines (alprazolam, midazolam, and triazolam) Cisapride Ergot alkaloids Rifapentine St John's wort Voriconazole	Anticonvulsants (carbamazepine, phenobarbital, and phenytoin) Buprenorphine Ethinyl estradiol HMG-CoA reductase inhibitors (atorvastatin and simvastatin) Macrolides (clarithromycin) Methadone Protease inhibitors (amprenavir, atazanavir, indinavir, lopinavir-ritonavir, nelfinavir, ritonavir, and saquinavir) Rifampin and rifabutin Warfarin
Nevirapine	Ketoconazole Rifampin and rifapentine St John's wort	Anticonvulsants (carbamazepine, phenobarbital, and phenytoin) Buprenorphine Calcium channel blockers (diltiazem, nifedipine, verapamil) Clarithromycin Methadone Oral contraceptives (do not use as sole method of contraception) Protease inhibitors (amprenavir, atazanavir, indinavir, lopinavir-ritonavir, nelfinavir, ritonavir, and saquinavir) Rifabutin
Etravirine	Anticonvulsants (carbamazepine, phenobarbital, and phenytoin) Protease inhibitors (except ritonavir-boosted darunavir, lopinavir, and saquinavir) Rifampin and rifapentine St John's wort	Clarithromycin Cyclosporine, sirolimus, and tacrolimus Diazepam Digoxin Methadone Voriconazole, itraconazole, and posaconazole

precursor polypeptide chains into smaller, functional proteins, thus allowing maturation of the HIV virion
  b. Inhibition of HIV-1 protease results in the release of structurally disorganized and noninfectious viral particles
  c. All PIs are metabolized by CYP450 system, and they also affect this system
    1) Drug interactions are a major issue
    2) Ritonavir is the most potent inhibitor of CYP450
  3) All currently licensed PIs, with the exception of nelfinavir, are commonly prescribed with low-dose ritonavir
    a) So-called boosting
    b) Allows for a more favorable pharmacokinetic profile (higher serum concentration) and more convenient dosing regimens
  4) General characteristics of currently available PIs are listed in Table 36.4
  d. All PIs and drug interactions

Table 36.4
General Characteristics of Current Protease Inhibitors

Drug Name (Alias)	Dosing and Adjustments	Metabolism	Toxic or Adverse Effects
Atazanavir (ATZ)	ATZ 300 mg plus RTV 100 mg once daily. Take with food. No dose adjustment for renal insufficiency. Dose adjustment for hepatic impairment required	CYP3A4 substrate and inhibitor	Indirect hyperbilirubinemia; prolonged PR interval, including symptomatic first degree AV block; nephrolithiasis; hyperglycemia; fat maldistribution; possible increased bleeding episodes in patients with hemophilia
Darunavir (DRV)	Treatment-naive patients: DRV 800 mg plus RTV 100 mg once daily. Antiretroviral-experienced patients: DRV 600 mg plus RTV 100 mg twice daily. Take with food. No dose adjustment for renal insufficiency required	CYP3A4 substrate and inhibitor	Rash, hepatotoxicity, diarrhea, nausea, headache, hyperlipidemia, increased serum transaminase, hyperglycemia, fat maldistribution, possible increased bleeding episodes in patients with hemophilia
Fosamprenavir (FPV)	FPV 1,400 mg twice daily or FPV 1,400 mg plus RTV 100-200 mg once daily (not recommended for treatment-experienced patients). FPV 700 mg plus RTV 100 mg twice daily. Take without regard to meals. No dose adjustment for renal insufficiency required. Dose adjustment for hepatic impairment required	CYP3A4 substrate, inhibitor, and inducer	Rash, diarrhea, nausea, vomiting, headache, hyperlipidemia, increased serum transaminase, nephrolithiasis, hyperglycemia, fat maldistribution, possible increased bleeding episodes in patients with hemophilia
Indinavir (IDV)	IDV 800 mg plus RTV 100-200 mg twice daily. Take without regard to meals. No dose adjustment for renal insufficiency required. Dose adjustment for hepatic impairment required	CYP3A4 substrate and inhibitor	Nephrolithiasis, GI intolerance, nausea, indirect hyperbilirubinemia, hyperlipidemia, headache, asthenia, blurred vision, dizziness, rash, metallic taste, thrombocytopenia, alopecia, hemolytic anemia, hyperglycemia, fat maldistribution, possible increased bleeding episodes in patients with hemophilia
Lopinavir-ritonavir (LPV-RTV)	LPV-RTV 400 mg/100 mg twice daily or LPV-RTV 800 mg/200 mg once daily (once daily not recommended for treatment-experienced or pregnant women). Take without regard to meals. No dose adjustment for renal insufficiency required	CYP3A4 substrate and inhibitor	GI intolerance, nausea, vomiting, diarrhea, asthenia, hyperlipidemia (especially hypertriglyceridemia), increased serum transaminases, hyperglycemia, fat maldistribution, possible increased bleeding episodes in patients with hemophilia

(continued)

Table 36.4
(continued)

Drug Name (Alias)	Dosing and Adjustments	Metabolism	Toxic or Adverse Effects
Nelfinavir (NFV)	1,250 mg twice daily or 750 mg 3 times daily Take with food No dose adjustment for renal insufficiency required	CYP2C19 and CYP3A4 substrate and inhibitor Has an active metabolite	Diarrhea, hyperlipidemia, hyperglycemia, fat maldistribution, possible increased bleeding episodes in patients with hemophilia, increased serum transaminase
Ritonavir (RTV)	Current use only as a pharmacokinetic enhancer for other protease inhibitors: 100-400 mg daily in 1-2 divided doses Take with food No dose adjustment for renal insufficiency required	CYP3A4 and CYP2D6 substrate and inhibitor	GI intolerance, nausea, vomiting, diarrhea, paresthesias (circumoral and extremities), hyperlipidemia (especially hypertriglyceridemia), hepatitis, asthenia, taste perversion, hyperglycemia, fat maldistribution, possibly increased bleeding episodes in patients with hemophilia
Saquinavir (SQV)	SQV 1,000 mg plus RTV 100 mg twice daily Take within 2 h after a meal No dose adjustment for renal insufficiency required	CYP3A4 substrate and inhibitor	GI intolerance, nausea, diarrhea, headache, increased serum transaminase, hyperlipidemia, hyperglycemia, fat maldistribution, possibly increased bleeding episodes in patients with hemophilia
Tipranavir (TPV)	TPV 500 mg plus RTV 200 mg twice daily Take without regard to meals No dose adjustment for renal insufficiency required	CYP3A4 substrate and inducer (but when combined with RTV, the net effect is inhibition)	Hepatotoxicity (including clinical hepatitis), rash, intracranial hemorrhages, hyperlipidemia (especially hypertriglyceridemia), hyperglycemia, fat maldistribution, possibly increased bleeding episodes in patients with hemophilia

Abbreviations: AV, atrioventricular; CYP, cytochrome P450; GI, gastrointestinal tract.

Adapted from Panel on Antiretroviral Guidelines for Adults and Adolescents. Guidelines for the use of antiretroviral agents in HIV-1-infected adults and adolescents. Department of Health and Human Services. December 1, 2009; 1-161. [cited 2010 Nov 29]. Available from: http://www.aidsinfo.nih.gov/ContentFiles/AdultandAdolescentGL.pdf.

1) PIs are associated with significant drug interactions since they are metabolized by CYP450 and they also inhibit CYP450
   a) This characteristic of PIs is further modified by differences in the magnitude of inhibition and by differences in the isoenzymes affected by individual PIs
   b) Therefore, even though PIs share many similar drug interactions, differences between specific PIs may be clinically important
2) Additionally, some drug interactions are not based on interaction with CYP450
   a) For example, atazanavir levels, unlike those of other boosted PIs, are significantly reduced when coadministered with gastric acid–reducing agents (ie, proton pump inhibitors or H_2 receptor antagonists)
3) Box 36.2 and Table 36.5 summarize clinical considerations related to PIs and drug interactions
6. Fusion inhibitor
   a. Enfuvirtide (T-20)
      1) The only currently FDA-approved fusion inhibitor
      2) A linear 36–amino acid peptide homologous to a segment of the heptad repeat 2 (HR2) region of gp41
         a) Binds to the heptad repeat 1 (HR1) region of gp41
         b) Blocks the formation of the 6-helix bundle necessary for fusion of the virus and host cell membranes

> **Box 36.2**
> **Drugs That Should Not Be Coadministered With Any Protease Inhibitor**
>
> Antiarrhythmics (amiodarone, propafenone, bepridil, quinidine, and flecainide)
> Anticonvulsants (phenytoin, carbamazepine, and phenobarbital)
> Benzodiazepines (alprazolam, midazolam, and triazolam)
> Ergot alkaloids (eg, dihydroergotamine, ergotamine)
> Gastrointestinal tract motility agents
> Lipid-lowering drugs (simvastatin and lovastatin)
> Pimozide
> Rifampin
> St John's wort

Table 36.5
Select Drugs That Require Caution, Monitoring, or Dose Adjustment When Coadministered With Protease Inhibitors

Drug or Class	Comment
Antacids	Staggered administration by at least 1 h
Anticonvulsants	Monitor toxicity and serum concentration Do not use phenytoin with lopinavir-ritonavir or carbamazepine with indinavir
Antidepressants	Concentrations of tricyclic antidepressants are increased Monitor for toxicity May require dose adjustment
Antimycobacterials	Rifampin is contraindicated Rifabutin dose needs to be adjusted
Azole antifungals	Concentrations of ketoconazole, itraconazole, and voriconazole are increased Monitor for toxicity Dose adjustment may be necessary Voriconazole is contraindicated with high-dose ritonavir (>400 mg twice daily)
Calcium channel blockers	Require dose adjustment and monitoring
Erectile dysfunction agents	Serum levels of phosphodiesterase inhibitors are increased Lower doses and a greater dosing interval for erectile dysfunction agents is recommended
H_2 blockers	Staggered administration with atazanavir and perhaps with fosamprenavir and tipranavir-ritonavir
Lipid-lowering agents	Lovastatin and simvastatin are contraindicated Careful monitoring with atorvastatin
Methadone	Most protease inhibitors (except atazanavir and indinavir) reduce methadone levels Monitor for withdrawal
Oral contraceptives	Alternative method of contraception is recommended except with atazanavir or indinavir
Proton pump inhibitors	Avoid with atazanavir and indinavir
Warfarin	Induction and inhibition of warfarin metabolism have been noted Monitor international normalized ratio

3) Has no activity against HIV-2
4) Is administered as a subcutaneous injection twice daily
  b. Adverse events
    1) Injection site reactions: most common
    2) Bacterial pneumonia (both gram-positive and gram-negative bacteria)
    3) Systemic hypersensitivity reactions: rash, fever, nausea or vomiting, chills, rigors, hypotension, and elevated liver enzymes
  c. Enfuvirtide is indicated for ART when previous therapy has failed
  d. Optimal time to include enfuvirtide in a regimen
    1) When there are at least 2 drugs that retain antiviral activity
    2) When CD4 cell counts are greater than 100/μL
    3) When plasma HIV-1 RNA levels are less than 10,000 copies/mL
  e. No significant drug interactions are expected with enfuvirtide since it is not a substrate, inhibitor, or inducer of CYP450 enzymes
7. Chemokine receptor CCR5 antagonist
  a. Approximately 1% of whites have a homozygous deletion in the *CCR5* gene (CCR5Δ32)
    1) Lack CCR5 molecules on $CD4^+$ cell surface
    2) Relatively normal immune function
    3) Homozygous carriers of the Δ32 mutation are resistant to HIV-1 infection because the mutation prevents functional expression of the CCR5 chemokine receptor normally used by HIV-1 to enter $CD4^+$ T cells
  b. Approximately 10% to 15% of whites have a heterozygous deletion in the *CCR5* gene (CCR5Δ32)
    1) Fewer CCR5 molecules on $CD4^+$ cell surface
    2) Normal immune function
    3) Heterozygous carriers of the Δ32 mutation have reduced susceptibility to HIV infection and delayed onset of AIDS

c. Maraviroc
   1) The only agent that is FDA approved
   2) Current use: for treatment-experienced patients with detectable viral loads and multidrug-resistant virus
   3) Among treatment-experienced patients, approximately 50% to 60% have CCR5 virus
      a) Maraviroc binds to CCR5 and induces conformational changes that lead to inhibition of the binding of CCR5 to gp120
      b) This prevents CCR5-mediated virus cell fusion and subsequent cell entry of M-tropic HIV-1
      c) Maraviroc has no efficacy against T-tropic or dual-tropic virus—it is effective only in patients with CCR5 virus
      d) Therefore, coreceptor tropism assay is required before use of maraviroc
         i) Tropism assay should be done as close to treatment initiation as possible
         ii) In clinical trials, 8% of participants who had CCR5-tropic virus at screening were discovered to have dual-tropic virus 4 to 6 weeks later at baseline (treatment initiation) evaluation
   4) Maraviroc is a substrate for CYP450, but it does not inhibit or induce CYP450
   5) Oral bioavailability of maraviroc: 23% to 33%
   6) Excretion of maraviroc
      a) Fecal: approximately 76%
      b) Renal: approximately 20%, so no need for adjustment in renal failure
   7) Dosing of maraviroc
      a) Maraviroc neither inhibits nor induces CYP450, but it is a substrate for the CYP450 3A4 isozyme (CYP3A4) and therefore has significant drug interactions with drugs that are CYP3A4 inhibitors or inducers, so dosing reflects this
      b) When given concomitantly with tipranavir-ritonavir, nevirapine, an NRTI, or enfuvirtide: 300 mg orally twice daily
      c) When given concomitantly with PIs (except tipranavir-ritonavir) or delavirdine: 150 mg orally twice daily
      d) When given concomitantly with efavirenz, etravirine, or rifampin: 600 mg orally twice daily
      e) Taken with or without food
   8) Adverse events with maraviroc
      a) Most common: diarrhea, nausea, headache, and fatigue
      b) Cough, fever, and upper respiratory tract infection
      c) Rash
      d) Aspartate aminotransferase and alanine aminotransferase elevations
      e) Creatine kinase elevation
      f) Myalgia
      g) Abdominal pain
      h) Dizziness
      i) Orthostatic hypotension (at a dosage of 600 mg twice daily)
      j) Hepatotoxicity with allergic features (rash, eosinophilia, IgE)
      k) Increased risk of myocardial infarction
8. Integrase inhibitor
   a. Raltegravir: the only FDA-approved integrase inhibitor
      1) Inhibits the catalytic activity of HIV-1 integrase, thus inhibiting the insertion of HIV-1 DNA into the host cell genome
      2) Metabolized by uridine diphosphate glucuronosyltransferase–mediated glucuronidation
         a) The coadministration of raltegravir with rifampin reduces plasma concentrations of raltegravir
         b) Therefore, the dose of raltegravir should be increased to 800 mg twice daily during coadministration with rifampin
      3) Does not inhibit or induce CYP450 enzymes
      4) Is not a substrate for CYP450 enzymes
   b. Dosing of raltegravir
      1) Administer 400 mg orally twice daily
      2) May be administered without regard to food
   c. Adverse effects of raltegravir
      1) Diarrhea
      2) Headache
      3) Nausea
      4) Fever
      5) Creatine kinase elevation

B. Guidelines on the Use of ART for HIV Infection
1. The Panel on Antiretroviral Guidelines for Adults and Adolescents, convened by the US Department of Health and Human Services, has been formulating guidelines for the use of antiretroviral agents in HIV-1–infected adults and adolescents since the early days of highly active antiretroviral therapy (HAART)
2. There is a general consensus for treating patients with symptoms ascribed to HIV infection
3. Asymptomatic patients
   a. Recommendations of when to start ART are based on estimates of the risks of AIDS or death, as determined primarily by CD4 T-cell count
   b. Historically, several reasons have contributed to the decision to defer therapy for patients with early HIV disease
      1) Long-term drug toxicity
      2) Reduced quality of life
      3) Potential for drug resistance
      4) Potential limitation of future treatment options when virologic failure occurs
   c. However, currently available drugs and drug combinations are better tolerated, easier to adhere to, and more effective
   d. Furthermore, data from recent studies show survival benefits of starting ART in patients with higher CD4 cell counts
4. ART should be initiated in all patients who have a CD4 cell count less than 350/μL
   a. Strength of recommendation: A1, which means that the strength is strong (A) and that 1 or more randomized trials with clinical outcomes or validated laboratory end points have provided supporting evidence
5. ART is recommended for all patients with CD4 cell counts between 350 and 500/μL
   a. The panel was divided on the strength of this recommendation: 55% voted for a strong recommendation (A) and 45% voted for a moderate recommendation (B)
   b. The quality of the evidence to support this recommendation was II (ie, from nonrandomized trials or cohort studies)
6. ART for patients with CD4 cell counts greater than 500/μL
   a. The panel was evenly divided in its opinion: half favored starting ART at this stage of HIV disease, and half considered the evidence to date inconclusive and viewed initiation of ART at this stage as optional
7. As with previous recommendations, the presence of certain conditions should trigger initiation of ART regardless of the CD4 cell count
   a. Pregnancy
   b. HIV-associated nephropathy
   c. Hepatitis B virus (HBV) coinfection when treatment of HBV is indicated
8. A more rapid initiation of ART in asymptomatic patients may be considered in other situations
   a. Rapidly decreasing CD4 cell counts (eg, an annual decrease >100/μL)
   b. Higher viral loads (eg, >100,000 copies/mL)
9. Additional conditions in which early ART may confer benefit
   a. Cardiovascular disease
      1) Untreated HIV infection may be associated with an increased risk of cardiovascular disease
      2) Some studies have suggested an improvement in endothelial function after ART
      3) In contrast, some antiretroviral drugs have been associated with an increased risk of cardiovascular disease
   b. Non-AIDS malignancies
      1) Non-AIDS malignancy is more frequent in HIV-infected subjects than in matched controls without HIV infection
      2) Low CD4 cell counts have been associated with an increased risk of malignancy both for malignancies defined by AIDS and for those not defined by AIDS
      3) A protective effect of ART for AIDS-defining malignancies has been demonstrated in some studies
   c. Neurocognitive decline
      1) HIV infection has been associated with neurocognitive decline
      2) Higher CD4 cell counts have been associated with a lower risk of neurocognitive decline
      3) ART has been associated with a significant decline in the incidence of symptoms of neurocognitive decline and with improvement in the symptoms
   d. Age
      1) Older age has been associated with a less robust immunologic recovery

e. Prevention of HIV transmission
   1) The level of plasma viremia is directly proportional to the HIV transmission risk
   2) Lower plasma viremia is associated with a lower concentration of HIV in genital secretions
   3) The introduction of ART in serodiscordant heterosexual couples has resulted in a decreased rate of HIV transmission
10. Underlying principles in the decision-making process of when to start ART
    a. Patients should understand the benefits and risks of therapy
    b. Patients should understand the importance of adhering to the regimen
    c. Patients should be willing and able to commit to lifelong treatment
11. Testing for HIV drug resistance should be performed for all persons with HIV infection when they enter into care regardless of whether therapy will be initiated immediately
    a. Rate of primary HIV resistance ranges from 6% to 16% in the United States and Europe
    b. If therapy is deferred, testing should be repeated when ART is initiated
    c. A genotypic assay is usually adequate and generally preferred for antiretroviral-naive persons
C. Regimens for Initial ART: 3 Categories
   1. Preferred regimens
      a. Have optimal and durable virologic efficacy in randomized controlled trials
      b. Are easy to use
      c. Have favorable tolerability and toxicity profiles
      d. Current regimens categorized as preferred regimens for first-line ART
         1) Efavirenz plus tenofovir plus emtricitabine
         2) Ritonavir-boosted atazanavir plus tenofovir plus emtricitabine
         3) Ritonavir-boosted darunavir plus tenofovir plus emtricitabine
         4) Raltegravir plus tenofovir plus emtricitabine
   2. Alternative regimens
      a. Effective regimens
      b. Have potential disadvantages when compared with preferred regimens
      c. Current regimens categorized as alternative regimens
         1) Efavirenz plus abacavir plus lamivudine
         2) Efavirenz plus zidovudine plus lamivudine
         3) Nevirapine plus zidovudine plus lamivudine
         4) Ritonavir-boosted atazanavir plus abacavir plus lamivudine
         5) Ritonavir-boosted atazanavir plus zidovudine plus lamivudine
         6) Fosamprenavir (once or twice daily) plus abacavir plus lamivudine
         7) Fosamprenavir (once or twice daily) plus zidovudine plus lamivudine
         8) Fosamprenavir (once or twice daily) plus tenofovir plus emtricitabine
         9) Ritonavir-boosted lopinavir (once or twice daily) plus abacavir plus lamivudine
         10) Ritonavir-boosted lopinavir (once or twice daily) plus zidovudine plus lamivudine
         11) Ritonavir-boosted lopinavir (once or twice daily) plus tenofovir plus emtricitabine
         12) Saquinavir plus tenofovir plus emtricitabine
   3. Acceptable regimens
      a. Currently lack efficacy data from large clinical trials, or are less effective or more toxic than the preferred and alternative regimens
      b. Current regimens categorized as acceptable regimens
         1) Efavirenz plus didanosine plus lamivudine
         2) Efavirenz plus didanosine plus emtricitabine
         3) Unboosted atazanavir plus abacavir plus lamivudine
         4) Unboosted atazanavir plus zidovudine plus lamivudine
D. HIV Drug-Resistance Testing to Guide Therapy
   1. Two main types of commercial assays are available to assess antiretroviral drug resistance
      a. Genotypic assays
         1) Sequence the reverse transcriptase and protease genes
         2) Identify mutations known to confer decreased drug susceptibility
         3) Test results
            a) Interpretation is based on knowledge of the mutations

selected for by different antiretroviral drugs
      b) Results are usually available within 1 to 2 weeks
   b. Phenotypic assays
      1) Measure the concentration of antiretroviral drugs required to inhibit viral replication
      2) Method
         a) A laboratory clone of HIV is created
         b) This recombinant virus incorporates the patient's HIV-1 genes encoding the viral targets of antiretroviral drugs
         c) The recombinant virus is then cultured in the presence of increasing concentrations of antiretroviral drugs to determine the 50% inhibitory concentration (IC_{50}), which is the concentration required to inhibit replication by 50%
         d) A fold increase in IC_{50} (reported as *fold resistance*) is calculated as the ratio of the IC_{50} of HIV-1 derived from the patient and the IC_{50} of reference HIV-1 wild-type viruses
   c. Both genotypic and phenotypic resistance assays have several limitations (Box 36.3)

2. In clinical practice, the use of resistance assays is recommended for several circumstances
   a. To determine antiretroviral regimen for initial treatment
   b. To guide antiretroviral drug selection after virologic failure
   c. To optimize ART in pregnant women to prevent perinatal transmission
3. Genotypic resistance testing is the preferred resistance test in most situations, including when the first or second antiretroviral regimen fails
4. Patients who have considerable ART experience
   a. Resistance pattern may be complex and difficult to interpret
   b. Phenotypic testing may provide additional and complementary information to what is provided by genotypic testing

E. Postexposure Prophylaxis
   1. Occupational exposure to HIV
      a. Potentially infectious material
         1) Blood
         2) Tissue, cells, cultures, mediums, or solutions
         3) Semen
         4) Vaginal secretions
         5) Bloody body fluids
         6) Saliva in dental setting
         7) Other body fluids: cerebrospinal, synovial, pleural, pericardial, peritoneal, amniotic
      b. Material that is not considered infectious (unless contaminated with blood)
         1) Sweat
         2) Tears
         3) Urine
         4) Vomitus
         5) Nasal secretions
         6) Saliva
         7) Feces
      c. Factors that affect risk of transmission
         1) Type of exposure
         2) Type of body fluid
         3) Type of organism
         4) Volume of exposed fluid entering the body
         5) Concentration of virus in fluid
      d. Average risk of exposure
         1) HBV
            a) Positive for hepatitis B e antigen (HBeAg): 22.0% to 30.0%
            b) Negative for HBeAg: 1.0% to 6.0%

Box 36.3

Limitations of HIV Drug-Resistance Testing

Limitations of genotypic assays
  Require ≥500-1,000 copies/mL of HIV-1 RNA
  Inability to detect minority variants (<10%-20% of the circulating virus population)
  Results available in 1-2 wk
  Interpretation of results often requires expert opinion
  Interpretation of mutations in patients with complex treatment history may be difficult
Limitations of phenotypic assays
  Require ≥500-1,000 copies/mL of HIV-1 RNA
  Inability to detect minority variants (<10%-20% of the circulating virus population)
  Results available in ≥2-3 wk
  The fold increase in IC_{50} that is associated with drug failure is not always clear
  Less sensitive than genotypic assays in detecting mixtures of resistant and wild-type viruses
  More expensive than genotypic assays

Abbreviations: HIV, human immunodeficiency virus; IC_{50}, 50% inhibitory concentration.

2) Hepatitis C virus (HCV): 1.8%
3) HIV
   a) Needlestick: 0.3%
   b) Mucus: 0.09%
e. Factors associated with increased risk of transmission
   1) Visible contamination of device (eg, needle) with patient's blood
   2) Needle having been placed directly into vein or artery
   3) Hollow-bore (versus solid) needle
   4) Deep injury
   5) Advanced disease in the source patient
f. Postexposure management
   1) Wound management
      a) Clean wounds with soap and water
      b) Flush mucous membranes with water
      c) Do not use antiseptics, disinfectants, or bleach
   2) Assessment of infection risk
      a) Type of exposure
      b) Type of body substance
      c) Status of source person
      d) Baseline laboratory tests
         i) Exposed health care worker: antibody to hepatitis B surface antigen (anti-HBs), anti-HCV, anti-HIV
         ii) Index patient: hepatitis B surface antigen (HBsAg), anti-HCV, anti-HIV
   3) Type and severity of exposure
   4) Bloodborne infection status of source person
   5) Treatment (postexposure prophylaxis [PEP]) (Tables 36.6 and 36.7)
      a) Postexposure prophylaxis should be started as soon as possible and no later than 72 hours after exposure
      b) For most HIV exposures, a 4-week regimen of 2 antiretroviral drugs is recommended
      c) Addition of a third drug, usually a PI, is recommended for exposures with an increased risk of

Table 36.6
Recommended HIV Postexposure Prophylaxis (PEP) for Percutaneous Injuries

Exposure Type	Infection Status of Source				
	HIV-Positive, Class 1[a]	HIV-Positive, Class 2[a]	Source With Unknown HIV Status[b]	Unknown Source[c]	HIV-Negative
Less severe[d]	Recommend basic 2-drug PEP	Recommend expanded ≥3-drug PEP	Generally, no PEP warranted; however, consider basic 2-drug PEP[e] for source with HIV risk factors[f]	Generally, no PEP warranted; however, consider basic 2-drug PEP[e] in settings in which exposure to HIV-infected persons is likely	No PEP warranted
More severe[g]	Recommend expanded 3-drug PEP	Recommend expanded ≥3-drug PEP	Generally, no PEP warranted; however, consider basic 2-drug PEP[e] for source with HIV risk factors[f]	Generally, no PEP warranted; however, consider basic 2-drug PEP[e] in settings in which exposure to HIV-infected persons is likely	No PEP warranted

Abbreviation: HIV, human immunodeficiency virus.

[a] HIV-positive, class 1: asymptomatic HIV infection or known low viral load (eg, <1,500 RNA copies/mL). HIV-positive, class 2: symptomatic HIV infection, AIDS, acute seroconversion, or known high viral load. If drug resistance is a concern, obtain expert consultation. Initiation of PEP should not be delayed pending expert consultation, and, because expert consultation alone cannot substitute for face-to-face counseling, resources should be available to provide immediate evaluation and follow-up care for all exposures.
[b] For example, deceased source person with no samples available for HIV testing.
[c] For example, a needle from a sharps disposal container.
[d] For example, solid needle or superficial injury.
[e] The recommendation "consider PEP" indicates that PEP is optional; a decision to initiate PEP should be based on a discussion between the exposed person and the treating clinician about the risks and benefits of PEP.
[f] If PEP is offered and administered and the source is later determined to be HIV-negative, PEP should be discontinued.
[g] For example, large-bore hollow needle, deep puncture, visible blood on device, or needle used in patient's artery or vein.

Adapted from Centers for Disease Control and Prevention. Updated U.S. Public Health Service guidelines for the management of occupational exposures to HIV and recommendations for postexposure prophylaxis. MMWR. 2005;54(No. RR-9):1-17.

Table 36.7

Recommended HIV Postexposure Prophylaxis (PEP) for Mucous Membrane Exposures and Nonintact Skin[a] Exposures

Exposure Type	Infection Status of Source				
	HIV-Positive, Class 1[b]	HIV-Positive, Class 2[b]	Source With Unknown HIV Status[c]	Unknown Source[d]	HIV-Negative
Small volume[e]	Consider basic 2-drug PEP[f]	Recommend basic 2-drug PEP	Generally, no PEP warranted[g]	Generally, no PEP warranted	No PEP warranted
Large volume[h]	Recommend expanded 2-drug PEP	Recommend expanded ≥3-drug PEP	Generally, no PEP warranted; however, consider basic 2-drug PEP[f] for source with HIV risk factors[g]	Generally, no PEP warranted; however, consider basic 2-drug PEP[f] in settings in which exposure to HIV-infected persons is likely	No PEP warranted

[a] For skin exposures, follow-up is indicated only if evidence exists of compromised skin integrity (eg, dermatitis, abrasion, or open wound).
[b] HIV-positive, class 1: asymptomatic HIV infection or known low viral load (eg, <1,500 RNA copies/mL). HIV-positive, class 2: symptomatic HIV infection, AIDS, acute seroconversion, or known high viral load. If drug resistance is a concern, obtain expert consultation. Initiation of PEP should not be delayed pending expert consultation, and, because expert consultation alone cannot substitute for face-to-face counseling, resources should be available to provide immediate evaluation and follow-up care for all exposures.
[c] For example, deceased source person with no samples available for HIV testing.
[d] For example, splash from inappropriately disposed blood.
[e] For example, a few drops.
[f] The recommendation "consider PEP" indicates that PEP is optional; a decision to initiate PEP should be based on a discussion between the exposed person and the treating clinician about the risks and benefits of PEP.
[g] If PEP is offered and administered and the source is later determined to be HIV-negative, PEP should be discontinued.
[h] For example, a major blood splash.

Adapted from Centers for Disease Control and Prevention. Updated U.S. Public Health Service guidelines for the management of occupational exposures to HIV and recommendations for postexposure prophylaxis. MMWR. 2005;54(No. RR-9):1-17.

transmission or when resistance to 1 of the recommended drugs is known or suspected
  d) Selection of antiretrovirals for PEP
    i) Zidovudine in combination with either lamivudine or emtricitabine
    ii) Tenofovir in combination with either lamivudine or emtricitabine
    iii) Lopinavir-ritonavir: the preferred third agent for expanded PEP
  e) Antiretroviral agents generally *not* recommended for PEP
    i) Nevirapine
    ii) Delavirdine
    iii) Abacavir
    iv) Zalcitabine
    v) Didanosine plus stavudine
  6) Follow-up testing with HIV serology at 6 weeks, 12 weeks, and 6 months
2. Nonoccupational exposure to HIV
  a. Similar to the rationale for occupational PEP, the rationale for nonoccupational PEP (nPEP) is based on results of animal studies, perinatal clinical trials, and studies of health care workers receiving prophylaxis after occupational exposures
  b. Several observational studies have provided additional information that nPEP might reduce the risk of infection after sexual HIV exposures
  c. Assessment of transmission risk
    1) HIV status of the potentially exposed person: check baseline HIV serology
    2) Timing and frequency of exposure
      a) nPEP is less likely to be effective if initiated more than 72 hours after HIV exposure
      b) nPEP should be used only for infrequent exposures
    3) Type of exposure and its associated transmission risk (Table 36.8 and Figure 36.7)
    4) HIV serostatus of source person
  d. Recommended regimens for nPEP prophylaxis of HIV infection
    1) Efavirenz plus lamivudine plus zidovudine
    2) Efavirenz plus lamivudine plus tenofovir

Table 36.8

Estimated Risk of Acquiring Human Immunodeficiency Virus

Exposure Route	Risk per 10,000 Exposures
Blood transfusion	9,000
Needle-sharing injection drug use	67
Percutaneous needle stick	30
Penile-vaginal intercourse	
Receptive	10
Insertive	5
Anal intercourse	
Receptive	50
Insertive	6.5
Oral intercourse	
Receptive	1
Insertive	0.5

Adapted from Centers for Disease Control and Prevention. Antiretroviral postexposure prophylaxis after sexual, injection-drug use, or other nonoccupational exposure to HIV in the United States: recommendations from the U.S. Department of Health and Human Services. MMWR. 2005;54(No. RR-2):1–20.

      3) Efavirenz plus emtricitabine plus zidovudine
      4) Efavirenz plus emtricitabine plus tenofovir
      5) Lopinavir-ritonavir plus lamivudine plus zidovudine
      6) Lopinavir-ritonavir plus emtricitabine plus zidovudine
  F. Recommendations for Use of Antiretroviral Drugs in Pregnancy
    1. Risk of perinatal transmission of HIV
      a. In the United States, 16% to 25% (<2% with highly active ART)
      b. Breast-feeding contributes 5% to 20% to the risk of HIV transmission
      c. Factors that affect the risk of perinatal transmission of HIV
        1) Maternal HIV RNA level
        2) CD4 cell count
        3) Chorioamnionitis
        4) Concurrent sexually transmitted infections
        5) Illicit drug use
        6) Cigarette smoking
        7) Unprotected sex with multiple partners
        8) Duration of ruptured membranes
        9) Invasive procedures
          a) Amniocentesis
          b) Placement of scalp electrodes
    2. Clinical scenario 1: pregnant woman who is infected with HIV-1 and is not receiving ART
      a. Considerations for initiation and choice of ART: generally the same as for persons who are not pregnant
      b. Caveats
        1) Women who require immediate initiation of therapy for their own health
          a) Treatment should begin as soon as possible, including in the first trimester of pregnancy
          b) Avoid the use of efavirenz during the first trimester
        2) Women who are receiving antiretroviral drugs solely for prevention of perinatal transmission
          a) Delaying initiation of prophylaxis until after the first trimester of pregnancy can be considered
        3) Zidovudine should be used as a component of the antiretroviral regimen whenever feasible
        4) Avoid nevirapine if CD4 cell count is greater than 250/μL
    3. Clinical scenario 2: woman who is infected with HIV-1 and is already receiving ART
      a. Continue therapy as long as tolerated and effective
      b. If pregnancy is identified during first trimester
        1) Avoid efavirenz during first trimester
        2) HIV drug-resistance testing should be performed if viremia is detectable (eg, >500-1,000 copies/mL) during therapy
        3) If nevirapine is already a component of therapy and the patient is virologically suppressed and is tolerating her regimen, use of nevirapine can be continued regardless of CD4 cell count
        4) Regardless of the antepartum antiretroviral regimen, zidovudine should be given during the intrapartum period (during labor) to the mother and after birth to the newborn
    4. Clinical scenario 3: pregnant woman who is infected with HIV-1 and has previously received ART or prophylaxis but is not currently receiving either

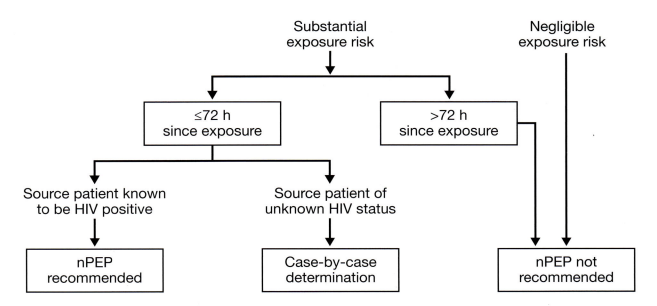

Figure 36.7. Algorithm for Evaluation and Treatment of Possible Nonoccupational HIV Exposures. HIV indicates human immunodeficiency virus; nPEP, nonoccupational postexposure prophylaxis. (From Centers for Disease Control and Prevention. Antiretroviral postexposure prophylaxis after sexual, injection-drug use, or other nonoccupational exposure to HIV in the United States: recommendations from the U.S. Department of Health and Human Services. MMWR. 2005;54[No. RR-2]:1-20.)

  a. Choose an effective regimen to prevent transmission to the newborn
  b. Obtain a comprehensive and accurate treatment history
  c. Perform HIV drug-resistance testing
  d. Initiate appropriate combination treatment, and avoid efavirenz in first trimester

5. Indications for cesarean delivery
  a. HIV-1 RNA levels that are more than 1,000 copies/mL near time of delivery
  b. HIV-infected woman presenting in late pregnancy near time of delivery with unknown HIV-1 RNA levels

Suggested Reading

Centers for Disease Control and Prevention. Antiretroviral postexposure prophylaxis after sexual, injection-drug use, or other nonoccupational exposure to HIV in the United States: recommendations from the U.S. Department of Health and Human Services. MMWR. 2005;54(No. RR-2):1–20.

Centers for Disease Control and Prevention. Updated U.S. Public Health Service guidelines for the management of occupational exposures to HIV and recommendations for postexposure prophylaxis. MMWR. 2005;54(No. RR-9): 1–17.

Panel on Antiretroviral Guidelines for Adults and Adolescents. Guidelines for the use of antiretroviral agents in HIV-1-infected adults and adolescents. Department of Health and Human Services. January 10, 2011; 1–174. [cited 2011 April 20]. Available from: http://aidsinfo.nih.gov/contentfiles/AdultandAdolescentGL.pdf.

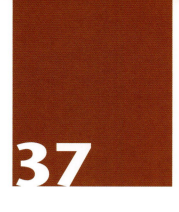

Anne M. Meehan, MB, BCh, PhD
Eric M. Poeschla, MD

HIV-Associated Opportunistic Infections and Conditions

I. Introduction
  A. Occurrence of Opportunistic Infections
    1. Early in the human immunodeficiency virus (HIV)/AIDS pandemic
      a. Opportunistic infections (OIs) accounted for most of the morbidity and mortality associated with HIV infection
      b. Introduction of effective primary and secondary antimicrobial prophylaxis regimens markedly decreased their incidence
    2. Later in the HIV/AIDS pandemic
      a. Advent of effective highly active antiretroviral therapy (HAART) further reduced OI mortality independently of antimicrobial prophylaxis
      b. HIV-associated OIs still occur
        1) When HIV is newly diagnosed
        2) When the course of care is in its early stages
        3) When HAART therapy fails
        4) When antimicrobial prophylaxis is stopped prematurely
  B. Immune Status
    1. Immune status of the patient is the critical factor in determining whether a specific OI occurs
      a. Tuberculosis, herpes zoster, bacterial pneumonia, and lymphoma can occur even at high CD4 cell counts (>200/μL)
      b. Pneumocystis pneumonia (PCP), esophageal candidiasis, and progressive multifocal leukoencephalopathy (PML) generally occur when CD4 cell counts are less than 200/μL
      c. Cerebral toxoplasmosis and miliary tuberculosis occur when CD4 cell counts are less than 100/μL
      d. Cryptococcosis, cytomegalovirus (CMV) retinitis, and atypical mycobacteriosis occur when CD4 cell counts are less than 50/μL
    2. Immune reconstitution with HAART
      a. May transiently worsen clinical manifestations of OIs: immune reconstitution syndromes
      b. So-called paradoxical reactions
        1) May necessitate administration of nonsteroidal anti-inflammatory drugs or corticosteroids to alleviate undue inflammation
        2) May be particularly troublesome in *Mycobacterium tuberculosis* infection, although it is unclear whether (and in

which patients) HAART should be delayed until an initial course of antituberculous treatment is completed
         c. Latent infections
            1) May also become clinically apparent at initiation of HAART
            2) Immune reconstitution inflammatory syndrome occurs in 5% to 10% of patients with a CD4 cell count less than 200/μL before antiretroviral treatment
      3. Sustained immune reconstitution
         a. CD4 cell count greater than 200/μL for more than 3 months
         b. Allows safe discontinuation of primary and secondary prophylaxis for PCP, cryptococcal meningitis, histoplasmosis, disseminated disease from *Mycobacterium avium-intracellulare* complex (MAC), cytomegalovirus retinitis (CD4 cell count >100/μL), and toxoplasma encephalitis
II. Pneumocystis Pneumonia
   A. Epidemiology
      1. Causative agent
         a. *Pneumocystis jiroveci*
         b. Previously classified as *Pneumocystis carinii*
         c. A ubiquitous fungus that infects most persons in early childhood
      2. PCP in immunocompromised hosts
         a. Generally from reactivation of latent organisms
         b. May also be from primary infections
      3. Typical predisposing factors
         a. CD4 cell count of 200/μL or less
         b. CD4 cells 15% or less
         c. Oral thrush
         d. Weight loss
         e. Recurrent bacterial pneumonia
         f. Higher viral load of HIV-1 RNA
      4. Characteristics of most PCP cases in the post-HAART era
         a. In persons who are unaware that they have HIV infection
         b. In persons not receiving medical care
         c. In patients who have advanced immunosuppression with CD4 cell counts less than 100/μL
   B. Clinical Manifestations
      1. Subacute onset
      2. Presentation: progressive dyspnea, fever, nonproductive cough, and chest discomfort
      3. Extrapulmonary disease may occur, especially with inhaled pentamidine prophylaxis
   C. Diagnosis
      1. Physical examination findings: usually nonspecific
         a. Fever
         b. Tachypnea
         c. Tachycardia
         d. Diffuse rales
      2. Arterial blood gas analyses: hypoxia with elevated alveolar-arterial gradient
      3. Lactate dehydrogenase level: an increase to more than 500 U/L is common but nonspecific
      4. Radiographic findings vary
         a. Chest radiograph: usually a butterfly-shaped pattern of diffuse, bilaterally symmetrical interstitial infiltrates appears to spread from the hilum
         b. Chest radiographic findings are normal in 10% to 25% of patients
         c. Pneumothoraces may occur
         d. Atypical chest radiograph findings: nodules, blebs, or asymmetrical disease
         e. Pleural effusion and cavitations are uncommon
            1) Should prompt consideration of an alternative diagnosis
            2) Cavitations can be a sequel to a severe episode
         f. High-resolution computed tomography (CT): characteristic ground-glass appearance
      5. Microbiologic findings
         a. Culture: *P jiroveci* cannot be routinely cultured
         b. Definitive diagnosis requires demonstration of the organism in specimen
            1) Induced sputum (60% sensitivity)
            2) Bronchoalveolar lavage fluid (90% sensitivity)
            3) Transbronchial biopsy
            4) Open lung biopsy
         c. Organisms remain detectable in clinical specimens for days or weeks after initiation of effective therapy
   D. Treatment
      1. Trimethoprim-sulfamethoxazole: treatment of choice (Table 37.1)
         a. Even when disease develops during prophylaxis with trimethoprim-sulfamethoxazole
         b. Dosing is based on the trimethoprim component and adjusted for renal function

Table 37.1

Drugs for Treating Pneumocystis Pneumonia

Drug	Dosage	Side Effects
TMP-SMX	5 mg/kg of TMP component every 8 h	Nausea, vomiting Rash
Pentamidine	4 mg/kg IV daily	Nephrotoxicity Abnormal glucose level Abnormal electrolyte levels Arrhythmias Pancreatitis
Clindamycin and	600 mg every 8 h	Diarrhea (*Clostridium difficile*)
Primaquine	15-30 mg daily	Hemolytic anemia (G6PD deficiency)
Dapsone and	100 mg daily	Hemolytic anemia (G6PD deficiency) Nausea, vomiting
TMP	5 mg/kg every 8 h	Rash
Atovaquone	750 mg every 8 h	Nausea, vomiting Rash
Trimetrexate and	45 mg/m² IV daily	
Leucovorin	20 mg/m² IV	
Prednisone	40 mg orally twice daily for 5 d (or when indicated: 40 mg daily for 5 d), then 20 mg daily for 11 d	

Abbreviations: G6PD, glucose-6-phosphate dehydrogenase; IV, intravenously; SMX, sulfamethoxazole; TMP, trimethoprim.

2. Adjunctive corticosteroids
   a. For patients with severe disease (defined by room air Po_2 <70 mm Hg or an alveolar-arterial gradient >35)
   b. Recommended duration of therapy: 21 days
3. Success of therapy is affected by several factors
   a. Medication used
   b. How many episodes have occurred
   c. Disease severity
   d. Extent of immunodeficiency
   e. When therapy is started
4. Mortality of up to 60% is associated with admission to intensive care unit and with use of mechanical ventilation
5. Clinical failure
   a. No improvement or decrease in respiratory function with therapy for 4 to 8 days
   b. Caused by drug-limiting toxicity or lack of drug efficacy
6. Second-line therapy
   a. Controversial
   b. Adding or switching to an alternative treatment regimen is appropriate
7. Early, reversible deterioration
   a. Typical in the first 3 to 5 days of treatment
   b. Caused by lysis of the organism in the lungs
8. For severe illness: intravenous (IV) pentamidine or clindamycin-primaquine is acceptable
9. For mild to moderate disease: atovaquone is sufficient
10. Secondary prophylaxis with trimethoprim-sulfamethoxazole or an alternative agent
    a. Should be lifelong or until immune reconstitution with HAART is sustained (ie, CD4 cell count >200/μL for 3 months)
    b. Prophylaxis should be promptly restarted if CD4 cell count decreases to less than 200/μL or if PCP recurs

III. Toxoplasma Encephalitis
   A. Epidemiology
      1. Causative agent: reactivation of latent tissue cysts of *Toxoplasma gondii*, an obligate intracellular protozoan

2. The most common cause of central nervous system (CNS) mass lesion in patients with AIDS
3. Environmental exposure (ingestion of water or food contaminated with oocysts) leads to lifelong human infection
4. Primary infection
   a. Rare
   b. Can lead to acute cerebral or disseminated disease
5. Seroprevalence
   a. In the United States: about 15%
   b. In European countries: 50% to 75%

B. Clinical Manifestations
   1. Clinical disease occurs with CD4 cell counts less than 100/μL
   2. Headache, focal neurologic signs, seizures, cranial nerve deficits, and sometimes fever

C. Diagnosis
   1. Physical examination findings: altered mental status, ataxia, tremor, and focal motor deficits may be apparent
   2. Anti-*Toxoplasma* antibodies: infected patients are almost universally (85%-90%) seropositive
   3. Absence of IgG makes the diagnosis unlikely
   4. Disseminated multifocal infection: affects the retina and lungs
   5. CT or magnetic resonance imaging of the brain: multiple ring-enhancing lesions with associated edema are usually noted
   6. Diagnostic criteria
      a. Compatible clinical syndrome
      b. One or more mass lesions on imaging studies
      c. Demonstration of the organism on tissue samples
         1) Requires brain biopsy
         2) Demonstration of organisms with hematoxylin-eosin or immunoperoxidase staining
   7. Polymerase chain reaction (PCR) detection of the organism in cerebrospinal fluid (CSF)
      a. Specific but insensitive
      b. Generally becomes negative after treatment has started
   8. Differential diagnosis of toxoplasma encephalitis (ie, CNS mass lesion in patient with AIDS)
      a. CNS lymphoma
      b. *Mycobacterium* infection
      c. Fungal infection
      d. Bacterial abscess
      e. Progressive multifocal leukoencephalopathy

D. Treatment
   1. Indications for empirical antitoxoplasmosis therapy
      a. Significant cellular immune deficiency due to HIV (CD4 cell count ≤100/μL)
      b. Positive toxoplasma serology
      c. Multiple ring-enhancing cranial lesions
   2. Empirical therapy allows deferral of biopsy in many cases, since treatment response is often reasonably prompt
   3. Therapeutic agents
      a. Initial preferred regimen
         1) Pyrimethamine 100 to 200 mg loading dose and then 50 to 100 mg daily for 6 weeks, *plus* leucovorin 10 to 20 mg daily and sulfadiazine 4 to 8 g daily
         2) Alternatives to sulfadiazine: clindamycin 600 mg daily, azithromycin 1,200 mg daily, or atovaquone 1,500 mg daily
      b. Pyrimethamine
         1) Penetrates brain parenchyma well (inflammation is not required)
         2) No parenteral formulation for pyrimethamine exists: if IV therapy is warranted, parenteral trimethoprim-sulfamethoxazole or IV clindamycin is indicated
         3) Therapy should be continued for 6 weeks (induction phase)
   4. Course of therapy
      a. If clinical improvement is not apparent in 14 days, the diagnosis is questionable and a brain biopsy is indicated
      b. Treatment should lead to a decrease in number, size, and contrast enhancement of lesions on imaging
      c. Lifelong suppressive therapy with lower-dose primary agents is warranted to prevent relapse
   5. Immune reconstitution with HAART
      a. Indications for discontinuation of secondary prophylaxis
         1) Patient has successfully completed initial therapy
         2) Patient remains asymptomatic and has a sustained increase in CD4 cell count to more than 200/μL for 6 months
      b. Follow-up brain imaging should be considered before therapy is stopped
      c. Decreased CD4 cell count
         1) If less than 200/μL: indication to restart prophylaxis
         2) If less than 100/μL with positive *Toxoplasma* serology: primary

prophylaxis is indicated (preferably with trimethoprim-sulfamethoxazole)
IV. Cryptococcosis
  A. Epidemiology
    1. Causative agent: *Cryptococcus neoformans*
      a. Ubiquitous round oval yeast
      b. Acquired by inhalation of yeast forms from the environment
    2. Disease occurs primarily in patients with CD4 cell counts less than 100/μL
  B. Clinical Manifestations
    1. Disease usually occurs as meningoencephalitis in patients with AIDS
    2. CNS involvement should be suspected and ruled out in the case of a nonneurologic presentation of cryptococcal disease
    3. Disease can also occur in lung (eg, cryptococcomas, cryptococcal pneumonia), skin, bone, and genitourinary tract
  C. Diagnosis
    1. Symptoms are nonspecific
      a. Fever, malaise, headache, or encephalopathy signs and symptoms (altered mentation, lethargy, personality changes, or memory loss)
      b. Classic meningismus occurs in only about 25% of patients
    2. If focal neurologic signs or obtundation is present, ophthalmoscopy and brain imaging are necessary before CSF examination
    3. Brain imaging is nonspecific, with ventricular enlargement and atrophy being most common
    4. Lumbar puncture findings
      a. Increased opening pressure (>200 mm water)
      b. Mildly increased serum protein level
      c. Low or normal glucose level
      d. Distinct lack of inflammation (ie, few lymphocytes and multiple organisms)
      e. India ink preparation of CSF
        1) Positive in 70% of cases
        2) Has been supplanted by the availability of rapid, sensitive, and specific cryptococcal antigen testing
          a) CSF cryptococcal antigen testing may be negative in nonmeningeal cryptococcosis
          b) Serum cryptococcal antigen testing results are positive in 99% of patients with cryptococcal meningitis
      f. CSF cultures are usually positive (blood cultures may be positive as well)
  D. Treatment
    1. Untreated cryptococcal meningitis is fatal
      a. Increased intracranial pressure
      b. Poor prognostic signs: altered mental status initially and high fungal burden
    2. Treatment phases: induction therapy, follow-up therapy, and long-term therapy
      a. Induction therapy
        1) Amphotericin B 0.7 to 1 mg/kg IV daily for 2 weeks
        2) Preferably, amphotericin B is given in combination with flucytosine 100 mg orally daily
          a) Amphotericin B in combination with flucytosine leads to a mycologic response of 70% and mortality of less than 10%
          b) Flucytosine decreases risk of relapse
          c) Flucytosine may lead to bone marrow failure
            i) Especially in patients with renal failure
            ii) Blood level monitoring (with peak serum levels <100 mg/mL) is helpful in preventing bone marrow toxicity
      b. Follow-up therapy: fluconazole 400 mg daily alone for 8 weeks or until CSF cultures are sterile
      c. Long-term therapy (secondary prophylaxis): fluconazole 200 mg daily
        1) Secondary prophylaxis may be discontinued if patient remains asymptomatic and CD4 cell count is greater than 200/μL for more than 6 months
        2) Secondary prophylaxis should be reinitiated if the CD4 cell count decreases to less than 200/μL
    3. Routine primary prophylaxis is not recommended for several reasons
      a. Cost
      b. Potential for resistance emerging
      c. Drug interactions
    4. Elevated intracranial pressures
      a. May require daily lumbar punctures or shunting
      b. Acetazolamide has anecdotal support but is of unproven benefit and is not recommended
    5. Follow-up CSF examination to show clearance of the organism is not required if clinical resolution occurs

6. Optimal therapy after treatment failure
   a. Unclear
   b. Voriconazole may have activity
7. Change in serum cryptococcal antigen level is not helpful in management

V. Cytomegalovirus Infection
   A. Epidemiology
      1. Causative agent: CMV, a double-stranded DNA gammaherpesvirus
      2. Approximately 60% of the US adult population has serologic evidence of prior infection with CMV
      3. Disease is generally associated with reactivation of latent infection in immunocompromised hosts
      4. In HIV-positive persons, CMV disease occurs with CD4 cell counts less than 50/μL
   B. Clinical Manifestations
      1. Chorioretinitis
         a. After HAART, 5% of patients with AIDS have retinitis
         b. Accounts for 80% to 90% of CMV end-organ disease
      2. Gastrointestinal tract disease
         a. CMV enterocolitis: diarrhea, weight loss, abdominal pain, anorexia, and fever
         b. CMV esophagitis: causes odynophagia
      3. Pneumonitis
      4. CNS disease
   C. Diagnosis
      1. Diagnosis is clinical
      2. Chorioretinitis diagnosis should be made promptly with a thorough eye examination by an experienced ophthalmologist
         a. Patients with chorioretinitis present with decreased visual acuity, floaters, or visual field loss
         b. On examination, large yellow-white granular areas with perivascular exudates and hemorrhages may occur at the periphery or center of the retina
         c. Progression to bilateral disease or blindness (or both) can occur if untreated
         d. Main differential diagnosis: toxoplasmic chorioretinitis
      3. Enterocolitis: evidence of patchy colitis on endoscopy
      4. Esophagitis
         a. Generally, distal ulceration is visible on endoscopy
         b. Biopsy: CMV inclusion bodies and inflammation
         c. Ophthalmic examination should be performed to rule out chorioretinitis
   D. Treatment
      1. Goal: halt vision loss but cannot reverse existing damage
      2. Treatment phases: induction phase and maintenance phase
      3. CMV chorioretinitis treatment
         a. IV ganciclovir, valganciclovir, IV foscarnet, and IV cidofovir are all effective
         b. Factors affecting choice of therapy from among these drugs
            1) Location and severity of the disease (eg, sight threatening)
            2) Presence of concomitant medications with overlapping toxicity (eg, bone marrow suppression, renal toxicity)
            3) Presence of comorbid conditions (eg, renal insufficiency, electrolyte abnormalities, anemia)
            4) If lesions threaten vision, an intraocular ganciclovir implant with systemic anti-CMV therapy is used
            5) Considerations related to foscarnet
               a) A pyrophosphate analogue with in vitro activity against all herpesviruses and HIV
               b) Retains activity against ganciclovir-resistant virus
               c) Requires daily infusions
               d) Is nephrotoxic
               e) Causes painful penile ulcers
      4. HAART
         a. Affects the prognosis of CMV retinitis
         b. Immune reconstitution may lead to inflammatory uveitis, papillitis, and vitreitis
         c. Treatment may require corticosteroids
      5. Routine primary prophylaxis in CMV-seropositive persons is not recommended
         a. Lack of proven benefits
         b. Treatment-associated toxicities
         c. Cost
      6. Secondary prophylaxis: may be discontinued if CD4 cell count is greater than 100/μL for 6 months
      7. Maintenance therapy for CMV esophagitis: may be indicated especially after relapse

VI. Tuberculosis
   A. Epidemiology
      1. Causative agent: *Mycobacterium tuberculosis* (MTB)
      2. Accounts for approximately 11% of deaths worldwide among AIDS patients
      3. Overall incidence is decreasing because of improved infection control and better diagnosis of HIV-1 and MTB

4. Disease may be from primary infection or reactivation
5. Latent MTB infection
    a. More likely to progress to active disease in HIV-positive persons, with an annual risk of 7% to 10%
    b. Lifetime risk among HIV-negative patients: 5% to 10%
B. Clinical Manifestations
    1. Depend on the patient's degree of immunodeficiency
    2. Presentation of patients with CD4 cell counts greater than 350/µL: similar to that of immunocompetent patients
        a. Disease is mostly confined to the lung, with upper cavitary disease and fibronodular infiltrates
        b. Histopathology shows caseating granulomas
        c. Extrapulmonary disease includes pericardial, pleuritic, and meningeal involvement
    3. Presentation of severely immunocompromised patients
        a. Tuberculosis has an atypical radiographic appearance
            1) Infiltrates may be seen in the lower or middle lobes
            2) Infection may manifest as interstitial or miliary infiltrates
            3) Cavitation is less common
        b. Even when patients have a normal chest radiograph, sputum smear and culture results can be positive
        c. Patients may present with severe systemic manifestations with high fevers, rapid progression, and sepsis syndrome
        d. Granulomas may be absent or poorly formed
C. Diagnosis
    1. Tuberculin skin test (TST)
        a. TST is positive for most patients who have pulmonary disease and CD4 cell counts greater than 200/µL
        b. For patients who have lower CD4 cell counts, the TST has limited diagnostic value
    2. Chest radiograph
    3. Sputum samples for smear and culture (results may be negative)
        a. Aspiration or biopsy of extrapulmonary sites of infection may be necessary
        b. Yield of MTB stain and culture from extrapulmonary sites may be higher among HIV-1 infected patients because the high organism burden reflects the lack of an effective immune response to limit the organism spread
        c. Drug susceptibility testing and adjustment of treatment based on results is mandatory
    4. Blood cultures may be positive in disseminated disease
D. Treatment
    1. Treatment of HIV-positive patients who have active tuberculosis is complex
    2. Protease inhibitors and nonnucleoside reverse transcriptase inhibitors (NNRTIs) have substantial interactions with the rifamycin drug group
        a. Rifamycins induce the cytochrome P450 system, thereby decreasing the levels of active antiretroviral drug in the system
        b. Protease inhibitors and NNRTIs are substrates for and may induce or inhibit the cytochrome P450 system
        c. Compared with rifampin, rifabutin has less cytochrome P450 inducer activity and should be considered a practical choice
    3. Monitoring for drug-induced adverse events is required, as for patients who are not infected with HIV-1
        a. Liver and kidney function
        b. Platelet count
        c. Ophthalmologic examination (if treatment includes ethambutol)
    4. Antituberculous treatment guidelines follow the same principles as for patients without HIV infection
    5. Regimen for drug-susceptible tuberculosis
        a. Six-month regimen
            1) Initial phase: isoniazid, rifampin or rifabutin, pyrazinamide, and ethambutol administered for 2 months
            2) Continuation phase: isoniazid and rifampin (or rifabutin) for 4 additional months
        b. Extension of treatment
            1) Isoniazid and rifampin (or rifabutin) should be administered for an additional 3 months (for a total of 9 months) if there was cavitary lung disease or if cultures were positive for MTB after the first 2 months of therapy
            2) Tuberculosis in the CNS or in bone and joints may require 9 to 12 months of treatment
        c. Adjuvant corticosteroids: required for CNS and pericardial tuberculosis

6. Other therapeutic considerations
   a. Directly observed therapy is recommended for the treatment of tuberculosis in patients with HIV infection
   b. Intermittent dosing (ie, 2 or 3 times weekly) of the antitubercular regimen is possible but with certain caveats
      1) Twice weekly dosing should not be used in the initial 8-week phase of therapy
      2) Twice weekly dosing should not be used in the continuation phase of therapy if the CD4 cell count is less than 100/μL
   c. Once-weekly isoniazid-rifapentine in the continuation phase of therapy should not be used for any patient with HIV infection
   d. Antiretroviral therapy (ART) during MTB treatment
      1) All HIV-infected patients with active tuberculosis should receive ART
      2) For patients with a CD4 cell count less than 200/μL, ART should be initiated within 2 to 4 weeks after the start of tuberculosis therapy
      3) For patients with a CD4 cell count of 200 to 500/μL, ART should be initiated within 2 to 4 weeks, or at least by 8 weeks, after the start of tuberculosis therapy
      4) For patients with a CD4 cell count greater than 500/μL, ART should be initiated within 8 weeks after the start of tuberculosis therapy
      5) Coadministration of rifampin and protease inhibitors is not recommended
      6) If a protease inhibitor–based regimen is used, rifabutin is the preferred rifamycin
   e. *Paradoxical reaction*: temporary worsening of symptoms, signs, or radiographic manifestations after HIV-1 therapy has been started
      1) Diagnosed only after a thorough work-up has ruled out other causes
      2) Short course of corticosteroids may be considered if symptoms are severe

VII. Latent Tuberculosis Infection
   A. Screening
      1. Screening for latent tuberculosis infection (LTBI) should be performed when HIV infection is diagnosed
         a. TST: considered positive for HIV-infected persons if induration is greater than 5 mm
         b. Interferon gamma release assay (IGRA): more specific than TST
   B. Treatment
      1. Treatment regimens for LTBI in HIV-infected persons
         a. Isoniazid daily for 9 months
         b. Isoniazid twice weekly for 9 months
         c. Rifampin or rifabutin alone for 4 months
      2. Treatment in the event of close contact
         a. Patients should be treated even if TST and IGRA results are negative
         b. Active tuberculosis must be ruled out first

VIII. *Mycobacterium avium-intracellulare* Complex Infection
   A. Epidemiology
      1. Causative agents: MAC includes *Mycobacterium avium* and *Mycobacterium intracellulare*
      2. Isolated from diverse environmental sources
   B. Clinical Manifestations
      1. Different from indolent pulmonary syndromes common in other populations
      2. Most cases occur as disseminated infections in HIV patients who generally are in a state of advanced immunocompromise (CD4 cell count <50-100/μL)
      3. Lymph node abscesses, skin lesions, and osteomyelitis
      4. Hectic fever, drenching night sweats, anorexia, weight loss, abdominal pain, and diarrhea are common
   C. Diagnosis
      1. Physical examination: wasting and hepatosplenomegaly
      2. Laboratory evaluations often show profound anemia and an elevated alkaline phosphatase level
      3. Diagnosis is made by blood culture, which is highly sensitive
         a. Organism usually grows within 1 to 2 weeks in the Bactec system
         b. Rapidly confirmed by probe hybridization specific for *M avium* and *M intracellulare*
      4. Rarely, bone marrow examination or lymph node biopsy is needed: granulomas are typically not seen
   D. Treatment
      1. Institution of effective HAART
      2. In addition, at least 2 drugs because monotherapy leads to resistance
         a. Clarithromycin: the preferred first agent
            1) Azithromycin is an acceptable alternative if clarithromycin cannot be used
            2) Features of both clarithromycin and azithromycin

a) Good intracellular penetration into macrophages
b) High activity
c) Ease of administration (once or twice daily)
d) Relatively benign side-effect profiles
b. Ethambutol: the preferred second agent
c. Depending on the severity of disease, a third or fourth drug may be required
1) Rifabutin: usually recommended as the third drug
a) Its toxic effects require monitoring (uveitis, arthralgias, and skin discoloration)
b) Its drug interactions, especially with protease inhibitors, can be limiting
2) Either amikacin or streptomycin is used if a fourth drug is needed
3. Criteria for discontinuation of anti-MAC therapy
a. Completion of at least 12 months of therapy
b. No MAC-related signs and symptoms
c. CD4 cell count increases to more than 100/μL for at least 6 months
4. Treatment should be restarted if the CD4 cell count decreases to less than 100/μL
5. Primary prophylaxis
a. Indicated when CD4 cell count is less than 50 cells/μL
1) Preferred: azithromycin 1,200 mg weekly
2) An alternative: clarithromycin 500 mg twice daily
3) Acceptable when macrolides cannot be used: rifabutin 300 mg daily
b. Can be stopped if the CD4 cell count increases to more than 100/μL for more than 3 months
6. An immune reconstitution syndrome similar to that seen with MTB can occur

IX. Cryptosporidiosis
A. Epidemiology
1. Causative agent: *Cryptosporidium* species
a. Intestinal parasites that infect gastrointestinal tract epithelium
b. Sporozoites invade jejunal and terminal ileal epithelium
c. Humans are infected by ingestion of water and food contaminated with oocysts
d. Oocysts are resistant to chlorine treatment and filtration
2. Infection leads to diarrhea in both immunocompetent and immunocompromised hosts

B. Clinical Manifestations
1. Four patterns of disease in patients with AIDS
a. Asymptomatic carriage
b. Self-limited diarrhea lasting less than 2 months
c. Chronic diarrhea lasting more than 2 months
d. Fulminant diarrhea with daily stool volume of more than 2 L
2. Chronic and fulminant diarrhea occur almost always with CD4 cell counts less than 100/μL
3. Extraintestinal manifestations of cryptosporidiosis
a. Sclerosing cholangitis
b. Pancreatitis
c. Pulmonary involvement
C. Diagnosis
1. Identification of the organism in stool or biopsy specimens
2. A modified acid-fast stain: most frequently used to identify oocysts
3. Direct immunofluorescence and enzyme-linked immunosorbent assays improve sensitivity
D. Treatment
1. There is no established consistently effective and specific therapy for cryptosporidiosis
2. Mainstay of treatment: immune reconstitution with HAART
3. Antidiarrheal agents (eg, loperamide) may provide symptomatic relief
4. Treatment of dehydration and electrolyte disturbances (which can be severe) with oral rehydration agents or intravenous fluids is indicated
5. Nitazoxanide is approved by the US Food and Drug Administration for immunocompetent children aged 1 to 11 years

X. Candidiasis
A. Epidemiology
1. Causative agent: *Candida* species
2. Yeast-forming normal fungal inhabitants of the gastrointestinal tract
3. Cause various infections in immunosuppressed persons
4. Oropharyngeal candidiasis
a. An important indicator of immunosuppression
b. Generally occurs with CD4 cell counts of 200/μL or less
B. Clinical Manifestations
1. Patients may complain of taste disturbance or tongue burning

2. Esophageal involvement
   a. Odynophagia
   b. Retrosternal discomfort
   c. Nausea
C. Diagnosis
   1. Plaques are visible on tongue and oral mucosa
      a. Painless, white, and nonadherent
      b. Distinguished from oral hairy leukoplakia by scraping: candidal plaques are removed, but oral hairy leukoplakia lesions are not
   2. Fever
      a. Generally not classically associated with oropharyngeal candidiasis
      b. Should prompt evaluation for other opportunistic infections
   3. Symptoms alone are suggestive enough to warrant empirical treatment with oral fluconazole
D. Treatment
   1. Fluconazole: the drug of choice
   2. Initial episodes can be treated with topical nystatin, clotrimazole, or miconazole
   3. Therapy is continued for at least 14 to 21 days
   4. Failure to improve clinically with antifungal therapy necessitates evaluation with endoscopy and biopsy to differentiate the characteristic white plaques of candidiasis from other lesions (eg, CMV infection or herpes simplex virus esophagitis)
   5. HAART should be instituted as appropriate

XI. Progressive Multifocal Leukoencephalopathy
A. Epidemiology
   1. Causative agent: the JC virus, a single-stranded DNA papovavirus
   2. PML is a demyelinating disease
   3. Infection with JC virus is ubiquitous
      a. Most primary infections are asymptomatic
      b. Reactivation with immunosuppression leads to demyelination and PML
         1) PML may occur at CD4 cell counts greater than 200/µL
         2) PML may occur in patients who are receiving antiretroviral therapy
B. Clinical Manifestations
   1. Depend on location of the lesion in the CNS
   2. Cognitive disorders, paresis, and visual and speech defects occur
C. Diagnosis
   1. Depends on compatible clinical scenario, radiographic findings, and positive PCR testing for JC virus
   2. Magnetic resonance imaging: useful in demonstrating increased T2 signal in affected white matter
   3. CSF PCR testing for JC virus: specificity of 95% and a sensitivity of 80%
D. Treatment
   1. There is no established, specific therapy for PML
   2. Treatment consists of immune reconstitution with HAART
      a. If patients are not receiving antiretroviral therapy, HAART should be immediately initiated
      b. If patients are receiving HAART but without virologic suppression, therapy should be modified and optimized to achieve virologic suppression

XII. HIV-Associated Malignancies
A. Kaposi Sarcoma
   1. Epidemiology
      a. Causative agent: human herpesvirus 8, also known as Kaposi sarcoma–associated herpesvirus
      b. Kaposi sarcoma is the most common HIV-associated malignancy
         1) It is an AIDS-defining diagnosis
         2) It is most commonly seen in men who have sex with men
   2. Clinical manifestations
      a. Vary widely
      b. Skin lesions: the most common manifestations, often mistaken for benign vascular lesions
      c. Intraoral lesions are common
      d. Lungs and organs of the gastrointestinal tract
         1) Most commonly affected visceral organs
         2) Can be affected without skin lesions
   3. Diagnosis
      a. Requires biopsy
      b. Whorls of spindle-shaped cells and abnormal proliferation of small blood vessels are seen
   4. Treatment
      a. Depends on site and extent of involvement
      b. Local therapy (eg, radiotherapy, intralesional chemotherapy, cryotherapy)
      c. Systemic therapy (eg, chemotherapy, interferon alfa): liposome-encapsulated anthracycline chemotherapeutic agents enable delivery of high doses of effective drug with fewer side effects

    d. Antiretroviral therapy
        1) Recommended for all HIV-infected patients with Kaposi sarcoma
        2) Has resulted in a substantial reduction in the incidence of Kaposi sarcoma
        3) Has been associated with a reduction in tumor burden and disease progression
B. Non-Hodgkin Lymphoma
    1. Epidemiology
        a. Non-Hodgkin lymphoma is a heterogeneous group of malignancies
        b. Occurs in HIV-infected persons with various levels of immune function
            1) Vast majority of non-Hodgkin lymphomas in patients with HIV are of B-cell origin
            2) Intermediate- or high-grade B-cell non-Hodgkin lymphoma is an AIDS-defining diagnosis
                a) Occurs much more commonly (increased risk is as high as 200-fold) among HIV-infected patients than in the general population
                b) May become even more frequent with the aging of the HIV-infected population
    2. Clinical manifestations
        a. Constitutional symptoms: fever, night sweats, and weight loss
        b. Lymphadenopathy
        c. Extranodal involvement
            a) CNS, bone marrow, gastrointestinal tract, and liver
            b) Involvement of the brain can be as an isolated disease (primary CNS lymphoma) or as leptomeningeal involvement from the spread of lymphoma elsewhere
    3. Treatment
        a. Optimal treatment of HIV-associated non-Hodgkin lymphoma has not been well defined
        b. Most patients should receive standard-dose chemotherapy, PCP prophylaxis, and growth factor support
        c. HAART is an essential component of the strategy
C. Primary CNS Lymphoma
    1. Epidemiology
        a. Primary CNS lymphoma has a higher incidence in HIV-infected persons than in the general population
        b. It occurs most often in the advanced stages of AIDS at a median CD4 cell count of less than $50/\mu L$
        c. It is almost always associated with Epstein-Barr virus
    2. Clinical manifestations
        a. Nonspecific
        b. Headache, confusion, lethargy, personality changes, memory loss, focal neurologic deficits, and seizure
    3. Diagnosis
        a. Brain imaging studies: single or multiple contrast-enhancing lesions, which may be difficult to distinguish from those of toxoplasmosis
        b. Biopsy: required for definitive diagnosis
        c. PCR testing of CSF for Epstein-Barr virus: usually positive
    4. Treatment
        a. Options are limited
        b. Whole-brain radiotherapy has been the primary treatment
        c. Median survival time: 2 to 5 months
        d. HAART may improve prognosis

Suggested Reading

Brooks JT, Kaplan JE, Holmes KK, Benson C, Pau A, Masur H. HIV-associated opportunistic infections: going, going, but not gone: the continued need for prevention and treatment guidelines. Clin Infect Dis. 2009 Mar 1;48(5):609–11.

Brooks JT, Kaplan JE, Masur H. What's new in the 2009 US guidelines for prevention and treatment of opportunistic infections among adults and adolescents with HIV? Top HIV Med. 2009 Jul-Aug;17(3):109–14.

Kaplan JE, Benson C, Holmes KH, Brooks JT, Pau A, Masur H; Centers for Disease Control and Prevention (CDC); National Institutes of Health; HIV Medicine Association of the Infectious Diseases Society of America. Guidelines for prevention and treatment of opportunistic infections in HIV-infected adults and adolescents: recommendations from CDC, the National Institutes of Health, and the HIV Medicine Association of the Infectious Diseases Society of America. MMWR Recomm Rep. 2009 Apr 10;58(RR-4):1–207.

John W. Wilson, MD
Michelle A. Elliott, MD

38

Infections in Patients With Hematologic Malignancies

I. General Approach
   A. Approach to Patients With Hematologic Malignancies and Infection
      1. Define and characterize the patient's immunologic competence (or specific immunologic defect)
      2. Define the patient's residential environment (eg, living at home or in a nursing home, recent hospitalization)
      3. Define the syndrome: characterize the type, location, and progress of the infection
      4. Define the pathogen: the identity of the pathogen(s) may be suspected or confirmed
      5. Define the treatment: medical or surgical or both
   B. Management of Patients With Hematologic Malignancies and Infection
      1. Requires knowledge of general infectious diseases and factors pertaining to the hematologic malignancy
         a. Pathophysiology of the hematologic malignancy
         b. Types of antineoplastic chemotherapy used in treatment
         c. Immunologic effects of both the malignancy and the associated chemotherapy
         d. Complications and toxicities of both the malignancy and the associated chemotherapy (can complicate antimicrobial therapy or masquerade as infection)
      2. Requires early recognition and treatment of opportunistic and nonopportunistic infections
II. Principles of Chemotherapy in Hematology
   A. Select Antineoplastic Chemotherapeutic Agents
      1. Classification of agents is shown in Box 38.1
      2. Indications for agents are listed in Table 38.1
   B. Select Chemotherapy Toxicities and Associated Syndromes
      1. Myelosuppression
         a. Most cytotoxic chemotherapeutic agents produce marked myelosuppression
         b. Exceptions include L-asparaginase, vincristine, all-*trans* retinoic acid (ATRA), rituximab
      2. Cardiotoxicity
         a. Acute: electrocardiographic changes and dysrhythmia
         b. Subacute: myocarditis and pericarditis
         c. Chronic: cardiomyopathy and congestive heart failure
         d. Specific drugs

> **Box 38.1**
>
> **Classification of Select Chemotherapeutic Agents Used in Hematology**
>
> Alkylating agents
>   Bendamustine
>   Busulfan
>   Carmustine (BCNU)
>   Chlorambucil
>   Cisplatin
>   Cyclophosphamide
>   Dacarbazine (DTIC)
>   Ifosfamide
>   Melphalan
>   Nitrogen mustard (mechlorethamine)
>   Procarbazine
> Antimetabolites
>   Asparaginase
>   Azacytidine
>   Azathioprine
>   Cytosine arabinoside (cytarabine, Ara-C)
>   Hydroxyurea
>   6-Mercaptopurine
>   Methotrexate
>   Purine nucleoside analogues: 2-chlorodeoxyadenosine (2-CdA, cladribine), clofarabine, deoxycoformycin (pentostatin), fludarabine, nelarabine
>   6-Thioguanine
> Antitumor antibiotics
>   Anthracenedione (mitoxantrone)
>   Anthracyclines: daunorubicin, doxorubicin, idarubicin
>   Bleomycin
> Mitotic spindle inhibitors
>   Vinca alkaloids: vinblastine, vincristine, vinorelbine
> Monoclonal antibodies
>   Alemtuzumab (Campath, anti-CD52)
>   Rituximab (anti-CD20)
> Molecularly targeted agents
>   Imatinib mesylate (Gleevec)
>   Nilotinib
>   Desatinib
> Differentiating agents
>   All-*trans* retinoic acid (ATRA)
>   Arsenic trioxide (ATO)

      1) Anthracyclines: entire class (doxorubicin most common; mitoxantrone less common)
      2) Occasional: cyclophosphamide and iphosphamide
  3. Pulmonary toxicity
    a. Early: interstitial and alveolar infiltrates, edema, and eosinophilia
    b. Late: pulmonary fibrosis
    c. Specific drugs
      1) Bleomycin: dose dependent and nonresponsive to corticosteroids
      2) Carmustine (BCNU): often used for bone marrow transplant (BMT) conditioning
      3) Busulfan: less frequent pulmonary toxicity than with BCNU
      4) Others: cyclophosphamide, methotrexate, and chlorambucil
  4. Renal and metabolic toxicity
    a. Methotrexate: related to drug precipitate in renal tubules and collecting ducts
    b. Cisplatin and cyclophosphamide
    c. Chemotherapy-associated tumor lysis syndrome: tumor cellular breakdown with associated hyperkalemia, hyperphosphatemia, hyperuricemia, and hypocalcemia
  5. Gastrointestinal tract toxicity
    a. Breakdown of oral, esophageal, and intestinal tissue barriers: oral mucositis, esophagitis, enteritis, and colitis
    b. Common with most myelosuppressive agents
    c. High risk with methotrexate (especially with higher doses) and anthracyclines (eg, doxorubicin, idarubicin)
  6. Hepatotoxicity
    a. Venoocclusive disease (sinusoidal obstruction syndrome)
      1) Injury of the sinusoidal endothelial cells of hepatic venules in stem cell recipients, leading to sinusoidal obstruction, fibrosis, and hepatocellular necrosis
      2) Marked by weight gain, ascites, hyperbilirubinemia, and tender hepatomegaly
      3) Usually occurs before day 21 after hematopoietic stem cell infusion (see "Infections in Hematopoietic Stem Cell Transplant Patients" section)
    b. High-dose conditioning preceding hematopoietic stem cell transplant (HSCT), including total body irradiation (TBI), busulfan, and cyclophosphamide
    c. Gemtuzumab: used in acute myelogenous leukemia therapy (especially in patients proceeding to transplant)
  7. Peripheral neuropathy
    a. Vinca alkaloids (vincristine)
    b. Cisplatin
    c. Thalidomide
    d. Disease-associated neuropathy with multiple myeloma, amyloidosis, or chronic graft-vs-host disease (GVHD) (less common)
  8. Other
    a. ATRA syndrome

Table 38.1
Common Chemotherapy Treatment of Hematologic Malignancies

Hematologic Malignancy	Agent or Regimen
AML (non-APL)	*Induction*: "3+7" approach is commonly used with anthracycline (idarubicin or daunorubicin) in combination with cytarabine *Consolidation*: high-dose cytarabine *Relapse*: high-dose cytarabine, MEC
APL[a]	*Induction*: ATRA with an anthracycline (eg, idarubicin) with or without cytarabine *Consolidation*: ATRA with an anthracycline with or without cytarabine *Maintenance*: ATRA, daily oral 6-mercaptopurine, weekly oral methotrexate *Relapse*: ATO

ALL	*Induction*: regimen of 4 or 5 drugs—vincristine, prednisone, anthracycline, and cyclophosphamide with or without L-asparaginase
	Consolidation: multiple cycles of multiagent regimen, which may include cytarabine, an anthracycline, vincristine, corticosteroid (prednisone or dexamethasone), etoposide, L-asparaginase, or high-dose methotrexate
	CNS prophylaxis or disease management: systemic high-dose methotrexate, intrathecal methotrexate, intrathecal cytarabine, cranial or craniospinal radiotherapy
	Maintenance: daily oral 6-mercaptopurine, weekly oral methotrexate
	Example of a specific regimen and its modifications: hyper-CVAD (B- and T-cell ALL)
	    Imatinib or dasatinib added in Ph+ ALL
	    Rituximab added in B-cell ALL or Burkitt-like leukemia or lymphoma
	Relapse or refractory ALL: clofarabine or nelarabine (T-cell ALL)

CLL	Chlorambucil Nucleoside analogues (fludarabine, cladribine, and pentostatin) often with cyclophosphamide and rituximab Bendamustine
CML	Imatinib mesylate (Gleevec) Dasatinib Nilotinib
Hairy cell leukemia	2-Chlorodeoxyadenosine (2-CdA, cladribine) Pentostatin
Hodgkin disease	ABVD (doxorubicin [Adriamycin], bleomycin, vinblastine, dacarbazine) Radiotherapy
NHL	CHOP (often with rituximab in CD20+ NHL) CVP (often with rituximab in CD20+ NHL) Radiotherapy
Multiple myeloma	Melphalan and prednisone Thalidomide or revlimid with dexamethasone Bortezomib (Velcade) with or without dexamethasone Radiotherapy

Allogeneic HSCT, AML, ALL, MDS, aplastic anemia	*Myeloablative conditioning regimens*:
	    TBI and cytoxan
	    Busulfan and cytoxan
	    Cytoxan and anti-thymocyte globulin

Allogeneic HSCT, AML, ALL, MDS	*Nonmyeloablative conditioning regimens*:
	    Fludarabine and melphalan
	    Fludarabine and busulfan
	    Fludarabine and TBI

Autologous HSCT, multiple myeloma, Hodgkin disease, NHL	*Myeloablative conditioning regimens*:
	    Melphalan
	    BEAM and CBV

Abbreviations: ALL, acute lymphoblastic leukemia; AML, acute myelogenous leukemia; APL, acute promyelocytic leukemia; ATO, arsenic trioxide; ATRA, all-*trans* retinoic acid; BEAM, carmustine, etoposide, cytarabine, and melphalan; HSCT, hematopoietic stem cell transplant; CBV, cyclophosphamide, carmustine, and etoposide; CHOP, cyclophosphamide, doxorubicin, vincristine, and prednisone; CLL, chronic lymphocytic leukemia; CML, chronic myelogenous leukemia; CNS, central nervous system; CVP, cyclophosphamide, vincristine, and prednisone; hyper-CVAD, hyperfractionated cyclophosphamide, vincristine, doxorubicin, and dexamethasone; MDS, myelodysplastic syndrome; MEC, mitoxantrone, etoposide, and cytarabine; NHL, non-Hodgkin lymphoma; Ph+, Philadelphia chromosome positive; TBI, total body irradiation.

[a]APL is the AML subtype that most commonly is associated with coagulopathy due to disseminated intravascular coagulation and fibrinolysis.

1) A potentially life-threatening cardiorespiratory distress syndrome in patients with acute promyelocytic leukemia treated with ATRA
2) Typically patients present with fever, weight gain, respiratory distress, interstitial pulmonary infiltrates, pleural and pericardial effusion, episodic hypotension, and acute renal failure
3) Treatment includes high-dose dexamethasone
  b. Engraftment syndrome
   1) Fever, rash, and often pulmonary infiltrates (usually as a complication of autologous HSCT) developing at the time of initial neutrophil recovery
   2) Usually occurs 7 to 11 days after autologous HSCT
   3) Responds well to high-dose corticosteroids

III. Immune System Dysfunction and Associated Infections
  A. Common Infections
   1. Common pathogens associated with specific immunologic deficiencies are listed in Table 38.2
  B. Common Contributing Factors to Specific Immunologic Deficiencies
   1. Neutropenia
    a. Cytotoxic chemotherapy
    b. Conditioning regimen (high-dose chemotherapy and TBI) before HSCT
    c. Marrow failure: aplastic anemia, myelodysplastic syndrome (MDS), and secondary causes (eg, irradiation, infection, drugs)
    d. Marrow involvement in hematologic malignancy: acute myelogenous leukemia, acute lymphoblastic leukemia, MDS, non-Hodgkin and Hodgkin lymphoma, multiple myeloma, and chronic lymphocytic leukemia
    e. Cyclic neutropenia
   2. Neutrophil dysfunction
    a. Chronic granulomatous disease
    b. Leukocyte adhesion deficiency
   3. Abnormal cell-mediated immunity
    a. Lymphoproliferative disease (Hodgkin and non-Hodgkin lymphoma, hairy cell leukemia, and T-cell chronic lymphocytic leukemia)
    b. Human immunodeficiency virus/AIDS and human T-lymphotropic virus 1
    c. Drug associated: purine nucleoside analogues (fludarabine, cladribine, and pentostatin), calcineurin inhibitors (cyclosporine and tacrolimus), corticosteroids, and monoclonal antibody agents (alemtuzumab [Campath])
    d. Chronic GVHD
   4. Abnormal humoral immunity
    a. Plasma cell proliferative diseases (multiple myeloma and Waldenström macroglobulinemia)
    b. Lymphoproliferative disease (Hodgkin and non-Hodgkin lymphoma, hairy cell leukemia, and chronic lymphocytic leukemia)
    c. Hereditary immunoglobulin deficiencies: primary hypogammaglobulinemia, IgA deficiency, and common variable immune deficiency
    d. Splenectomy or functional asplenia
    e. Nephrotic syndrome
    f. Chronic GVHD
   5. Functional or anatomical asplenia
    a. Surgical splenectomy: diagnostic (staging), therapeutic, or trauma
    b. Sickle cell disease
  C. Special Considerations for Patients With Functional or Anatomical Asplenia
   1. Thrombocytosis and leukocytosis may occur after splenectomy
    a. Platelet and white blood cell values usually peak within 10 days and then normalize gradually
   2. Delayed or long-term major risks with splenectomized patients
    a. Recurrent bacterial infections with encapsulated bacteria are often fulminant
    b. Postsplenectomy sepsis (PSS)
     1) *Streptococcus pneumoniae*: most common organism in PSS (50%-90% of cases)
     2) *Haemophilus influenzae* type b: second most common with most cases in children younger than 15 years
     3) *Neisseria meningitidis*: third most common cause of PSS
     4) *Capnocytophaga canimorsus*: after dog bites and scratches
     5) *Salmonella* species: not common role in PSS, but more common in children with asplenia or sickle cell disease
   3. Malaria (*Plasmodium* species) and babesiosis (*Babesia*): more severe or life threatening
   4. Vaccines
    a. Should be administered to all patients with functional or anatomical asplenia

Table 38.2

Pathogens Associated With Specific Immunologic Deficiencies

Deficiency	Bacteria	Fungi	Viruses	Parasites
Neutropenia (<500 cells/μL)	Viridans streptococci Aerobic gram-negative bacteria (Enterobacteriaceae and Pseudomonas) Staphylococcus aureus Coagulase-negative staphylococci Bacteroides species Clostridium species	Aspergillus species Zygomycetes Other filamentous fungi Candida species	Herpes simplex virus	
Decreased cell-mediated immunity	Listeria species Salmonella species Nocardia species Legionella species Mycobacteria species Bartonella species Brucella Rhodococcus equi	Candida species Pneumocystis jiroveci (pneumocystis pneumonia) Cryptococcus Histoplasma Coccidioides Penicillium marneffei	Cytomegalovirus Herpes simplex virus Varicella-zoster virus Epstein-Barr virus JC virus	Toxoplasma Strongyloides Cryptosporidium
Hypogammaglobulinemia	Streptococcus pneumoniae Haemophilus influenzae type b Neisseria meningitidis		Enteroviruses	Giardia
Complement deficiencies	S pneumoniae H influenzae S aureus Enterobacteriaceae N meningitidis			
Asplenia	S pneumoniae H influenzae N meningitidis Capnocytophaga Salmonella species			Plasmodium species (malaria) Babesia species

b. Give at least 2 weeks before elective splenectomy to optimize antibody response or give after surgical recovery from urgent splenectomy
c. Pneumococcal vaccine
d. *Haemophilus influenzae* type b vaccine
e. Meningococcal vaccine

IV. Infections in Hematopoietic Stem Cell Transplant Patients
A. Immunologic Function and Specific Infections
1. Can be broadly categorized into specific time periods during and after transplant (Figure 38.1)
2. Timing and categorization of immune function and infection development after HSCT can be variable owing to several factors
   a. Underlying hematologic malignancy and condition
   b. Previous chemotherapies or radiotherapy
   c. Delayed cellular engraftment
   d. GVHD (acute or chronic) and its treatment
B. Preengraftment Period
1. Period extends from the date of transplant conditioning to neutrophil recovery (ie, the first of 3 consecutive days with an absolute neutrophil count >500 cells/μL)
   a. Typically day 0 to approximately days 10 to 30 after stem cell infusion
   b. Duration of period varies, depending on several factors
      1) Quantity of hematopoietic stem cells infused

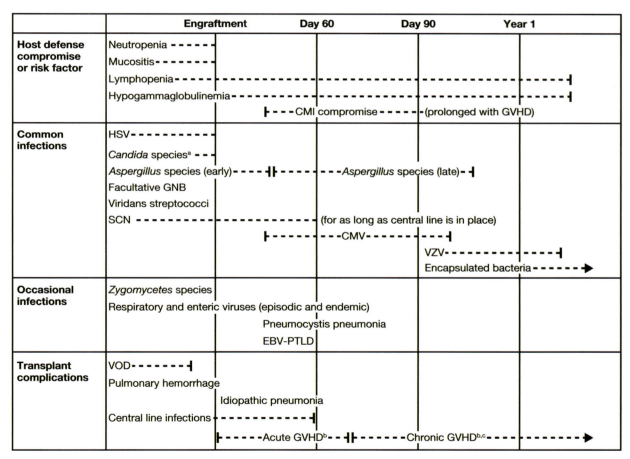

Figure 38.1. Infections and Immunosuppression After Hematopoietic Stem Cell Transplant (HSCT). CMI indicates cell-mediated immunity; CMV, cytomegalovirus; EBV, Epstein-Barr virus; GNB, gram-negative bacilli; GVHD, graft-vs-host disease; HSV, herpes simplex virus; PTLD, posttransplant lymphoproliferative disease; SCN, coagulase-negative staphylococcus; VOD, venoocclusive disease; VZV, varicella-zoster virus. Superscript letters indicate the following: [a]Candidal infections (predominantly not *Candida albicans*) due to fluconazole prophylaxis. [b]Almost exclusively in allogeneic HSCT; GVHD can prolong CMI suppression. [c]Chronic GVHD can be quite prolonged and variable in some allogeneic HSCT patients.

2) Source (bone marrow, peripheral blood, or umbilical cord blood)
3) Type of GVHD prophylaxis
2. Clinical and laboratory characteristics
   a. Leukopenia, neutropenia, and thrombocytopenia are present
   b. Patients are commonly receiving prophylactic antimicrobials, which vary between medical center protocols (eg, oral penicillin, levofloxacin, fluconazole, acyclovir)
   c. Oral, esophageal, and enteric mucositis are common
   d. Venoocclusive disease may occur during this period
      1) Marked by hepatomegaly, right upper quadrant pain, weight gain, jaundice, and ascites
      2) Most common during the first 3 weeks after hematopoietic stem cell infusion
      3) Increased levels of serum transaminases and bilirubin, especially conjugated (direct) bilirubin
      4) Also called sinusoidal obstructive syndrome and may resemble Budd-Chiari syndrome
      5) In severe venoocclusive disease, confusion, bleeding, and renal and cardiopulmonary failure may develop
3. Infection complications
   a. Herpes simplex virus: predictably reactivates in 80% of seropositive patients
   b. Gram-positive and gram-negative bacteremia: often associated with mucosal disruption or intravascular catheter infections (viridans streptococci, coagulase-negative staphylococci, *Staphylococcus aureus*, enterococci, the Enterobacteriaceae, *Pseudomonas aeruginosa*, etc)
   c. *Candida* infections: later onset and more common in patients with prolonged neutropenia due to slow engraftment
   d. Intravascular catheter infections: coagulase-negative staphylococci, *S aureus*, etc

C. Postengraftment Period
   1. Period extends from neutrophil recovery to day 100 after hematopoietic stem cell infusion
      a. Early B- and T-cell recovery, although abnormal cellular function should be expected for 18 months
   2. Clinical and laboratory complications
      a. Acute GVHD
         1) Occurs almost exclusively in allogeneic HSCT patients as donor T lymphocytes attack the recipient patient's tissues and organ systems
         2) Clinical presentation is variable: can include rash, nausea and vomiting, hepatitis (especially increased levels of conjugated bilirubin and alkaline phosphatase), enteritis or colitis with diarrhea (can be severe and measured in liters)
      b. Cellular immune dysfunction
   3. Infection complications (from approximately day 31 to days 90-100)
      a. Cytomegalovirus (CMV) disease
         1) CMV reactivation is much more common than primary CMV disease (with the use of irradiated and leukocyte-poor blood products)
         2) CMV disease is often associated with GVHD and TBI (eg, CMV pneumonia)
         3) Must distinguish between viral reactivation without clinical disease (detectable viremia or antigenemia by polymerase chain reaction or antigen-detection testing, respectively) and CMV disease (defined organ or tissue involvement, such as CMV pneumonia, CMV hepatitis, or CMV colitis)
      b. Late-onset aspergillosis: seen during this period especially in patients with GVHD and those receiving high-dose corticosteroids
      c. Other complications, such as idiopathic pneumonia syndrome: diffuse alveolar injury with variable degrees of respiratory compromise
         1) Noninfectious in origin and possibly related to conditioning chemotherapy regimen or TBI
         2) Typically patients present in the first few weeks or in the second or third month after transplant
         3) More common in allogeneic BMT patients

D. Late-Risk Period
   1. Period extends from approximately day 100 until the immune system has fully recovered (usually 18-36 months after BMT)
   2. Clinical and laboratory complications
      a. Chronic GVHD
      b. Significant cellular *and* humoral immune dysfunction due to chronic GVHD or its treatment

1) First-line therapy includes prednisone with or without a calcineurin inhibitor such as cyclosporine or tacrolimus
2) Median duration of immunosuppressive therapy for chronic GVHD is 23 months
3. Infection complications (after approximately day 90)
a. Varicella-zoster virus
b. Encapsulated bacterial infections (eg, *Streptococcus pneumoniae*)
c. *Aspergillus* species

V. Common Infection Syndromes in Hematology Patients
A. Neutropenia and Fever
1. *Neutropenia*: less than 500 cells/μL
2. *Fever*: isolated oral temperature greater than 38.3°C or sustained temperature of 38.0°C for more than 1 hour
3. Risk factors associated with increased risk of bacterial and fungal infections in patients with neutropenia
a. Severe (≤100 cells/μL) and prolonged duration of neutropenia (eg, >10 days)
b. Multiple impaired immunologic components: compromised neutrophil count or function, cell-mediated immunity, immunoglobulin count or function, asplenia
c. Severe mucositis, enteritis, or colitis
d. Prolonged use of central intravenous catheters
e. Extensive antimicrobial exposure with secondary risks
1) Drug-resistant bacteria
2) *Clostridium difficile* and antibiotic-associated colitis
3) Invasive candidiasis
4. Common sites of infection in febrile patients with neutropenia
a. Mouth and pharynx (25%)
b. Lower respiratory tract (25%)
c. Skin, soft tissue, intravenous catheters (15%)
d. Gastrointestinal tract (15%)
e. Perineal region (10%)
f. Urinary tract (5%-10%)
g. Nose and sinuses (5%)
5. Bacterial infections during neutropenia
a. Since the late 1980s, infections caused by gram-positive bacteria (eg, coagulase-negative staphylococci, *S aureus*, *Enterococcus* species, and viridans streptococci) have been more commonly encountered than those caused by gram-negative bacteria (eg, *P aeruginosa* and the Enterobacteriaceae, including *Escherichia coli*, *Klebsiella* species, and *Citrobacter* species)
1) Although less virulent, coagulase-negative staphylococci are the most commonly encountered gram-positive bacteria and the most common cause of nosocomial bloodstream infections
2) If treatment is delayed during neutropenia, *S aureus* and viridans streptococci can cause rapid clinical deterioration
3) The Enterobacteriaceae and *P aeruginosa* are highly virulent in the neutropenic host and are among the most frequent causes of patient death
4) Although infections caused by gram-positive bacteria are more common, the ratio of gram-negative to gram-positive bacteria causing infections in patients with fever and neutropenia is increasing
b. Factors possibly contributing to the shift toward infections caused by gram-positive bacteria
1) More myelosuppressive or cytotoxic antineoplastic chemotherapy regimens, resulting in more prolonged and severe neutropenia
2) Higher prevalence of chemotherapy-associated enteric and oral mucositis (especially with high-dose cytosine-arabinoside therapy for acute leukemias)
3) Increased use of long-dwelling intravenous catheters
4) Antibacterial prophylaxis with a fluoroquinolone or trimethoprim-sulfamethoxazole
6. Principles of neutropenic fever management are outlined in Boxes 38.2 and 38.3
a. Empirical antibacterial therapy for a febrile patient with neutropenia must be started *promptly*, before blood culture results are available
1) Any empirical regimen must include activity against the Enterobacteriaceae and *P aeruginosa*
2) Untreated infections with aerobic gram-negative bacilli can rapidly cause septic shock and death in a neutropenic patient
b. Considerations for initial inclusion of vancomycin in empirical antimicrobial regimen

Box 38.2

Management of Patients With Fever and Neutropenia

Definitions
- *Neutropenia*: <500 neutrophils/μL
- *Fever*: isolated temperature ≥38.3°C or ≥38.0°C for ≥1 h

Considerations for antimicrobial agent selection
- Potential sources of infection and commonly associated bacteria (if evident from history, clinical examination, or radiologic and laboratory data)
- Current or recently received antimicrobial prophylaxis and therapy
- Medication allergies
- Concurrent organ dysfunction
- Hospital or unit-specific data for frequency of select bacteria and antimicrobial susceptibility patterns

Empirical antibacterial therapy
- Monotherapy
  - Preferred: cefepime or meropenem (or imipenem)
  - Alternative: piperacillin-tazobactam or ceftazidime
- Combination drug therapy
  - In combination with 1 of the monotherapy drugs, give an aminoglycoside or (if patient is not receiving fluoroquinolone prophylaxis) a fluoroquinolone

Important special circumstances
- Considerations for including vancomycin initially in empirical therapy
  - Clinically apparent intravenous catheter infections (commonly caused by coagulase-negative staphylococci, which are typically methicillin resistant or β-lactam resistant)
  - Substantial chemotherapy-associated mucosal damage (higher risk of viridans streptococci infections, which occasionally are penicillin resistant or β-lactam resistant)
  - Blood cultures are positive for bacteria that appear to be gram-positive before identification and susceptibility testing
  - Patient is receiving (or recently received) fluoroquinolone prophylaxis (associated with increased rate of gram-positive bacterial infections)
  - Known patient colonization with methicillin-resistant *Staphylococcus aureus* (MRSA) or penicillin- or cephalosporin-resistant *Streptococcus pneumoniae*
  - Patient is clinically or hemodynamically unstable
- Considerations for including coverage for oral or enteric pathogens
  - Coverage for anaerobic bacteria (ie, metronidazole, meropenem or imipenem, or piperacillin-tazobactam) for the following suspected conditions:
    1. Perirectal soft tissue infection or abscess
    2. Typhlitis or neutropenic colitis
    3. Necrotizing gingivitis
    4. Anaerobic bacteria isolated in culture
  - For diarrhea, consider the following:
    1. Empirical oral metronidazole for suspected *Clostridium difficile* infection pending stool assay result
    2. Cytomegalovirus colitis in allogeneic bone marrow transplant patients, especially with coinciding graft-vs-host disease

Empirical antimicrobial dual therapy (against gram-negative bacillus)
- Positive blood culture for gram-negative bacillus pending identification and susceptibility results (especially in hospitals with high rates of resistant gram-negative bacteria and in patients who are receiving or recently received fluoroquinolone prophylaxis)
- Patient clinically or hemodynamically unstable

Outpatient therapy
- May be considered for patients at low risk of infection-related complication (eg, age <60 y; absolute neutrophil count ≥100 cells/μL; duration of neutropenia relatively short (<1 wk) with expected recovery within 10 d; malignancy in remission; temperature <39°C; other than fever, no focus of bacterial infection or symptoms and signs (such as rigors and hypotension) suggesting systemic infection
- Oral amoxicillin-clavulanate *plus* ciprofloxacin

---

1) Clinically suspected intravenous catheter-related infections
2) Known colonization with penicillin- and cephalosporin-resistant pneumococci or methicillin-resistant *S aureus* (MRSA)
3) Positive blood culture results for gram-positive bacteria before final identification and susceptibility testing
4) Hemodynamically unstable patient
5) Recent or current antimicrobial prophylaxis with a fluoroquinolone
6) Significant mucositis and high institutional rates of penicillin-resistant viridans streptococci

c. Empirical vancomycin therapy should be discontinued in 72 hours if no resistant gram-positive bacteria have been isolated

> **Box 38.3**
>
> **Evaluation of Response to Empirical Therapy After 3-5 Days**
>
> Patient is responding to therapy (fever is resolving with clinical improvement)
>   Infectious cause identified
>   Discontinue vancomycin therapy (if started) if cultures are negative for resistant gram-positive bacteria
>   Antimicrobial should be the most appropriate one according to susceptibility data
>   Duration of therapy depends on infection syndrome, recovery of neutrophils, and the identified bacterial or fungal pathogen (duration of therapy for filamentous fungal infection is typically weeks to months)
>   Depending on expected duration of neutropenia and patient's infection risk factors, consider continuing broad-spectrum therapy against gram-negative bacteria
>   Infectious cause not identified
>   Discontinue vancomycin therapy (if started) if cultures are negative for resistant gram-positive bacteria
>   Continue antimicrobial therapy until recovery of neutrophils ≥500 cells/μL for 2 consecutive days and patient is afebrile for ≥48 h
>   If neutropenia is expected to be quite prolonged and the patient is clinically improved, consider changing to an oral route of administration for hospital discharge or eventually stopping the use of antibiotics (after 2 wk) if the patient can continue to be closely monitored and does not have mucositis, ulcerations, catheter site infection, or any plans for immediate invasive procedures or additional ablative chemotherapy
> Patient has no response to therapy, fever persists, or clinical condition worsens
>   Infectious cause not identified
>   If patient's condition is stable despite continuation of fever, consider stopping vancomycin therapy
>   Decide whether to change or add antimicrobial therapy on the basis of patient's clinical status and any new clinical, laboratory, or radiologic findings that support potential infectious causes
>   If vancomycin is not already being used, consider administering it after 2-3 d
>   If patient is febrile for 5-7 d, consider adding antifungal agent (with activity against filamentous fungi) such as voriconazole, caspofungin, or an amphotericin product
>   If patient is clinically unstable
>   Broaden antimicrobial coverage to cover resistant gram-negative and gram-positive bacteria and anaerobes
>   Consider adding antifungal therapy for yeast and filamentous fungi
> Additional considerations for prolonged fever when no infectious cause has been identified for a clinically stable patient
>   Drug fever (antimicrobial or other medication)
>   Tumor fever and other noninfectious causes of fever

        in culture and the patient is clinically stable
    d. Consider subsequent addition of vancomycin when a patient with neutropenia is not responding to initial antibacterial therapy and no pathogen has been isolated
B. Bloodstream Infections
   1. Bacteria
     a. Bacteria associated with the highest mortality: enteric gram-negative bacteria and *P aeruginosa*
     b. More common bloodstream isolates: gram-positive bacteria
       1) Viridans streptococci (especially *Streptococcus mitis*, *Streptococcus oralis*, *Streptococcus salivarius*, and *Streptococcus milleri*)
         a) Toxic shock–like syndrome in 10% of neutropenic patients
         b) Usual source is oral flora when chemotherapy-associated mucositis or stomatitis is present
         c) Resistance to penicillin and second- and third-generation cephalosporins is increasing, so that vancomycin should be considered until susceptibility results are available
       2) *Staphylococcus aureus*
         a) Highly virulent bacteria
         b) Increasing rates of nosocomial and community-acquired MRSA infections
       3) *Staphylococcus epidermidis* and other coagulase-negative staphylococci: commonly associated with line and other foreign body infections
       4) Vancomycin-resistant enterococci (commonly *Enterococcus faecium*)
       5) *Bacillus cereus*
         a) Often associated with line infections
         b) Penicillin resistant
       6) *Corynebacterium jeikeium*
         a) Common line-associated pathogen
         b) Penicillin resistant
       7) *Leuconostoc* species
         a) Gram-positive coccus
         b) Commonly mistaken for viridans streptococcus
         c) Resistant to vancomycin
     c. Anaerobic bacteria
       1) *Clostridium septicum*
         a) Enteric pathogen
         b) Associated with neutropenic colitis (typhlitis), colonic malignancy, and other bowel disorders
       2) *Lactobacillus* species

a) Commensal organism of mouth, gastrointestinal tract, and genitourinary tract
b) Resistant to vancomycin
3) *Leptotrichia buccalis*: usually associated with oral stomatitis
2. Fungi
a. Yeast
1) *Candida* species: common sources include intravenous catheters and alimentary tract
a) *Candida albicans*: fourth most common isolate from blood cultures with positive results
b) *Candida glabrata*: may be susceptible, dose-dependent susceptible, or resistant to fluconazole
c) *Candida krusei*: resistant to fluconazole
d) *Candida parapsilosis*
i) Commonly associated with line infections
ii) Echinocandin minimum inhibitory concentration is slightly higher than with other *Candida* species (clinical relevance is unclear)
2) *Cryptococcus neoformans*
a) Respiratory tract is typical source
b) Need to perform lumbar puncture to evaluate for central nervous system disease
c) *Cryptococcus gatti* (also known as *C neoformans* var *gatti*) emerged as a human pathogen in the Pacific Northwest (including Vancouver Island), surrounding areas within Canada, and the northwestern United States
i) Higher likelihood for development of cryptococcomas in brain, lung, and other tissues
ii) Slower response to antifungal therapy
iii) Infection also occurs in immunocompetent patients
C. Respiratory Tract Infections
1. Bacterial infection: community-acquired or nosocomial pathogens
2. Fungal pneumonitis: *Aspergillus* species, agents of mucormycosis, and other filamentous fungi
a. Hemoptysis is common owing to the angioinvasive tendency of *Aspergillus* and the agents of mucormycosis
b. Novel pathogens that should be considered
1) *Aspergillus* species (*Aspergillus fumigatus*, *Aspergillus versicolor*, *Aspergillus flavus*, *Aspergillus terreus*, and others)
a) Morphology: septate hyphae branching at 45° angles
b) Angioinvasive: involvement of blood vessels with tissue infarction
c) Multiple organ systems can be infected: lungs, sinus, central nervous system, etc
d) Susceptibility to amphotericin B: *A terreus* is typically resistant and *A flavus* has variable susceptibility
2) The agents of mucormycosis (*Rhizopus* species, *Absidia* species, *Cunninghamella* species, *Rhizomucor* species, *Syncephalastrum* species, *Mucor* species, *Saksenaea* species, and *Apophysomyces* species)
a) Morphology: broad, nonseptate (or rarely septate) hyphae with short, stubby, and typical right-angle branching
b) Angioinvasive disease with extensive tissue infarction and often black, necrotic lesions
c) Staining
i) Gomori methenamine silver stain: variable
ii) Hematoxylin-eosin and periodic acid-Schiff stains: may be more reliable for identifying hyphae
d) Growth in culture may be hindered by the highly fragile nature of aseptate hyphae in processed or ground tissue specimens
3) Other common pulmonary filamentous fungi: *Scedosporium apiospermum*, the asexual form (anamorph) of *Pseudallescheria boydii*
c. Clinical considerations
1) Isolation of *Aspergillus* species or other filamentous fungi in sputum samples
a) Can reflect airway colonization in an immunocompetent host (especially with chronic obstructive pulmonary disease and bronchiectasis)

b) Should be considered *pathogenic* in patients with neutropenia (typically not discounted as colonization in these hosts)
2) A sputum culture positive for *Aspergillus* in patients with leukemia or soon after HSCT has a positive predictive value of 80% to 90%
3) A negative sputum fungal culture does not exclude the diagnosis of invasive pulmonary aspergillosis or mucormycosis
   a) Results of sputum stains and cultures can be negative in up to 70% of patients with confirmed invasive pulmonary aspergillosis
   b) With the exception of *Fusarium* species, blood cultures are rarely positive for mold infections
d. Radiologic findings are variable
   1) Bronchopneumonia and subpleural nodules (solitary or multiple)
   2) Cavitation: more common with neutrophil recovery or postengraftment phase (BMT)
   3) Halo sign (in early-stage disease): a zone of ground-glass attenuation of alveolar hemorrhage surrounding an inflammatory focus of fungal infection
   4) Air crescent sign (in late-stage disease): a crescent-shaped air-filled lucency adjacent to nodule or focus of fungal infection
      a) Develops with tissue necrosis and usually correlates with recovery from neutropenia

D. Fungal Sinus Infections
   1. Clinical considerations
      a. More common after chemotherapy in patients who have prolonged neutropenia
      b. Infection is acquired through inhalation of fungal spores into nasal mucosa and paranasal sinuses
      c. Tissue necrosis of nasal septum and turbinates
      d. High potential for rapid spread of fungal disease through palate and cribriform plate to orbit and brain: requires urgent medical care
      e. Treatment includes prompt surgical (nasal endoscopic) intervention with systemic antifungal therapy
   2. Common pathogens that should be considered
      a. The agents of mucormycosis (especially *Rhizopus* species)
      b. *Aspergillus* species
      c. Other molds
   3. Complications
      a. Cavernous sinus thrombosis
      b. Orbital invasion, requiring enucleation
      c. Invasion of cerebral tissue resulting in high patient mortality

E. Gastrointestinal Tract Infections
   1. Oral stomatitis and esophagitis
      a. Common effect after chemotherapy
      b. Common pathogens include herpes simplex virus (reactivation) and *Candida*
      c. In severe cases, the patient's ability to maintain adequate oral hydration and nutrition can be significantly impaired
   2. Typhlitis (neutropenic colitis)
      a. Occurs in patients after receiving cytotoxic chemotherapy with subsequent profound and prolonged neutropenia
      b. The symptoms are variable but can include fever, diarrhea, and pain in the right lower abdominal quadrant
      c. The cecum is typically involved with extension along ascending colon
      d. Cecal or colonic inflammation can lead to tissue necrosis and microbial bowel-wall translocation or perforation
      e. Enteric organisms, including *Clostridium septicum*, are typically involved
   3. *Clostridium difficile* colitis
      a. Antimicrobial-associated diarrhea: common in hematology patients
      b. Sigmoid colon is a common site, but other colonic regions may be involved
      c. High toxin-producing strain (from bacterial regulatory gene deletion) is becoming more prevalent in hospitals and communities

F. Hepatobiliary Infections
   1. Hepatosplenic candidiasis (chronic disseminated candidiasis)
      a. A distinct form of chronic *Candida* infection
         1) Most commonly seen in patients treated for acute leukemia or after allogeneic stem cell transplant
         2) Primarily involves the liver and spleen and occasionally the kidneys
      b. Most common species is *C albicans*; others include *Candida tropicalis*, *C parapsilosis*, *C glabrata*, and *C krusei*
   2. Risk factors
      a. Prolonged neutropenia

            b. Enteric mucosal disruption (eg, chemotherapy associated)
            c. Use of broad-spectrum antibacterial agents
            d. Intravenous catheters
        3. Clinical presentation
            a. Symptoms are often vague and nonspecific
            b. Patients may present during period of neutropenia or during neutrophil recovery
                1) Fever develops during period of neutropenia or upon neutrophil recovery
                2) Fever nonresponsive to antibacterial therapy
                3) Findings upon neutrophil recovery
                    a) New fever or continuation or progression of fever
                    b) Elevation of alkaline phosphatase level
                    c) New or worsening right upper abdominal quadrant pain, nausea, and anorexia
        4. Radiologic findings with abdominal computed tomography, magnetic resonance imaging, or ultrasonography
            a. Liver and splenic lesions may or may not be visible during neutropenic period
            b. Lesions usually become more prominent and visible during neutrophil recovery
                1) Multiple small round hypoechoic or low attenuated lesions scattered throughout liver and spleen
                2) Lesions may later calcify
                3) Lesions may persist despite successful therapy because of focal scarring and chronic inactive granulomatous changes during healing
        5. Diagnosis
            a. Predominantly a clinical diagnosis in the appropriate setting with supportive radiologic findings
            b. Liver biopsy
                1) May show granulomas or microabscesses
                2) Results of fungal stains and cultures for *Candida* are commonly negative
                3) Biopsy is often problematic because of high prevalence of thrombocytopenia and subsequent bleeding risk of procedure
            c. Blood culture results are usually negative
        6. Antifungal therapy
            a. Duration is individualized and prolonged—usually for months
            b. Amphotericin product, echinocandin, or fluconazole can be used
            c. Because of the necessity for prolonged antifungal therapy, patients with stable hematopoietic stem cells on treatment (no radiologically new or expanding lesions and clinical stability) may receive additional chemotherapy or proceed to HSCT with close monitoring
    G. Novel Cutaneous Infections
        1. Bacterial infections
            a. Most common causes are staphylococci and streptococci infections, including intravenous catheter associated and community acquired
            b. Ecthyma gangrenosum
                1) Predominantly occurs in patients with neutropenia
                2) Most common cause is *P aeruginosa*
                3) Less common causes include *Klebsiella* species, *Serratia* species, *Aeromonas hydrophila*, *E coli*, and some fungi
                4) Clinical presentation typically includes solitary or multiple hemorrhagic and necrotic lesions that form 1 or more gangrenous ulcers with a gray-black eschar with surrounding erythematous rim
        2. Fungal infections
            a. *Fusarium* species
                1) Typically a disseminated infection
                2) Multiple painful papules that become necrotic
                3) Skin lesions commonly present in the extremities
            b. Agents of mucormycosis
                1) Disseminated disease or localized infection through inoculation or trauma
                2) Erythematous lesions with central, commonly black, tissue necrosis
            c. *Aspergillus* species
                1) Disseminated disease or localized infection
                2) Rapidly progressive erythema with necrotic, ulcerated center
                3) Can resemble pyoderma gangrenosum
            d. *Candida* species
                1) Typically causes disseminated infection
                2) Various clinical cutaneous manifestations
                    a) May appear as macronodular lesions (nodules that are 0.5-1 cm, pink or red, and single or widely distributed)
                    b) May appear as intertrigo

c) Occasionally resembles ecthyma gangrenosum and purpura fulminans
e. *Cryptococcus neoformans*
1) Extrapulmonary disseminated disease
2) Various types of skin lesions
a) Nodular or maculopapular lesions
b) Ulcerations
f. Dematiaceous fungi
1) Agents of phaeohyphomycosis (hyphomycosis caused by dark-walled fungi)
2) Cutaneous and subcutaneous dematiaceous (dark-walled) fungal infections
a) May begin as erythematous nodule
b) Typical initial cyst development followed by progressive tissue destruction and necrosis

VI. Intravascular Catheter Infections
A. General Principles
1. Hematology patients (especially patients receiving therapy for leukemia and allogeneic BMT) compose one of the largest patient groups requiring long-term central intravenous and tunneled catheter placement
a. These patients require repetitive chemotherapy and blood product replacement (eg, red blood cell and platelet transfusions), and maintenance of a functional intravascular line is often crucial
b. Catheter infections are quite common in this patient group, and management depends on the specific catheter in place, type of infection, and causative pathogen
2. Intravascular catheters
a. Nontunneled central venous catheters
1) Pose a higher risk of line infection than do surgically implanted or tunneled cuffed catheters, subcutaneous central venous ports (ie, Groshong catheters), and peripherally inserted central catheters (PICCs)
2) Most common pathogens: coagulase-negative staphylococci, *S aureus, Candida* species, and enteric gram-negative bacilli
b. Surgically placed, tunneled, and other long-term intravascular catheters (includes Hickman, Broviac, and Palindrome catheters; subcutaneous central ports; and PICCs)
1) Almost universal use in the treatment of most leukemias and in patients receiving allogeneic HSCT
2) Most common pathogens: coagulase-negative staphylococci, enteric gram-negative bacilli, *S aureus*, and *P aeruginosa*
c. Primary sources of catheter-related infections
1) Skin flora at exit site of catheter
2) Contamination of the catheter hub
3) Contamination of the infused solution
4) Secondary hematogenous organism seeding of the intravascular line
B. Management of Infected Intravascular Catheters
1. Short-term catheters
a. Generally, the recommendation is to remove the catheter and treat for 7 to 14 days with antimicrobial therapy
b. For uncomplicated infections with coagulase-negative staphylococci and when immediate line removal is not feasible, retain the catheter and treat with systemic and antimicrobial intraluminal lock therapy for 10 to 14 days
2. Long-term catheters
a. Complicated infection
1) Subcutaneous tunnel infection or port abscess
a) Remove catheter
b) Administer antimicrobial therapy for 7 to 10 days
2) Patients with endocarditis or severe sepsis
a) Remove catheter
b) Administer antimicrobial therapy for 4 to 6 weeks for endocarditis and for 6 to 8 weeks for osteomyelitis
b. Uncomplicated infection
1) Coagulase-negative staphylococci
a) Can attempt line salvage with 10 to 14 days of systemic and intraluminal antimicrobial lock therapy
b) Remove the catheter if bacteremia is persistent or if patient is deteriorating clinically
2) *Staphylococcus aureus*
a) Generally, the recommendation is to remove the catheter and treat for 4 to 6 weeks with antimicrobial therapy

b) Can consider shorter duration of antimicrobial therapy if patient meets the following criteria
   i) Patient has prompt clearing of bloodstream after starting antimicrobial therapy
   ii) Patient has no evidence of endocarditis, infected thrombosis, or other metastatic complication of *S aureus* infection
   iii) Patient is immunocompetent or not diabetic
   iv) Patient has no prosthetic intravascular device
c) In very select cases of uncomplicated, transient, and low-grade *S aureus* catheter-associated bloodstream infection when immediate line removal is not feasible, line salvage can be considered with a combination of systemic and intraluminal antimicrobial lock therapy

3) *Enterococcus* species
   a) Can attempt line salvage with 7 to 14 days of systemic and intraluminal antimicrobial lock therapy
   b) Remove the catheter if bacteremia is persistent or if patient is deteriorating clinically

4) Gram-negative bacilli
   a) Can attempt line salvage with 10 to 14 days of systemic and intraluminal antimicrobial lock therapy
   b) Remove the catheter if bacteremia is persistent or if patient is deteriorating clinically

5) *Candida* species
   a) Remove the catheter and treat with antifungal therapy for 14 days beyond the first negative blood culture

3. Indications for removal of long-term catheter in catheter-associated bloodstream infection
   a. Line-associated intravascular infected thrombosis
   b. Subcutaneous tunnel infection or port abscess
   c. Endocarditis or severe sepsis
   d. Blood cultures persistently positive beyond 72 hours despite administration of antimicrobial therapy to which the isolated organisms are susceptible
   e. Infection caused by *S aureus*, *P aeruginosa*, fungi, or mycobacteria
   f. Consider line removal for select, less virulent but more drug-resistant pathogens (eg, *Bacillus* species, *Micrococcus* species, *Propionibacterium* species) if contamination has been excluded

Suggested Reading

Freifeld AG, Bow EJ, Sepkowitz KA, Boeckh MJ, Ito JI, Mullen CA, et al. Clinical practice guideline for the use of antimicrobial agents in neutropenic patients with cancer: 2010 update by the Infectious Diseases Society of America. Clin Infect Dis. 2011 Feb;52(4):e56–93.

Marr KA. Fungal infections in oncology patients: update on epidemiology, prevention, and treatment. Curr Opin Oncol. 2010 Mar;22(2):138–42.

Mermel LA, Allon M, Bouza E, Craven DE, Flynn P, O'Grady NP, et al. Clinical practice guidelines for the diagnosis and management of intravascular catheter-related infection: 2009 Update by the Infectious Diseases Society of America. Clin Infect Dis. 2009 Jul 1;49(1):1–45. Errata in: Clin Infect Dis. 2010 Feb 1;50(3):457. Clin Infect Dis. 2010 Apr 1;50(7):1079. Dosage error in article text.

Person AK, Kontoyiannis DP, Alexander BD. Fungal infections in transplant and oncology patients. Infect Dis Clin North Am. 2010 Jun;24(2):439–59.

Wingard JR, Hsu J, Hiemenz JW. Hematopoietic stem cell transplantation: an overview of infection risks and epidemiology. Infect Dis Clin North Am. 2010 Jun;24(2):257–72.

Raymund R. Razonable, MD

Infections in Transplant Recipients

I. General Principles
   A. Importance of Infections
      1. Most common complication of organ transplant
      2. Caused by bacteria, fungi, viruses, and parasites
         a. Nosocomial or health care–associated pathogens (*Staphylococcus aureus*, enterococci, *Pseudomonas aeruginosa*, and others)
         b. Opportunistic pathogens (cytomegalovirus [CMV], *Aspergillus fumigatus*, *Pneumocystis jiroveci*, polyomaviruses BK virus and JC virus, and others)
         c. Community-acquired pathogens (*Streptococcus pneumoniae* and respiratory viruses)
   B. Determinants of Risk of Infection After Transplant
      1. Epidemiologic exposures (exposure history for both donor and recipient)
      2. Net state of immunosuppression
         a. Antirejection immunosuppressive drugs
         b. Graft-vs-host disease (GVHD) prophylaxis and treatment
         c. Cytotoxic chemotherapy
         d. Immunomodulating viruses
         e. Inherent defects in innate and adaptive immunity
   C. Pharmacologic Immunosuppression
      1. Essential for prevention of acute allograft rejection (in solid organ transplant) or GVHD (in allogeneic hematopoietic stem cell transplant)
      2. Impairs the ability to mount an adequate immune response during infection
      3. Leads to generally more severe infections
      4. Leads to atypical manifestations of infections
   D. Prevention of Infection
      1. Major goal in management of transplant patients
      2. Detailed risk assessment before transplant
         a. Detailed history taking
         b. Infectious disease serologic testing
      3. Vaccination
         a. Updated for all at-risk patients before and after transplant
         b. Vaccination with live viruses is avoided after transplant
      4. Antibacterial, antiviral, and antifungal prophylaxis
         a. Antibacterial prophylaxis during period of neutropenia in allogeneic stem cell transplant recipients
         b. Antiherpetic and anti-CMV prophylaxis to all at-risk patients

c. Antifungal prophylaxis to lung recipients, allogeneic hematopoietic stem cell transplant recipients, and selected liver and kidney recipients
     1) Prevention of *Aspergillus* species infection in lung and high-risk allogeneic hematopoietic stem cell transplant recipients
     2) Prevention of *Candida* species infections during neutropenia
  E. Early Diagnosis of Infection
     1. Key to successful treatment
     2. Routine surveillance testing
        a. Culture of blood and other body fluids
        b. Stool or rectal cultures to detect colonization with vancomycin-resistant enterococci
     3. Culture of explanted and implanted tissues and organs
     4. Molecular surveillance tests
        a. CMV polymerase chain reaction (PCR) and pp65 antigenemia assays
        b. BK virus PCR testing of urine and plasma, and decoy cell detection in urine (in kidney transplant recipients)
  F. Treatment of Infections
     1. Should be initiated as early as possible
     2. Empirical therapy: administered as soon as infection is suspected and after appropriate samples for cultures have been collected
     3. Pathogen-specific therapy: provided as soon as the cause is established
     4. Decreased doses for pharmacologic immunosuppression should complement antimicrobial therapy
        a. Monitor for the development of acute graft rejection
        b. Monitor drug levels of cyclosporine, tacrolimus, and others
     5. Surgical drainage and débridement: essential components to therapy
        a. Drainage of infected fluid collections (ie, infected hematoma and abdominal abscesses)
        b. Débridement of surgical site infections
        c. Removal of infected intravascular and urinary catheters
II. Risk Factors for Infection After Transplant
  A. Epidemiologic Exposures
     1. Major sources of pathogens after organ and tissue transplant are listed in Box 39.1
     2. Endogenous source: transplant recipient may harbor latent, active, or subclinical infection
        a. Assess epidemiologic exposures of potential transplant recipients
        b. Recommended screening tools to evaluate potential recipients and donors before transplant are listed in Box 39.2
        c. Pathogens generally screened: herpes simplex virus (HSV)-1 and HSV-2, varicella-zoster virus (VZV), Epstein-Barr virus (EBV), CMV, human T-lymphotropic virus (HTLV)-1 and HTLV-2, hepatitis viruses, *Mycobacterium tuberculosis*, *Toxoplasma gondii* (in heart transplant recipients), and *Treponema pallidum*
        d. Specialized screening tests (for selected patients): *Coccidioides immitis*, *Strongyloides stercoralis*, or *Trypanosoma cruzi*
        e. Most active infections do not absolutely contraindicate transplant

---

Box 39.1

Epidemiologic Exposures and Examples of Associated Pathogens in the Evaluation of Transplant Patients With Infectious Syndromes

Community-acquired infections
  Residence in endemic areas
    Mycobacterium tuberculosis
    Strongyloides stercoralis
    Blastomyces dermatitidis
    Histoplasma capsulatum
    Coccidioides immitis
    Trypanosoma cruzi
  Exposure to index cases
    M tuberculosis
    Respiratory viruses (influenza virus, parainfluenza virus, respiratory syncytial virus, adenoviruses)
  Ingestion of contaminated water and food
    Salmonella species
    Campylobacter jejuni
    Listeria monocytogenes
    Giardia lamblia
  Environmental source
    Aspergillus fumigatus
    Nocardia asteroides
    Sporothrix schenckii
  Vector borne
    West Nile virus
    Tick-borne diseases
Nosocomial infections
  Contaminated air
    A fumigatus
  Contaminated water
    Legionella pneumophila
  Hand contact
    Methicillin-resistant *Staphylococcus aureus*
    Vancomycin-resistant enterococci
    Drug-resistant gram-negative bacilli

Adapted from Razonable RR, Paya CV. Infections in transplant patients. In: Schlossberg D, editor. Clinical infectious disease. New York (NY): Cambridge University Press; c2008. p. 611–23. Used with permission.

Box 39.2

Suggested Screening Tools in the Evaluation of Donors and Recipients Before Transplant

Human immunodeficiency virus (HIV) antibody[a]
Herpes simplex virus (HSV)-1 and HSV-2 antibodies
Cytomegalovirus (CMV) antibody[a]
Epstein-Barr virus (EBV) antibody panel[a]
Varicella-zoster virus (VZV) antibody
Toxoplasma antibody (in heart recipients)
Rapid plasma reagin test for syphilis
Human T-lymphotropic virus (HTLV)-1 and HTLV-2 antibodies
Hepatitis C virus (HCV) antibody[a]
Hepatitis B virus (HBV) serology[a]
Purified protein derivative (tuberculin) (PPD) skin testing
Strongyloides serology (with stool examination for ova and parasites for transplant candidates from areas where *Strongyloides* is endemic)
Coccidioides serology (for transplant candidates from areas where *Coccidioides* is endemic)
Trypanosoma cruzi (for donors and recipients from areas where *T cruzi* is endemic)
West Nile virus (nucleic acid testing for living donors)

[a] Donors should be tested for these pathogens at the minimum.

Adapted from Razonable RR, Paya CV. Infections in transplant patients. In: Schlossberg D, editor. Clinical infectious disease. New York (NY): Cambridge University Press; c2008. p. 611–23. Used with permission.

1) Infection should be adequately controlled before transplant
2) Examples of common active infections before transplant
    a) Ascending bacterial cholangitis and spontaneous bacterial peritonitis (liver transplant candidates)
    b) Pacemaker and other cardiac device–associated infections (heart transplant candidates)
    c) Hemodialysis and other vascular catheters (kidney transplant candidates)
    d) Bacterial and fungal lung infections (lung transplant candidates)
    e) Vascular access infections and bacteremia (bone marrow transplant candidates)
3. Donor-transmitted infections: allograft donor may harbor latent, active, or subclinical infection
    a. Screening tools are used to assess epidemiologic exposures and risk factors involving transplant donors (Box 39.2)
    b. Routine screening is not indicated for unusual infections unless there are epidemiologic clues
        1) Examples of donor-transmitted infections: CMV, EBV, *T gondii*, hepatitis B virus (HBV), hepatitis C virus (HCV), and human immunodeficiency virus (HIV)
        2) Examples of unusual infections: *Histoplasma capsulatum*, *Cryptococcus neoformans*, lymphocytic choriomeningitis virus, rabies virus, and West Nile virus
4. Exogenous source: the environment of the hospital or the community
    a. Health care environment
        1) A main source of infectious pathogens
        2) Procedures and practices that increase the risk of infection (Box 39.3)
            a) Transplant surgery
                i) Prolonged and complicated surgery
                ii) Involvement of areas of high microbial load (gastrointestinal tract in liver and intestinal transplant)

Box 39.3

Risk Factors for Acquiring Infections After Solid Organ Transplant

Preoperative period
  Lack of pathogen-specific immunity
  Severity of underlying clinical illness
  Fulminant hepatic failure
  Renal insufficiency
  Anemia
  Prior fungal infection (ie, endemic mycosis)
  Prior bacterial or fungal colonization (*Aspergillus* species or *Pseudomonas aeruginosa* in a patient with cystic fibrosis)
Intraoperative period
  Presence of pathogens in the transplant allograft
  Prolonged operative time
  Complicated surgical procedure
  Profound blood loss and infusion of large volume of blood products
  Choledochojejunostomy
Postoperative period
  Prolonged hospitalization
  Prolonged duration of stay in intensive care unit
  Prolonged antibiotic use
  Renal insufficiency
  Gastrointestinal tract and biliary complications
  Vascular complications
  Corticosteroid use and treatment of allograft rejection
  Immunosuppressive drugs
  CMV and HHV-6 reactivation
  Reoperation within 1 mo after transplant
  Retransplantation

Abbreviations: CMV, cytomegalovirus; HHV, human herpesvirus.

Adapted from Razonable RR, Paya CV. Infections in transplant patients. In: Schlossberg D, editor. Clinical infectious disease. New York (NY): Cambridge University Press; c2008. p. 611–23. Used with permission.

iii) Surgical reexploration (retransplant, bleeding, and other vascular complications)
iv) Type of biliary duct anastomosis (eg, choledochojejunostomy)
b) Indwelling urinary catheters
i) Bacterial (*Escherichia coli*) urosepsis
ii) Fungal (*Candida glabrata*) urinary infections
c) Intravascular catheters
i) Bacteremia due to methicillin-resistant *S aureus* (MRSA)
ii) *Candida albicans* fungemia
d) Endotracheal tubes and mechanical ventilation: pneumonia due to drug-resistant organisms such as *P aeruginosa*
e) Antibiotic use: *Clostridium difficile*–associated colitis
f) Blood transfusion: West Nile virus (nucleic acid testing of donated blood products is recommended)
g) Hospital construction and renovations: *Aspergillus* species infections
h) Water supply: *Legionella pneumophila* pneumonia
i) Numerous gram-positive and gram-negative bacteria may be acquired in hospitals, including multidrug-resistant *P aeruginosa*, vancomycin-resistant enterococci, and MRSA
b. Community-acquired infections (natural transmission)
1) Seasonal infections with respiratory viruses, such as influenza virus, parainfluenza, metapneumovirus, and respiratory syncytial virus
2) Pneumonia due to *S pneumoniae*, *Haemophilus influenzae*, *Mycoplasma pneumoniae*, and *Chlamydia* species
3) Community-onset skin and soft tissue infections due to *Staphylococcus* species and streptococci
4) Community-onset opportunistic pathogens: *Pneumocystis jiroveci*, *Listeria monocytogenes*, *T gondii*, and *C neoformans*
B. Main Factors Influencing the Net State of Immunosuppression
1. Pharmacologic immunosuppression
   a. Prevent allograft rejection (solid organ transplant recipients) and GVHD (allogeneic hematopoietic stem cell transplant recipients)
   b. Most intense level during the first 3 months after transplant
   c. Drugs associated with increased risk of infections
      1) Mycophenolate mofetil: CMV, HCV
      2) Prednisone: *P jiroveci*, CMV, human herpesvirus (HHV)-6, fungi
      3) Alemtuzumab: CMV, *C neoformans*
      4) Muromonab-CD3 (OKT3): CMV, EBV
   d. The combined effect of multiple drugs further enhances the risk
2. Immunomodulating viruses
   a. Virus reactivation is common with immunosuppressive drugs: paradoxically enhances the overall state of immunosuppression
   b. Viruses with immunomodulating properties: CMV and HHV-6
      1) CMV and HHV-6 infections increase the risk of bacterial and fungal opportunistic infections
      2) CMV and HHV-6 accelerate the course of posttransplant HCV
III. Timing of Infections After Transplant
  A. Temporal Patterns
    1. Timing of infections after solid organ transplant is shown in Figure 39.1
    2. Timing of infections after allogeneic hematopoietic stem cell transplant is shown in Figure 39.2
    3. Natural course and epidemiology of transplant infections is influenced by antimicrobial prophylaxis
       a. Example: CMV disease
         1) Generally occurs 2 to 3 months after solid organ transplant and within 100 days after allogeneic hematopoietic stem cell transplant
         2) Antiviral prophylaxis delays the onset of CMV disease to 3 to 6 months after solid organ transplant and to more than 100 days after allogeneic hematopoietic stem cell transplant
       b. Example: fluconazole prophylaxis leads to emergence of infections caused by fluconazole-resistant *Candida* species
  B. After Solid Organ Transplant
    1. First month: 3 major sources of infections
       a. Endogenous infection (present in the recipient before transplant)
         1) Bacterial peritonitis in liver recipients

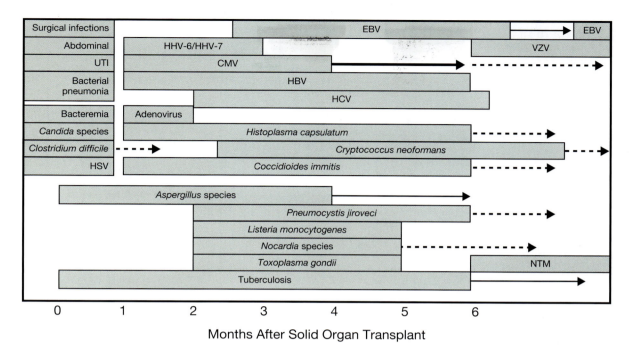

Figure 39.1. Timeline of Infections After Solid Organ Transplant. Thin-shafted arrow indicates persistent but lower risk; thick-shafted arrow, persistent but intermediate risk; broken-line–shafted arrow, episodic. CMV indicates cytomegalovirus; EBV, Epstein-Barr virus; HBV, hepatitis B virus; HCV, hepatitis C virus; HHV, human herpesvirus; HSV, herpes simplex virus; NTM, nontuberculous mycobacteria; UTI, urinary tract infection; VZV, varicella-zoster virus. (Adapted from Razonable RR, Paya CV. Infections in transplant patients. In: Schlossberg D, editor. Clinical infectious disease. New York [NY]: Cambridge University Press; c2008. p. 611–23. Used with permission.)

2) Vascular line–related bacteremia in renal transplant recipients
3) Infected cardiac device in heart transplant recipients
4) Reactivation of latent HSV in HSV-seropositive transplant recipient
   a) Common viral opportunistic pathogen
   b) Antiviral prophylaxis (acyclovir or valganciclovir) reduces the incidence of HSV
b. Donor-transmitted infection (transmitted from the allograft)
   1) CMV, EBV, HIV, and HCV
   2) *Histoplasma capsulatum* and *C neoformans*
   3) Various bacterial and fungal pathogens
c. Infections related to surgery and hospitalization
   1) Constitute most infections during the first month
   2) Risk factors (Box 39.3)

a) Surgical site infections due to *Staphylococcus* species, *Streptococcus* species, or nosocomially acquired pathogens
b) Catheter-associated urinary tract infections with gram-negative bacteria such as *E coli*, gram-positive bacteria such as enterococcus, and fungi such as *C albicans*
c) Nosocomial and ventilator-associated pneumonia due to drug-resistant *P aeruginosa*, *Acinetobacter* species, *S aureus*, and others
d) Vascular catheter–associated bacteremia with gram-positive bacteria such as coagulase-negative staphylococci
e) Intra-abdominal infections and abscesses in patients who require abdominal reexploration

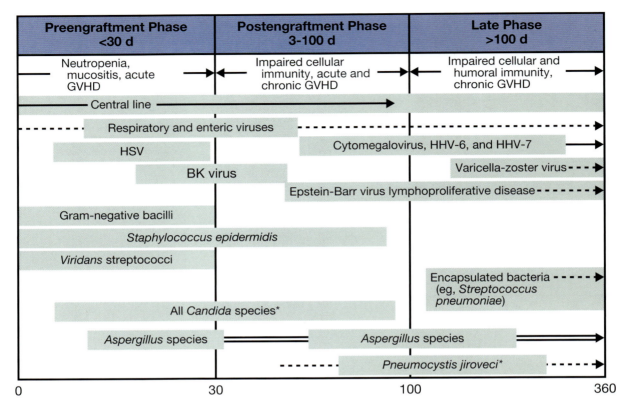

Figure 39.2. Timeline of Infections After Allogeneic Hematopoietic Stem Cell Transplant. Asterisk indicates without standard prophylaxis. Single-shafted arrow indicates continuous risk; double-shafted arrow, low incidence; broken-line–shafted arrow, episodic and endemic. GVHD indicates graft-vs-host disease; HHV, human herpesvirus; HSV, herpes simplex virus. (Adapted from Razonable RR, Paya CV. Infections in transplant patients. In: Schlossberg D, editor. Clinical infectious disease. New York [NY]: Cambridge University Press; c2008. p. 611–23. Used with permission.)

      (ie, hepatic artery thrombosis, portal vein thrombosis, biliary leakage, or retransplant)
    3) Prolonged hospitalization: increased risk of nosocomial pneumonia, urinary infections, bacteremia, and antibiotic-related *C difficile* diarrhea
2. Second to sixth month
  a. Most opportunistic infections occur during this period
  b. Two major types of infection
    1) Infection with immunomodulating virus: CMV, EBV, or HHV-6
      a) Without antiviral prophylaxis, viruses in the Betaherpesvirinae subfamily (CMV, HHV-6, and HHV-7) reactivate to cause disease
      b) Antiviral prophylaxis delays the onset of CMV disease to 3 to 6 months after transplant
    2) Infections resulting from impaired cell-mediated immunity
      a) Examples: CMV, EBV, *L monocytogenes*, *A fumigatus*, and *P jiroveci*
      b) Prophylaxis with trimethoprim-sulfamethoxazole to prevent *P jiroveci* infection also protects against bacterial infections caused by agents such as *Nocardia* species
      c) Invasive aspergillosis
        i) Most commonly due to *A fumigatus*
        ii) At-risk patients: patients with fulminant hepatitis,

epidemiologic exposure, prolonged neutropenia, or profound immunosuppression
  d) Infections with endemic fungi (eg, *H capsulatum, C immitis*) and *C neoformans*
3. After the sixth month
  a. Three categories of transplant recipients
    1) Patients with good allograft function and minimal immunosuppression: risk of infection is similar to that for nonimmunocompromised persons in the community
    2) Patients with chronic viral hepatitis: patients have an accelerated clinical course that progresses to allograft failure and a need for retransplant
    3) Patients with poor allograft function due to recurrent allograft rejection or chronic dysfunction
       a) Patients are generally overimmunosuppressed
       b) Patients remain at high-risk of opportunistic infections
       c) Examples of agents causing infections: *P jiroveci, L monocytogenes, C neoformans, Nocardia asteroides,* CMV, *Aspergillus* species
  b. Typical infections during this late period
    1) Endemic mycoses from fungi such as *H capsulatum* and *C immitis*
    2) Varicella zoster infection: peaks at 9 to 12 months after transplant
    3) EBV-related posttransplant lymphoproliferative disorder: severity ranges from infectious mononucleosis-like illness to fulminant and malignant non-Hodgkin lymphoma
    4) CMV infection may occur despite prolonged valganciclovir prophylaxis
C. After Hematopoietic Stem Cell Transplant
  1. Preengraftment period (0-30 days after transplant)
    a. Two major risk factors
      1) Neutropenia
      2) Disruption in mucocutaneous barrier
        a) Mucositis (gastrointestinal tract)
        b) Vascular access catheters
    b. Agents causing common infections
      1) *Candida* species
        a) Most prevalent fungal infection
        b) Fluconazole prophylaxis prevents many *C albicans* infections but could lead to *C glabrata* infections
      2) *Aspergillus* species
        a) Risk increases with duration of neutropenia
        b) Voriconazole or posaconazole prophylaxis prevents infection
      3) Herpes simplex virus
        a) Often complicates severe mucositis
        b) Acyclovir prophylaxis prevents infection
      4) Viridans streptococci
        a) May cause severe systemic infection and sepsis (mortality may be high)
        b) Septic shock is a common presentation
        c) Prophylaxis with trimethoprim-sulfamethoxazole or a fluoroquinolone is associated with increased risk of viridans streptococcal bacteremia and sepsis
      5) Other agents causing infections
        a) Gram-positive bacteria such as *S aureus* and coagulase-negative staphylococci
        b) Gram-negative bacteria such as *E coli* and *P aeruginosa*
        c) Fungi such as *C albicans*: entry into the bloodstream through indwelling vascular catheters
  2. Postengraftment period (30-100 days after transplant)
    a. Characterized by severe impairment in cell-mediated immunity
    b. Graft-vs-host disease
      1) With engraftment, the risk of GVHD is increased
      2) Immunosuppressive drugs to prevent GVHD (eg, cyclosporine, mycophenolate mofetil, methotrexate, prednisone) increase the risk of infections
    c. Pathogens causing classic infections during this period
      1) Cytomegalovirus
        a) Infection manifests as febrile syndrome or tissue-invasive disease (CMV pneumonia is associated with high mortality)
        b) CMV could delay engraftment of donor cells
        c) Anti-CMV prophylaxis delays the onset of CMV disease to beyond 100 days after transplant
        d) Anti-CMV prophylaxis with ganciclovir or valganciclovir is generally not used: myelosuppressive properties may delay engraftment

e) With preemptive therapy, use CMV PCR testing or pp65 antigenemia assay to monitor CMV reactivation and guide treatment
   2) Other pathogens during this period
      a) Fungi such as *Aspergillus* species, *Fusarium* species, *Mucor*, *Rhizopus* species, and *P jiroveci*
      b) Viruses such as HHV-6 and adenovirus
3. Late period (>100 days after transplant)
   a. Patients with persistent impairment in cell-mediated and humoral immunity
      1) Viruses causing common infections: CMV, VZV, and EBV
      2) Fungi causing common infections: *Aspergillus* species and *P jiroveci*
   b. Patients with adequate immune reconstitution
      1) Infections with community-acquired respiratory viruses such as influenza, parainfluenza, and respiratory viruses
      2) Infections with encapsulated bacteria such as *S pneumoniae* and *H influenzae*

IV. Specific Infectious Agents
   A. Bacterial
      1. Prevention of bacterial infections in solid organ transplant recipients (Table 39.1)
         a. Perioperative antibacterial prophylaxis with cefazolin or cefotaxime: prevents surgical site infections at time of transplant
         b. Oral selective bowel decontamination solution
            1) Contains mixture of antibiotics such as colistin, gentamicin, and nystatin
            2) Selective pressure to the intestinal flora to reduce colonization with gram-negative bacilli and fungi, while sparing the anaerobic organisms
            3) Reduces the incidence of bacterial (and fungal) infections
      2. Prevention of bacterial infections in hematopoietic stem cell transplant recipients (Table 39.1)
         a. Antibacterial prophylaxis with penicillin in combination with a fluoroquinolone: prevention of bacterial infections while patient has severe mucositis
            1) Fluoroquinolones and trimethoprim-sulfamethoxazole increase risk of infection and sepsis due to viridans streptococci
            2) Empirical treatment of febrile neutropenia: intravenous vancomycin and broad-spectrum cephalosporins or carbapenems
         b. Use of intravenous immunoglobulins
            1) For prevention of bacterial infections (sinopulmonary infections with *S pneumoniae*)
            2) For severe hypogammaglobulinemia during the first 100 days after transplant
   B. Viral
      1. Cytomegalovirus
         a. Main cause of morbidity and mortality after transplant
         b. Infection occurs usually within 3 months after transplant, but in both solid organ and hematopoietic stem cell transplant recipients, antiviral prophylaxis has delayed the onset of infection
         c. Direct and indirect effects
            1) Direct effects (CMV disease)
               a) CMV syndrome: febrile illness with myelosuppression
               b) CMV tissue-invasive disease: any organ system may be affected
                  i) CMV pneumonitis (common in lung and bone marrow transplants)
                  ii) Gastrointestinal tract disease (most common end-organ involvement)
                  iii) Hepatitis (liver recipients)
                  iv) Retinitis (rare)
                  v) Encephalitis (rare)
            2) Indirect effects
               a) Acute allograft rejection
               b) Other opportunistic infections such as invasive fungal disease and EBV–posttransplant lymphoproliferative disease (PTLD)
               c) Chronic allograft dysfunction
                  i) Transplant vascular sclerosis (heart transplant)
                  ii) Bronchiolitis obliterans (lung transplant)
                  iii) Vanishing bile duct syndrome (liver transplant)
                  iv) Tubulointerstitial fibrosis (chronic allograft nephropathy)
               d) GVHD after bone marrow transplant
         d. Risk factors for CMV disease
            1) CMV-mismatch status
               a) CMV-seropositive donor and CMV-seronegative recipient

Table 39.1
Examples of Antimicrobial Prophylactic Strategies After Transplant

Prophylactic Agent	Indication	Dosage	Comments
Cefotaxime	Perioperative prophylaxis	1 g every 8 h IV for 48 h	Adjustments are based on resistance patterns
Cefazolin	Perioperative prophylaxis	1 g every 8 h IV for 48 h	Adjustments are based on resistance patterns
Trimethoprim-sulfamethoxazole	*Pneumocystis jiroveci*	80 or 160 mg of trimethoprim component orally once daily	May also protect against *Nocardia* species, *Listeria* species, and other bacteria
Levofloxacin	Antibacterial prophylaxis	500 mg once daily until engraftment	Prophylaxis against bacterial pathogens in patients receiving allogeneic hematopoietic stem cell transplant
Penicillin V potassium	Antibacterial prophylaxis	Dose and duration variable	Prophylaxis against bacterial pathogens in patients receiving allogeneic hematopoietic stem cell transplant
Acyclovir	Herpes simplex virus	200 mg orally 3 times daily for 28 d	Withheld when ganciclovir or valganciclovir is used. Valacyclovir may be used if available
Valganciclovir	Cytomegalovirus	900 mg once daily. Duration is variable (often 3 mo)	Used as prophylaxis or preemptive therapy. May protect against HHV-6, HSV, VZV
Ganciclovir	Cytomegalovirus	1 g orally 3 times daily. Duration is variable (often 3 mo)	Used as prophylaxis or preemptive therapy. May protect against HHV-6, HSV, VZV
Fluconazole	*Candida* species	400 mg orally daily for 28 d	Administered to solid organ transplant patients with complicated and prolonged surgery or profound blood loss. Prophylaxis during period of neutropenia after allogeneic stem cell transplant
Voriconazole	Mycelial fungi	200 mg orally 2 times daily	Antifungal prophylaxis in patients at high risk of *Aspergillus* species infections (eg, lung transplant recipients and allogeneic hematopoietic stem cell transplant recipients with graft-vs-host disease)
Amphotericin B	*Aspergillus* species	0.2 mg/kg daily	Administered to patients with fulminant hepatic failure
Oral selective bowel decontamination solution	Gram-negative bacilli and fungi	Variable	Selective pressure favoring anaerobic environment, with goal of decreasing risk of fungal and bacterial infection
Hepatitis B immune globulin	Hepatitis B virus	10,000 international units daily for first week and then every 4 wk	Maintain serum level of hepatitis B immune globulin >100 international units. May be used in combination with lamivudine. Role of other agents (eg, adefovir) not yet defined

Abbreviations: HHV, human herpesvirus; HSV, herpes simplex virus; IV, intravenous; VZV, varicella-zoster virus.

Adapted from Razonable RR, Paya CV. Infections in transplant patients. In: Schlossberg D, editor. Clinical infectious disease. New York (NY): Cambridge University Press; c2008. p. 611–23. Used with permission.

(CMV D+/R−): highest risk after solid organ transplant
b) CMV-seropositive recipient (CMV R+): high risk after allogeneic hematopoietic stem cell transplant
c) CMV-seronegative donor and CMV-seronegative recipient (CMV D−/R−): lowest risk of CMV disease
2) Immunosuppressive regimens that increase the risk of CMV: muromonab-CD3, antithymocyte globulin, antilymphocyte globulin, alemtuzumab, and mycophenolate mofetil
3) Risk according to transplant type
   a) Lung or intestinal transplant presents greater risk than pancreas, liver, or heart transplant, which presents greater risk than kidney transplant
   b) Allogeneic transplant presents greater risk than autologous hematopoietic stem cell transplant
e. Diagnostic methods for CMV disease
   1) Viral culture: poor sensitivity but high specificity
   2) Serology: impaired antibody production after transplant

3) Histopathology: document tissue-invasive CMV disease
4) CMV pp65 antigenemia assay: detection of late viral antigen in leukocytes suggests active infection
5) Molecular diagnostic tests (eg, PCR assay): rapid, sensitive, and quantitative properties are useful in prognostication and monitoring of treatment

f. Prevention of CMV disease
1) Antiviral prophylaxis
   a) Administration of antiviral drugs (most commonly valganciclovir) to all patients at risk of CMV disease
   b) Usual duration of prophylaxis is 3 months, but can be prolonged in highest-risk patients (eg, CMV D+/R− lung recipients)
2) Preemptive therapy
   a) Administration of antiviral drugs (most commonly valganciclovir) to patients with evidence of asymptomatic CMV infection such as a positive result for pp65 antigenemia or CMV DNAemia
   b) Preferred in allogeneic bone marrow transplant patients to avoid myelosuppressive effect of valganciclovir that could delay engraftment
3) Use of leukocyte-reduced or CMV-seronegative red blood cells or leukocytes: prevents transfusion-associated CMV infection

g. Treatment of CMV disease
1) Intravenous ganciclovir, 5 mg/kg every 12 hours
   a) Drug of choice
   b) Dosage adjusted for renal function
2) Valganciclovir, 900 mg orally twice daily
   a) Dosage adjusted for renal function
   b) Effective in patients with nonsevere CMV disease
3) Main adverse effect of intravenous ganciclovir and valganciclovir: bone marrow suppression (leukopenia, thrombocytopenia, and anemia)
   a) Resolves with discontinuation of antiviral drug therapy
   b) Granulocyte growth factors may be needed occasionally
4) Alternative treatment regimens: for patients who cannot tolerate ganciclovir or who have ganciclovir-resistant CMV
   a) Cidofovir or foscarnet
      i) Inhibits CMV DNA polymerase
      ii) Adverse effects: nephrotoxicity and electrolyte imbalances
   b) Maribavir and leflunomide: experimental therapies
5) Viral load monitoring: assess response to treatment
6) Duration of antiviral treatment: at least 2 weeks but should be given until CMV is cleared from blood and tissues

2. Herpes simplex virus
a. Usually infection results from reactivation of endogenous latent virus
b. Rarely donor transmitted
c. Orolabial and genital ulcers: most common manifestation
d. Systemic or disseminated disease may occur: hepatitis, pneumonitis, and esophageal disease
e. Onset of disease: within first month after transplant
f. Incidence has decreased with antiviral prophylaxis
1) All HSV-seropositive patients should receive oral acyclovir
2) Ganciclovir is also effective against HSV-1 and HSV-2
3) In hematopoietic stem cell transplant recipients, acyclovir prophylaxis is administered from the start of conditioning therapy until engraftment occurs or mucositis resolves
g. Diagnosis of mucocutaneous HSV disease
1) Mainly based on clinical grounds
2) PCR testing shows HSV DNA and confirms the diagnosis
h. Treatment of HSV: acyclovir, valacyclovir, or famciclovir

3. Varicella-zoster virus
a. Usually a reactivation disease: more than 90% of adult transplant recipients have VZV antibodies
1) Most common manifestation: dermatomal zoster (monodermatomal or multidermatomal)
2) Disseminated disease may occur (if severe immunocompromise)
3) Incidence: about 10% of transplant patients
4) Onset of disease: typically 9 to 12 months after transplant

b. Diagnosis: clinical grounds with typical vesicular lesions
   1) Localized disease: lesions in a dermatomal distribution
   2) Disseminated disease: lesions in a widespread distribution
c. Treatment
   1) Serious disease: intravenous acyclovir
   2) Limited disease: oral acyclovir, famciclovir, or valacyclovir
d. Varicella vaccine
   1) VZV-seronegative transplant candidates should receive the vaccine to prevent primary varicella infection after transplant
   2) To avoid potential exposure, all family members, household contacts, and health care workers should receive the vaccine
   3) In hematopoietic stem cell transplant, vaccination should be completed at least 6 weeks before transplant
4. Epstein-Barr virus
   a. EBV causes most PTLDs (80%-90%)
   b. Types of lymphoproliferation
      1) Nodal or extranodal
      2) Symptomatic or subclinical
      3) Localized or disseminated
      4) Monoclonal or polyclonal
      5) True malignancies containing chromosomal malignancies
   c. Two patterns
      1) Early PTLD: occurs within 12 months after transplant
      2) Late PTLD: occurs more than 12 months after transplant (small percentage of late cases are EBV negative)
   d. Risk factors for EBV-PTLD
      1) EBV D+/R− mismatch: primary EBV infection is the most clearly defined risk factor
      2) Pediatric transplant recipients (mainly EBV-seronegative and at risk of primary EBV infection)
      3) CMV disease: CMV D+/R− status
      4) Use of muromonab-CD3 as immunosuppressive regimen
      5) Overimmunosuppression (high dose and prolonged duration)
   e. Incidence varies among organ transplant types
      1) Highest: small-bowel and lung transplant recipients
      2) Lowest: kidney transplant recipients
   f. Diagnosis of EBV-PTLD
      1) Confirmed by histopathology of specimens obtained by excisional biopsy
      2) Surveillance (eg, EBV PCR testing)
         a) Low or absent EBV viral load: very good negative predictive value
         b) Specificity of higher EBV load: modest
         c) Viral load trends: better predictive value than single viral load measurements
   g. Treatment of PTLD: no reliable strategy
      1) Decrease immunosuppression
      2) Rituximab: anti-CD20 therapy (for CD20+ tumors)
      3) Cytotoxic chemotherapy (for CD20− tumors)
      4) Surgery: debulk large tumors or remove single or isolated tumors
      5) Radiotherapy
   h. Prevention: best method of management
      1) Know donor and recipient EBV serologic status for all transplant patients, with EBV PCR surveillance for patients with a mismatch
      2) Main strategy: decrease immunosuppression by avoiding or minimizing use of lymphocyte-depleting drugs (eg, muromonab-CD3)
      3) Antiviral chemoprophylaxis (acyclovir and ganciclovir) has theoretical value but no proven benefit for established disease
      4) Preemptive therapy: immunoglobulins, antiviral drugs, rituximab, and EBV-specific T cells
5. Human herpesviruses 6 and 7
   a. Reactivation causes disease after transplant (>95% HHV-6 and HHV-7 seropositivity by age 5 years)
   b. Clinical disease: direct and indirect effects
      1) Direct: HHV-6 causes febrile illness, rash, bone marrow suppression, hepatitis, pneumonitis, and encephalitis
      2) Indirect: HHV-6 and HHV-7 interact with CMV and have potent immunomodulating effects
   c. Diagnosis: serology, culture, immunohistochemistry, and nucleic acid testing
   d. Treatment
      1) Insufficient data

2) HHV-6 appears to be susceptible to ganciclovir, cidofovir, and foscarnet
3) HHV-7 is resistant to ganciclovir in vitro
6. Polyomaviruses: BK virus and JC virus
   a. JC virus infections
      1) Very rare
      2) Clinical disease: progressive multifocal leukoencephalopathy
   b. BK virus infections
      1) Mainly in recipients of kidney transplants and hematopoietic stem cell transplants
      2) Clinical disease
         a) Kidney transplant recipients
            i) Tubulointerstitial nephritis and ureteral stenosis
            ii) Indicated by unexplained increase in serum creatinine level and impairment in renal function
         b) Hematopoietic stem cell transplant recipients: hemorrhagic cystitis
      3) Diagnosis of BK virus–associated nephropathy
         a) Kidney biopsy
         b) Decoy cells in urine
         c) BK virus PCR testing of urine and plasma
      4) Treatment
         a) Specific antiviral treatment of BK virus is not available
         b) Mainstay of treatment: decrease immunosuppression
         c) Cidofovir and leflunomide: off-label and experimental therapies
      5) Prevention of BK virus disease
         a) Surveillance testing to identify infection early and prevent progression to kidney allograft failure
         b) Two methods for surveillance
            i) Detection of decoy cells in urine
            ii) Nucleic acid testing of urine and blood specimens to detect BK virus DNA
7. Human parvovirus B19
   a. Occurs rarely after solid organ and hematopoietic stem cell transplant
   b. Clinical manifestation
      1) Infects and lyses erythroid precursor cells
      2) Causes refractory anemia
   c. Diagnosis
      1) Serology: limited value because patient may not be able to mount good immune response after transplant
      2) Bone marrow examination to demonstrate pure red cell aplasia
      3) PCR tests to demonstrate human parvovirus B19 DNA in clinical specimens
   d. Treatment: intravenous immunoglobulin (but dose and duration are undefined)
8. Hepatitis B virus
   a. Risk factors
      1) Blood transfusion (risk: 1 in 63,000)
      2) Lack of pretransplant HBV vaccination
         a) HBV screening (antibodies against hepatitis B surface antigen) in transplant recipients
         b) All HBV-susceptible transplant recipients should be vaccinated
   b. Severe liver failure due to HBV: indication for liver transplant
      1) Increased risk of HBV progression after transplant
      2) Prevention of HBV recurrence after transplant
         a) Hepatitis B immune globulin with high titers against HBV (eg, 10,000 international units daily for first week and then at 4-week intervals): can lead to emergence of surface antigen mutants
         b) Lamivudine: can lead to tyrosine-methionine-aspartate-aspartate (YMDD) mutants
         c) Adefovir dipivoxil: may be used against lamivudine-resistant HBV
9. Hepatitis C virus
   a. Chronic liver disease due to HCV: main indication for liver transplant
   b. With immunosuppressive drugs, the clinical course of HCV is more aggressive and accelerated after transplant
   c. Treatment of recurrent HCV hepatitis after liver transplant
      1) Interferon-alfa or peginterferon, alone or in combination with ribavirin: currently approved treatment for chronic hepatitis C
      2) High degree of intolerance and adverse effects accompany use of interferon (eg, tachyarrhythmias, somnolence, fatigue, headache, depression, leukopenia, thrombocytopenia) and ribavirin (eg, anemia)

C. Fungal Infections
1. Colonization is common
   a. Potential transplant recipients may be colonized with yeasts and mycelial fungi
   b. Lung transplant candidates with bronchiectasis and cystic fibrosis are often colonized with fungi (eg, *Aspergillus* species)
2. Isolation of fungi in culture: may herald onset of invasive fungal infection after transplant
   a. Need to distinguish between colonization and true infection
      1) Factors that indicate true infection
         a) Compatible clinical manifestations
         b) Radiographic signs
      2) Confirmation of true infection
         a) Biopsy specimens: identify fungal pathogen
         b) PCR assays and detection of fungal antigens (mannan and galactomannan)
   b. Most common fungal pathogens in transplant recipients
      1) *Candida* species
      2) *Aspergillus* species
      3) *Cryptococcus neoformans*
   c. Less common fungal pathogens
      1) *Fusarium* species, *Rhizopus* species, *Mucor* species, other molds, and *P jiroveci*
      2) Fungi associated with endemic mycoses: *H capsulatum* and *C immitis*
3. Risk factors for fungal infection after transplant
   a. *Candida* species (most common fungal pathogen): surgical procedures, indwelling urinary and intravascular catheters, and broad-spectrum antibacterial use
   b. *Aspergillus* species: prior colonization with *Aspergillus* species, fulminant hepatic failure, prolonged duration of neutropenia, and severe immunocompromise
   c. *Cryptococcus neoformans*, endemic mycoses, zygomycosis, dermatophytes, hyalohyphomycosis, and phaeohyphomycosis: usually after the sixth month after transplant
4. Antifungal strategies
   a. Therapeutic: treat established infection
   b. Preemptive: administer antifungal drug when clinical and laboratory markers indicate that transplant patient has high risk of invasive fungal disease
   c. Prophylactic: administer antifungal drug to prevent infection in all transplant patients
5. Liver transplant recipients
   a. *Candida* species and *Aspergillus* species: high risk of infection
   b. For fulminant hepatitis: antifungal prophylaxis (eg, low-dose amphotericin B or triazoles)
   c. Oral fluconazole: administered for up to 4 weeks to certain liver transplant recipients
      1) Patients who will undergo retransplantation or reoperation
      2) Patients who had prolonged surgical time or profound blood loss
6. Lung transplant recipients
   a. Risk factors
      1) Hyperacute rejection, acute graft failure, ischemic bronchial segments, anastomotic dehiscence, or retransplantation
      2) *Aspergillus* species colonization or CMV infection
   b. Therapeutic recommendation: administration of antifungal drug with activity against *Aspergillus* species and other mycelial fungi
      1) Itraconazole has been used widely
      2) Voriconazole use is becoming more common
      3) Aerosolized amphotericin B is used occasionally
      4) Itraconazole and voriconazole
         a) Drug interactions occur, especially with calcineurin inhibitors
         b) Systemic levels of the drugs should be monitored
7. Heart transplant recipients
   a. Risk factors: isolation of *Aspergillus* species in respiratory and other body secretions
   b. Infections of ventricular assist devices often involve *Candida* species and should be treated aggressively before transplant
8. Kidney and pancreas transplant recipients
   a. Pancreas transplant patients have high rates of invasive infections caused by *Candida* species
   b. Risk factors: anastomotic leaks, microbial translocation through the wall of the gastrointestinal tract, older donors and recipients, and retransplantation
   c. Prevention among patients at high risk
      1) Anti-*Candida* prophylaxis with fluconazole

2) Duration of prophylaxis is not defined but is often for 4 to 12 weeks after transplant
9. Allogeneic hematopoietic stem cell transplant recipients
   a. Risk factors: neutropenia and mucositis
      1) Fluconazole prophylaxis prevents invasive disease with fluconazole-susceptible *Candida* species during neutropenia (within 30 days after transplant)
      2) Autologous hematopoietic stem cell transplant patients often do not have prolonged neutropenia and so generally have lower risk of invasive fungal infections
   b. Indications for antifungal prophylaxis
      1) Hematologic malignancy (leukemia or lymphoma)
      2) Prolonged neutropenia or severe mucositis
      3) Receipt of fludarabine or cladribine
10. Hospital construction and renovations
    a. High incidence of invasive mold infections, particularly with aspergillosis
    b. Transplant patients should avoid areas of construction or renovations
11. Treatment of established fungal infection: depends on which pathogen is isolated
12. *Pneumocystis jiroveci*
    a. Major cause of opportunistic pneumonia after transplant
    b. Clinical manifestation
       1) Subacute
       2) Low-grade fever, progressive dyspnea, hypoxemia, and nonproductive cough
       3) Extrapulmonary disease is rare
       4) Coinfection with CMV and *Aspergillus* species may occur
    c. Prevention
       1) Trimethoprim-sulfamethoxazole
       2) Aerosolized or intravenous pentamidine and dapsone are alternatives
       3) Duration of prophylaxis: usually 3 to 6 months after transplant, but it may be prolonged if patients have prolonged immunosuppression (eg, chronic GHVD)
    d. Diagnosis of *P jiroveci* pneumonia: demonstration of organism, by smear or PCR testing, in lung and respiratory secretions
    e. Treatment of *P jiroveci* pneumonia
       1) Trimethoprim-sulfamethoxazole
       2) Add corticosteroids if patient is severely ill and hypoxemic
       3) Alternative therapies: pentamidine, atovaquone-dapsone-trimethoprim, primaquine-clindamycin, and pyrimethamine-sulfadiazine
D. Parasitic Infections
   1. *Toxoplasma gondii*
      a. Clinical presentation
         1) Fever and lymphadenopathy
         2) Manifestations of tissue-invasive infection, including pneumonia, heart failure, and neurologic manifestations
         3) Extensive involvement in the brain, heart, lungs, and lymphoid organs
      b. Diagnosis: serology, biopsy specimens, and PCR testing
      c. Prevention of toxoplasmosis
         1) For heart transplant recipient with *Toxoplasma* D+/R− serologic status
         2) Prophylaxis: pyrimethamine and sulfadiazine for 3 months followed by lifelong prophylaxis with trimethoprim-sulfamethoxazole
         3) Alternative regimens
            a) Dapsone with pyrimethamine
            b) Trimethoprim-sulfamethoxazole
            c) Atovaquone
      d. Choices for treatment of established toxoplasmosis
         1) Pyrimethamine in combination with a sulfonamide (ie, sulfadiazine)
         2) Clindamycin
   2. *Trypanosoma cruzi*
      a. Causes Chagas disease (also called American trypanosomiasis)
      b. Often a reactivation disease that causes heart failure and brain abscesses in transplant recipients
      c. Treatment
         1) Benznidazole with decreased immunosuppression and long-term therapy with nifurtimox
         2) Treatment often fails to eradicate the parasite
   3. *Strongyloides stercoralis*
      a. Nematode whose larvae tend to disseminate in immunocompromised patients
         1) Larvae accumulate in lungs and cause Löffler syndrome or eosinophilic pneumonia
         2) Peripheral eosinophilia is often present
      b. Hyperinfection syndrome
         1) Larvae penetrate gut

2) Cause bacteria and fungi to translocate
3) Results in systemic bacterial and fungal infections
4) Associated with pneumonitis, abdominal crisis, eosinophilic meningitis, and septic shock
5) Diagnostic clue: polymicrobial bloodstream infection with *Candida* species, gram-negative organisms such as *E coli*, enterococci, and other gut-derived bacteria
6) Gram-negative bacterial septic shock is often the cause of death
   c. Treatment
   1) Thiabendazole, ivermectin, and albendazole
   2) Therapy for superimposed infections complements *Strongyloides* therapy
V. Other Measures to Prevent Transplant Infections
   A. Environment
      1. Rooms for hematopoietic stem cell transplant patients should have more than 12 air exchanges per hour and point-of-use high-efficiency (>99%) particulate air (HEPA) filters that remove particles 0.3 μm or larger in diameter
      2. Use of HEPA filters should be considered for transplant patients during periods of hospital construction or renovation
   B. Food Safety
      1. Avoid consumption of raw or undercooked meat, including beef, poultry, pork, lamb, and venison or other wild game
      2. Avoid consumption of raw or undercooked eggs or foods that contain raw or undercooked ingredients
      3. Avoid consumption of raw or undercooked seafood, such as sushi, sashimi, oysters, and clams
   C. Immunizations
      1. All transplant patients should have updated immunizations before and after transplant
      2. Patients should avoid live vaccines after transplant
      3. Susceptible liver transplant candidates should receive hepatitis A vaccine and hepatitis B vaccine
      4. Hematopoietic stem cell transplant recipients should receive diphtheria, pertussis, and tetanus (DPT) or tetanus and diphtheria toxoids (Td), inactivated polio, *H influenzae*, and hepatitis B vaccines in 3 doses at 12, 14, and 24 months after transplant
      5. Measles, mumps, and rubella (MMR) vaccine contains live virus
         a. Contraindicated during the first 24 months after hematopoietic stem cell transplant
         b. Should be administered at 24 months or later, after the patient is immunocompetent
      6. Lifelong seasonal influenza vaccination should be given beginning at 6 months after hematopoietic stem cell transplant, and close contacts should receive seasonal influenza vaccines
      7. Pneumococcal vaccine is recommended at 12 and 24 months after hematopoietic stem cell transplant or later, after the patient is immunocompetent

Suggested Reading

Center for International Blood and Marrow Transplant Research (CIBMTR); National Marrow Donor Program (NMDP); European Blood and Marrow Transplant Group (EBMT); American Society of Blood and Marrow Transplantation (ASBMT); Canadian Blood and Marrow Transplant Group (CBMTG); Infectious Disease Society of America (IDSA); Society for Healthcare Epidemiology of America (SHEA); Association of Medical Microbiology and Infectious Diseases Canada (AMMI); Centers for Disease Control and Prevention (CDC). Guidelines for preventing infectious complications among hematopoietic cell transplant recipients: a global perspective. Bone Marrow Transplant. 2009 Oct;44(8): 453–558.

Special issue: AST infectious diseases guidelines 2nd edition. Am J Transplant. 2009 Dec;9 Suppl 4:S1–281.

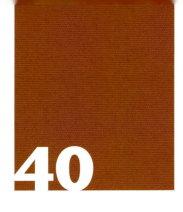

Rodney L. Thompson, MD
Priya Sampathkumar, MD

Health Care–Associated Infections

I. Introduction
   A. Definitions
      1. *Health care–associated infection* (*HAI*): infection that occurs in hospitals, nursing homes, clinics, or home health care programs
      2. *Nosocomial infection*: infection acquired in acute care settings
   B. Infection Control Departments
      1. Constituted to prevent and control infectious complications
      2. Prevention and control require combinations of education and training, procedures and policies, surveillance and reporting, and interventions that include isolation and teamwork
      3. Resistant organisms make treatment more difficult and outcomes less successful
   C. Common Nosocomial Infections
      1. Urinary tract infections
      2. Surgical site infections (SSIs)
      3. Bloodstream infections (BSIs)
      4. Ventilator-associated pneumonia (VAP)
II. Nosocomial Urinary Tract Infections
   A. Clinical Importance
      1. Urinary tract infections are the most common HAI, accounting for 40% of all HAIs
      2. Primarily related to presence of an indwelling catheter
      3. Up to 25% of hospitalized patients have a urinary catheter
   B. Definitions
      1. *Catheter-associated urinary tract infection* (*CAUTI*): urinary tract infection occurring in the presence of a urinary catheter
      2. CAUTI rates are reported as
      $$\frac{\text{Number of CAUTIs}}{\text{Number of catheter-days}} \times 1{,}000$$
      3. *Bacteriuria*: growth of more than 100 colony-forming units (CFU) of a clinically significant pathogen from a catheterized urine specimen
   C. Clinical Features of CAUTI
      1. Catheter-associated bacteriuria and either local symptoms (lower abdominal or flank pain) or systemic symptoms (fever, nausea, and vomiting)
         a. Resistant organisms are common in the intensive care unit (ICU): *Candida* species, *Enterococcus*, and *Pseudomonas*
         b. Morbidity is low and treatment of bacteriuria is generally unnecessary
      2. Bacteremia complicates CAUTI in up to 4% of cases
      3. Prevention strategies for CAUTI are listed in Box 40.1

> **Box 40.1**
>
> **Prevention of Catheter-Associated Urinary Tract Infection**
>
> Avoid using urinary catheters whenever possible, and consider alternatives to indwelling urinary catheters (eg, condom catheters in men, intermittent catheterization)
>
> Always insert a catheter aseptically, maintain a sterile closed drainage system, and properly secure the catheter after insertion to prevent movement and urethral traction during use
>
> Bladder irrigation, antibacterial instillation in the drainage bag, rigorous meatal cleaning, and use of meatal lubricants and creams have not been clearly shown to prevent bacteriuria and should not be used
>
> Do not change indwelling catheters or urinary drainage bags at arbitrarily fixed intervals
>
> Assess the need for the catheter daily, and remove the catheter when it is no longer needed

   D. Indications for a Urinary Catheter
      1. Perioperative use for selected surgical patients and procedures
         a. Genitourinary tract operation
         b. Procedure expected to require prolonged surgical time
         c. Surgical patient with urinary incontinence
         d. Patient with need for intraoperative hemodynamic monitoring
         e. Patient expected to receive large volume of diuretics during surgery
      2. Urine output monitoring in critically ill patients
      3. Management of acute urinary retention and urinary obstruction
      4. Assistance in pressure ulcer healing for incontinent patients
      5. As an exception, at patient request to improve comfort (eg, end-of-life comfort care)
III. Surgical Site Infections
   A. Clinical Importance
      1. SSIs are usually caused by organisms introduced at surgery and are generally caused by organisms present on skin or colonized tracts of the patient
      2. Shedding from staff with resultant SSI is unusual but possible
         a. Health care workers (HCWs) colonized with methicillin-resistant *Staphylococcus aureus* (MRSA) or group A streptococci can transmit these organisms to the patient in the operating room
         b. A single case of early group A streptococci SSI requires screening of the surgical team
   B. Classification of Surgical Wounds
      1. Surgical procedures are classified by wound type, which is an indicator of intrinsic wound contamination
      2. Likelihood of an SSI increases as wound class increases from I to IV (Box 40.2)
         a. Type I surgical procedures
            1) Enter through uninfected skin
            2) Respiratory, gastrointestinal, and genitourinary tracts are not entered
            3) There is no break in sterile technique
            4) Example: resection of an intracranial tumor
            5) Expected infection rate: 1% to 5%
         b. Type II surgical procedures
            1) Respiratory, gastrointestinal, or genitourinary tract is entered in a controlled manner
            2) Infection rates are higher because of the normal flora in the tracts
            3) Example: elective colon resection in patient with bowel preparation
            4) Expected infection rate: 8% to 11%
         c. Type III surgical procedures
            1) Fresh accidental wounds
            2) Wounds in which the surgeon encounters nonpurulent inflammation or gross spillage from the gastrointestinal tract
            3) Example: bowel perforation during splenectomy
            4) Expected infection rate: 15% to 20%
         d. Type IV surgical procedures
            1) Involve old trauma wounds with devitalized tissue

> **Box 40.2**
>
> **Surgical Wound Classification**
>
> Class I/clean
>   An uninfected operative wound in which no inflammation is encountered and the respiratory, alimentary, genital, or uninfected urinary tract is not entered; clean wounds are primarily closed and, if necessary, drained with closed drainage
> Class II/clean-contaminated
>   An operative wound in which the respiratory, alimentary, genital, or urinary tract is entered under controlled conditions and without unusual contamination
> Class III/contaminated
>   Open, fresh, accidental wounds; operations with major breaks in sterile technique (eg, open cardiac massage) or gross spillage from the gastrointestinal tract; and incisions in which acute, nonpurulent inflammation is encountered
> Class IV/dirty-infected
>   Old traumatic wounds with retained devitalized tissue and those that involve existing clinical infection or perforated viscera
>
> Adapted from Guideline for prevention of surgical site infection, 1999. Infect Control Hosp Epidemiol. 1999;20(4) 247–78.

2) Procedures in which the surgeon encounters pus or other evidence of infection
3) Example: open drainage of an intra-abdominal abscess
4) Expected infection rate: greater than 25%

C. Risk Stratification
1. Assessment of patient risk is difficult: many factors increase infection rates in various types of operations
2. The common epidemiologic risk assessment used by the National Healthcare Safety Network (NHSN) of the Centers for Disease Control and Prevention includes 3 components
   a. Wound class
   b. American Society of Anesthesiologists (ASA) score (an estimate of patient's condition)
   c. Duration of surgery (an estimate of the complexity of the operation)
3. A point value (either 0 or 1) is assigned for each primary risk factor
   a. Wound classes I and II are assigned 0 points, and classes III and IV are assigned 1 point
   b. ASA scores of 1 or 2 are assigned 0 points, and ASA scores of 3 or more are assigned 1 point
   c. Duration of surgery greater than 75 percentile for like procedures (published by the NHSN) is assigned 1 point
4. Risk index score is determined by adding the points for the 3 risk factors
   a. There are 4 possible scores: 0, 1, 2, or 3
   b. Risk of SSI increases as the score increases
5. Low SSI rates are considered a marker of institutional quality
   a. State and national groups look at SSI rates for assessment of care for consumers, payers, and regulators (eg, Medicare, National Quality Forum)
   b. Intrahospital comparisons are difficult because of various patient risks, different criteria for diagnosis of infection, and inconsistent surveillance efforts

D. SSI Classification
1. When an SSI is diagnosed, wound depth must be assessed
2. Wound depth determines morbidity (Figure 40.1)
   a. Superficial incisional SSI involves only the skin and the subcutaneous tissue divided by the incision

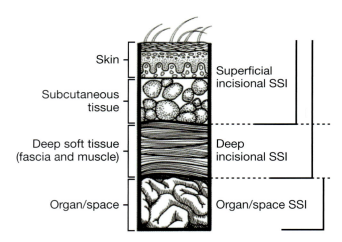

Figure 40.1. Classification of Surgical Site Infections. Cross-sectional drawing of abdominal wall shows the surgical site infection (SSI) classification system of the Centers for Disease Control and Prevention. (Adapted from Guideline for prevention of surgical site infection, 1999. Infect Control Hosp Epidemiol. 1999;20[4]:247–78.)

   b. Deep incisional SSI involves deep soft tissues of the incision, extending below the fascia but not including an organ or space
   c. Organ/space SSI involves an organ or space within the body that was entered during surgery
      1) Examples: peritoneal cavity, joint, cranium
      2) Associated with the most morbidity and mortality

E. Microbiology of SSI
1. Microbiology of SSI reflects the type of surgery undertaken
2. Location of procedure
   a. Skin: organisms such as *Staphylococcus aureus* or coagulase-negative staphylococci
   b. An internal tract entered during surgery: organisms such as gram-negative bacilli, anaerobes, and *Enterococcus*
3. Classification of procedure
   a. Type I: SSI tends to be caused by 1 pathogen, usually a skin microorganism
   b. Types II through IV: SSI tends to be polymicrobial

F. Treatment of SSI
1. Superficial collections: drainage may be sufficient
2. Cellulitis and complicated infections: appropriate antibiotics are needed
3. Deep incisional SSIs and organ/space SSIs: drainage and antibiotics are the optimal treatment

G. Surgical Prophylactic Antibiotics
1. Appropriate use of prophylactic antibiotics can decrease the rate of SSIs
   a. Given on time
   b. Given for the shortest time needed
   c. Active against the common organisms causing SSI
2. Current surgical quality indicators
   a. Prophylactic antibiotic given within 1 hour of incision (or within 2 hours if a long infusion time is required, such as for vancomycin and ciprofloxacin)
   b. Selected agents should be supported by national guidelines for the procedure
      1) For most type I operations: cefazolin is selected unless there is a risk of MRSA or unless patient allergies make vancomycin necessary
      2) For type II operations: anaerobic coverage is often provided
   c. Duration of antibiotic use should not exceed 24 hours postoperatively (or 48 hours for cardiac surgery)
   d. These process indicators are made public by the Centers for Medicare and Medicaid Services as evidence of quality

IV. Health Care–Associated Bloodstream Infections
A. Definitions
1. Health care–associated BSIs may be primary or secondary
   a. *Primary BSIs*
      1) Caused by either intravenous devices or indeterminate factors
      2) In acute care, intravenous device–related BSIs are the most common, especially in the ICU
   b. *Secondary BSIs*
      1) Occur secondary to a documented focus of infection
      2) Source may be an SSI, pneumonia, urinary tract infection, or another type of infection
2. *Central venous catheter (CVC)-associated BSI*: a primary BSI when a CVC is in place
3. Clinical definition of *catheter-related BSI*: a bacteremia or fungemia in a patient who has an intravascular catheter and who meets other specific criteria
   a. At least 1 blood culture with positive results from a peripheral vein sample
   b. Clinical manifestations of infection (ie, fever, chills, or hypotension)
   c. No apparent source for the BSI except the catheter
   d. One of the following culture results
      1) Positive results on semiquantitative culture (>15 CFU/catheter segment) or quantitative culture (>10^3 CFU/catheter segment), with the same pathogen (species and antibiogram) isolated from the catheter segment and peripheral blood
      2) Simultaneous quantitative blood cultures with results indicating a CVD to peripheral blood ratio of 5:1 or more
      3) Differential period of positivity of more than 2 hours for CVC culture compared with peripheral blood culture
4. *Exit site infection*: erythema or induration within 2 cm of the catheter exit site, without concomitant BSI and purulence
5. *Tunnel infection*: tenderness, erythema, or site induration more than 2 cm from the catheter site along the subcutaneous tract of a tunneled (eg, Hickman or Broviac) catheter, without concomitant BSI
6. *Pocket infection*: purulent fluid in the subcutaneous pocket of a totally implanted intravascular catheter, with or without spontaneous rupture and drainage or necrosis of the overlaying skin and without concomitant BSI

B. Risks
1. Risk of BSI from a CVC depends on multiple factors
   a. Site of placement (listed in descending order of risk): femoral, internal jugular, subclavian
   b. Type of catheter: risk is greater with nontunneled than with tunneled
   c. Circumstances at time of catheter placement: risk is greater with emergency placement than with elective placement
   d. Number of catheter lumens: risk is greater with multiple lumens than with a single lumen
   e. Frequency of catheter manipulation
   f. Duration of use
   g. Parenteral nutrition
   h. Patient-related factors: underlying disease, severity of illness
2. Dialysis catheters and temporary lines in the femoral site have the highest risk of infection
3. BSI rates are reported as
$$\frac{\text{Number of BSIs}}{\text{Number of line-days}} \times 1{,}000$$

C. Duration of Catheter Use

1. Intravenous tunneled devices or subcutaneous ports
   a. Can often be used for relatively long intervals (weeks to years) before infection occurs
   b. Ultimately these may become contaminated intraluminally during line manipulations
   c. "Lock therapy" and systemic treatment of the BSI may help to salvage infected devices if the organism is fully sensitive
2. Peripherally inserted central catheter (PICC) lines
   a. When used in outpatients, PICC lines are relatively resistant to infections and can be left in for weeks
   b. When used in the ICU, PICC lines seem to become infected relatively frequently
D. Pathogens and Management
   1. Common organisms in health care–associated BSIs of all types include coagulase-negative staphylococci, *S aureus*, gram-negative bacilli, including *Pseudomonas* and *Candida*
   2. Some institutions have reported short-term eradication of BSIs through several steps
      a. Careful attention to sterile technique
      b. Use of full barrier precautions at the time of line placement
      c. Daily assessment for removal of unnecessary devices
   3. Intravascular access is used widely at care locations and at patients' homes
      a. Surveillance is required in home health care situations, in nursing homes, and in other locations
      b. Various management plans have been developed
         1) Catheter site care with chlorhexidine
         2) Antibiotic-impregnated catheters
         3) Daily observation of the catheter site
V. Ventilator-Associated Pneumonia
   A. Definition
      1. *VAP*: pneumonia in a patient receiving mechanical ventilation (by endotracheal tube or tracheostomy) currently or within the previous 48 hours
      2. According to the 2009 NHSN definition, there is no minimum period that the ventilator must be in place for the pneumonia to be considered ventilator associated
   B. Clinical Importance
      1. VAP develops in 10% to 20% of patients receiving mechanical ventilation for more than 48 hours
      2. Compared with similar patients without VAP, patients who have VAP are twice as likely to die, have longer lengths of stay in the ICU, and incur higher hospital costs
   C. Diagnosis
      1. Epidemiologic definition of VAP does not require positive culture results or other microbiology data, but it does require that certain criteria all be met
         a. Radiographic changes noted on 2 or more serial chest radiographs
         b. At least 1 of the following signs of infection: fever; leukopenia or leukocytosis; or mental status changes in patients older than 70 years
         c. At least 2 signs of respiratory compromise: increased secretions or purulent secretions, worsening cough or dyspnea, worsening gas exchange, or rales or bronchial breath sounds
      2. VAP surveillance is challenging and labor intensive
      3. Accurate diagnosis of VAP can be difficult because ICU patients who have multiple comorbidities may have multiple reasons for chest radiographic changes
      4. VAP rate
         a. VAP rate is reported as number of cases of VAP/1,000 ventilator-days
         b. VAP rates are highest in burn, trauma, and surgical ICUs and lowest in medical and coronary care ICUs
   D. Prevention Strategies
      1. Active surveillance for VAP
      2. Adherence to hand hygiene guidelines
      3. Use of noninvasive ventilation whenever possible
      4. Minimizing the duration of ventilation
      5. Education about VAP for HCWs who care for patients receiving ventilation
   E. Ventilator Bundle
      1. The Institute for Healthcare Improvement (IHI) has suggested that process improvements can be a powerful infection prevention tool when they are bundled together
      2. Several ICUs have adopted the IHI Ventilator Bundle and shown sustained decreases in the VAP rate
      3. Key components of the IHI Ventilator Bundle
         a. Elevation of the head of the bed
         b. Daily sedation vacations and assessment of readiness to extubate
         c. Peptic ulcer disease prophylaxis
         d. Deep vein thrombosis prophylaxis
VI. Multidrug-Resistant Organisms
   A. Resistance
      1. Resistance rates vary around the world
      2. The number of microorganisms with resistance to common antibiotics is increasing

a. Some microorganisms have undergone mutations and are stable and resistant (eg, MRSA, vancomycin-resistant enterococci)
b. Other organisms have inducible resistance that develops during treatment with a specific agent (eg, *Pseudomonas*, *Enterobacter*)
c. There are many mechanisms of resistance in health care settings

B. Control
1. Primary mode of transmission is by the hands of HCWs
2. Control focuses on hand hygiene, appropriate use of barriers (eg, gloves, gowns), and antibiotic stewardship
3. Admission screening and isolation has been advocated as a way to decrease the number of multidrug-resistant organisms
   a. Universal: screen all admissions
   b. Targeted: screen admissions to ICUs or to other units with high-risk patients or screen certain patients (eg, the elderly, transfers from long-term care facilities)
   c. Vancomycin-resistant enterococci screening of diarrheal stools submitted for *Clostridium difficile* testing can identify carriers who are at high risk of transmission

C. *Clostridium difficile*
1. *Clostridium difficile*–associated diarrhea is growing in importance as a health care–associated infection
2. Transmission of *C difficile* between patients may occur by hands or from the environment or fomites
   a. Isolation, environmental cleaning, and antibiotic management have all been used to control this pathogen
   b. Recently, hypertoxin-producing strains have spread in hospitals and regions, causing severe disease and death
3. Special efforts are required to control outbreaks, including enhanced cleaning to kill *C difficile* spores, which are relatively resistant to routinely used cleaning agents

VII. Viral Infections and Outbreaks
A. Clinical Importance
1. Viral infections in health care settings are important causes of morbidity in patients and staff and can be fatal in patient groups
2. Influenza A outbreaks are associated with increased mortality among elderly and immunocompromised hosts
   a. These patients, their health care providers, and family members should receive influenza vaccination
   b. HCW influenza vaccination rates remain low (about 42%) despite a Joint Commission requirement that all accredited health care facilities provide influenza vaccinations on site and at no charge to all employees

B. Recent Outbreaks
1. Pertussis and mumps outbreaks have occurred in recent years in the United States and elsewhere
2. HCWs have been infected, and they have infected patients
3. Vaccine from childhood has a short protective duration: adult vaccine is now available and recommended

Suggested Reading

Anderson DJ, Kaye KS, Classen D, Arias KM, Podgorny K, Burstin H, et al. Strategies to prevent surgical site infections in acute care hospitals. Infect Control Hosp Epidemiol. 2008 Oct;29 Suppl 1:S51–61.

Calfee DP, Salgado CD, Classen D, Arias KM, Podgorny K, Anderson DJ, et al. Strategies to prevent transmission of methicillin-resistant *Staphylococcus aureus* in acute care hospitals. Infect Control Hosp Epidemiol. 2008 Oct;29 Suppl 1:S62–80.

Coffin SE, Klompas M, Classen D, Arias KM, Podgorny K, Anderson DJ, et al. Strategies to prevent ventilator-associated pneumonia in acute care hospitals. Infect Control Hosp Epidemiol. 2008 Oct;29 Suppl 1:S31–40.

Dubberke ER, Gerding DN, Classen D, Arias KM, Podgorny K, Anderson DJ, et al. Strategies to prevent *Clostridium difficile* infections in acute care hospitals. Infect Control Hosp Epidemiol. 2008 Oct;29 Suppl 1:S81–92.

Lo E, Nicolle L, Classen D, Arias KM, Podgorny K, Anderson DJ, et al. Strategies to prevent catheter-associated urinary tract infections in acute care hospitals. Infect Control Hosp Epidemiol. 2008 Oct;29 Suppl 1:S41–50.

Marschall J, Mermel LA, Classen D, Arias KM, Podgorny K, Anderson DJ, et al. Strategies to prevent central line-associated bloodstream infections in acute care hospitals. Infect Control Hosp Epidemiol. 2008 Oct;29 Suppl 1:S22–30. Erratum in: Infect Control Hosp Epidemiol. 2009 Aug;30(8):815.

O'Grady NP, Alexander M, Burns LA, Dellinger EP, Garland J, Heard SO, et al; the Healthcare Infection Control Practices Advisory Committee (HICPAC) (Appendix 1). Guidelines for the prevention of intravascular catheter-related infections. Clin Infect Dis. 2011 May;52(9):e162–193. Epub 2011 Apr 1.

Yokoe DS, Mermel LA, Anderson DJ, Arias KM, Burstin H, Calfee DP, et al. A compendium of strategies to prevent healthcare-associated infections in acute care hospitals. Infect Control Hosp Epidemiol. 2008 Oct;29 Suppl 1:S12–21.

Kristi L. Boldt, MD

Obstetric and Gynecologic Issues Related to Infectious Diseases

I. Introduction
   A. Infection in Pregnancy
      1. Infection is the most common complication during pregnancy and the postpartum period
   B. Antibiotic Therapy in Pregnancy
      1. Choices are limited
      2. Must take into account several factors
         a. Effect of pregnancy on serum levels
         b. Distribution of antibiotics
         c. Placental transfer
         d. The fetus
         e. The newborn
         f. Excretion in milk
         g. The breast-feeding infant
      3. Antimicrobial therapy is selected on the basis of experience and guidelines
         a. US Food and Drug Administration pregnancy category definitions (Tables 41.1 and 41.2)
         b. Teratogen Information System (TERIS) rating system
         c. REPROTOX system from the Reproductive Toxicology Center
II. Urinary Tract Infection
   A. Epidemiology
      1. Urinary tract infection (UTI): most common medical complication during pregnancy
      2. UTI is more common in females, especially during pregnancy because of physiologic and anatomical changes
      3. Organisms
         a. *Escherichia coli* (90%)
         b. *Proteus mirabilis*
         c. *Klebsiella pneumoniae*
         d. Enterococci
         e. Group B streptococci (GBS)
         f. *Staphylococcus saprophyticus*
   B. Asymptomatic Bacteriuria
      1. Affects 2% to 11% of pregnant women
      2. Associations
         a. Sickle cell trait
         b. Low socioeconomic status
         c. Poor prenatal care
         d. Age
      3. Increased risks with untreated asymptomatic bacteriuria (ASB)
         a. Acute pyelonephritis (up to 65%)
         b. Preterm labor
         c. Low-birth-weight infants
      4. If ASB is treated, the rate of complications is 0% to 5%
      5. Pathogenesis
         a. Bacterial products stimulate the immune system

Table 41.1
US Food and Drug Administration Categories for Drug Use in Pregnancy[a]

Category	Description
A	Adequate, well-controlled studies in pregnant women have not shown an increased risk of fetal abnormalities
B	Animal studies have revealed no evidence of harm to the fetus; however, there are no adequate, well-controlled studies in pregnant women *or* Animal studies have shown an adverse effect, but adequate, well-controlled studies in pregnant women have not shown a risk to the fetus
C	Animal studies have shown an adverse effect, and there are no adequate, well-controlled studies in pregnant women *or* No animal studies have been conducted, and there are no adequate, well-controlled studies in pregnant women
D	Adequate, well-controlled or observational studies in pregnant women have shown a risk to the fetus; however, the benefits of therapy may outweigh the potential risk
X	Adequate, well-controlled or observational studies in animals or pregnant women have shown positive evidence of fetal abnormalities. The use of the product is contraindicated in women who are or may become pregnant

[a] The US Food and Drug Administration (FDA) is reviewing the study of medication exposure in pregnancy since currently many high-quality data are required before a drug is classified in category A. As a result, many drugs that would be classified in category A in other countries are classified in category C by the FDA.

Adapted from Code of Federal Regulations Title 21: 21CFR201.57. Silver Spring (MD): US Food and Drug Administration. Updated 2010 Apr 1 [cited 2011 Jan 5]. Available from: http://www.accessdata.fda.gov/scripts/cdrh/cfdocs/cfcfr/CFRSearch.cfm?fr=201.57.

Table 41.2
Safety and Toxicity of Selected Antimicrobial Agents During Pregnancy

Antimicrobial Agent	Possible Fetal Toxicity	FDA Pregnancy Category
Aminoglycosides	Ototoxicity (not described with gentamicin) Nephrotoxicity, especially if combined with cephalosporins	C
Amoxicillin-clavulanate	Increased risk of necrotizing enterocolitis in newborn	Unknown
Cephalosporins	Possible teratogenicity: cefaclor, cephalexin, cephradine	B
Chloramphenicol	Gray baby syndrome	C
Fluoroquinolones	Animal studies: arthropathy in developed bone and cartilage	C
Lindane	Potential neurotoxin	C
Sulfonamides[a]	Compete with bilirubin Possible hyperbilirubinemia in neonates	C
Tetracyclines	In second and third trimester, bind with calcium Discoloration of deciduous teeth, enamel hypoplasia, and inhibition of bone growth	D
Trimethoprim[a]	Folate antagonist Possible increase in neural tube and cardiac defects in first trimester	C

Abbreviation: FDA, US Food and Drug Administration.

[a] Avoid administering in first trimester or if patient has high risk of preterm delivery. Outcome depends on resistance in community.

      b. Immune system triggers prostaglandin production
        1) Interleukin 1
        2) Interleukin 6
        3) Tumor necrosis factor
        4) Platelet-activating factor
  6. Screening is cost-effective
  7. Treatment should prevent 70% to 80% of cases (Table 41.3)
  8. Among pregnant women with bacteriuria, 10% to 15% have evidence of chronic pyelonephritis within 10 to 12 years after delivery
C. Acute Pyelonephritis
  1. Affects 1% to 2% of all pregnant women
  2. Recurrence rate: 10% to 18% during same pregnancy
  3. Serious threat to well-being of fetus and mother
  4. Similar causative organisms as with ASB and cystitis
  5. Treatment
      a. Aggressive antimicrobial treatment (Table 41.4) and supportive therapy
      b. Treatment helps to avoid maternal complications that can result from bacterial endotoxin-induced tissue damage
        1) Hypotension
        2) Anemia
        3) Renal dysfunction

Table 41.3
Suggested Regimens for the Treatment of Asymptomatic Bacteriuria and Cystitis

Antimicrobial Agent	Regimen	FDA Pregnancy Category
Nitrofurantoin, long acting[a,b]	100 mg orally 2 times daily for 7 d	B
Trimethoprim-sulfamethoxazole[b]	160 mg-800 mg orally 2 times daily for 3 d	C
Cephalexin	500 mg orally 4 times daily for 3 d	B
Amoxicillin[c]	500 mg orally 4 times daily for 3 d	B

Abbreviation: FDA, US Food and Drug Administration.

[a] *Proteus* is not sensitive.
[b] Avoid administering in first trimester or if patient has high risk of preterm delivery. Outcome depends on resistance in community.
[c] Check susceptibilities before prescribing β-lactam monotherapy.

Table 41.4
Suggested Initial Empirical Antimicrobial Regimens for the Treatment of Pyelonephritis in Pregnancy and Lactating Mothers

Antimicrobial Agent	Regimen	FDA Pregnancy Category
Ampicillin and gentamicin	Ampicillin: 2 g IV every 6 h; gentamicin; see below	C
Gentamicin	2 mg/kg load, then 1.7 mg/kg in 3 divided doses	C
Ceftriaxone	1 g IV or IM daily	B
Cefazolin	1-2 g IV every 6-8 h	B

Abbreviations: FDA, US Food and Drug Administration; IM, intramuscularly; IV, intravenously.

Table 41.5
Suggested Suppressive Therapy Regimens for Recurrent Urinary Tract Infection or Pyelonephritis

Antimicrobial Agent	Regimen	FDA Pregnancy Category
Nitrofurantoin	100 mg orally at bedtime	B
Trimethoprim-sulfamethoxazole	160 mg-800 mg orally at bedtime	C
Cephalexin	250 mg orally at bedtime	B

Abbreviation: FDA, US Food and Drug Administration.

        4) Respiratory insufficiency akin to acute respiratory distress syndrome
        5) Septic shock
      c. When patient is clinically stable and afebrile for 48 hours, switch to oral antimicrobial therapy for 2 weeks
      d. Follow-up test of cure: to ensure eradication of the bacteria
    D. Suppressive Therapy
      1. Possible indications for suppressive therapy (Table 41.5)
        a. Recurrent UTI
        b. One or more episodes of pyelonephritis
      2. Duration of suppressive therapy: remainder of pregnancy until 2 weeks after delivery
  III. Bacterial Vaginosis
    A. Clinical Importance
      1. Most common cause of vaginitis in both pregnant and nonpregnant women
      2. Adverse outcomes in pregnancy
        a. Premature rupture of the membranes
        b. Preterm labor
        c. Preterm birth
        d. Intra-amniotic infection
        e. Postpartum endometritis
    B. Treatment
      1. Symptomatic disease in pregnant women should be treated (Box 41.1)
      2. It is not clear whether screening for and treating bacterial vaginosis in pregnant women can reliably decrease the incidence of pregnancy complications
      3. Results of investigations: treatment may decrease the risk of prematurity among pregnant women who have bacterial vaginosis and a high risk of preterm deliveries
      4. High-risk pregnant women who have asymptomatic bacterial vaginosis may need evaluation and treatment
  IV. Preterm Labor and Premature Rupture of Membranes
    A. Clinical Importance
      1. Responsible for two-thirds of all premature deliveries

---

Box 41.1
Recommended Regimens for Bacterial Vaginosis in Pregnant Women[a]

Metronidazole 500 mg orally 2 times daily for 7 d
or
Metronidazole 250 mg orally 3 times daily for 7 d
or
Clindamycin 300 mg orally 2 times daily for 7 d

[a] Vaginal clindamycin cream and metronidazole vaginal gels are not routinely used during pregnancy.

Adapted from Centers for Disease Control and Prevention. Sexually transmitted diseases treatment guidelines, 2006. MMWR. 2006; 55(RR-11):1–94.

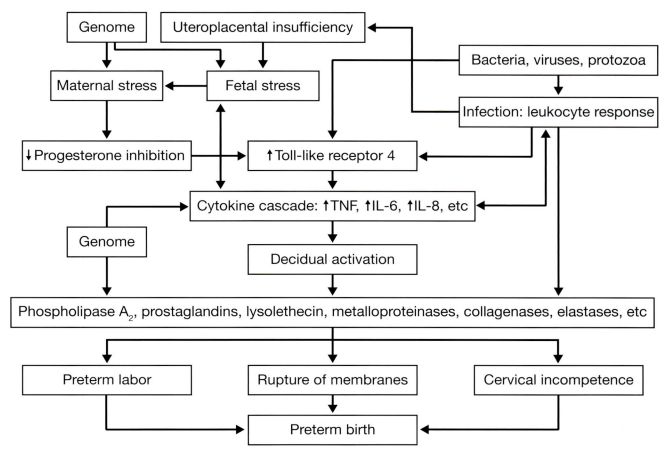

Figure 41.1. Relation of infection and host response to preterm labor, preterm premature membrane rupture, and premature cervical dilation. IL indicates interleukin; TNF, tumor necrosis factor. (Adapted from Newton ER. Preterm labor, preterm premature rupture of membranes, and chorioamnionitis. Clin Perinatol. 2005 Sep;32[3]:571–600. Used with permission.)

2. Strong association between infection and earlier preterm births (<32 weeks' gestation) (Figure 41.1)

V. Intra-amniotic Infection: Chorioamnionitis and Amnionitis
  A. Incidence of Subclinical Histologic Chorioamnionitis
    1. At 24 to 28 weeks: 50%
    2. At 28 to 32 weeks: 30%
    3. At 33 to 36 weeks: 20%
    4. At more than 37 weeks: 10%
  B. Probability of Intra-amniotic Infection and Premature Rupture of Membranes
    1. At less than 28 weeks: 40%
    2. At 28 to 34 weeks: 20%
    3. At more than 37 weeks: 5%
  C. Clinical Importance
    1. Occurs in 0.5% to 10% of term pregnancies
    2. Complicates up to 50% of preterm deliveries
    3. Causes 10% to 40% of peripartum maternal febrile morbidity
    4. Associated with increased maternal morbidity
      a. Uterine atony
      b. Pelvic abscesses
      c. Endometritis
      d. Wound infection
      e. Blood transfusions
    5. Associated with increased fetal morbidity
      a. Early neonatal sepsis and pneumonia (20%-40%)
      b. Neonatal seizures
  D. Source of Infection
    1. Typically: lower genital tract bacteria ascending with the onset of labor or with rupture of membranes
    2. Infrequently: extragenital sources of bacteria from the urinary tract or periodontal disease
    3. Occasionally: hematogenous or transplacental infection occurs as exemplified by fulminant listeriosis
    4. Sometimes: invasive obstetrical procedures (eg, amniocentesis, cerclage placement)

E. Risk Factors for Intra-amniotic Infection
   1. Preterm labor
   2. Rupture of membranes longer than 12 hours
   3. GBS colonization
   4. Long labor
   5. Low parity
   6. Young age
   7. Bacterial vaginosis
   8. Preexisting lower genital tract infections
   9. Low socioeconomic status
   10. Immunocompromised status
   11. Multiple vaginal examinations in labor
   12. Internal fetal or uterine pressure monitoring
   13. Long duration of monitoring
F. Diagnosis of Clinical Infection
   1. Usually maternal fever greater than 38°C and at least 2 of the following criteria
      a. Maternal tachycardia
      b. Uterine tenderness
      c. Fetal tachycardia
      d. Malodorous amniotic fluid
   2. Diagnostic testing is summarized in Table 41.6
G. Therapy
   1. Initiation of parenteral antibiotic therapy
      a. As soon as diagnosis of intra-amniotic infection (IAI) is entertained unless delivery is imminent
      b. Prevents neonatal and maternal complications
   2. Considerations for antibiotic selection
      a. Bioavailability to the fetus
      b. Spectrum broad enough to encompass the pathogenic organisms responsible
   3. Recommendations
      a. Rule out sexually transmitted infections
      b. Sample urinary tract, endocervix, and amniotic fluid for culture
      c. Often the choice of drugs remains empirical
   4. Specific therapeutic agents
      a. Most extensively tested regimen: ampicillin (2 g every 6 hours) in combination with gentamicin (1.5 mg/kg every 8 hours)
         1) Ampicillin: drug of choice for fetal therapy
            a) Targets both GBS and *E coli*
            b) Lacks coverage for selected enterococci and penicillin-resistant bacteroides
         2) Aminoglycoside: drug of choice for maternal therapy
         3) Administration of ampicillin in combination with an aminoglycoside covers many pathogens, including resistant enterococci
      b. Clinical deterioration
         1) Expedited delivery is required
         2) Also, addition of anaerobic coverage: metronidazole or clindamycin
            a) Especially recommended if patient is undergoing cesarean delivery
            b) Cesarean delivery when patient has clinical chorioamnionitis or IAI greatly increases the risk of maternal complications, such as endometritis or wound infections

Table 41.6
Diagnostic Tests for Intra-amniotic Infection

Test	Abnormal Finding	Comment
Maternal WBC count	$\geq 15.0 \times 10^9$/L with preponderance of leukocytes	Labor or corticosteroids may elevate WBC count
Amniotic fluid glucose	$\leq 10\text{-}15$ mg/dL	Excellent correlation with positive amniotic fluid culture and clinical infection
Amniotic fluid interleukin	≥ 7.9 ng/mL	Excellent correlation with positive amniotic fluid culture and clinical infection
Amniotic fluid leukocyte esterase	$\geq 1+$	Good correlation with positive amniotic fluid culture and clinical infection
Amniotic fluid Gram stain	Any organism in an oil-immersion field	Allows identification of particularly virulent organism such as group B streptococci. Very sensitive to inoculum effect. Cannot identify pathogens such as mycoplasmas
Amniotic fluid culture	Growth of aerobic or anaerobic microorganism	Results are not immediately available for clinical management
Blood cultures	Growth of aerobic or anaerobic microorganism	Positive in 5%-10% of patients. Usually of no value for clinical decisions unless patient is at increased risk of bacterial endocarditis, is immunocompromised, or has a poor response to initial treatment

Abbreviation: WBC, white blood cell.

Adapted from Gabbe SG, Niebyl JR, Simpson JL. Obstetrics: normal and problem pregnancies. 5th ed. New York: Churchill Livingstone; c2007. Used with permission.

VI. Major Perinatal Infections and Infectious Agents
   A. Key Points
      1. Summarized in Table 41.7
      2. Details are reviewed elsewhere in this chapter or in other chapters
   B. Cytomegalovirus
      1. Epidemiology
         a. Cytomegalovirus (CMV): most common cause of perinatal infections
         b. Routine maternal serologic screening for CMV is not recommended
         c. During pregnancy, 0.1% to 4% of women have seroconversion
         d. In immunocompetent women, most maternal CMV infections are asymptomatic
         e. Among women of childbearing age, 50% to 85% have previously been infected with CMV
      2. Infection outcomes
         a. Primary infection
            1) Like other DNA viruses, CMV becomes latent after primary infection
            2) Naturally acquired immunity does not prevent reactivation with viral shedding or exogenous reinfection with another strain
            3) Cannot accurately predict the neonatal sequelae of primary infection
            4) Among pregnant women who acquire primary CMV, 40% to 50% of the fetuses become infected
            5) Greatest risk of congenital infection: third trimester
            6) Greatest risk of severe fetal injury: maternal infection in first trimester
         b. When infection occurs intrapartum or during breast-feeding, sequelae are rarely serious
         c. Recurrent or reactivated CMV infection
            1) Women with recurrent or reactivated CMV infection are 70% less likely to transmit the disease to their offspring
            2) Offspring infected from recurrent maternal CMV infections
               a) At birth, nearly 100% are asymptomatic
               b) After 5 years, at least 8% have a major sequela, usually nothing more severe than hearing loss
      3. Detection of maternal infection
         a. Acute infection in immunocompetent adults is frequently asymptomatic
         b. Assays of IgM and IgG titers should be performed
            1) Optimal diagnostic testing
               a) Detection of CMV-specific IgG antibodies in a previously seronegative woman
               b) Would require routine screening, which is not currently practical or recommended
            2) Caution should be used when interpreting positive results because the specificity of the test affects results
            3) High levels of CMV-specific IgM titers are suggestive of a primary infection, especially when sequential titers decrease rapidly
            4) Low levels that decrease slowly may be related to primary infection with an onset months earlier, possibly before pregnancy
            5) A small number of women have persistent IgM levels
            6) IgG avidity testing is often useful to distinguish primary from nonprimary infection
         c. Because of the limitations of serologic testing in the diagnosis of CMV, additional testing of at-risk women may be appropriate
            1) Tissue culture
            2) Viral DNA and RNA testing
      4. Management
         a. Identification of women who should be offered invasive fetal testing (Figure 41.2)
   C. Group B Streptococci (*Streptococcus agalactiae* Serotypes)
      1. A leading infectious cause of morbidity and death among US newborns: 0.4 infant cases per 1,000 live births
      2. Conditions associated with GBS
         a. Chorioamnionitis
         b. Premature labor and rupture of membranes
         c. Endometritis
         d. Bacteremia
         e. Wound and urinary tract infections
      3. Early-onset newborn disease
         a. Younger than 7 days
         b. Bacteremia, generalized sepsis, pneumonia, or meningitis
      4. Late-onset newborn disease
         a. Aged 7 to 89 days
         b. Often bacteremia without a focus, meningitis (35%), and some focal infections

Table 41.7
Summary of Etiology, Diagnosis, and Management of Major Perinatal Infections

Agent or Condition	Complications — Maternal Disease	Complications — Fetal/Neonatal Susceptibility	Diagnosis — Maternal	Diagnosis — Fetal/Neonatal	Management — Maternal	Management — Fetal/Neonatal
CMV	1%–4% seroconversion in pregnancy. Majority are symptomatic. 15% have mononucleosis-like symptoms. Periodic reactivation with shedding. Maternal immunity does not prevent congenital infection	0.2%–2% of newborns. Susceptible at all trimesters. 85%–90% asymptomatic at birth. Problems subsequently develop in 10%–15%. 5%–15% overtly affected at birth: jaundice, chorioretinitis, hearing loss, hydrocephalus or microcephaly, IUGR, hepatosplenomegaly. 30% die early in life. Many are severely handicapped mentally and physically	Detection of antibody	Amniocentesis, culture, and PCR testing of amniotic fluid and fetal blood. Ultrasonography. Negative testing does not preclude infection	Prevention and education are important. Ganciclovir for severe infection	Counseling based on available data. Even though infection rate is high in first half of pregnancy, majority of fetuses develop normally. Some evidence suggests that maternal and fetal treatment with ganciclovir may be helpful. More studies are needed
Group B streptococci	UTI. Chorioamnionitis. PTL/PROM. Bacteremia. Endomyometritis. Wound infection	Early-onset disease: sepsis, pneumonia, meningitis, death	Rectovaginal culture in selective media	Culture	Intrapartum antibiotic prophylaxis	Prevention with intrapartum prophylaxis is key for early-onset disease. Treat with ampicillin or penicillin
Hepatitis A	1/1,000 acute infections in pregnancy. Serious complications are rare	None	Detection of IgM antibodies or anti-HBc (IgM)	Not applicable	Supportive care. Prevention: hepatitis A vaccine if at risk or exposed (vaccine is safe in pregnancy)	Administer immune globulin to neonate if mother has acute infection at delivery
Hepatitis B	1/1,000–2/1,000 acute infections in pregnancy. 5/1,000–15/1,000 chronic infections	Perinatal transmission is high without immunoprophylaxis, especially if HbeAg positive or if infection began in third trimester. Majority of transmission is intrapartum	Detection of surface antigen		Prevention: HBIG + HBV for susceptible household contacts; HBV for mothers at risk (HBV is safe in pregnancy)	Passive and active immunization prevents 90%–95% of infections: HBIG plus HBV immediately after delivery, followed by 2 more injections of HBV within the first 6 mo (can still breast-feed). Active immunization of all newborns is recommended

Hepatitis C	50% have chronic liver disease	7%–8% Infection from vertical transmission is probably proportional to titer of maternal virus Increased risk of infection if mother is HIV positive	Detection of antibody	Supportive care	No immunoprophylaxis is available Many recommend no breast-feeding since antibodies to hepatitis C are not protective
Hepatitis D	Requires hepatitis B for replication Chronic disease is more severe than other hepatitis	Vertical transmission is documented	Detection of hepatitis D antigen in hepatic tissue or serum IgM antibody to hepatitis D virus	Supportive care	Same as for hepatitis B
Hepatitis E	Rare Usually self-limited and does not become chronic High maternal mortality rate	Vertical transmission has been reported		Supportive care	
Herpes simplex	Infects 22% of pregnant women 2% are acutely infected during pregnancy Often disease is subtle; may be disseminated; rarely postpartum endometritis	1/3,200 births 50% of infections are disseminated or CNS infections 30% mortality 40% long-term neurologic sequelae	Clinical examination Culture PCR testing Type-specific serologic tests	Clinical examination Culture PCR testing	Acyclovir or valacyclovir for severe primary infection and suppression	Cesarean delivery when mother has overt infection or prodromal symptoms
Listeriosis	More susceptible Sporadic form more common than epidemic form Contamination of food and food products Many are asymptomatic or have flulike illness Rarely death	Transplacental infection Early onset: diffuse sepsis with multiorgan involvement and high rates of stillbirth and neonatal mortality Late onset: meningitis with sequelae and 40% mortality rate	High clinical suspicion Gram stain Cervical and blood cultures Amniotic fluid culture	Clinical suspicion Cultures and Gram stain	Ampicillin and gentamicin	Ampicillin
Parvovirus infection	1/400 pregnancies 25% are asymptomatic One-third have mild rash-like illness	Depends on trimester Fetal loss Anemia Hydrops High-output cardiac failure Myocarditis Death	Detection of antibody	Ultrasonography	Supportive care	Intrauterine transfusion for severe anemia

(*continued*)

Table 41.7
(continued)

Agent or Condition	Complications		Diagnosis		Management	
	Maternal Disease	Fetal/Neonatal Susceptibility	Maternal	Fetal/Neonatal	Maternal	Fetal/Neonatal
Rubella (German measles)	Mild febrile illness Up to 25% of women are susceptible	Congenital rubella syndrome	Sometimes difficult to confirm Detection of antibody	Ultrasonography Viral RNA in chorionic villous, amniotic fluid, or fetal blood	Prevention: vaccination before pregnancy	No treatment Pregnancy termination for affected fetus
Rubeola (measles)	Otitis media Hepatitis Pneumonia Encephalitis	Abortion Preterm delivery Minimal risk for IUGR, microcephaly, and oligohydramnios	Detection of antibody	Ultrasonography	Prevention: vaccination before pregnancy	If delivered within 7-10 d of maternal infection, give immunoglobulin
Syphilis	Aortitis Neurosyphilis	Congenital infection	Serology Dark-field examination	Ultrasonography	Penicillin	Penicillin
Toxoplasmosis	Majority are asymptomatic Occasionally mononucleosis-like illness or diffuse lymphadenopathy	All trimesters, but prognosis is worse if in first trimester Chorioretinitis CNS infection	Detection of seroconversion, but IgM may remain positive for up to 2 y	Amniocentesis or cordocentesis PCR testing Detection of IgM or IgA antibodies in the infant	Sulfadiazine Alternatives: pyrimethamine or spiramycin	Treatment up to 1 y with pyrimethamine plus sulfadiazine plus leucovorin
Varicella-zoster (chickenpox)	5% have pneumonia Encephalitis	Congenital infection: chorioretinitis, cerebral atrophy Cutaneous and bony leg lesions Hydronephrosis 0.4% ≤13 wk 2% between 13 and 20 wk 0% >20 wk	Clinical examination Detection of antibody	Ultrasonography	VZIG and acyclovir for prophylaxis or treatment	VZIG or ZIG prophylaxis if maternal infection <5 d before delivery

Abbreviations: CMV, cytomegalovirus; CNS, central nervous system; HBc, hepatitis B core antigen; HBeAg, hepatitis B e antigen; HBIG, hepatitis B immune globulin; HBV, hepatitis B vaccine; HIV, human immunodeficiency virus; IUGR, intrauterine growth restriction; PCR, polymerase chain reaction; PROM, premature rupture of membranes; PTL, preterm labor; UTI, urinary tract infection; VZIG, varicella-zoster immune globulin; ZIG, zoster immune globulin.

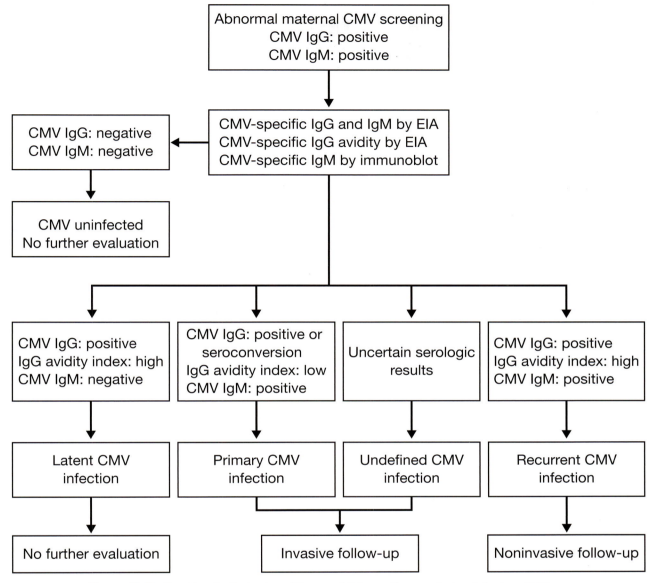

Figure 41.2. Algorithm for Evaluation of Suspected Primary Cytomegalovirus Infection. CMV indicates cytomegalovirus; EIA, enzyme immunoassay. (Adapted from Cunningham FG, Leveno KJ, Bloom SL, Hauth JC, Rouse DJ, Spong CY. Infectious diseases. In: Cunningham FG, Leveno KJ, Bloom SL, Hauth JC, Rouse DJ, Spong CY, editors. Williams obstetrics. 23rd ed. New York: McGraw-Hill Medical; c2010. Used with permission.)

5. 2010 National GBS Prevention Guidelines (Table 41.8, Boxes 41.2 and 41.3)
   a. Centers for Disease Control and Prevention (CDC), American Academy of Pediatrics, and American Congress of Obstetricians and Gynecologists recommend universal prenatal screening
   b. Helps decrease the number of early-onset GBS infections in neonates
6. Colonization
   a. Can be transient, intermittent, or chronic
   b. At least 20% to 30% of all pregnant women are carriers
D. Herpes Simplex Virus
   1. Large increase in herpes simplex virus (HSV) genital infections
      a. HSV type 1 (HSV-1) genital infections are developing in more people

Table 41.8
Indications and Nonindications for Intrapartum Antibiotic Prophylaxis to Prevent Early-onset Group B Streptococcal (GBS) Disease

Intrapartum GBS Prophylaxis Indicated	Intrapartum GBS Prophylaxis Not Indicated
Previous infant with invasive GBS disease	Colonization with GBS during a previous pregnancy (unless an indication for GBS prophylaxis is present for current pregnancy)
GBS bacteriuria during any trimester of the current pregnancy[a]	GBS bacteriuria during previous pregnancy (unless an indication for GBS prophylaxis is present for current pregnancy)
Positive GBS vaginal-rectal screening culture in late gestation[b] during current pregnancy[a]	Negative vaginal and rectal GBS screening culture in late gestation[b] during the current pregnancy, regardless of intrapartum risk factors

Unknown GBS status at the onset of labor (culture not done, incomplete, or results unknown) and any of the following:
  Delivery at <37 wk of gestation[c]
  Amniotic membrane rupture ≥18 h
  Intrapartum temperature ≥38.0°C[d]
  Intrapartum NAAT[e] positive for GBS
	Cesarean delivery performed before onset of labor on a woman with intact amniotic membranes, regardless of GBS colonization status or gestational age

Abbreviation: NAAT, nucleic acid amplification tests.

[a] Intrapartum antibiotic prophylaxis is not indicated in this circumstance if a cesarean delivery is performed before onset of labor on a woman with intact amniotic membranes.

[b] Optimal timing for prenatal GBS screening is at 36-37 weeks' gestation.

[c] Recommendations for the use of intrapartum antibiotics for prevention of early-onset GBS disease in the setting of threatened preterm delivery are presented in Figures 5 and 6 of the reference cited below.

[d] If amnionitis is suspected, broad-spectrum antibiotic therapy that includes an agent known to be active against GBS should replace GBS prophylaxis.

[e] NAAT testing for GBS is optional and might not be available in all settings. If intrapartum NAAT is negative for GBS but any other intrapartum risk factor (delivery at <37 weeks' gestation, amniotic membrane rupture at ≥18 hours, or temperature ≥38.0°C) is present, then intrapartum antibiotic prophylaxis is indicated.

Adapted from Centers for Disease Control and Prevention. Prevention of perinatal group B streptococcal disease. MMWR. 2010;59(No. RR-10):1–32.

    b. Increase reflects changes in sexual practices
2. Viral shedding
    a. HSV-1 infections, like HSV type 2 (HSV-2) infections, exhibit viral shedding
    b. HSV-1 genital infections do not shed virus as frequently
3. Neonatal infection
    a. Neonates may become infected with HSV-1 but usually exhibit the mild form of disease
    b. Neonatal herpes

Box 41.2
Group B Streptococci Specimen Collection

Collect a rectovaginal specimen with 1 swab by taking a sample from the distal posterior vagina (15 seconds) and then dragging the swab over the perineum and partially inserting the swab into the rectum
Place the swab in a nonnutritive transport medium
Inoculate swab into a broth medium such as Todd-Hewitt broth supplemented with gentamicin and nalidixic acid
Incubate for 18-24 hours
Subculture the broth onto sheep blood agar
Read results after 18-48 hours

Adapted from Centers for Disease Control and Prevention. Prevention of perinatal group B streptococcal disease. MMWR. 2010; 59(No. RR-10):1–32.

Box 41.3
Regimens for Intrapartum Antimicrobial Prophylaxis for Perinatal GBS Disease Prevention

Recommended
    Penicillin G 5 million units IV for an initial dose, then 2.5-3 million units IV every 4 h until delivery
Alternative
    Ampicillin 2 g IV for an initial dose, then 1 g IV every 4 h until delivery
If penicillin allergic
    Patients not at high risk of anaphylaxis
        Cefazolin 2 g IV for an initial dose, then 1 g IV every 8 h until delivery
    Patients at high risk of anaphylaxis
        GBS susceptible to clindamycin
            Clindamycin 900 mg IV every 8 h until delivery
        GBS resistant to clindamycin or susceptibility unknown
            Vancomycin 1 g IV every 12 h until delivery

Abbreviations: GBS, group B streptococci; IV, intravenously.

Adapted from Centers for Disease Control and Prevention. Prevention of perinatal group B streptococcal disease. MMWR. 2010; 59(No. RR-10):1–32.

1) The most severe complication of HSV infection
   a) Skin, eye, and mouth infections with limited involvement of other systems: 45%
   b) Central nervous system (CNS) disease: 30%
   c) Disseminated disease: 25%
2) Usually contracted by contact with infected genital secretions during labor
     c. Risk of neonatal infection
        1) Highest when maternal primary disease occurs in the third trimester
        2) Infection also occurs when patients have recurrent HSV or are shedding HSV at delivery
  4. Postnatal acquisition of HSV may occur from orolabial herpes or from infection at a nongenital site (eg, finger [herpetic whitlow], breast)
  5. Treatment
     a. Treatment of neonates: no recent advances for disseminated or CNS disease
     b. Treatment of women who have a recognized primary or first episode of HSV infection during pregnancy
        1) Short-term administration of acyclovir or valacyclovir
        2) Then administration of suppressive doses until delivery
     c. Treatment of pregnant women who have frequent recurrences: many gynecologists administer suppressive therapy from 36 weeks (or earlier) until delivery to reduce the chance of shedding at delivery
  6. Prevention
     a. Best strategy is to prevent primary disease and also decrease the risk of maternal shedding at time of delivery
     b. Invasive monitoring or artificial rupture of membranes during delivery should be avoided
     c. If there is evidence of active infection or prodromal symptoms, cesarean delivery is recommended
     d. Other suggested methods to prevent the acquisition of HSV by pregnant women
        1) Appropriate education
        2) Universal screening in pregnancy of the woman with or without her partner
        3) Advise all pregnant women to abstain from all forms of sexual contact in third trimester
        4) In HSV-discordant couples in which the woman is seronegative, encourage safe sexual practices and administer antivirals for suppression in the partner
  E. Human Parvovirus B19
     1. Epidemiology
        a. Infections are more common in winter and spring
        b. Infection gives lifelong immunity in immunocompetent patients
        c. Approximately 60% of childbearing women are immune
     2. Acute infection
        a. Usually from close contact with children who have erythema infectiosum (fifth disease)
        b. Occurs in 1 in 400 pregnancies
        c. Risk of vertical transmission depends on the trimester
        d. Overall, transmission is about 33%
        e. Infection in early pregnancy may result in fetal loss
     3. Transplacental infection in second or third trimester
        a. May result in fetal anemia, high-output cardiac failure, hydrops, or, rarely, myocarditis
        b. Hydrops
           1) Develops in approximately 3%
           2) Spontaneous resolution occurs in about one-third
        c. Without transfusion, risk of death: 30%
        d. Close fetal surveillance is usually done for 8 to 12 weeks after maternal infection is diagnosed
     4. Diagnosis (Figure 41.3)
  F. Rubella (German Measles)
     1. The causative virus is one of the most teratogenic agents known
     2. Often maternal illness is not obvious
     3. Incidence of congenital infection varies with timing of maternal infection (Table 41.9)
     4. Congenital rubella (Box 41.4)
        a. Neonates with congenital rubella may shed the virus for many months
        b. Should not be exposed to susceptible infants or others
        c. Extended rubella syndrome
           1) May not develop until second or third decade of life
           2) Develops in many asymptomatic neonates
           3) Involves progressive panencephalitis and type 1 diabetes mellitus
  G. Syphilis
     1. Clinical importance

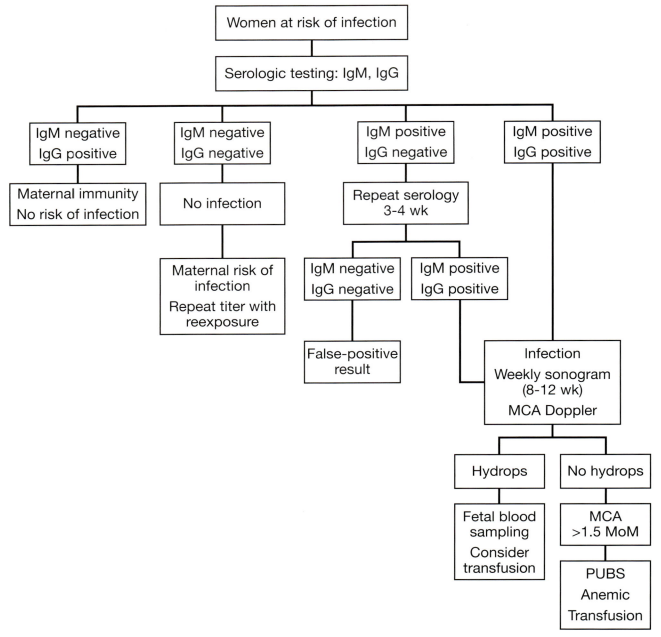

Figure 41.3. Diagnostic Algorithm for Human Parvovirus B19 Infection. MCA indicates middle cerebral artery; MoM, multiples of the median; PUBS, percutaneous umbilical blood sampling. (Adapted from Ramirez MM, Mastrobattista JM. Diagnosis and management of human parvovirus B19 infection. Clin Perinatol. 2005 Sep;32[3]:697–704. Used with permission.)

- a. Incidence of syphilis is increasing
- b. CDC guidelines for serologic testing for syphilis
  1) Test all pregnant women
  2) Test during pregnancy and before infant is discharged from hospital
- c. Absence of adequate treatment during pregnancy
  1) Results in miscarriage, stillbirth, and perinatal demise
  2) Stigmata in 40% of surviving infants
- d. Fetal infections in utero
  1) Not a time-limited event
  2) Even adequate maternal therapy may result in congenital syphilis

Table 41.9
Timing of Maternal Infection and Incidence of Congenital Infection

Timing of Maternal Infection	Incidence of Congenital Infection
First 12 wk (organogenesis)	80%
13-14 wk	54%
End of second trimester	25%
Third trimester	Infection is unlikely

Box 41.4
Congenital Rubella Syndrome

One or more of the following:
  Sensorineural deafness
  Eye defects, including glaucoma and cataracts
  Heart disease, including patent ductus arteriosus, peripheral pulmonary stenosis
  Pigmentary retinopathy
  CNS: microcephaly, delayed development, mental retardation, and meningoencephalitis
  Purpura
  Hepatosplenomegaly and jaundice
  Radiolucent bone disease

Abbreviation: CNS, central nervous system.

Box 41.5
Recommendations for Decreasing the Risk of Primary Toxoplasmosis Infection Among Pregnant Women

Avoid consumption of undercooked meat: cook all meat until it is no longer pink and the juices run clear
Always wear gloves while handling raw meat, and wash hands thoroughly afterward
Thoroughly wash all utensils that have contacted undercooked meat
Wash all uncooked vegetables thoroughly
Wear gloves when gardening or working in the soil (roaming cats may have deposited their feces), and wash hands immediately after contact with soil
If possible, keep cats indoors throughout pregnancy, and do not feed cats uncooked meat
Wear gloves while changing cat litter, and wash hands immediately afterward

Adapted from Kravetz JD, Federman DG. Toxoplasmosis in pregnancy. Am J Med. 2005 Mar;118(3):212–6. Used with permission.

---

    2. Treatment
       a. Same as for nonpregnant women
         1) Penicillin
         2) Desensitization of penicillin-allergic patients is optimal
       b. Efficacy
         1) Adequacy of eradication of established fetal disease with effective maternal therapy is unknown
         2) Therapy for maternal syphilis in second and third trimesters is more likely to be suboptimal for fetus
       c. Jarisch-Herxheimer reaction
         1) Occurs in up to 45% of pregnant women receiving penicillin for treatment of syphilis, particularly for primary and secondary disease
         2) May result in uterine contractions and decreased fetal movement
         3) Typically occurs within 2 to 8 hours after treatment and resolves within 24 hours
  H. Toxoplasmosis
    1. Seroprevalence of *Toxoplasma*-seropositive women of childbearing age in the United States: 22.5%
       a. Routine screening is not recommended in the United States
       b. If maternal infection is detected, it is unclear as to whether prenatal treatment is effective in preventing congenital toxoplasmosis
    2. Recommendations for decreasing the risk among pregnant women are listed in Box 41.5
    3. Congenital toxoplasmosis is relatively uncommon in the United States
    4. Maternal infection is transmitted transplacentally to the fetus and, depending on trimester, can cause various congenital problems
    5. Intrauterine diagnosis via amniocentesis or cordocentesis has inherent procedural risks
  I. Varicella-zoster Virus
    1. Causative agent of chickenpox, which in pregnancy may be relatively severe
    2. Varicella-zoster immunoglobulin (VZIG)
       a. Prevents or attenuates varicella infection in susceptible women if given within 96 hours of viral exposure
       b. VZIG or zoster immune globulin (ZIG) prophylaxis in infants reduces the risk
    3. Neonatal exposure to active maternal infection within 5 days of delivery, before maternal antibody has formed, may result in death, morbidity (CNS), or disseminated disease
    4. Primary varicella infection may reactivate in older or immunocompromised persons, resulting in herpes zoster (shingles)
  J. Human Immunodeficiency Virus Infection During Pregnancy in the United States
    1. Human immunodeficiency virus (HIV) infection is now considered a chronic disease owing to recent advances in HIV diagnosis and management

2. Considerations for providers caring for pregnant women infected with HIV type 1 (HIV-1)
   a. Antiretroviral treatment of maternal HIV-1 infection to prolong and improve the quality of the mother's life
   b. Antiretroviral chemoprophylaxis to decrease the risk of perinatal HIV-1 transmission
   c. Antiretroviral therapy should be offered to all HIV-infected pregnant women (unlike the recommendations for nonpregnant patients)
3. Epidemiology
   a. Worldwide, 47% of HIV-infected persons are women
   b. In the United States, 27% of HIV-infected persons are women
   c. Among US women, 79% of new infections are attributed to heterosexual intercourse
   d. Mother-to-child transmission (MTCT) of HIV: data and risk factors are summarized in Box 41.6
4. Treatment

Box 41.6

Mother-to-Child Transmission (MTCT) of HIV

Rate of MTCT without prophylaxis
   In developed countries: 14%-33%
   In developing countries: up to 43%
   Total transmission antepartum: 25%-40%
   Total transmission intrapartum: 60%-75%
MTCT with breast-feeding
   Rate of MTCT with breast-feeding: 5%-15%
   Risk of MTCT when mother is infected prenatally: 14%
   Risk of MTCT when HIV virus is acquired postnatally (primary infection): 29%
Risk factors for MTCT
   Viral load (HIV RNA level)
   Genital tract viral load
   CD4 cell count (decreases in pregnancy regardless of HIV status)
   Clinical stage of HIV
   Smoking cigarettes
   Poor nutritional status
   Vitamin A deficiency
   Substance abuse
   STDs and other coinfections
   Route of delivery
   Invasive fetal monitoring
   Breast-feeding
   Preterm delivery
   Placental disruption
   Duration of membrane rupture

Abbreviations: HIV, human immunodeficiency virus; STD, sexually transmitted disease.

Box 41.7

HIV Testing Recommendations of ACOG, AAP, and CDC

Universal opt-out approach to testing for HIV infection as part of the routine battery of prenatal blood tests
Repeat offer of HIV testing in the third trimester to women in areas with high prevalence of HIV, to women known to be at high risk of HIV infection, and to women who declined testing earlier in pregnancy, as allowed by state laws and regulations
Use of conventional HIV testing for women who are candidates for third-trimester testing
Use of rapid HIV testing (20-40 minutes) in labor for women with undocumented HIV status
   If a rapid HIV test result is positive, initiate antiretroviral prophylaxis (with consent) without waiting for the results of the confirmatory test

Abbreviations: AAP, American Academy of Pediatrics; ACOG, American Congress of Obstetricians and Gynecologists; CDC, Centers for Disease Control and Prevention; HIV, human immunodeficiency virus.

Adapted from ACOG Committee on Obstetric Practice. ACOG committee opinion number 304, November 2004. Prenatal and perinatal human immunodeficiency virus testing: expanded recommendations. Obstet Gynecol. 2004 Nov;104(5 Pt 1):1119–24. Used with permission.

---

   a. Most HIV transmission (50%-70%) is thought to occur intrapartum, so treatment is focused on identifying HIV-infected women as early as possible in their pregnancy (Box 41.7)
   b. Prevention of MTCT of HIV (Box 41.8)
      1) Antiretroviral medications given to women with HIV perinatally and to their newborns in the first weeks of life decrease the vertical transmission rate from 25% to 2% or less
      2) Even maternal prophylaxis given during labor and delivery or neonatal prophylaxis given within 24 to 48 hours of delivery can substantially decrease rates of infection in infants
   c. Antiretroviral medications in pregnancy
      1) Risk-benefit considerations
         a) Benefits of antiretroviral therapy for the pregnant woman
         b) Risk of adverse events to the woman, fetus, and newborn
      2) Standard combination highly active antiretroviral therapy (HAART)
         a) Recommended for all pregnant women
         b) Whichever regimen is chosen, if possible it should include a zidovudine chemoprophylaxis regimen similar to that used in the

Box 41.8
Prevention of MTCT of HIV

Antiretroviral therapy to prevent MTCT is recommended for all pregnant women, regardless of virologic, immunologic, or clinical parameters

A decrease in HIV RNA levels to less than 1,000 copies/mL and the use of antiretroviral therapy appear to have an independent effect on reducing perinatal transmission

In antiretroviral-naive pregnant women, initiation of antiretroviral therapy may be delayed until after 12 weeks' gestation to avoid the period of greatest vulnerability of the fetus to potential teratogenic effects and because nausea and vomiting in early pregnancy may affect optimal adherence to the regimen and absorption of antiretroviral medications

If the patient is already taking antiretroviral medication, therapy should be continued through the first trimester

  An exception would be if the patient were taking medication associated with teratogenesis (eg, efavirenz or hydroxyurea)

  If the patient cannot tolerate her medications owing to nausea and vomiting, antiretroviral therapy should be discontinued so as to not promote resistance

If clinical, virologic, or immunologic indications exist for initiation of therapy in nonpregnant persons, many experts recommend initiating therapy regardless of gestational age

Abbreviations: HIV, human immunodeficiency virus; MTCT, mother-to-child transmission.

Data from Panel on Treatment of HIV-Infected Pregnant Women and Prevention of Perinatal Transmission. Recommendations for use of antiretroviral drugs in pregnant HIV-1-infected women for maternal health and interventions to reduce perinatal HIV transmission in the United States. Updated 2010 May 24 [cited 2011 Jan 5]; p 1–117. Available from: http://aidsinfo.nih.gov/ContentFiles/PerinatalGL.pdf.

Table 41.10
Modified Pediatric AIDS Clinical Trials Group (PACTG) 076 Zidovudine (ZDV) Regimen

Time of ZDV Administration	Regimen
Antepartum	Oral administration of 300 mg ZDV twice daily, initiated at 14-34 wk of gestation and continued throughout pregnancy
Intrapartum	During labor, intravenous administration of ZDV in a 1-h initial dose of 2 mg/kg body weight, followed by a continuous infusion of 1 mg/kg body weight hourly until delivery
Postpartum	Oral administration of ZDV to the newborn (ZDV syrup at 2 mg/kg body weight every 6 h) for the first 6 wk of life, beginning at 8-12 h after birth[a]

[a] Intravenous dosage for infants who cannot tolerate oral intake is 1.5 mg/kg body weight intravenously every 6 hours.

Adapted from Panel on Treatment of HIV-Infected Pregnant Women and Prevention of Perinatal Transmission. Recommendations for use of antiretroviral drugs in pregnant HIV-1-infected women for maternal health and interventions to reduce perinatal HIV transmission in the United States. Updated 2010 May 24 [cited 2011 Jan 5]; p 1–117. Available from: http://aidsinfo.nih.gov/ContentFiles/PerinatalGL.pdf.

Pediatric AIDS Clinical Trial Group 076 (PACTG 076) study (Table 41.10)
  i) In clinical trials, this zidovudine regimen has shown the greatest reductions in MTCT
  ii) Intrapartum and neonatal components of the zidovudine regimen should be administered no matter which antiretroviral regimen was used antepartum
3) Nucleoside/nucleotide analogue reverse transcriptase inhibitors (NRTIs)
  a) Combivir (combination preparation of zidovudine and lamivudine [3TC])
    i) The recommended nucleoside backbone
    ii) Excellent transplacental penetration
    iii) No need for dose adjustment
    iv) Macrocytic anemia and hepatic dysfunction are common and should be monitored for through pregnancy
  b) Mitochondrial fatty acid oxidation disorder in mother or fetus in late pregnancy
    i) May cause acute fatty liver of pregnancy and HELLP (*h*emolysis, *e*levated *l*iver enzymes, and *l*ow *p*latelet count) syndrome
    ii) May increase susceptibility to antiretroviral-associated mitochondrial toxicity
  c) Lactic acidosis with hepatic steatosis syndrome
    i) An NRTI toxicity that probably results from mitochondrial toxicity
    ii) Pregnancy can mimic early symptoms of lactic acidosis with hepatic steatosis syndrome
    iii) Other disorders of liver metabolism may occur during pregnancy

iv) Physicians administering NRTIs to HIV-1–infected pregnant women should watch for early signs of this syndrome
  (a) Hepatic enzymes and electrolytes should be assessed more frequently during the last trimester of pregnancy
  (b) Thoroughly evaluate new symptoms
v) Pregnant women should not receive didanosine with stavudine: the combination may cause fatal hepatic steatosis and lactic acidosis
4) Nonnucleoside reverse transcriptase inhibitors (NNRTIs)
 a) Nevirapine
  i) No need for dose adjustment
  ii) In preventing MTCT (PMTCT) trials, nevirapine was a favorable NNRTI and was safe in pregnancy
  iii) Recently, nevirapine has been associated with an increased risk of hepatitis in women who have a CD4 cell count of 250 to 350/μL
  iv) First 18 weeks of treatment with nevirapine: increased hepatic transaminase levels (alanine aminotransferase and aspartate aminotransferase) may be associated with rash or systemic symptoms
 b) Avoid administration of efavirenez: possibility of neural tube defects
5) Protease inhibitors
 a) Recommended agents
  i) Lopinavir-ritonavir (twice daily dosing)
  ii) Nelfinavir
 b) Increased doses may be required in the third trimester
 c) Complications
  i) Hyperglycemia, new-onset diabetes mellitus, exacerbation of existing diabetes mellitus, and diabetic ketoacidosis
  ii) Whether protease inhibitors increase the risk of pregnancy-associated hyperglycemia is unknown (since pregnancy itself increases the risk of hyperglycemia)
  iii) Glucose level should be monitored closely
 d) Methylergonovine maleate (used to manage postpartum hemorrhage) should not be coadministered with protease inhibitors or other cytochrome P450 3A4 isozyme (CYP3A4) inhibitors
6) Antepartum monitoring related to HIV infection and medications
 a) Data are inconclusive as to whether HIV infection or the use of HAART in pregnancy increases adverse pregnancy outcomes
 b) Suggested testing is listed in Box 41.9
 c) Evaluation and appropriate prophylaxis as indicated
  i) Opportunistic infections

Box 41.9

Suggested Testing for HIV-Positive Women Antepartum

Baseline laboratory tests
  HIV-1 viral load
  CD lymphocyte count
  CD4 cell percentage
  Complete blood cell count with differential leukocyte count
  Hepatic function panel and electrolytes
  Glucose
  Cholesterol panel
Additional testing if not already done as part of routine prenatal screening
  Sexually transmitted infections: *Chlamydia* infection, gonorrhea, syphilis
  Hepatitis B
Further screening
  Hepatitis A
  Hepatitis C
  Herpes simplex virus
  Tuberculosis
  Toxoplasmosis
  Cytomegalovirus
Periodic testing
  Viral loads every month until virus is undetectable; then every trimester[a]
  Levels should be determined at 34-36 wk to allow discussions for mode of delivery
  CD4 cell counts every trimester
  Resistance testing if indicated
  Monitoring for therapeutic toxicity

Abbreviations: HIV, human immunodeficiency virus; HIV-1, HIV type 1.

[a] Whether the risk of transmission is zero below a certain HIV-1 RNA threshold is unknown, but zidovudine has been effective in reducing transmission at all maternal viral loads.

> **Box 41.10**
>
> **Special Considerations for Mode of Delivery**
>
> Maternal HIV viral load >1,000 copies/mL
>   ACOG has chosen this threshold
>   Scheduled cesarean delivery is recommended as an adjunct to prevent HIV transmission to newborn
> Maternal HIV viral load <1,000 copies/mL
>   Unclear benefit of cesarean delivery
>   In this group, the rate of HIV transmission is already low, so it is unlikely that scheduled cesarean delivery would reduce HIV transmission further
>   In this group, the risk of cesarean delivery may outweigh the risk of HIV transmission by vaginal delivery (<2%)
>   If a patient is receiving effective antiretroviral therapy and has an undetectable viral load, the risk of HIV transmission is low (≤2%) regardless of mode of delivery
> Complications of cesarean delivery
>   Complications, especially postpartum infections, are approximately 5-7 times higher after cesarean delivery with labor or membrane rupture compared with vaginal delivery
>   Complications after scheduled cesarean delivery are intermediate between those of vaginal delivery and urgent cesarean delivery
> Membrane rupture
>   If vaginal delivery is chosen, the duration of ruptured membranes should be minimized because the HIV transmission rate increases with longer duration of membrane rupture (but no cutoff value for duration of membrane rupture has been defined)
>   The additive risk and the critical duration of ruptured membranes are unknown for perinatal HIV transmission in women who are receiving HIV therapy and who have low viral loads
>   Management of women who are scheduled for cesarean delivery and who present with ruptured membranes must be individualized on the basis of duration of rupture and progress of labor
>   If the woman presents after 4 hours of membrane rupture, it is less likely that cesarean delivery would affect HIV transmission
>   Data from International Perinatal HIV Group indicate that the risk of perinatal transmission increases by 2% for every 1-hour increase in duration of membrane rupture in HIV women with ≤24 hours of membrane rupture
> If the decision is made to perform a scheduled cesarean delivery to prevent HIV transmission, ACOG recommends that it be done at 38 weeks of gestation, but the increased risk at 38 weeks rather than 39 weeks must be balanced against the potential risk of labor or membrane rupture between 38 and 39 weeks of gestation
> Patients scheduled for cesarean delivery should receive intravenous zidovudine beginning 3 hours before surgery
>
> Abbreviations: ACOG, American Congress of Obstetricians and Gynecologists; HIV, human immunodeficiency virus.
>
> Data from Panel on Treatment of HIV-Infected Pregnant Women and Prevention of Perinatal Transmission. Recommendations for use of antiretroviral drugs in pregnant HIV-1-infected women for maternal health and interventions to reduce perinatal HIV transmission in the United States. Updated 2010 May 24 [cited 2011 Jan 5]; p 1–117. Available from: http://aidsinfo.nih.gov/ContentFiles/PerinatalGL.pdf.

      ii) Immunizations (eg, influenza, pneumococcal, and hepatitis B vaccines)
    d. Considerations for mode of delivery are summarized in Box 41.10
VII. Puerperal Infection and Fever
   A. Infection
     1. The most common puerperal complication
     2. Includes endometritis, septic pelvic thrombophlebitis, ovarian vein thrombosis, pelvic abscess, wound infection, mastitis, breast abscess, and urinary tract infections
   B. Fever
     1. Mnemonic (7 *W*'s) for causes of fever is shown in Box 41.11
   C. Acute Postpartum Endometritis
     1. The most common cause of puerperal fever
     2. *Endometritis*: infection of the decidua
     3. *Endomyometritis*: infection extending into the myometrium
     4. *Parametritis*: infection extending into the parametrium
     5. Epidemiology
       a. Incidence
         1) After vaginal birth: less than 3%
         2) With scheduled cesarean delivery, without labor or rupture of membranes: 5% to 15%
         3) With cesarean delivery after labor or rupture of membranes, with no antibiotic prophylaxis: 30% to 65%
         4) With cesarean delivery and antibiotic prophylaxis: 15% to 20%
       b. Risk factors are listed in Box 41.12
     6. Causative organisms
       a. Polymicrobial
       b. Genital tract anaerobes, aerobes, and mycoplasmas including GBS, anaerobic streptococci, and gram-negative bacilli such as *Bacteroides* and *Prevotella* species
     7. Diagnosis
       a. Fever: usually 38°C or higher within 36 hours after delivery

> **Box 41.11**
>
> **The *7 W*'s: Causes of Fever After Vaginal or Operative Delivery**
>
> Wind: pneumonia, atelectasis
> Water: urinary tract
> Walk: phlebitis, deep vein thrombosis
> Wound: incision (abdominal or pelvic)
> Wonder drug
> Pregnancy-associated fever
>   Womb: endometritis
>   Wonderbra: mastitis

> **Box 41.12**
> **Risk Factors for Endometritis**
>
> Operative delivery
> Prolonged rupture of membranes or labor
> Multiple vaginal examinations
> Internal fetal or uterine monitoring
> Preexisting infection (eg, intra-amniotic infection, gonorrhea, preexisting colonization with group B streptococci, bacterial vaginosis)
> Maternal diabetes
> Anemia
> Immunodeficiency disorder
> Corticosteroid therapy
> Manual removal of the placenta
> Low socioeconomic status
> Young age
> Smoking in current pregnancy
> Presence of meconium

       b. Malaise
       c. Uterine or abdominal tenderness
       d. Malodorous, discolored lochia
       e. Exclusion of other causes of fever by physical examination and a limited number of laboratory tests, such as white blood cell count, urinalysis, and urine culture
   8. Treatment
       a. Low threshold for treatment: reduce acute and long-term concerns such as infertility and chronic pelvic pain
       b. Empirical parenteral antibiotic therapy
          1) Polymicrobial coverage
          2) In selection, consider that patient may be breast-feeding
          3) Traditionally start with clindamycin and gentamicin
             a) If patient has no response within 24 hours, reassess and add ampicillin
          4) With antibiotic therapy, defervescence occurs in approximately 90% of patients within 48 to 72 hours
             a) When the patient has been afebrile and asymptomatic for approximately 24 to 48 hours, parenteral antibiotic therapy should be discontinued
             b) Unless there are complicating factors, the patient does not require further oral antibiotic therapy
       c. Major causes of treatment failure
          1) Antibiotic resistance
          2) Wound infection
   9. Prevention
       a. Antibiotic prophylaxis for all women undergoing cesarean delivery, especially if their risk of infection is high
       b. Usual prophylaxis
          1) First-generation cephalosporin before incision or at time of cord clamping
          2) Clindamycin is an alternative for patients allergic to cephalosporins
D. Septic Pelvic Thrombophlebitis and Ovarian Vein Thrombosis
   1. Pathogenesis
       a. Infection may cause seeding of the venous circulation with pathogenic organisms
       b. Organisms may damage the vascular epithelium
       c. Damaged vascular epithelium initiates thrombosis
       d. Subsequently, the clot itself becomes infected
       e. Infection occurs in 2 forms: ovarian vein thrombosis and septic pelvic thrombophlebitis (SPT)
   2. Epidemiology
       a. Rare: 1 in 569 to 1 in 2,000 deliveries
       b. Occurs in 0.5% to 2% of patients with endometritis or wound infections
       c. More than 87% of cases are associated with cesarean delivery or febrile abortion
   3. Ovarian vein thrombosis
       a. More common than SPT
       b. Involves acute thrombosis of 1 or both ovarian veins
       c. Clinical features
          1) Moderate fever, disproportionate tachycardia, and abdominal pain
          2) Begins from 48 to 96 hours up to 1 month after delivery or surgery
          3) Pain often localizes to side of affected vein (usually the right) and may involve the back
          4) May be associated with nausea, vomiting, and abdominal distension
          5) In 67% of patients, a ropy, tender 2- to 8-cm mass extends laterally and cephalad from the uterus
          6) Tenderness on pelvic examination
       d. Diagnosis
          1) Leukocytosis
          2) Radiologic imaging is reasonably reliable (computed tomography is less expensive than magnetic resonance imaging and results are equivalent)
          3) Differential diagnosis is shown in Box 41.13

> **Box 41.13**
> **Differential Diagnosis of Ovarian Vein Thrombosis**
> Appendicitis
> Pyelonephritis
> Pelvic abscess
> Enterocolitis
> Broad ligament hematoma
> Operative injury to ureters or bowel
> Urolithiasis
> Endometritis
> Adnexal torsion

4. Septic pelvic thrombophlebitis
   a. Clinical features
      1) "Enigmatic fever": spiking fever despite antimicrobial therapy in a postpartum patient being treated for endometritis
      2) Pain is usually absent
   b. Diagnosis
      1) A clinical diagnosis
      2) Negative imaging result does not exclude SPT in smaller vessels
      3) Differential diagnosis is shown in Box 41.14
5. Treatment of SPT and ovarian vein thrombosis
   a. Broad-spectrum antibiotics and heparinization
      1) In SPT, the efficacy of heparin has recently been questioned
      2) Response to therapy may not be apparent for up to 7 days
      3) If no response to therapy, occasionally surgery may be needed, depending on the clinical picture and the relative certainty of the diagnosis
      4) Continuation of anticoagulation after patient is discharged is unnecessary in most cases
   b. Management of complicating infections (eg, abscesses, multiple septic emboli) during treatment is critical because they occasionally cause death
E. Pelvic Abscess
   1. Since the introduction of antibiotics, pelvic abscesses rarely occur in postpartum patients (unlike in gynecologic patients) in developed countries
   2. Management in postpartum patients is similar to management in gynecologic patients
F. Postpartum Wound Infections
   1. A cause of complications
      a. Complicates 0.1% of episiotomies, and up to 1% to 2% of episiotomies are complicated by extensions of wound infections
      b. Overall, 3% to 15% of cesarean deliveries are complicated by wound infections
      c. Among endometritis cases after cesarean delivery, 3% to 5% are complicated by wound infections
      d. Wound infection is the most common cause of treatment failure of endometritis
   2. Incidence is less than 2% with the use of prophylactic preoperative antibiotics
   3. Necrotizing fasciitis: an uncommon complication of abdominal wound infection, but it has also been reported with episiotomies
G. Mastitis
   1. Occurs in 1% to 5% of lactating women and in less than 1% of nonlactating women
   2. Sporadic mastitis usually occurs 2 to 4 weeks post partum and only rarely antepartum
   3. More than 10% may lead to breast abscesses, especially if therapy is delayed
   4. Etiology
      a. Staphylococci: most common pathogen, especially where mastitis is endemic
      b. Also common: coagulase-negative staphylococci and groups A and B streptococci
      c. *Candida* species have been implicated
      d. Less commonly reported: *Streptococcus faecalis*, *Haemophilus* species, *E coli*, and *K pneumoniae*
   5. Diagnosis
      a. Usually clinical
      b. High fever, malaise, localized erythema, induration, and palpable heat
   6. Treatment
      a. Penicillinase-resistant antibiotic: dicloxacillin or a cephalosporin for 10 to 14 days
      b. Unless mother has very high fever or an abscess, she may continue to breast-feed
      c. Candidiasis
         1) From limited study results, treatment of both mother and infant may be indicated

> **Box 41.14**
> **Differential Diagnosis of Septic Pelvic Thrombophlebitis**
> Any cause of postpartum fever
> Drug fever
> Viral syndrome
> Collagen vascular disease
> Pelvic abscess

2) For mother: oral fluconazole for extended time along with topical antifungals
   3) For infant: oral solutions
   d. Abscess: prompt incision and drainage are indicated

Suggested Reading

American College of Obstetricians and Gynecologists. 2010 compendium of selected publications. Washington (DC): American College of Obstetricians and Gynecologists; c2010.

Brown ZA, Gardella C, Wald A, Morrow RA, Corey L. Genital herpes complicating pregnancy. Obstet Gynecol. 2005 Oct;106(4):845–56. Review. Errata in: Obstet Gynecol. 2006 Feb;107(2 Pt 1):428. Obstet Gynecol. 2007 Jan;109(1):207.

Centers for Disease Control and Prevention. Prevention of perinatal group B streptococcal disease. MMWR 2010;59 (RR-10):1–32.

Lazzarotto T, Guerra B, Lanari M, Gabrielli L, Landini MP. New advances in the diagnosis of congenital cytomegalovirus infection. J Clin Virol. 2008 Mar;41(3):192–7. Epub 2007 Dec 4.

Panel on Treatment of HIV-Infected Pregnant Women and Prevention of Perinatal Transmission. Recommendations for use of antiretroviral drugs in pregnant HIV-1-infected women for maternal health and interventions to reduce perinatal HIV transmission in the United States. May 24, 2010; pp 1–117. [cited 2011 Jan 5]. Available from: http://aidsinfo.nih.gov/ContentFiles/PerinatalGL.pdf.

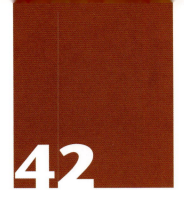

Thomas G. Boyce, MD

42

Pediatric Infectious Diseases

I. Childhood Immunizations
   A. Types of Vaccines
      1. Live-attenuated vaccines: generally provide long-lasting immunity
      2. Inactivated vaccines: often require booster doses
         a. Inactivated whole organisms
         b. Inactivated toxins (toxoids)
         c. Subcellular fragments (subunit vaccines)
            1) Purified surface antigen
            2) Capsular polysaccharide (with or without conjugation to a protein carrier)
               a) Effects of protein conjugation
                  i) T-cell–dependent immune response
                  ii) Development of immune memory
                  iii) Boosting of immune response with subsequent doses
               b) Protein conjugation allows administration of vaccine to children younger than 2 years
   B. Vaccines Given Routinely During Childhood
      1. Hepatitis B vaccine
         a. Purified surface antigen
         b. Given at birth and at 1 and 6 months of age
      2. Diphtheria and tetanus toxoids and acellular pertussis (DTaP) vaccine
         a. Diphtheria and tetanus are toxoids, and pertussis is a toxoid plus subunit vaccine
         b. Given at 2, 4, 6, and 15 to 18 months of age
         c. A booster is given between 4 and 6 years of age
      3. *Haemophilus influenzae* type b (Hib) vaccine
         a. Polysaccharide capsule (with a protein conjugate)
         b. Given at 2, 4, 6, and 12 to 15 months of age
      4. Pneumococcal vaccine
         a. Polysaccharide capsule (with a protein conjugate)
         b. Given at 2, 4, 6, and 12 to 15 months of age
      5. Inactivated poliovirus vaccine (IPV)
         a. Inactivated whole organism
         b. Given at 2, 4, and 6 to 18 months
         c. A booster is given between 4 and 6 years of age
      6. Rotavirus vaccine
         a. Live-attenuated human-bovine reassortant vaccine
         b. Administered orally
         c. Given at 2, 4, and 6 months of age

7. Measles, mumps, and rubella (MMR) vaccine
   a. All 3 are live-attenuated vaccines
   b. Given at 12 to 15 months and at 4 to 6 years of age
8. Varicella virus vaccine
   a. Live-attenuated vaccine
   b. Given at 12 to 18 months and at 4 to 6 years of age
9. Meningococcal vaccine
   a. Polysaccharide capsule (with a protein conjugate)
   b. Contains serotypes A, C, W135, and Y
   c. Given at 11 to 12 years of age
   d. Recommended for incoming college freshmen if they did not receive it earlier in adolescence
10. Tetanus toxoid, reduced diphtheria toxoid, and acellular pertussis (Tdap) vaccine for adolescents and adults
    a. Toxoid and subunit vaccine
    b. Given at 11 to 12 years of age
    c. Boosters are recommended every 10 years
11. Influenza vaccines
    a. Inactivated subunit vaccine (purified hemagglutinin): given intramuscularly to children older than 6 months
    b. Live-attenuated influenza vaccine: given intranasally to children older than 2 years
12. Hepatitis A vaccine
    a. Inactivated whole organism
    b. Given at 12 and 18 months of age
13. Human papillomavirus (HPV) vaccine
    a. Subunit vaccine (viruslike particle)
    b. Three-dose series given to girls at 11 to 12 years of age

II. Infectious Diseases in Children
   A. Acute Otitis Media
      1. Risk factors
         a. Younger than 2 years
         b. Day care attendance
         c. Lack of breast-feeding
         d. Exposure to environmental tobacco smoke
         e. Allergic rhinitis
         f. Recent viral upper respiratory infection
         g. Cleft palate
      2. Frequency: responsible for more than 20 million antibiotic prescriptions yearly in the United States
      3. Etiology
         a. *Streptococcus pneumoniae*
         b. *Haemophilus influenzae* (non-type b)
         c. *Moraxella catarrhalis*
      4. Complications
         a. Mastoiditis
         b. Meningitis
         c. Conductive hearing loss
      5. Treatment
         a. First-line: amoxicillin
         b. Second-line: amoxicillin-clavulanate, cefdinir, ceftriaxone
   B. Croup (Laryngotracheobronchitis)
      1. Epidemiology
         a. Most common cause of upper airway obstruction in young children
         b. Outbreaks in the fall and early winter
         c. Occurs most commonly in children 6 months to 3 years old
      2. Etiology
         a. Parainfluenza virus (most common cause)
         b. Respiratory syncytial virus (RSV)
         c. Influenza virus
         d. Adenovirus
         e. Human metapneumovirus
      3. Clinical manifestations
         a. Mild prodrome of low-grade fever, rhinorrhea
         b. Sudden onset of barking cough, inspiratory stridor, and suprasternal retractions
      4. Treatment
         a. Maintenance of an adequate airway, administration of humidified air or oxygen
         b. Moderate or severe cases are treated with nebulized epinephrine or corticosteroids (or both)
   C. Bronchiolitis
      1. Epidemiology
         a. Most common cause of hospitalization among infants during the winter months
         b. Peak incidence is in children 3 to 6 months old
      2. Risk factors for severe bronchiolitis
         a. Prematurity
         b. Bronchopulmonary dysplasia
         c. Cyanotic congenital heart disease
      3. Etiology
         a. RSV: most common cause
         b. Parainfluenza virus
         c. Influenza virus
         d. Adenovirus
         e. Human metapneumovirus
      4. Clinical manifestations
         a. Prodrome of copious rhinorrhea
         b. Cough, wheezing, and intercostal retractions
         c. Tachypnea and inability to feed
         d. Hypoxia or hypercapnea (or both)
         e. Apnea in very young infants

5. Treatment
   a. Oxygen
   b. Mechanical ventilation in severely affected infants
   c. Inhaled ribavirin is usually reserved for immunocompromised hosts
   d. β-Agonists and corticosteroids are generally ineffective
6. Prevention
   a. Children at high risk of severe disease are given palivizumab monthly during the winter
   b. Palivizumab: a humanized monoclonal antibody to RSV given by intramuscular injection

D. Urinary Tract Infection
1. Epidemiology
   a. Urinary tract infection (UTI) is a common bacterial infection
   b. Affects about 8% of girls and 2% of boys in the first 6 years of life
2. Risk factors
   a. Female: UTI rates are higher among girls than boys
   b. Not circumcised: the incidence of UTI is approximately 10-fold higher among uncircumcised boys than among circumcised boys
   c. Fever: the likelihood of UTI increases with the severity and duration of fever
   d. Anatomical abnormality: any anatomical abnormality that inhibits the ability to empty the bladder increases the risk of UTI
   e. Reflux: vesicoureteral reflux is a risk factor for pyelonephritis in children with UTI
3. Etiology
   a. *Escherichia coli*: most common
   b. Other Enterobacteriaceae
   c. *Pseudomonas aeruginosa*
   d. *Enterococcus* species
   e. *Staphylococcus saprophyticus* (adolescents)
4. Clinical manifestations
   a. Fever may be the only symptom, particularly in a young infant
   b. Vomiting, bedwetting, foul-smelling urine
   c. Among febrile infants with UTI, 60% have evidence of pyelonephritis by scintigraphy
5. Diagnosis
   a. Urinalysis and urine culture
   b. Urine specimen obtained by catheterization or bladder puncture
   c. Bagged specimens are not reliable
   d. Pure growth of more than 50,000 colony-forming units per milliliter from a catheterized specimen is suggestive of UTI
6. Treatment
   a. Infants and older children who are vomiting are usually treated with intravenous antibiotics initially: cefotaxime alone or ampicillin in combination with gentamicin
   b. Older children who appear healthy can be treated with an oral agent, such as trimethoprim-sulfamethoxazole or cefdinir
   c. Definitive therapy is based on susceptibility testing
7. Evaluation for predisposing conditions
   a. With their first documented UTI, children should generally undergo renal ultrasonography and voiding cystourethrography
   b. Exclude anatomical abnormalities and vesicoureteral reflux

E. Sexually Transmitted Diseases in Prepubertal Children and Suspicion of Child Sexual Abuse
1. Diagnosis of a sexually transmitted disease in a child is suggestive of sexual abuse, unless the disease is likely to have been perinatally acquired

F. Gastrointestinal Tract Infections
1. Frequency and importance
   a. Among hospitalized children younger than 5 years, 13% have a discharge diagnosis of diarrhea
   b. The rate of diarrhea among children in day care is 2- to 3-fold higher than among children not in day care
   c. There is a key difference in the approach to diarrhea in children as compared with adults
      1) In children, empirical antibiotic therapy is avoided
      2) Rationale: children have a relatively higher incidence of *E coli* O157:H7 infection, for which antibiotics are contraindicated
2. Clinical patterns
   a. Acute inflammatory diarrhea
      1) Characterized by mucosal invasion and usually involves the large intestine
      2) Stools contain blood, pus, and mucus
      3) Fever and abdominal cramps are common
      4) Most common causes are bacteria
         a) *Campylobacter jejuni*
            i) Acquired from undercooked poultry, unpasteurized milk, and (as a zoonosis) cats or dogs with diarrhea
            ii) Treatment: usually with a macrolide

- b) *Salmonella enterica*
    - i) Acquired from undercooked poultry, from undercooked eggs, and (as a zoonosis) from reptiles and amphibians
    - ii) Treatment: usually avoided
        - (a) Exceptions: neonates and immunocompromised hosts, in whom invasive disease can develop
        - (b) For those patients, a parenteral third-generation cephalosporin can be used
- c) *Shigella* species
    - i) Acquired from contaminated food or water (especially recreational water) or from person-to-person contact (especially in a day care facility)
    - ii) Treatment: usually with trimethoprim-sulfamethoxazole or an oral third-generation cephalosporin
- d) *Escherichia coli* O157:H7 (and other Shiga toxin–producing *E coli*)
    - i) Acquired from contaminated food (most commonly ground beef) or water (especially recreational water) or from person-to-person contact (especially in a day care facility)
    - ii) Antimicrobial therapy: contraindicated because it increases the incidence of hemolytic uremic syndrome (HUS)
        - (a) Overall, HUS occurs in 5% to 10% of children with *E coli* O157:H7 infection
        - (b) HUS is the most common cause of acute renal failure in children
- e) *Clostridium difficile*
    - i) Caused by overgrowth of colonic microflora in patients exposed to antibacterial agents
    - ii) Treatment
        - (a) Discontinue use of the offending agent
        - (b) Administer oral metronidazole (preferred) or oral vancomycin
    - iii) Interpretation of a positive test for *C difficile* toxin in the stools of children younger than 12 months is difficult: one-third to one-half of children that age without diarrhea have colonies of toxin-producing strains of *C difficile*
  - b. Acute noninflammatory diarrhea
    1) Characterized by mucosal hypersecretion or decreased absorption without mucosal invasion and usually involves the small intestine
    2) Stools are watery (without blood or pus)
    3) Vomiting is common
    4) Fever is variable
    5) Most common causes are viruses
        - a) *Rotavirus*
        - b) Caliciviruses (including *Norovirus*)
        - c) Enteric adenovirus
        - d) *Astrovirus*
    6) Occasionally, toxin-producing bacteria are the cause
        - a) Enterotoxigenic *E coli*: especially in travelers who have returned from developing countries
        - b) *Staphylococcus aureus*: preformed heat-stabile toxin
        - c) *Clostridium perfringens*: heat-labile toxin produced in vivo
        - d) *Bacillus cereus*: 1 heat-stabile toxin and 1 heat-labile toxin
        - e) *Vibrio* species: if suspected, ask microbiology laboratory to culture stools on thiosulfate citrate bile salts sucrose (TCBS) agar
  - c. Chronic diarrhea
    1) Most common infectious causes are parasites
        - a) *Giardia lamblia* (most common): treatment options include metronidazole, furazolidone, and nitazoxanide
        - b) *Cryptosporidium parvum*: treatment is with nitazoxanide
        - c) *Cyclospora cayetanensis*: treatment is with trimethoprim-sulfamethoxazole
        - d) *Entamoeba histolytica*: treatment is with metronidazole followed by paromomycin or iodoquinol
- G. Classic Rash Illnesses of Childhood
  1. Scarlet fever
     a. Diffuse, erythematous rash with a texture of fine sandpaper
     b. Caused by concomitant pharyngitis with strains of Group A streptococci that produce pyrogenic exotoxin

2. Measles
   a. Maculopapular to confluent erythematous rash accompanied by high fever
   b. Prodrome of conjunctivitis, coryza, cough, and Koplik spots
   c. Effectively controlled in the United States by vaccination
3. Rubella
   a. Postnatally, a mild illness with pink, maculopapular rash on trunk and posterior cervical adenopathy
   b. Importance is in preventing infection in utero
   c. Effectively controlled in the United States by vaccination
4. Chickenpox
   a. Caused by infection with varicella-zoster virus (VZV)
   b. Before implementation of vaccine, chickenpox was a universal infection of childhood
   c. Clinical features
      1) Starts with fever
      2) Rash progresses from macules to papules to vesicles to crusts
      3) Classic vesicular lesion is described as a dewdrop on a rose petal
5. Fifth disease
   a. Caused by infection with human parvovirus B19
   b. Causes springtime outbreaks among school-aged children
   c. Rash
      1) Diffuse erythema on the face ("slapped-cheek" appearance)
      2) Slightly raised, serpiginous, lacelike rash on extremities
6. Roseola infantum
   a. Caused by infection with human herpesvirus 6
   b. Clinical features
      1) Classic: high fever without a focus for several days in children in the first 2 years of life
      2) Upon defervescence, a fine, maculopapular rash develops on the trunk

III. Bone and Joint Infections in Children
   A. Osteomyelitis
      1. Usually from hematogenous seeding of the metaphysis of a long bone
      2. Peak incidence is in young children
      3. More than 50% involve the tibia or femur
      4. Patients present with fever, pain, and point tenderness
      5. Laboratory test results
         a. White blood cell (WBC) count: often normal
         b. Erythrocyte sedimentation rate (ESR): usually increased
         c. C-reactive protein (CRP) level: usually increased
      6. Etiology
         a. *Staphylococcus aureus*: most common
         b. Group B streptococcus: neonates
         c. *Salmonella*: patients with sickle cell anemia
         d. *Pseudomonas*: after puncture wound to the foot
      7. Confirm diagnosis with bone scan or magnetic resonance imaging
      8. Definitive diagnosis: Gram stain and culture of needle aspirate from bone
      9. Treatment
         a. Antibiotics (initially intravenously) for 4 weeks
         b. If a subcortical abscess is present, it should be drained surgically
   B. Septic Arthritis
      1. Usually from hematogenous seeding of the synovial space
      2. Can be a complication of osteomyelitis in young infants if the infection breaks through the cortex into the joint
      3. Peak incidence is in young children
      4. Joint involvement (in decreasing order of frequency): knee, hip, ankle, elbow, and, rarely, other joints
      5. Patients present with fever, pain, and limited motion (pseudoparalysis in young infants)
      6. Laboratory test results: WBC count, ESR, and CRP level are usually increased
      7. Etiology
         a. *Staphylococcus aureus*: most common
         b. Group B streptococcus: neonates
         c. *Streptococcus pneumoniae*, Group A streptococcus, *Kingella kingae*
         d. *Neisseria gonorrhoeae* in sexually active adolescents
         e. *Borrelia burgdorferi*: Lyme arthritis
      8. Ultrasonography of the joint (eg, hip) can be useful to determine whether fluid is present
      9. Definitive diagnosis: needle aspiration of the joint (usually WBC count >25×10^9/L in septic arthritis)
      10. Treatment
         a. Open irrigation and drainage of the joint
         b. Antibiotics (intravenously initially) for 3 to 4 weeks

IV. Infections of the Fetus and Newborn
    A. Definitions
        1. *Congenital infections*: infections existing at birth (acquired in utero)
        2. *Perinatal infections*: acquired during the birth process (intrapartum period) or shortly after birth (neonatal period)
    B. Congenital and Perinatal Infections
        1. Mnemonic *CHEAP TORCHES*: the most important congenital and perinatal infections
            a. Chickenpox (varicella, VZV)
            b. Hepatitis B virus (HBV) and hepatitis C virus (HCV)
            c. Enteroviruses
            d. AIDS (human immunodeficiency virus [HIV] infection)
            e. Parvovirus (human parvovirus B19)
            f. Toxoplasmosis
            g. Other (Group B streptococcus, *Listeria monocytogenes*, *Candida* species, *Mycobacterium tuberculosis*, lymphocytic choriomeningitis virus)
            h. Rubella
            i. Cytomegalovirus (CMV)
            j. Herpes simplex virus (HSV)
            k. Everything else sexually transmitted (*Neisseria gonorrhoeae*, *Chlamydia trachomatis*, *Ureaplasma urealyticum*, HPV)
            l. Syphilis
        2. Timing of transmission of some congenital and perinatal infections is shown in Table 42.1
    C. Cytomegalovirus
        1. Epidemiology
            a. Most common congenital infection in the United States (affects 1% of all live births)
            b. Risk of transmission: much greater if primary infection occurs during pregnancy (transmission rate, 40%) than if previous infection reactivates (transmission rate <1%)
            c. Transmission early in pregnancy results in more severe disease
        2. Clinical manifestations
            a. Most infants with congenital CMV are asymptomatic
            b. Prematurity
            c. Intrauterine growth retardation
            d. Petechial or purpuric rash
            e. Jaundice, hepatosplenomegaly
            f. Neurologic abnormalities (seizures, microcephaly, periventricular intracranial calcifications)
        3. Sequelae
            a. Sequelae are more common in infants who are symptomatic at birth
            b. Sensorineural hearing loss
            c. Mental retardation
            d. Seizures
            e. Chorioretinitis
        4. Diagnosis: viral isolation in first 3 weeks of life (eg, urine culture)
        5. Treatment
            a. If asymptomatic: no treatment necessary
            b. If symptomatic: intravenous ganciclovir may be given for 6 weeks (in 1 study, this regimen decreased the progression of hearing loss from 68% to 21%)
    D. Herpes Simplex Virus
        1. Epidemiology
            a. Infection rate: 1 infection per 3,000 live births
            b. Type: 75% of isolates are HSV-2, and 25% are HSV-1
            c. Risk of transmission to the infant
                1) With reactivated maternal infection: less than 2%
                2) With primary maternal infection: 50%
        2. Risk factors for neonatal HSV

Table 42.1
Timing of Transmission of Some Congenital and Perinatal Infections

Pathogen or Disease	Timing of Transmission[a]		
	Intrauterine (Congenital)	Intrapartum	Neonatal
Toxoplasmosis	+++	+/–	–
Rubella	+++	+/–	+
Parvovirus	+++	+/–	+
Syphilis	+++	+	–
Cytomegalovirus	+++	++	++
Lymphocytic choriomeningitis virus	+++	+/–	+/–
Human immunodeficiency virus	++	+++	++
Varicella-zoster virus	++	+++	++
Herpes simplex virus	+	+++	++
Enterovirus	+/–	+++	++
Hepatitis B	+/–	+++	++
Hepatitis C	+/–	+++	+
Tuberculosis	+	++	+++

[a] Plus signs and minus signs indicate the following about the period of transmission: +++, most common; ++, less common; +, uncommon; +/–, questionable; –, not transmitted during this period.

a. Primary maternal infection: most important risk factor
   b. Vaginal delivery
   c. Prolonged rupture of membranes
   d. Use of scalp electrodes
   e. Prematurity
   f. *Absence* of visible lesions in the maternal genital tract (women with visible lesions are more likely to undergo cesarean section, which is protective)
  3. Clinical manifestations
   a. Skin, eye, and mucous membrane disease
    1) Usual age at onset: 7 to 14 days
    2) Grouped vesicles on a red base
    3) Conjunctivitis (dendritic keratitis)
    4) Low mortality, but 75% of untreated patients will progress to central nervous system (CNS) disease or disseminated disease
   b. CNS disease
    1) Usual age at onset: 14 to 21 days
    2) Fever, lethargy, seizures
    3) Cerebrospinal fluid (CSF) pleocytosis with negative Gram stain results
    4) Mortality with treatment: 15%
    5) Neurologic sequelae in 50% of survivors
   c. Disseminated disease
    1) Usual age at onset: 5 to 10 days
    2) Sepsis syndrome
    3) Liver dysfunction
    4) Pneumonia
    5) Mortality with treatment: 50%
    6) Long-term sequelae in 40% of survivors
  4. Diagnosis
   a. Viral culture or polymerase chain reaction (PCR) testing: vesicles, mouth, eyes, rectal swab, or CSF
   b. Serology and Tzanck preparation are not useful
  5. Treatment
   a. Skin, eye, and mucous membrane disease: intravenous acyclovir for 14 days
   b. CNS disease: intravenous acyclovir for 21 days
   c. Disseminated disease: intravenous acyclovir for 21 days
  6. Prevention
   a. Cesarean section for women with HSV lesions
   b. Use of acyclovir in pregnant women with HSV: commonly given, but there are no data
   c. For infants born to mothers with HSV lesions: HSV cultures at 24 and 48 hours after birth
 E. Toxoplasmosis
  1. Epidemiology
   a. Infection rate: 1 in 1,000 to 1 in 10,000 live births
   b. Little or no risk of transmission of infection if a mother had a prior infection
   c. Risk of transmission in primary maternal infection
    1) Highest risk in the third trimester, but most disease is asymptomatic
    2) Lower risk earlier in gestation, but high rate of symptomatic disease in the infant if infection does occur
  2. Clinical manifestations
   a. Most infants with congenital toxoplasmosis are asymptomatic
   b. Chorioretinitis
   c. Neurologic abnormalities (seizures, hydrocephalus, microcephaly, diffuse intracranial calcifications, and mental retardation)
   d. Jaundice and hepatosplenomegaly
  3. Diagnosis
   a. Nonspecific tests
    1) Radiography of the skull or computed tomography of the head
    2) Retinal examination
    3) Complete blood cell count (CBC), liver enzymes, and CSF studies
   b. Specific tests
    1) *Toxoplasma* IgM
    2) *Toxoplasma* IgG (increasing titer)
    3) *Toxoplasma* PCR test on CSF
    4) Mouse inoculation
    5) Cell culture
  4. Treatment
   a. All children younger than 1 year should be treated to prevent CNS disease and progressive chorioretinitis
   b. Pyrimethamine, sulfadiazine, and folinic acid for 1 year
 F. Human Parvovirus B19
  1. Maternal infection, especially during the second trimester, can result in nonimmune fetal hydrops
  2. Diagnosis: parvovirus IgM or PCR testing
  3. Intrauterine red blood cell transfusions can prevent fetal loss
 G. Human Immunodeficiency Virus
  1. Routes of transmission to neonates
   a. In utero (20% of cases)
   b. Intrapartum (50% of cases)

c. Postpartum by breast milk (30% of cases among breast-feeding infants of HIV-infected mothers)
2. Risk factors for transmission
    a. Maternal factors
        1) High viral load (most important factor)
        2) Low CD4 count
        3) Primary maternal infection
        4) AIDS
    b. Perinatal factors
        1) Rupture of membranes for more than 4 hours
        2) Chorioamnionitis
        3) Prematurity
        4) Vaginal delivery
3. Zidovudine
    a. Compared with placebo, zidovudine decreased rate of transmission from 26% to 8%
    b. Zidovudine is given in 3 phases
        1) Orally starting at 14 weeks of gestation
        2) Intravenously during labor
        3) Orally to the infant for the first 6 weeks of life
4. Rate of transmission
    a. If the pregnant woman receives highly active antiretroviral therapy: less than 3%
    b. If complete viral suppression is achieved: less than 1%
5. Cesarean section is reserved for women with viral loads of more than 1,000 copies/mL
6. Clinical manifestations of HIV infection in infants
    a. *Pneumocystis* pneumonia: most common AIDS-defining condition in infants
    b. Lymphadenopathy
    c. Hepatosplenomegaly
    d. Persistent oral candidiasis
    e. Failure to thrive
    f. Developmental delay
    g. Parotitis
    h. Recurrent infections (especially with *S pneumoniae*)
H. Rubella
  1. Owing to efficacy of vaccine, rubella (and congenital rubella syndrome) is now rare in the United States
  2. Transmission is highest early in gestation, causing persistent infection of the placenta and target organs
  3. Infants are born with multiple malformations, such as purpura, deafness, cataracts, heart defects, and mental retardation
  4. Diagnosis: IgM in serum, a 4-fold increase in IgG in serum, or viral isolation from nasal secretions, urine, or blood
  5. No specific therapy is available
I. Syphilis
  1. Clinical features of congenital syphilis
      a. At birth, 60% are asymptomatic
      b. Placental and umbilical cord abnormalities
      c. Stillbirth, prematurity, intrauterine growth retardation
      d. Hepatomegaly and increased liver enzyme values
      e. Anemia and thrombocytopenia
      f. Generalized lymphadenopathy
      g. Maculopapular, copper-colored skin rash, often involving palms and soles
      h. Symmetrical osteochondritis
      i. Abnormal CSF profile (increased leukocytes and protein concentration)
  2. Evaluation
      a. No newborn should be dismissed from the hospital without determination of the mother's serologic status for syphilis
      b. Initial evaluation of infant born to a mother with a history of syphilis
          1) Careful physical examination
          2) Quantitative nontreponemal syphilis test (eg, rapid plasma reagin test)
          3) Indications for further evaluation of the infant
              a) Maternal titer has not decreased despite therapy
              b) Infant's titer is 4-fold greater than mother's titer
              c) Infant is symptomatic
              d) Maternal syphilis was inadequately treated (eg, nonpenicillin regimen)
              e) Maternal syphilis was treated less than 1 month before delivery
      c. Further evaluation of the infant if any of the above factors are present
          1) Complete blood cell count
          2) CSF examination for cell count, protein, and quantitative VDRL test
          3) Long-bone radiography
  3. Treatment
      a. Preferred: aqueous crystalline penicillin G intravenously for 10 to 14 days
      b. Alternative: penicillin G procaine intramuscularly for 10 days
V. Clinical Approaches to Selected Situations
    A. Evaluation of Children Who Are Immigrants, Refugees, or Internationally Adopted

1. Complete history and physical examination
2. Immunization status (consider resuming primary series or measuring titers)
3. Tuberculin skin test
4. Stool examination for ova and parasites
5. Serologic testing
   a. HBV serology: hepatitis B surface antigen (HBsAg), antibody to HBsAg (anti-HBs), and antibody to hepatitis B core antigen (anti-HBc)
   b. HCV antibody
   c. HIV antibody
   d. Serologic test for syphilis
6. Complete blood cell count
7. Nutritional assessment
8. Developmental assessment
9. Vision, hearing, and dental screening

B. Evaluation of Febrile Neonates and Young Infants
1. Febrile children in the first 2 to 3 months of life are difficult to evaluate
   a. Fever (or hypothermia) may be the only clue to a serious bacterial infection (eg, bacteremia, meningitis, UTI)
   b. Risk of serious bacterial infection in an infant increases with increasing height of the fever, with increasing WBC counts, and with younger age of the infant
2. Neonatal sepsis is categorized into 2 forms
   a. Early-onset sepsis
      1) Defined as septicemia in the first 7 days of life
      2) Usually manifests within the first 24 hours of life
      3) Mortality is higher than for infants with late-onset disease
      4) Less likely to have a focus of infection
      5) Clinical signs and symptoms commonly associated with early-onset sepsis
         a) Fetal distress before delivery
         b) Meconium staining of the amniotic fluid
         c) Respiratory distress after birth
         d) Persistent tachycardia
         e) Hypothermia or hyperthermia
         f) Apnea or bradycardia
         g) Hypotension
   b. Late-onset sepsis
      1) Defined as septicemia occurring after the first 7 days of life
      2) More likely to have a focus of infection (eg, meningitis, cellulitis, UTI)
      3) Clinical signs and symptoms commonly associated with late-onset sepsis
         a) Jaundice
         b) Poor feeding
         c) Lethargy and decreased tone
         d) Vomiting, abdominal distention, diarrhea
         e) Fever
         f) Cool or mottled skin
3. Common causes of neonatal sepsis
   a. Group B streptococcus
   b. *Escherichia coli* and other Enterobacteriaceae
   c. Herpes simplex virus
   d. *Streptococcus pneumoniae*
   e. *Staphylococcus aureus*
   f. *Listeria monocytogenes*
   g. *Enterococcus* species
4. Most physicians agree that a child who has a fever (38°C) in the first month of life should be hospitalized and undergo an evaluation for sepsis
   a. Sepsis evaluation in a neonate with fever
      1) CBC with differential blood count
      2) Blood culture
      3) Catheterization for urinalysis and urine culture
      4) Lumbar puncture
         a) CSF analyzed for glucose, protein, cell count and differential count, Gram stain, and culture
         b) CSF analyzed for HSV with PCR testing in selected infants
      5) Chest radiography is often appropriate
   b. Empirical antimicrobial therapy for the neonate hospitalized with fever
      1) Ampicillin and gentamicin are used most commonly
      2) Ampicillin and cefotaxime may be used
      3) Acyclovir may be added if HSV is suspected
         a) CSF pleocytosis with negative Gram stain results
         b) Elevated liver enzyme values
         c) Decreased platelet count
         d) Vesicular rash
         e) Known perinatal exposure to HSV
      4) After 48 hours, if culture results are negative and the child is afebrile and appears well, the use of antibiotics can be discontinued and the child can be dismissed to home
5. The approach to the febrile infant older than 1 month is less uniform
6. For infants 28 to 90 days old, many physicians use the Rochester Criteria to determine whether a child is at low risk of

serious bacterial infection and thus can be managed safely with careful follow-up as an outpatient
- a. Patient considerations
  - 1) Looks healthy and physical examination findings are normal
  - 2) Was born at 37 weeks' gestation or later
  - 3) Was dismissed from the birth hospital at the same time as the mother (or before)
  - 4) Has not received antibiotics for this illness
  - 5) Does not have an underlying condition
- b. Diagnostic considerations
  - 1) WBC count: 5.0 to 15.0×10^9/L
  - 2) Band cell count: less than 1.5×10^9/L
  - 3) Urinalysis: less than 10 WBCs per high-power field

C. Prevention of Early-Onset Group B Streptococcal Infection
  1. Intrapartum antibiotic prophylaxis (IAP)
     a. Screening for Group B streptococcal (GBS) infection in pregnant women
        1) All pregnant women should undergo rectovaginal culture at 35 to 37 weeks' gestation
        2) Culture should be incubated in selective broth medium
     b. Treatment of GBS-positive mothers
        1) Mothers whose cultures are positive for GBS should be given IAP
        2) Antibiotic of choice: penicillin
        3) Patients allergic to penicillin should receive cefazolin or clindamycin
     c. Indications for IAP in women who did not undergo GBS screening (because they presented in labor before 35 to 37 weeks' gestation or because screening was omitted)
        1) Delivery before 37 weeks
        2) Rupture of membranes for more than 18 hours
        3) Intrapartum temperature greater than 38°C
     d. Other indications for IAP
        1) GBS bacteriuria during the current pregnancy
        2) Previous delivery of an infant with GBS disease
  2. Approach to newborn whose mother received IAP
     a. If suspected chorioamnionitis was the rationale for IAP
        1) Evaluate for sepsis (CBC, blood culture, possibly lumbar puncture)
        2) Treat empirically with intravenous antibiotics
     b. If the newborn appears ill
        1) Evaluate for sepsis (CBC, blood culture, possibly lumbar puncture)
        2) Treat empirically with intravenous antibiotics
     c. If the child appears well, but gestational age is less than 35 weeks
        1) Perform a limited evaluation (CBC and blood culture)
        2) Observe in hospital for at least 48 hours
     d. Indications for observing for at least 48 hours
        1) Gestational age older than 35 weeks
        2) Mother received IAP more than 4 hours before delivery because she was a GBS carrier
        3) Child appears well

Suggested Reading

Fisher RG, Boyce TG. Moffet's pediatric infectious diseases: a problem-oriented approach. 4th ed. Philadelphia (PA): Lippincott Williams and Wilkins; c2005.

Long SS, Pickering LK, Prober CG. Principles and Practice of Pediatric Infectious Diseases, 3rd ed. Philadelphia (PA): Churchill Livingstone/Elsevier; c2008.

Pickering, LK. Red Book: 2009 Report of the Committee on Infectious Diseases. 28th ed. Elk Grove Village (IL): American Academy of Pediatrics; c2009.

Abinash Virk, MD

43

Travel Medicine

I. Introduction
   A. International Travel
      1. Travel between developing countries and developed countries is increasing every year
         a. Reasons for this increase include ease of travel, more affluence, business, philanthropy, and immigration
         b. United Nations World Tourism Organization (UNWTO) provides travel and tourism data
            1) Approximately 880 million passengers arrived at international airports in 2009
               a) Leisure or vacation: 50% (about 400 million)
               b) Business: 16% (about 125 million)
               c) Visiting friends and relatives or traveling for religious purposes or health treatment: 26% (about 200 million)
            2) In 2006, a record 842 million passengers arrived at international airports
         c. Tourism is expected to continue growing at an annual rate of approximately 4%
      2. Travel destinations
         a. Europe and the Americas are the most popular
         b. Other geographic regions are gaining international travel interest
            1) The increase in travel to Africa has outpaced the increase for all other regions by almost twice, with the rate of growth reaching 8.1% in 2006
            2) Popular travel destinations in Africa: South Africa, Botswana, Kenya, Tanzania, and Morocco
            3) Asian and Pacific Rim countries continue to hold substantial travel interest
            4) Travel to the Middle East has kept pace with travel growth despite the political instability there
      3. More people are traveling to destinations that present higher risks of infectious diseases
         a. Knowledge of prevention of preventable diseases becomes increasingly important
         b. Management of posttravel illness becomes increasingly important
   B. Pretravel Preventive Strategies
      1. Individual risk assessment of acquisition of health problems during travel is necessary
      2. Exacerbation of a preexisting medical problem
         a. Quick review of preexisting medical history should identify any active issues that should be dealt with before travel

b. Examples: coronary artery disease, uncontrolled hypertension, asthma, diabetes mellitus, dental abscesses
3. Acquisition of a new problem
   a. The bulk of the pretravel assessment and counseling is centered on preventing the acquisition of new problems
      1) Example: deep vein thrombosis (DVT) during long-haul flight
      2) Example: human immunodeficiency virus (HIV) infection from sexual exposure at destination
   b. Risk assessment and decision making for preventive counseling
      1) Destination details (exact locations in countries)
      2) Duration of travel
      3) Purpose of travel
      4) Accommodations
      5) Activities planned

II. General Advice for All International Travelers
   A. Insect Bite Precautions
      1. Clothing for travelers to higher-risk areas
         a. Long-sleeved shirts and long pants
         b. While hiking in the bush or areas with more insects, travelers should tuck their pant legs into their socks
         c. Hikers should wear boots instead of open sandals
      2. Ticks
         a. Patients should check their body for ticks regularly
         b. Remove ticks completely with tweezers when discovered
      3. Mosquitoes
         a. Mosquitoes that transmit malaria bite from dusk to dawn
         b. Mosquitoes that transmit diseases such as dengue fever bite during the day
      4. Use of bed nets: advised for travel to countries where malaria is endemic
      5. Insect repellents
         a. Insect repellents should be used on skin
         b. Repel mosquitoes, ticks, fleas, and other insects
         c. In the United States, repellents with either of 2 active ingredients (diethyltoluamide [DEET] or picaridin) are considered effective
            1) Repellents with DEET (many products are available)
               a) DEET is safe and effective at concentrations of 20% to 50% for adults and for children older than 2 months
                  i) No added repellency is noted with concentrations greater than 50%
                  ii) DEET concentrations of 30% to 50% are effective for 6 to 8 hours
               b) For international travel, DEET-containing repellents have an advantage since they last longer than repellents with picaridin
               c) Sunscreen should be applied on the skin before repellent (otherwise the sunscreen may be less effective)
            2) Repellents with picaridin (many products are available)
               a) Picaridin is better tolerated on the skin than DEET
               b) Picaridin may be an option for persons who have allergy or intolerance to DEET-containing products
               c) Picaridin is available in 7% and 15% concentrations
                  i) Lasts for 2 to 4 hours
                  ii) Requires more frequent application
      6. Insecticide
         a. Insecticide (permethrin) should be used on clothing
            1) For persons who are traveling to higher-risk areas, children, or persons who attract mosquitoes
            2) Applied to clothing, shoes, tents, mosquito nets, and other equipment for greater protection
            3) Available commercially as a spray or liquid or in pretreated clothing from outdoor supply stores
            4) Clothing that is properly soaked with permethrin is effective for up to 4 weeks and 5 to 6 washes
            5) Bednets soaked with permethrin are effective for several months
         b. DEET on the skin in combination with permethrin impregnated into clothing significantly decreases insect bites: repels insects and prevents bites by mosquitoes, chiggers, tsetse flies, ticks, and other insects
   B. Deep Vein Thrombosis Prevention While Flying
      1. An association of DVT with air travel is present but small
         a. Incidence increases in persons with risk factors
         b. Overall risk of DVT: 2.7% to 6%

c. One study showed that DVT developed in the calf in about 10% of long-haul airline travelers
2. Factors in DVT
   a. Immobilization (predominantly)
   b. Low humidity
   c. Relative dehydration
   d. Coach class seats
3. Incidence increases among persons with additional risk factors
   a. Previous DVT or pulmonary embolism
   b. Pregnancy
   c. Age older than 50 years
   d. Hormone replacement therapy
   e. Malignancy
   f. Obesity
   g. Thrombophilic defect (polycythemia and others)
   h. Recent surgery
   i. Cardiac failure
   j. Sedation
   k. Prothrombotic states such as factor V Leiden, deficiency of protein C or protein S, or lupus anticoagulant
4. Preventive measures
   a. General
      1) Regular leg exercises
      2) Short walks in the aisle every 2 to 3 hours
      3) Fluids
   b. Specific preventive strategies
      1) Aspirin: shows a minor decrease in DVT risk to 3.6%
      2) Below-knee compression stockings with 20 mm Hg pressure: decreases risk to 0.24%
      3) Low-molecular-weight heparin (LMWH): decreases DVT risk to 0%
   c. For persons with limited DVT risk, the best preventive measures are to exercise and use compression knee stockings
   d. For patients with multiple risk factors or significant risk factors, use of compression stockings in combination with subcutaneous LMWH may need to be considered
C. Animal Bite Prevention
1. Patients should avoid voluntarily petting dogs, cats, and other animals in countries outside the United States because of the risk of a bite and the transmission of rabies
2. An unprovoked animal that bites should always be considered rabid
   a. An unprovoked bite constitutes a medical emergency that requires immediate medical attention
   b. Patients should be advised of their need for rabies immunoglobulin and rabies vaccination depending on their preexposure rabies vaccination status (see rabies vaccine information in the "Vaccine-Preventable Diseases and Immunization" section)
D. Motion Sickness
1. Motion sickness can occur with any type of motion
2. Symptoms: drowsiness, tremulousness, headache, nausea, vomiting, increased salivation, and sweatiness
3. Habituation
   a. Occurs after 3 to 4 days of exposure to the movement
   b. After habituation, persons can get a rebound postdisembarkation illness as a result of compensatory mechanisms that are still operating
4. Persons at higher risk
   a. Women, especially during menstrual periods or pregnancy
   b. Persons with history of migraines
5. Persons at lower risk
   a. Children younger than 2 years
   b. Elderly persons
6. Preventive strategies
   a. Stabilizing the head and body and decreasing sensory stimuli that may aggravate the symptoms
   b. General measures
      1) Lean head on a headrest or lie down
      2) Occupy the most stable part of the vehicle (eg, in the front of the car, over the wings of a plane, in the midpoint of the ship)
      3) Avoid reading or focusing on objects close-up
      4) Focus on a distant stationary object
      5) Eat only small, low-fat meals
      6) Avoid alcoholic beverages and smoking
   c. Preventive medications
      1) Medications such as dimenhydrinate, meclizine, or scopolamine patches are helpful
      2) Patients should be warned about potential adverse effects of the medications
E. Jet Lag
1. Cause of jet lag
   a. Desynchronization of the body's circadian system (or desynchronization of the

physiologic response to light-dark cycles) from crossing many time zones
b. Traveler flying westward from Thailand to Chicago will feel the urge to sleep earlier on arrival than the local time in Chicago would dictate
c. Traveler flying eastward from Chicago to Thailand will feel quite awake on arrival even though it is nighttime in Thailand
2. Preventive strategies
a. Exposure to sunlight at the destination
1) After flying westward, it is advisable to remain in sunlight after arrival
2) After flying eastward, it is best to avoid sunlight during the morning but stay in the sunlight during the afternoon
b. Over-the-counter sedatives or prescribed sedatives such as zaleplon (Sonata), eszopiclone (Lunesta), and zolpidem (Ambien) may help in the first 2 to 3 nights after arrival
c. Melatonin
1) Efficacy for jet lag is controversial and the evidence is not conclusive
2) Two recent meta-analyses: 1 showed that melatonin is effective for jet lag, and the other did not
3) Melatonin probably helps but needs to be taken at the right time and at the right dose to be effective
F. Altitude Sickness
1. Cause of altitude sickness: inability to acclimate to decreased atmospheric pressure after reaching higher altitudes
2. Symptoms
a. Mild symptoms are common
b. Severe symptoms can occur from potentially life-threatening high-altitude pulmonary edema (HAPE) or high-altitude cerebral edema (HACE)
3. Preventive strategies
a. Ascend gradually if possible
b. Increase fluid intake
c. Avoid strenuous activities for the first few days
d. Avoid alcoholic and caffeinated drinks
e. Avoid medications that decrease breathing rate such as sleeping pills, tranquilizers, and narcotic-based pain relievers
4. Prescription medication
a. Acetazolamide is effective in preventing acute mountain sickness
1) Dosage: 125 to 250 mg every 12 hours starting 1 day before reaching the higher altitude and continued for 2 days after reaching it
2) Acetazolamide is a sulfonamide: can cause a cross-reaction in persons with allergy to sulpha-containing medications
b. Other medications may be given depending on the patient's understanding of self-management
1) Nifedipine for emergency treatment of HAPE
2) Dexamethasone for emergency treatment of HACE
G. Sexual Exposure While Traveling
1. Sexually transmitted diseases (eg, gonorrhea, HIV/AIDS, syphilis) can be acquired through unprotected sexual exposure
2. Travelers should be reminded to limit sexual contacts with strangers and to carry and use effective barrier protection
3. Persons who anticipate sexual contact while traveling
a. Should be counseled on prevention of sexually transmitted diseases
b. Should be advised to consider hepatitis A and hepatitis B vaccination before traveling
III. Vaccine-Preventable Diseases and Immunization
A. Basis for Specific Vaccine Recommendations
1. Prevalence of vaccine-preventable diseases at international destinations
2. Specific risk to the traveler of acquiring a vaccine-preventable disease
a. Planned activities
b. Cumulative exposure
c. Traveler's prior immunity to a disease
d. Host immune status
3. Considerations in risk-benefit assessment of giving a specific vaccine to a patient (vaccine safety and contraindications)
a. Age
b. Immune status
c. Prior disease immunity or vaccination
d. Pregnancy
B. Immunizations for International Travel
1. Routine (Table 43.1)
2. Recommended (Table 43.2)
3. Required (Table 43.3)
C. Routine Immunizations
1. All travelers should be up-to-date with their routine childhood and adult vaccinations based on age and health status (Table 43.1) (pediatric travel vaccine recommendations are not discussed in this text)

Table 43.1
Routine Vaccines for Adult Travelers

Vaccine	Vaccine Type and Efficacy	Indications	Boosters	Schedule	Contraindications[a]	Comments[b]
Influenza	Trivalent inactivated vaccine (TIV) Live-attenuated influenza vaccine (LAIV) Efficacy: 70%–90% in healthy persons; less in persons older than 65 y	Age >50 y Increased risk of severity: chronic disease (including diabetes mellitus), immunosuppression, pregnancy Travel to the tropics any month Travel to the Southern Hemisphere in its winter (April to September) Cruise travel Organized group travel	Annually	None	Egg type I hypersensitivity TIV: precaution if Guillain-Barré syndrome occurred within 6 wk after a previous dose of TIV LAIV: immunosuppression: age >50 y; pregnancy, chronic diseases (eg, asthma); adolescents receiving aspirin therapy	TIV is advised for pregnant women regardless of the stage of pregnancy Breast-feeding is not a contraindication
Pneumococcal	Inactivated, pneumococcal polysaccharide vaccine (PPV) Efficacy: 60%–70%	Age >65 y and healthy Any age with chronic liver, kidney, cardiac, or lung disease; diabetes mellitus; asplenia; sickle cell disease Smokers Immunocompromised	Once in 5 y for those with asplenia, diabetes mellitus, or chronic conditions or for persons older than 65 y who received the vaccine before age 65 y	Single dose		
Measles, mumps, and rubella (MMR)	Live-attenuated virus vaccine Efficacy: 95%	All unvaccinated persons with no evidence of immunity	None	2 doses at least 1 mo apart	Pregnancy and for 1 mo before pregnancy; immunosuppression; allergy to eggs	Give on same day as PPD skin test and other live-attenuated vaccines, or separate by 28 d
Varicella	Live-attenuated virus vaccine Efficacy: 95%	All unvaccinated persons with no evidence of immunity	None	2 doses at least 1 mo apart	Pregnancy, breast-feeding, immunosuppression	Give on same day as PPD skin test and other live-attenuated vaccines, or separate by 28 d
Shingles vaccine (Zostavax)	Live-attenuated virus vaccine Efficacy: 50%	Age ≥60 y	None	Single dose	Immunosuppression, pregnancy	Give on same day as PPD skin test and other live-attenuated vaccines, or separate by 28 d

(continued)

Table 43.1
(continued)

Vaccine	Vaccine Type and Efficacy	Indications	Boosters	Schedule	Contraindications[a]	Comments[b]
Tetanus and diphtheria with (Tdap) or without (Td) acellular pertussis	Inactivated toxoid Efficacy: 95%	All adults who have had primary series. For Tdap: patient should not have had a Td within 2 y	Td: every 10 y Tdap: no booster determination yet	Primary series: 3 doses 4-8 wk apart	Allergy to components Guillain-Barré syndrome ≤6 wk after receipt of a tetanus toxoid-containing vaccine is a precaution (weigh risks and benefits) for subsequent tetanus toxoid–containing vaccine	
Human papillomavirus (HPV) vaccine	Efficacy in women: 100% for cervical precancerous lesion Efficacy in men: 62%-89% for genital warts	All women aged 9-26 y Can consider for boys aged 9-26 y	Unknown	Primary series: 0, 2, and 6 mo	Allergic reaction to previous dose	

Abbreviation: PPD, purified protein derivative (tuberculin).

[a] Common contraindications to all vaccines include 1) allergic reaction to a previous dose or to components of individual vaccine and 2) ongoing acute illness (moderate to severe acute illness, fever, otitis, diarrhea, vomiting).

[b] Common comments for live virus vaccines: all are contraindicated in hosts who are immunocompromised or pregnant. Some contraindications for live vaccines are relative and need to be reviewed for individual patient and vaccines. Intervals between immune globulin products and live viral vaccines should be kept in mind. Live-attenuated vaccines are best given on the same day as a PPD skin test and other live-attenuated vaccines or separated by 28 days to prevent a decreased immune response to the second vaccine or the PPD.

Table 43.2

Recommended Vaccines for Adult Travelers

Vaccine	Vaccine Type and Efficacy	Indications	Boosters	Schedule	Contraindications[a]	Comments[b]
Cholera, oral (not available in the United States)	Killed whole-cell, recombinant B-subunit vaccine (Dukoral) Efficacy: 85%-90%	Travel for health care delivery; refugee assistance, and volunteer work where disease is epidemic	Every 2 y for persons aged >6 y	Age >6 y: 2 doses orally 7-42 d apart No accelerated schedule	Category C	Protection (67%) for traveler's diarrhea caused by heat-labile toxin of enterotoxigenic *Escherichia coli* (ETEC)
Hepatitis A	Inactivated viral antigen (Havrix or VAQTA) Efficacy: 70%-80% in 2 wk; >95% in 4 wk	All travelers to developing countries	None	1 dose followed by second in 6-12 mo No accelerated schedule	Category C Not contraindicated during lactation Allergies to components	Can be interchanged with each other or other hepatitis A vaccines
Hepatitis A immune globulin	Passive immunity Efficacy: 85%-90%	Rarely used now except for immunosuppressed persons leaving imminently for a high-risk area	Dose is repeated if patient has continued exposure and no immunity through vaccination	For a stay <3 mo: 0.02 mL/kg For a stay 3-5 mo: 0.06 mL/kg Intramuscular injection		Observe recommended intervals between immune globulin products and live viral vaccines
Hepatitis A and hepatitis B (combined vaccine)	Inactivated viral antigen (Twinrix) Efficacy: 100% protective hepatitis A antibody levels and 94% protective hepatitis B antibody levels after 3 doses	Prolonged stays in countries with high prevalence of hepatitis B for health care delivery, adoption, or medical tourism	None	Regular schedule: dose at 0, 1, and 6 mo Accelerated schedule: 0, 7, and 21 d plus booster at 1 y		
Hepatitis B	Inactivated viral antigen recombinant vaccine (Engerix-B or Recombivax HB) Efficacy: 95% protective after 3 doses	Prolonged stays in countries with high prevalence of hepatitis B for health care delivery, adoption, or medical mission	Boosters may be necessary in immuno-compromised patients with anti-HBs titer <10 mU/mL	Regular schedule: dose at 0, 1, and 6 mo Accelerated schedule: 0, 1, 2, and 12 mo or 0, 7, and 21 d and 12 mo	History of yeast allergy	Brands can be used interchangeably with each other Pregnancy is not a contraindication to vaccination
Japanese encephalitis	JE-VAX: inactivated viral vaccine for persons 16 y or younger JE-VAX: efficacy: 0% with 1 dose; 80% with 2 doses; 95% with 3 doses Ixiaro: new inactivated vaccine for persons 17 y or older	Prolonged (>4 wk) travel to Southeast Asian countries where disease is prevalent, especially rural areas	Single booster in at least 3 y if ongoing exposure	JE-VAX: regular schedule: 0, 7, and 30 d JE-VAX: accelerated schedule: 0, 7, and 14 d Ixiaro: 0 and 28 d Ixiaro: accelerated schedule: not determined	Pregnancy JE-VAX: with allergic predisposition (eg, urticaria, atopy), need risk-benefit assessment Ixiaro: does not carry the risk of anaphylaxis	JE-VAX: administer last vaccine dose 10 d before departure in case of rare delayed hypersensitivity reaction (estimated incidence in US citizens: 15-62 per 10,000)

(*continued*)

Table 43.2
(continued)

Vaccine	Vaccine Type and Efficacy	Indications	Boosters	Schedule	Contraindications[a]	Comments[b]
Poliovirus	Injectable inactivated poliovirus (IPV)	Traveling to country with ongoing wild poliovirus transmission	Single booster as adult if >10 y since completion of primary series	Primary series: doses at 0, 2, and 8-14 mo Accelerated schedule: doses at 0, 1, and 2 mo (≥4 wk apart)	Category C Risk-benefit assessment needed in pregnancy Not contraindicated during lactation	Oral polio vaccine no longer used in the United States
Rabies	Inactivated viral vaccine (many types and brands)	Prolonged travel into areas where rabies is endemic and access to rabies immune globulin is poor; expected animal exposures (eg, veterinarian)	Unknown duration of protection (possibly ≥3 y) May need serology to determine need for boosters	Regular schedule: 0, 7, and 28 d Accelerated schedule: 0, 7, and 21 d		
Tick-borne encephalitis (not available in the United States)	Inactivated viral vaccine Efficacy: seroconversion rates of about 100% after 3 doses	Prolonged stay and working in the woods in parts of Europe	Every 3-5 y	Regular schedule: day 0, 4-12 wk, and 9-12 mo	Category C Pregnancy Breast-feeding	
Typhoid	1) Live-attenuated bacterial vaccine (capsule): TY21a (Vivotif); efficacy 50%-80%	Travel to areas with high prevalence of typhoid, especially for prolonged stays, rural travel, health care delivery, or adventurous eating habits	5 y	4 capsules: 1 orally every other day on days 0, 2, 4, and 6	Category C Contraindicated if patient is concurrently receiving antibiotics or antimalarials Inflammatory bowel disease Immunosuppression	Capsules must be refrigerated and taken on an empty stomach with a cool liquid
	2) Polysaccharide vaccine (injectable): efficacy 63%-96%		Every 2-3 y	None	Category C Allergy to vaccine components	

Abbreviation: anti-HBs, antibody to hepatitis B surface antigen.

[a] Common contraindications to all vaccines include 1) allergic reaction to a previous dose or to components of individual vaccine and 2) ongoing acute illness (moderate to severe acute illness, fever, otitis, diarrhea, vomiting).

[b] Common comments for live virus vaccines: all are contraindicated in hosts who are immunocompromised or pregnant. Some contraindications for live vaccines are relative and need to be reviewed for individual patient and vaccines. Intervals between immune globulin products and live viral vaccines should be kept in mind. Live-attenuated vaccines are best given on the same day as a purified protein derivative (tuberculin) (PPD) skin test and other live-attenuated vaccines or separated by 28 days to prevent a decreased immune response to the second vaccine or the PPD.

Table 43.3
Required Vaccines for Adult Travelers in Certain Geographic Areas

Vaccine	Vaccine Type and Efficacy	Indications	Boosters	Schedule	Contraindications[a]	Comments[b]
Yellow fever	Live-attenuated viral vaccine (YF-Vax) Efficacy: >98%	Travel into areas where yellow fever is endemic	Every 10 y	Single dose Should be administered ≥10 d before exposure to be considered effective	Pregnancy unless exposure is unavoidable; then risks and benefits need to be weighed Breast-feeding should be avoided (no data) Egg type I hypersensitivity Immunosuppression Thymus dysfunction	Life-threatening vaccine-associated viscerotropic disease: 1:300,000 risk if healthy; 1:30,000 risk if age >65 y Give on same day as PPD skin test and other live-attenuated vaccines, or separate by 28 d
Meningococcal (for meningococcal disease caused by Neisseria meningitidis)	2 vaccines are effective against groups A, C, Y, and W135, with efficacy of 85%–90% after 1–2 wk: 1) Polysaccharide vaccine (MPSV4) 2) Conjugated meningococcal vaccine (MCV4)	College students Travel to Saudi Arabia for Hajj pilgrimage Travel to "meningitis belt" of Africa (see text) Asplenic patients	Same dose MPSV4: every 3–5 y MCV4: every 5 y	Single dose	Category C Severe allergic reaction to any component of the vaccine, including diphtheria toxoid (for MCV4), or to dry natural rubber latex	

Abbreviation: PPD, purified protein derivative (tuberculin).

[a] Common contraindications to all vaccines include 1) allergic reaction to a previous dose or to components of individual vaccine and 2) ongoing acute illness (moderate to severe acute illness, fever, otitis, diarrhea, vomiting).

[b] Common comments for live virus vaccines: all are contraindicated in hosts who are immunocompromised or pregnant. Some contraindications for live vaccines are relative and need to be reviewed for individual patient and vaccines. Intervals between immune globulin products and live viral vaccines should be kept in mind. Live-attenuated vaccines are best given on the same day as a PPD skin test and other live-attenuated vaccines or separated by 28 days to prevent a decreased immune response to the second vaccine or the PPD.

2. In general, a previous reaction to a vaccine or its components contraindicates the use of that particular vaccine
3. Tetanus, diphtheria, and acellular pertussis vaccine
   a. Prevalence: tetanus, diphtheria, and pertussis occur worldwide
   b. Schedule and specific risk of disease acquisition to traveler
      1) All international travelers should have completed a primary series and be up-to-date for their age
      2) For adults who have completed the primary series, tetanus and diphtheria toxoids (Td) should have been given within 5 to 10 years before travel
      3) For prolonged or high-risk travel, Td should be boosted if the last one was given more than 5 years earlier
      4) Recently approved adult tetanus, diphtheria, and acellular pertussis (Tdap) can be given instead of the Td booster if the latest Td was given at least 2 years earlier
         a) Tdap is a 1-time booster
         b) Subsequent booster should be a Td booster in 10 years
   c. Vaccine safety and contraindications
      1) Relatively contraindicated for persons with a history of Guillain-Barré syndrome within 6 weeks or seizures within 3 days of a prior dose
      2) In those instances, risk-benefit assessment is required before proceeding with vaccination
4. Measles, mumps, and rubella vaccine
   a. Prevalence
      1) Many countries do not routinely vaccinate against measles, mumps, or rubella
      2) These diseases are common worldwide
   b. Specific risk of disease acquisition to traveler
      1) All travelers born after 1957 should have completed their primary measles, mumps, and rubella (MMR) series
      2) Persons born before 1957 are considered immune
      3) Immigrants to the United States from developing countries who are returning to their native country should have serologies done to ascertain immune status and need for vaccination
   c. Vaccine safety and contraindications
      1) Live-attenuated viral vaccine
      2) Contraindicated for persons with congenital or acquired immunocompromised state
         a) Corticosteroid use
         b) Chemotherapy
         c) Tumor necrosis factor α inhibitors
         d) HIV/AIDS
         e) Pregnancy
      3) Data do not show a causal link to autism
5. Influenza vaccine
   a. Prevalence
      1) Seasonal (winter) in temperate countries
      2) Nonseasonal and year-round in tropical countries
      3) Influenza is the most common vaccine-preventable disease in travelers
   b. Specific risk of disease acquisition to traveler
      1) Recommendations for influenza vaccine for travelers are the same as the usual recommendations for all persons
         a) Persons older than 50 years
         b) Persons at increased risk of complications
            i) Cardiopulmonary conditions: coronary artery disease, chronic obstructive pulmonary disease (COPD), asthma
            ii) Immunosuppression
            iii) Diabetes mellitus
            iv) Other debilitating chronic diseases
         c) All health care workers
         d) All who want to decrease their risk while traveling
      2) In addition, influenza vaccine is recommended for travelers to the Southern Hemisphere during winter there
   c. Vaccine safety and contraindications
      1) Contraindicated for persons with type I hypersensitivity to eggs
      2) Vaccine can be administered to people who have an intolerance to eggs but can eat them
      3) Nasal live-attenuated influenza vaccine is contraindicated for immunocompromised persons
6. Pneumococcal vaccine
   a. Prevalence
      1) Prevalent worldwide
      2) Risk of infection with drug-resistant strains is potentially higher for persons

traveling for prolonged duration in countries with high resistance rates
    b. Schedule and specific risk of disease acquisition to traveler
        1) Indications for pneumococcal 23-valent vaccine
            a) All healthy adults older than 65 years
            b) Persons with increased risk of invasive pneumococcal disease
                i) Asplenic patients
                ii) Persons with chronic cardiopulmonary diseases (coronary artery disease, COPD, asthma)
                iii) Immunosuppression
                iv) Persons with diabetes mellitus or other debilitating chronic diseases
        2) Healthy adults who received their first pneumococcal vaccine before the age of 65 years should receive a second dose after they turn 65 years but 5 years after the previous dose
        3) Similarly, asplenic patients should receive a second dose 5 years after the previous dose
    c. Vaccine safety and contraindications
        1) Pneumococcal vaccine is safe
        2) Most common adverse effect: local reaction
7. Varicella vaccine
    a. Prevalence
        1) Prevalent worldwide
        2) Primary varicella in developing countries occurs more often in older children and young adults
    b. Schedule and specific risk of disease acquisition to traveler
        1) A nonimmune person carries the risk of acquiring the disease while traveling if exposed
        2) People 13 years or older without laboratory-documented evidence of immunity against chickenpox should receive 2 doses of the varicella vaccine 4 to 8 weeks apart
    c. Vaccine safety and contraindications
        1) Live-attenuated vaccine
        2) Has 1,350 plaque-forming units (PFU)
        3) Contraindicated for all immunosuppressed persons (contraindications are similar to those for MMR vaccine)
8. Shingles vaccine
    a. Prevalence: worldwide
    b. Schedule and specific risk of disease acquisition to traveler
        1) In elderly, reactivation of childhood-acquired varicella-zoster virus (VZV) can cause dermatomal or disseminated varicella
        2) Live-attenuated vaccine for the prevention of herpes zoster
            a) Approved in 2006 for persons older than 60 years
            b) Given as a single 0.65-mL dose subcutaneously
            c) Dose contains at least 19,400 PFU (10-fold higher PFU of virus than the varicella vaccine) of the live-attenuated Oka/Merck strain of VZV
    c. Vaccine safety and contraindications
        1) Shown to be safe
        2) Most common adverse events reported to the Vaccine Adverse Event Reporting System (VAERS): injection site reaction, rash, and episodes of herpes zoster (although none had the Oka/Merck strain isolated from the samples tested)
        3) Live-attenuated vaccine
        4) Contraindicated in all immunosuppressed persons (contraindications are similar to those for MMR vaccine)
9. Human papillomavirus (HPV) vaccine
    a. Prevalence: HPV types 6, 11, 16, and 18 occur worldwide
    b. Schedule and specific risk of disease acquisition to traveler
        1) HPV infection is the most common viral sexually transmitted disease in the United States
        2) Two vaccines are available to protect females against the types of HPV that cause most cervical cancers
            a) Cervarix (HPV types 16 and 18)
            b) Gardasil (HPV types 6, 11, 16, and 18)
                i) Approved in 2006 for females aged 9 to 26 years
                ii) Approved in 2009 for males aged 9 to 26 years for prevention of genital warts caused by HPV types 6 and 11
                iii) Doses are given as intramuscular injections at 0, 2, and 6 months

iv) Efficacy in women
    (a) For prevention of cervical precancerous lesions caused by the targeted HPV types: 100% efficacy
    (b) For prevention of vulvar and vaginal precancerous lesions and genital warts caused by the targeted HPV types among women aged 16 to 26 years who are naive to the specific HPV vaccine types: nearly 100% efficacy
v) Efficacy in men
    (a) For prevention of genital warts related to HPV types 6, 11, 16, or 18 after 3 doses of vaccine in those with no prior HPV exposure: 89.4% efficacy
    (b) For prevention of genital warts related to HPV types 6, 11, 16, or 18 among males who received at least 1 vaccine dose (regardless of baseline DNA or serology): 67.2% efficacy
    (c) For prevention of genital warts related to any HPV type: 62.1% efficacy
c. Vaccine safety and contraindications
    1) Shown to be safe
    2) Adverse events
        a) Most common: local injection site symptoms
        b) Fever higher than 37.8°C in about 4%
        c) Serious adverse events in less than 0.1%
    3) Duration of immunogenicity: thought to be about 5 years

D. Recommended Travel Immunizations
    1. Hepatitis A vaccine
        a. Prevalence
            1) Endemic everywhere except North America, Western Europe, Great Britain, Scandinavia, Japan, Australia, and New Zealand
            2) Hepatitis A virus (HAV) infection is the second most frequent vaccine-preventable disease
        b. Schedule and specific risk of disease acquisition to traveler
            1) Spread by fecal-oral transmission, so risk exists for all travelers
                a) Risk increases with less stringent food and water precautions
                b) Mortality with HAV infection is low, but symptomatic hepatitis can last for weeks to months
                c) Public health implications upon return also need to be considered
            2) Inactivated vaccine induces HAV antibodies within 2 to 4 weeks after the initial dose
                a) Booster given 6 to 18 months later provides long-term immunity up to 20 to 25 years
                b) Boosters have been shown to be effective even when given as long as 8 years after the initial dose
                c) The schedule never needs to be restarted
            3) Testing for HAV immunity before vaccination should be considered for certain travelers
                a) Travelers born outside the United States and now traveling overseas
                b) Travelers who have a history of hepatitis or jaundice
        c. Vaccine safety and contraindications
            1) An extremely safe and immunogenic vaccine
            2) An inactivated vaccine
            3) Immune response may be inadequate in an immunocompromised host (ICH)
                a) For a high-risk traveler (such as an ICH) to an area where HAV infection is endemic, the immune response may be better after both doses are given
                b) If possible, an ICH should receive both doses before travel
                c) For an ICH traveling imminently (leaving in <2 weeks), immune globulin may be used to provide protection against HAV through passive transfer of antibodies
    2. Hepatitis B vaccine
        a. Prevalence
            1) Hepatitis B virus (HBV) is present worldwide
            2) Prevalence of hepatitis B surface antigen (HBsAg)-positive persons is much higher in some countries than others
                a) Countries and regions with high prevalence (HBsAg positivity >8%)

i) Countries in Africa
ii) Countries in Southeast Asia, including China, Korea, Indonesia, and the Philippines
iii) Countries in the Middle East (except Israel)
iv) South Pacific and western Pacific islands
v) Interior Amazon River basin
vi) Haiti and the Dominican Republic

b) Countries and regions with intermediate prevalence (HBsAg positivity, 2%-7%)
i) South Central and Southwest Asia, Japan, Russia, Israel
ii) Eastern and southern Europe
iii) Most areas surrounding the Amazon River basin, Honduras, and Guatemala

b. Schedule and specific risk of disease acquisition to traveler
1) Transmission of HBV: blood and body fluids
a) Risk to traveler is through medical or dental care, sexual exposure, needlestick exposure (tattoos or drug abuse), and health care delivery
b) Potential for exposure increases with duration of stay
2) Hepatitis B vaccine is recommended for repeated or prolonged (>4 weeks) travel to high- or intermediate-risk regions or for persons who are likely to engage in high-risk activities such as medical tourism or health care delivery
3) Standard dosing schedule: 0, 1, and 6 months
a) Adequate time should be allowed for the full series before travel
b) Engerix-B vaccine has an accelerated dosing schedule approved by the US Food and Drug Administration (FDA) for persons who are departing imminently and need HBV protection
4) Examples of accelerated schedules
a) Doses at 0, 1, and 2 months and a booster in 12 months
b) Doses at 0, 7, and 21 days and a booster in 12 months
5) Subsequent boosters are not generally needed: hepatitis B vaccine provides long-term immunity
6) Health care workers should have a seropositive response documented after completion of the primary series

c. Vaccine safety and contraindications
1) Hepatitis B vaccines are safe
2) There is no association of hepatitis B vaccine and neurologic diseases such as multiple sclerosis or Guillain-Barré syndrome

3. Typhoid vaccine
a. Prevalence
1) Acute bacterial illness caused by *Salmonella typhi* is more prevalent in countries with poor sanitation
2) Endemic in Central and South America, the Indian subcontinent, and sub-Saharan Africa

b. Schedule and specific risk of disease acquisition to traveler
1) Factors increasing risk
a) Prolonged stay
b) Rural travel
c) Low-budget travel
d) Less stringent food and water precautions where the disease is endemic
2) Oral and injectable typhoid vaccines are available
a) Oral vaccine: estimated efficacy of 60% to 96% that lasts for 5 years
b) Injectable vaccine: similar efficacy as oral vaccine but requires repeating in 2 years if patient has continued exposure

c. Vaccine safety and contraindications
1) Oral vaccine
a) Live-attenuated bacterial vaccine
b) Contraindications: ICH, pregnant women, or persons taking antibiotics
c) Mefloquine, chloroquine, and proguanil should not be administered concomitantly
i) Potential to decrease the vaccine immune response
ii) Administration should be separated by at least 48 hours
d) Vaccine is very well tolerated
e) Occasionally vaccine may cause mild gastric upset
2) Injectable typhoid vaccine
a) Safe
b) No major adverse effects

4. Japanese encephalitis vaccine
a. Prevalence

1) Mosquito-borne viral encephalitis is endemic in Asia (China, Korea, Indian subcontinent, and Southeast Asia)
2) More common in rural areas
b. Schedule and specific risk of disease acquisition to traveler
1) Risk for short-term (<4 weeks) or predominantly urban travelers is low
2) Risk is higher for travelers who go to rural areas or who stay for a prolonged duration (ie, those who expatriate for >4 weeks to a country with Japanese encephalitis virus)
a) These patients should receive the vaccine
b) These patients should use primary insect bite precautions
3) Two inactivated vaccines are available: JE-VAX and Ixiaro
a) Ixiaro: approved in 2009 by the FDA
b) JE-VAX
i) Originally manufactured by BIKEN (Osaka, Japan), but no longer actively manufactured
ii) Limited supplies are available through Sanofi Pasteur (Toronto, Ontario, Canada)
4) Vaccine dosing
a) JE-VAX
i) For persons 16 years or younger
ii) Doses at 0, 7, and 30 days
iii) Third dose can be accelerated to 14 days if time does not allow a regular schedule
iv) After receiving each dose, patients are observed for 30 minutes because of risk of anaphylaxis
v) After the last dose, patients are advised to not travel for 10 days
vi) Boosters are needed after 3 years for continued exposure
b) Ixiaro
i) For persons 17 years or older
ii) Doses at 0 and 28 days
iii) No established accelerated schedule
iv) A booster dose may be given before potential reexposure if the primary series was given more than 1 year earlier
5) Efficacy of the vaccine
a) JE-VAX
i) With 3 doses: more than 95% efficacy
ii) With 2 doses: 80% efficacy
b) Ixiaro: 94.6% seroconversion rate after 2 doses
c. Vaccine safety and contraindications
1) JE-VAX
a) Adverse effects: malaise, fever, headache, myalgia, and swelling at the injection site
b) Risk of anaphylaxis: reported rate is 180 to 640 cases per 100,000 vaccinees
c) Risk of anaphylaxis is potentially higher in persons with a history of urticaria, asthma, allergic rhinitis, or multiple allergies
d) Allergic reaction to a previous dose of JE-VAX is a contraindication for another dose of JE-VAX
2) Ixiaro
a) Adverse effects: headache and myalgia are the most common (>10%) systemic adverse events reported
b) Allergic reaction to a previous dose of Ixiaro is a contraindication for another dose of Ixiaro
5. Rabies vaccine
a. Prevalence
1) Worldwide except for a few countries that are rabies free
2) Endemic in the Indian subcontinent, China, Southeast Asia, Philippines, parts of Indonesia, Latin America, Africa, and the former Soviet Union
b. Schedule and specific risk of disease acquisition to traveler
1) Risk overseas is mainly from stray dogs and other stray animals (unlike in the United States, where the risk is mainly from bats, raccoons, and other wild animals)
2) Persons at higher risk
a) Expatriates
b) Persons involved in outdoor activities, especially in rural areas even if their trip is brief
c) Veterinarians working in areas were rabies is endemic
3) Many developing countries do not have an adequate supply of rabies immune globulin, so that an animal bite is a true medical emergency

4) High-risk travelers should receive the preexposure rabies vaccination series at 0, 7, and 21 or 28 days
   a) Series is usually effective for several years
   b) Continued exposure can be dealt with in different ways
      i) Rapid fluorescent focus inhibition test (RFFIT) to check for immune response: if less than 1:5 serum dilution, a booster can be given
      ii) Alternatively, a booster can be given without serology if primary series was given more than 3 years ago
   c. Vaccine safety and contraindications
      1) Many types of rabies vaccines
      2) Newer, modern cell culture vaccines are safe and are the most immunogenic
      3) Occasional "immune complex–like" illness is reported in persons receiving human diploid cell vaccine (HDCV)
      4) Older rabies vaccines derived from nerve tissue
         a) Can cause neuroparalytic reactions
         b) They are not available in the United States but can be found in developing countries
6. Cholera vaccine
   a. Prevalence
      1) Endemic in many parts of Africa
      2) Less common in Indian subcontinent, Southeast Asia, Middle East, and parts of Latin America
   b. Specific risk of disease acquisition to traveler
      1) Risk of cholera to travelers is extremely low
      2) Some risk exists for persons engaged in activities in refugee camps or in other areas of high transmission
      3) No cholera vaccine is available in the United States
      4) Vaccine available in other countries: Dukoral, a killed whole-cell, recombinant B-subunit oral cholera vaccine
         a) Contains formalin and heat-inactivated whole bacterial cells of the *Vibrio cholerae* O1 Inaba, Ogawa, and El Tor strains and a recombinant B-subunit of the toxin
         b) Efficacious (about 80%) for approximately 6 months
         c) This vaccine has also shown some protection against diarrhea caused by heat-labile enterotoxigenic *Escherichia coli* (ETEC)
            i) In a Bangladeshi population: 67%
            ii) In US students traveling in Mexico: 50%
      c. Vaccine safety and contraindications: minimal gastrointestinal adverse effects
7. Tick-borne encephalitis virus vaccine
   a. Prevalence
      1) Virus is endemic in forested areas in Eastern Europe and the former Soviet Union from April to August (also called spring-summer encephalitis virus)
      2) Virus is transmitted to humans by bites from infected *Ixodes* ticks
   b. Specific risk of disease acquisition to traveler
      1) Risk is highest among persons working outdoors, especially in the woods, during the peak transmission season
      2) Can be transmitted by consumption of unpasteurized dairy products
      3) Vaccine is available in Europe and Canada but not in the United States
      4) Travelers should be advised about personal protective measures such as insect repellents and protective clothing
   c. Vaccine safety and contraindications: allergic reaction can occur
E. Required Travel Immunizations
   1. Meningococcal vaccine
      a. Prevalence
         1) *Neisseria meningitidis* is endemic worldwide
            a) Outbreaks of *N meningitidis* meningitis occur annually in the dry belt of sub-Saharan Africa, including the following countries: Benin, Burkina Faso, Cameroon, Central African Republic, Chad, Côte d'Ivoire, Djibouti, Ethiopia, Gambia, Ghana, Guinea, Guinea-Bissau, Mali, Niger, Nigeria, Senegal, Somalia, Sudan, and Togo and occasionally Kenya, Tanzania, and Uganda
            b) Outbreaks also occur sporadically during the annual religious pilgrimage (Hajj and Umrah) to Mecca in Saudi Arabia

2) Incidence of meningococcal meningitis in the United States: 0.5 to 1.1 per 100,000
    a) In the general population: 0.5 to 1.1 per 100,000
    b) Among freshman living in dormitories: 2 to 5 per 100,000
3) Serogroups
    a) In the United States: serogroups B, C, Y, and W135 are prevalent
    b) In Africa: serogroups A and C are more common
    c) In the Americas and Europe: serogroups B and C are most common
    d) Serogroup W135 is associated with meningococcal disease epidemics in Saudi Arabia and Burkina Faso
b. Schedule and specific risk of disease acquisition to traveler
    1) Owing to meningococcal disease risk and crowding during the Hajj and Umrah pilgrimage to Mecca, meningococcal vaccine is required for entry to Saudi Arabia
    2) Travelers to sub-Saharan Africa during the dry season (December through June) should receive the vaccine, especially if they anticipate a prolonged stay, health care delivery, or extensive contact with local populations
    3) Two types of quadrivalent vaccine are available in the United States
        a) Both are effective against serogroups A, C, Y, and W135
        b) No vaccine offers protection against serogroup B
        c) Older polysaccharide vaccine (MPSV4): Menomune
            i) Provides immunity for approximately 3 years
            ii) Another dose should be considered for persons with continued or repeated exposure beyond 3 years
        d) Newer conjugated quadrivalent meningococcal vaccine (MCV4): Menactra and Menveo
            i) Better immunogenicity and expected to have immunity lasting for 5 years
            ii) Conjugated vaccine is preferred over polysaccharide vaccine
    4) Recommendations of the Centers for Disease Control and Prevention
        a) Vaccination for all incoming college freshmen owing to increased risk of transmission in dormitories
        b) Meningococcal vaccination is also advised for persons who have terminal complement deficiency or anatomical or functional asplenia and for persons who work with *N meningitidis* in the laboratory
c. Vaccine safety and contraindications
    1) Both types of vaccine are safe
    2) In 2005 and 2006, 8 cases of Guillain-Barré syndrome were reported within 6 weeks of receipt of MCV4
        a) Causality was not proven
        b) However, persons with a history of Guillain-Barré syndrome might be at increased risk of postvaccination Guillain-Barré syndrome
        c) Therefore, a history of Guillain-Barré syndrome is a relative contraindication to receiving MCV4
        d) If benefit from the receipt of the vaccine exceeds risk (eg, patient is going to Chad for 4 months for health care work and Menomune is not available), vaccination with MCV4 could be considered after discussion with the patient
        e) Alternatively, the older polysaccharide vaccine (Menomune) can be used if available
2. Yellow fever vaccine
    a. Prevalence
        1) Yellow fever is an acute viral hemorrhagic disease transmitted by the *Aedes aegypti* mosquito
        2) Occurs only in tropical climates of Africa and South America
        3) Transmission is seasonal
            a) During the rainy season in South America (January to March)
            b) During the late rainy and early dry seasons in Africa (July to October)
    b. Schedule and specific risk of disease acquisition to traveler
        1) Traveling to a country with endemic or epidemic yellow fever poses a risk of acquisition
            a) Risk is higher with prolonged travel, no vaccination, travel to forested regions, and appropriate season

- b) But risk exists almost everywhere in countries where yellow fever is endemic
- 2) Risk is higher in Africa than in tropical South America
  - a) A 2-week stay in West Africa without vaccination carries an estimated risk of illness of 50 per 100,000 and an estimated risk of death of 10 per 100,000
  - b) These risks are higher during the rainy season
  - c) These risks are estimated to be 10 times lower for travel in South America
- 3) Yellow fever vaccine is extremely effective
  - a) In more than 90% of the recipients, protective immunity develops within 10 days and in 99%, after 30 days
  - b) Immunity lasts for 10 years or longer
- 4) International Health Regulations
  - a) Proof of vaccination (a completed international certificate of vaccination) is required for travel to and from certain countries
  - b) The vaccination is considered valid for 10 years
- 5) World Health Organization (WHO) controls the production of yellow fever vaccine
  - a) Vaccine is administered only at approved yellow fever vaccination centers
  - b) Up-to-date information on country-specific requirements may be obtained through the CDC and WHO
- c. Vaccine safety and contraindications
  - 1) Yellow fever vaccine is a live-attenuated vaccine
    - a) Contraindicated in pregnant, immunosuppressed patients and in patients with a history of thymic dysfunction, thymoma, or thymectomy
    - b) Depending on the degree of exposure risk, these patients will need a yellow fever vaccine waiver before entry to countries where the disease is endemic if the risk from the activities at the travel destination is low, or they should be advised not to travel to high-risk areas
  - 2) Overall, yellow fever vaccine is safe
    - a) Mild symptoms occur in less than 25% of recipients: headache and low-grade fever
    - b) Severe adverse effects can occur, particularly in persons with congenital, iatrogenic, or age-related immunosuppression
  - 3) Two severe adverse effects from yellow fever vaccine are associated with first-time vaccinees
    - a) Yellow fever vaccine–associated neurotropic disease (YF-AND)
      - i) Has occurred more often in infants, but it can occur in adults
      - ii) Estimated incidence of YF-AND is 0.5 per 100,000 doses given
    - b) Yellow fever vaccine–associated viscerotropic disease (YF-AVD)
      - i) A multisystem organ infection with the vaccine strain of yellow fever virus
      - ii) Rare
      - iii) Recognized since the 1990s
      - iv) More than 30 cases worldwide, with a mortality rate of 58%
      - v) Thought to be related to the host response rather than to a change in the vaccine strain
      - vi) Risk of YF-AVD is higher in persons older than 60 years and is probably related to age-related immunosenescence
      - vii) A risk-benefit discussion should be conducted before administration of the vaccine
      - viii) CDC estimates for incidence of YF-AVD
        - (a) Overall: 0.3 to 0.5 per 100,000
        - (b) Among persons older than 60 years: 1.8 per 100,000

IV. Malaria Prevention
   A. Prevalence
   1. Malaria is transmitted in more than 100 countries worldwide
      a. Prevalent in Africa, Asia (including the Indian subcontinent, Southeast Asia, and the Middle East), some regions of Central America and South America, the island of Hispaniola (includes Haiti and the Dominican Republic), and areas of Eastern Europe and the South Pacific

b. Most of the world now has chloroquine-resistant *Plasmodium falciparum* malaria except in the Central American countries, Hispaniola, and parts of the Middle East
      1) Chloroquine-resistant *Plasmodium viviax* has been reported from Papua New Guinea
      2) Areas where Thailand borders Burma (Myanmar) and where Thailand borders Cambodia are home to mefloquine-resistant *P falciparum*
   2. Malaria is the most important cause of fever among travelers returning from tropical countries
B. Specific Risk of Disease Acquisition to Traveler
   1. Risk of malaria acquisition is highest with travel to Africa, with majority of disease from *P falciparum*
   2. Increased specific individual risk
      a. With perceived low risk of acquisition, as when US immigrants return to visit friends and relatives in countries where malaria is endemic
      b. With inappropriate or no chemoprophylaxis
      c. With poor adherence to personal protective measures
C. Medications
   1. Chloroquine: the recommended chemoprophylactic agent for travel to countries with chloroquine-sensitive malaria
   2. Common options for travel to countries with chloroquine-resistant malaria: mefloquine, Malarone (atovaquone-proguanil), or doxycycline
      a. Primaquine can be considered for patients for whom the other options are contraindicated, but glucose-6-phosphate dehydrogenase (G6PD) testing is required before use
      b. For areas where mefloquine resistance is common, Malarone or doxycycline is indicated
   3. Dosages are listed in Table 43.4
   4. Malarone and doxycycline must be taken with food
      a. Malarone is better absorbed when taken with a meal
      b. Doxycycline should be taken with a meal to avoid gastric or esophageal irritation
   5. For pregnant women traveling to countries where malaria is endemic, chloroquine and mefloquine are the only available and

Table 43.4

Commonly Used Medications for Malaria Chemoprophylaxis for Adults With Normal Renal Function

Feature	Chloroquine-Sensitive Areas	Chloroquine-Resistant Areas		
	Chloroquine	Mefloquine	Doxycycline	Atovaquone-proguanil
Formulation	Tablets and suspension	Tablets	Tablets	Tablets
Efficacy	>90% in sensitive areas	90%-100%	77%-99%	99%
Safe	Yes	Yes	Yes	Yes
Use in pregnancy	Review risks and benefits	Review risks and benefits	No	No
Schedule	500 mg (phosphate salt) once weekly; Start 1-2 wk before entering the malaria area; Then weekly while in the area and for 4 wk after exiting the malaria area	250 mg (salt) once weekly; Start 2 wk before entering the malaria area; Then weekly while in the area and for 4 wk after exiting the malaria area	100 mg daily; Start 1-2 d before entering the malaria area; Then weekly while in the area and for 4 wk after exiting the malaria area	100 mg daily; Start 1-2 d before entering the malaria area; Then weekly while in the area and for 7 d after exiting the malaria area
Major contraindications	Retinal or visual field changes; Hypersensitivity to 4-aminoquinoline compounds	Active or recent history of psychiatric disorders; Cardiac arrhythmias; Seizure disorder; Hypersensitivity to mefloquine or related compounds (eg, quinine, quinidine)	Pregnancy; Age <8 y; Hypersensitivity to doxycycline or tetracycline products	Pregnancy; Hypersensitivity to atovaquone or proguanil; Severe renal impairment (creatinine clearance <30 mL/min)

recommended options for malaria chemoprophylaxis
D. Medication Adverse Effects and Contraindications
1. Chloroquine
   a. Tolerated well in the short term
      1) Can cause nausea or emesis
      2) Has a bitter taste
   b. Possible longer-term use associations
      1) Tinnitus
      2) Chloroquine-induced retinopathy (blurred vision, loss of color differentiation, night blindness, and field defects)
      3) Prolonged QT interval
      4) Exacerbation of psoriasis
2. Mefloquine
   a. Gastrointestinal adverse effects
   b. Bizarre dreams
   c. Sleep disturbance
   d. Transient dizziness
   e. More serious adverse effects
      1) Lower seizure threshold
      2) Acute neuropsychotic adverse event
      3) Prolonged QT interval and arrhythmias
   f. Avoid use in persons with underlying history of seizures, prolonged QT interval or arrhythmias, and psychiatric diagnoses such as depression
   g. Fatal arrhythmias
      1) Can occur if halofantrine is taken concurrently with mefloquine, as might happen in a developing country while a traveler is treated for malaria
      2) Patients should be warned before travel
3. Malarone
   a. Safe overall
   b. Most common adverse events: abdominal pain, diarrhea, and nausea
4. Doxycycline
   a. Adverse effects: photosensitivity; gastritis, esophagitis, or ulcers if taken on an empty stomach (doxycycline is very acidic); yeast infections; or potentially *Clostridium difficile* colitis
   b. Gastrointestinal adverse effects can be decreased by taking doxycycline with food, but milk products decrease its absorption
5. Primaquine
   a. Hemolytic anemia in patients with G6PD deficiency
   b. Hemolytic anemia in the fetus if the fetus has G6PD deficiency
6. Pregnancy
   a. Use of Malarone should be avoided in pregnant and lactating women: limited data on fetal or infant toxicity
   b. Use of doxycycline or primaquine is contraindicated in pregnant women
E. Patient Education
1. It is extremely important to discuss signs and symptoms of malaria with travelers going to areas where malaria is endemic
2. Morbidity and mortality from malaria in the returned traveler is increased when diagnosis or treatment is delayed
   a. Reasons for delays
      1) Patient is not aware of the need to seek medical attention early
      2) Patient does not provide key travel information
      3) Medical personnel do not recognize malaria symptoms
   b. Knowledge of these issues is advantageous if patients return with a febrile illness
V. Traveler's Diarrhea
A. Prevalence
1. Traveler's diarrhea (TD) is the most common travel-associated illness
   a. Occurs often but is mostly a nuisance for travelers
   b. Occasionally results in serious adverse outcomes
      1) Confined to bed: approximately 20% to 30% of TD patients
      2) Need to change their schedule: 40%
      3) Hospitalization or death: less than 1%
2. TD is a constellation of diarrhea (with or without blood in the stool) and nausea with or without fever
   a. TD lasts for 3 to 5 days in most infected persons
   b. TD lasts for more than 2 weeks in 5% to 10%
   c. TD lasts for longer than 4 weeks in less than 3%
3. Incidence varies by geographic destination
   a. Incidence is highest (30%-50%) with travel to South Asia, Southeast Asia, the Middle East, Africa, Central America, and South America
   b. Risk is about 10% with travel to South Africa, Turkey, Greece, the Caribbean Sea, and Eastern European countries
   c. Risk is low with travel to Canada, Japan, Australia, and northern and western Europe

B. Etiology
1. Most common microbial cause of TD is bacterial (80%-85%), followed by parasitic and viral
2. Bacteria
   a. Most common bacterial cause of TD worldwide is ETEC
   b. Other bacteria causing TD: enteroaggregative *E coli*, *Campylobacter*, *Salmonella*, and *Shigella* species
   c. Cholera is an exceedingly rare cause of diarrhea among travelers, with risk limited to those working in extreme conditions (eg, involved in health care in a refugee camp with an ongoing cholera epidemic)
   d. Quinolone resistance among *Campylobacter* species is increasing, particularly in Southeast Asia
   e. Bloody TD is most often caused by *Campylobacter* or *Shigella* species, but it may be caused by amebiasis
3. Parasites
   a. Parasitic TD is more likely with prolonged travel and rural locations
   b. Most common parasites causing TD: *Giardia lamblia*, *Cryptosporidium parvum*, *Entamoeba histolytica*, and *Cyclospora cayetanensis*
C. Specific Risk of Disease Acquisition to Traveler
1. Risk of TD is highest with travel to developing countries that have poor sanitation and hygiene standards
2. Factors that increase risk of TD
   a. Younger age (<35 years): probably related to adventurous eating habits and low-budget travel
   b. Prolonged stay at destination (>60% after 30 days' stay; higher in the first 6 months of stay)
   c. Unrestricted food and water choices
      1) Eating food from street vendors, local families, rural locations, raw foods (vegetables, salads, precut fruit, meats, and seafood)
      2) Drinking iced beverages, tap water, raw milk, and fresh unpasteurized juices
      3) Eating foods that were made from liquids: ice cream, ice milk, and flavored ice
3. TD risk cannot be entirely eliminated, even with excellent adherence to pretravel counseling about food and water precautions
   a. Most studies indicate that adherence to recommended precautions is poor
   b. Risk of parasitic diarrhea (giardiasis and amebiasis) increases with prolonged stay in developing countries where disease is endemic
   c. Eating and drinking while trekking in Nepal has been associated with acquisition of TD caused by *Cyclospora*
D. General Measures and Medications
1. General advice for travelers on food and water precautions
   a. Avoid tap water and ice
   b. Avoid foods from vendors, small rural restaurants, and raw foods
   c. Limit consumption of cream and other milk products in rural locations (risk of listeriosis, brucellosis, and tuberculosis if unpasteurized milk is used)
   d. Food and drinks that are more likely to be safe: hot cooked foods, breads, hot drinks (tea or coffee), or carbonated drinks
2. Following the recommended food and water precautions may not always be possible since travelers may have no choice while traveling
3. Primary prevention of TD
   a. Rarely indicated and used
   b. May be justified for patients with severe immunocompromise or for persons with a critical business trip
4. Medications used for primary prevention: bismuth subsalicylate (BSS), rifaximin, or a fluoroquinolone
   a. Bismuth subsalicylate
      1) An insoluble salt of trivalent bismuth and salicylic acid
      2) Exerts its antidiarrheal effect by inhibiting bacteria-causing diarrhea, binding to toxins produced by *E coli*, and inhibiting gastrointestinal secretions
      3) Compared with placebo, BSS decreases TD incidence by 65%
   b. Rifaximin
      1) A newer nonabsorbable rifamycin derivative that is excreted unchanged in feces
      2) Has been shown to provide about 70% protection against TD compared with placebo
      3) Active against *E coli* diarrhea
      4) Less effective against *Shigella*, *Yersinia*, and *Campylobacter* diarrhea
      5) Dose for primary prevention: 200 mg orally 3 times daily
      6) Comparable in efficacy to ciprofloxacin for treatment of TD caused by

noninvasive pathogens but less so for invasive pathogens such as *Shigella* or *Campylobacter*
   c. Fluoroquinolones (ciprofloxacin or levofloxacin): provide 90% protection for TD
   d. Efficacy of probiotics for the prevention of TD: data are variable and inconclusive
5. Educating and empowering patients to self-manage TD while traveling is important
   a. Fluoroquinolones (ciprofloxacin or levofloxacin) used as a single dose with antimotility agents such as loperamide: extremely effective for mild to moderate diarrhea
   b. Azithromycin
      1) Alternative for TD self-treatment
      2) Usual dose: either 1 g as a single dose or 500 mg orally once daily for 3 days (single dose may cause more upper gastrointestinal adverse effects)
      3) For TD caused by multidrug resistant *Shigella*, azithromycin has a cure rate of 82% (compared with 89% with ciprofloxacin)
      4) Success rates for TD presumed to be caused by other bacteria are 86% (compared with 100% with ciprofloxacin; however, with increasing fluoroquinolone resistance, these data may change)
      5) Success rates are higher with azithromycin (62%) than with ciprofloxacin (48%) for *Campylobacter* TD
      6) Azithromycin is a possible alternative for management of TD in pregnant women since it is a category B drug
6. Management of posttravel diarrhea is beyond the scope of this section
E. Medication Adverse Effects and Contraindications
   1. Bismuth subsalicylate
      a. Patients should be warned that bismuth sulfide causes harmless black discoloration of stool, tongue, and teeth
      b. Patients receiving aspirin or warfarin therapy should avoid taking BSS since it may increase bleeding risk
      c. For children and young adults with viral infections, BSS should be avoided to prevent Reye syndrome
      d. BSS should be avoided in patients with renal insufficiency because it can accumulate and cause an encephalopathy
   2. Rifaximin
      a. Adverse effects are uncommon but include rash, angioneurotic edema, and urticaria
      b. Contraindications
         1) Children younger than 12 years
         2) Pregnancy
         3) Rifamycin allergy
   3. Fluoroquinolones
      a. Common adverse effects: nausea, diarrhea, or indigestion
      b. Less common adverse effects: prolonged QT interval and torsades de pointes, serum sickness–like reaction, musculoskeletal disorders (eg, tendon injury or rupture or rhabdomyolysis), skin rash (eg, Stevens-Johnson syndrome), elevated liver function tests, liver failure, headache, and seizures (by lowering the seizure threshold)
      c. All fluoroquinolones are contraindicated in pregnant or breast-feeding women
VI. Conclusion
   A. Risk Assessment for International Travel
      1. Risk assessment should be individualized
      2. Vaccination and other preventive recommendations should be based on individualized risk assessment and on the epidemiology of risk
   B. Epidemiologic Data
      1. Updated by the CDC and WHO
      2. Relevant information is available to providers online
      3. Other services are available to practitioners for more detailed programs to tailor recommendation for travelers

Suggested Reading

Centers for Disease Control and Prevention. Yellow Book [Internet]. 2010 edition. [cited 2010 Aug 16]. Available from: http://wwwn.cdc.gov/travel/default.aspx.

Hill DR, Ericsson CD, Pearson RD, Keystone JS, Freedman DO, Kozarsky PE, et al; Infectious Diseases Society of America. The practice of travel medicine: guidelines by the Infectious Diseases Society of America. Clin Infect Dis. 2006 Dec 15;43(12):1499–539. Epub 2006 Nov 8.

World Health Organization. International travel and health book [Internet]. 2010 edition. [cited 2010 Aug 16]. Available from: http://www.who.int/ith/en/.

Priya Sampathkumar, MD

44

Adult Immunizations

I. General Information About Vaccines
   A. Safety
      1. No vaccine is 100% effective or completely safe
      2. All vaccines are associated with risks and benefits that need to be balanced against each other
         a. Personal benefits: protection from illness, improved quality of life, and prevention of death
         b. Societal benefits: creation of herd immunity, prevention of disease outbreaks, and a decrease in health care costs
         c. Vaccination risks range from minor, local adverse events to rare, severe, and life-threatening problems
         d. Use of vaccines in pregnancy is summarized in Box 44.1
   B. Timing and Spacing of Vaccinations
      1. Commonly available vaccines for adults are listed in Box 44.2
      2. Vaccines are recommended for the youngest age group of people at risk of the disease for whom safety and efficacy data are available
      3. Detailed schedules are published by the Centers for Disease Control and Prevention (CDC) National Immunization Program for both adults and children (Figures 44.1-44.3)
      4. These schedules should be adhered to as much as possible
   C. Multidose Vaccine Series
      1. Do not shorten the recommended minimum intervals between doses
         a. Risks are associated with administering vaccines before the recommended minimum age or at intervals less than the recommended minimum interval
            1) Suboptimal response to the vaccine
            2) Increased local or systemic reactions

> **Box 44.1**
> **Vaccines in Pregnancy**
> Indicated
>   Hepatitis B
>   Influenza (inactivated)
>   Tetanus
> Contraindicated
>   Measles, mumps, and rubella
>   Varicella
>   Zoster
> Give If Benefits Outweigh Risks
>   Hepatitis A
>   Injectable polio
>   Meningococcal
>   Pneumococcal
>   Rabies
>   Typhoid

> **Box 44.2**
> **Commonly Available Adult Vaccines**
>
> Inactivated
>   Hepatitis A
>   Hepatitis B
>   Human papillomavirus
>   Influenza
>   Injectable polio
>   Injectable typhoid
>   Japanese encephalitis
>   Meningococcal
>   Pneumococcal conjugate vaccine
>   Rabies
>   Tetanus and diphtheria toxoids (Td)
>   Td and acellular pertussis (Tdap)
> Live Vaccines
>   Live attenuated influenza vaccine (LAIV)
>   Measles, mumps, and rubella
>   Monovalent mumps
>   Oral polio[a]
>   Oral typhoid
>   Varicella
>   Yellow fever
>   Zoster
>
> [a] Oral polio vaccine is no longer used in the United States.

    b. The CDC Advisory Committee on Immunization Practices (ACIP) recommends that vaccines be considered valid if they are given within 4 days before the minimum interval or age
        1) Exception: rabies vaccine
    c. Doses given 5 or more days before the minimum interval or age should not be considered valid
        1) Doses should be repeated, spaced after the invalid dose by the recommended minimum interval
2. Lengthening the recommended intervals between doses is acceptable
    a. If intervals between doses of a series are longer than recommended, it is not necessary to restart the series again or to give extra doses
3. Interchangeability of vaccines from different manufacturers
    a. It is not necessary to restart a series if the brand used previously is not available or is not known

Vaccine	Birth	1 mo	2 mo	4 mo	6 mo	12 mo	15 mo	18 mo	19-23 mo	2-3 y	4-6 y
Hepatitis B (HepB)	HepB	HepB			HepB						
Rotavirus (RV)			RV	RV	RV						
Diphtheria, tetanus, pertussis (DTaP)			DTaP	DTaP	DTaP		DTaP				DTaP
Haemophilus influenzae type b (Hib)			Hib	Hib	Hib	Hib					
Pneumococcal			PCV	PCV	PCV	PCV				PPSV	
Inactivated poliovirus (IPV)			IPV	IPV	IPV						IPV
Influenza					Influenza (yearly)						
Measles, mumps, rubella (MMR)						MMR					MMR
Varicella						Varicella					Varicella
Hepatitis A (HepA)						HepA (2 doses)				HepA series	
Meningococcal (MCV)										MCV	

🟨 Range of recommended ages except for certain high-risk groups
🟥 Range of recommended ages for certain high-risk groups

Figure 44.1. Recommended Immunization Schedule for Persons Aged 0 Through 6 years, United States, 2010. Detailed footnotes accompanying this figure are published at http://www.cdc.gov/vaccines/recs/schedules/downloads/child/2010/10_0-6yrs-schedule-pr.pdf. PCV indicates pneumococcal conjugate vaccine; PPSV, pneumococcal polysaccharide vaccine.

Vaccine	Age		
	7-10 y	11-12 y	13-18 y
Tetanus, diphtheria, pertussis (Tdap)		Tdap	Tdap
Human papillomavirus (HPV)		HPV (3 doses)	HPV series
Meningococcal (MCV)	MCV	MCV	MCV
Influenza	Influenza (yearly)		
Pneumococcal polysaccharide (PPSV)	PPSV		
Hepatitis A (HepA)	HepA series		
Hepatitis B (HepB)	HepB series		
Inactivated poliovirus (IPV)	IPV series		
Measles, mumps, rubella (MMR)	MMR series		
Varicella	Varicella series		

Range of recommended ages except for certain high-risk groups

Range of recommended ages for catch-up immunization

Range of recommended ages for certain high-risk groups

Figure 44.2. Recommended Immunization Schedule for Persons Aged 7 Through 18 Years, United States, 2010. Detailed footnotes accompanying this figure are published at http://www.cdc.gov/vaccines/recs/schedules/downloads/child/2010/10_7-18yrs-schedule-pr.pdf.

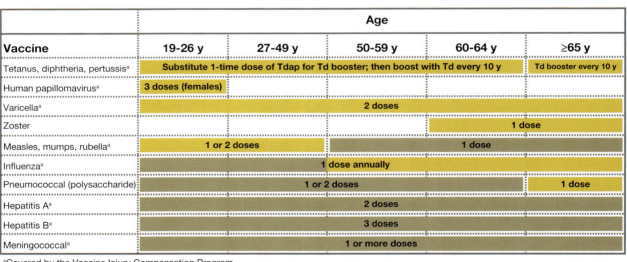

Vaccine	Age				
	19-26 y	27-49 y	50-59 y	60-64 y	≥65 y
Tetanus, diphtheria, pertussis[a]	Substitute 1-time dose of Tdap for Td booster; then boost with Td every 10 y				Td booster every 10 y
Human papillomavirus[a]	3 doses (females)				
Varicella[a]	2 doses				
Zoster				1 dose	
Measles, mumps, rubella[a]	1 or 2 doses		1 dose		
Influenza[a]	1 dose annually				
Pneumococcal (polysaccharide)	1 or 2 doses				1 dose
Hepatitis A[a]	2 doses				
Hepatitis B[a]	3 doses				
Meningococcal[a]	1 or more doses				

[a] Covered by the Vaccine Injury Compensation Program.

For all persons in this category who meet the age requirements and who lack evidence of immunity (eg, lack documentation of vaccination or have no evidence of prior infection)

Recommended if some other risk factor is present (eg, on the basis of medical, occupational, lifestyle, or other indications)

No recommendation

Figure 44.3. Recommended Immunization Schedule for Adults, United States, 2010. Detailed footnotes accompanying this figure are published at http://www.cdc.gov/vaccines/recs/schedules/downloads/adult/2010/adult-schedule.pdf. Td indicates tetanus and diphtheria toxoids; Tdap, tetanus, diphtheria, and acellular pertussis.

D. Administration of Multiple Vaccines During the Same Visit
  1. Each vaccine should be given in a separate syringe except for combination vaccines approved by the US Food and Drug Administration (FDA)
  2. Since inactivated vaccines do not interfere with the immune response to other inactivated vaccines or to live vaccines, an inactivated vaccine can be given at the same time or at any time before or after another inactivated vaccine or live vaccine
  3. If 2 live parenteral vaccines are needed (eg, varicella and yellow fever), administration should be on the same day or separated by at least 4 weeks
  4. Live oral vaccines (eg, oral typhoid, oral polio) can be given at any interval before or after inactivated or live parenteral vaccines
E. Spacing of Antibody-Containing Products and Vaccines
  1. If the product containing antibody is given first, wait a minimum of 3 months to give live vaccine
    a. Blood and blood products (immune globulin, whole blood, plasma, packed red cells, and platelets) can inhibit the immune response to live vaccines for 3 months or more
    b. Administration of live vaccines should therefore be delayed by a minimum of 3 months after administration of an antibody-containing product
    c. A longer wait may be necessary after administration of a hyperimmune product such as hepatitis A immunoglobulin or high-dose intravenous immunoglobulin
    d. Exceptions
      1) Yellow fever vaccination does not need to be delayed after blood product administration since blood products available in the United States are unlikely to contain clinically significant titers of yellow fever antibodies
      2) Zoster vaccine can be given at the same time as (or at any interval after) blood or other antibody-containing blood product
        a) The reason is that persons with a history of varicella maintain high levels of antibody to varicella-zoster virus indefinitely
        b) These levels are comparable to those found in donated blood and antibody-containing blood products
  2. For all other live vaccines, if the live vaccine is given first, the antibody-containing product should be deferred for at least 14 days after the live vaccine
    a. Usually vaccine virus replication and stimulation of immunity occurs 1 to 2 weeks after vaccination
    b. If an antibody-containing product is administered within 14 days of a live vaccine, either repeat the vaccine dose after the recommended interval or check serology to ensure that the vaccine worked
  3. Inactivated vaccines: administered simultaneously or separated by any interval from antibody-containing products
II. Specific Vaccines for Adults in the United States
  A. Hepatitis A Vaccine
    1. Characteristics
      a. Inactivated viral vaccine
      b. Schedule: 2 doses at 0 and 6 months, intramuscularly
      c. For combined hepatitis A and B vaccine (Twinrix), schedule is 3 doses at 0, 1, and 6 months
      d. Duration of protection: lifelong
      e. Very efficacious: protective efficacy is 94% to 100%
    2. Indications
      a. Persons with clotting factor disorders or chronic liver disease
      b. Men who have sex with men
      c. Users of illegal drugs
      d. Persons working in laboratories where they may be exposed to hepatitis A
      e. Persons traveling to countries where hepatitis A is endemic
      f. Any person who wants immunity to hepatitis A
      g. Recently added to vaccines recommended in childhood
    3. Side effects and precautions
      a. Injection site pain and induration
  B. Hepatitis B Vaccine
    1. Characteristics
      a. Inactivated vaccine
      b. Schedule: 3 doses at 0, 1, and 6 months, intramuscularly
      c. Duration of protection: several years
    2. Indications
      a. Chronic hemodialysis (use special formulation: 40-mcg dose instead of usual 20-mcg dose)
      b. Persons who receive clotting factor concentrates

c. Health care and public safety workers who have occupational exposure to blood
d. Injection drug users
e. Persons with more than 1 sex partner in the past 6 months
f. Men who have sex with men
g. Household contacts and sex partners of persons with chronic hepatitis B infection
h. Inmates of correctional facilities and residents and staff of institutions for the developmentally disabled
i. International travelers who will spend more than 6 months in countries that have a high prevalence of chronic hepatitis B virus infection
3. Side effects and precautions
a. Injection site pain and swelling
b. Systemic symptoms are rare

C. Human Papillomavirus Vaccine
1. Characteristics
a. There are more than 40 types of human papillomaviruses (HPVs)
1) HPV types 6 and 11: responsible for 90% of genital warts
2) HPV types 16 and 18: responsible for 70% of cervical cancers
b. Two types of HPV vaccine have been approved by the FDA
1) Quadrivalent vaccine (HPV4) (Gardasil) protects against HPV types 6, 11, 16, and 18
2) Bivalent vaccine (HPV2) (Cervarix) protects against HPV types 16 and 18
c. Quadrivalent vaccine
1) Noninfectious subunit vaccine
2) Consists of immunogenic viral proteins stripped free from whole virus particles (in this case, virus-like particles of the major capsid [L1] protein of HPV) and then purified from other irrelevant components, thereby decreasing the risk of adverse reactions and residual infectious virus
3) Approved for males and females 9 to 26 years old
4) Schedule: 3 doses at 0, 2, and 6 months, intramuscularly
5) Duration of protection: 4 years or more
6) Series should be started before sexual activity begins, but women who are sexually active should still be vaccinated
7) Does not provide protection against all types of HPV viruses that cause cervical cancer; therefore, patients should continue to receive routine screening for cervical cancer
d. Bivalent vaccine
1) Approved for use *only in females* 10 to 25 years old
2) Same schedule as for quadrivalent vaccine (ie, 0, 2, and 6 months)
2. Indications
a. Routine vaccination is recommended for adolescents 11 to 12 years old
b. HPV vaccination is also recommended for females 13 to 26 years old who previously have not received the vaccine
c. Vaccination can be given as early as age 9 at the discretion of the physician
3. Contraindication to HPV vaccine: pregnancy
4. Side effects and precautions
a. Injection site pain, redness, and itching
b. Mild to moderate fever

D. Influenza Vaccine
1. Characteristics
a. Typically contains 2 strains of influenza A virus and 1 strain of influenza B virus
b. A new vaccine incorporating the new virus strains needs to be administered annually because of antigenic drift in circulating viruses
c. Vaccine efficacy varies, depending on the age and immunocompetence of the vaccine recipient and on the degree of similarity between the vaccine virus and the circulating influenza viruses
d. Vaccine efficacy is lowest in persons who are elderly or immunocompromised
e. Two types of influenza vaccines are available (Table 44.1)
1) An inactivated vaccine administered as an intramuscular injection
2) A live attenuated influenza vaccine (LAIV) administered as an intranasal spray
f. Both vaccines contain the same viral antigens
g. Viruses for both vaccines are grown in eggs
2. Indications for annual vaccination
a. As of 2010, ACIP recommends that everyone older than 6 months receive an annual influenza vaccine
b. Vaccine is especially important for several groups
1) Women who will be pregnant during the influenza season

Table 44.1
Comparison of Live Attenuated Influenza Vaccine (LAIV) and Trivalent Inactivated Vaccine (TIV)

Factor	LAIV	TIV
Type of vaccine	Live, attenuated	Inactivated
Route	Intranasal spray	Intramuscular injection
Age group for which vaccine is approved	2-49 y	>6 mo
Contraindicated if person is immunosuppressed or has chronic health conditions	Yes	No
Contains egg proteins	Yes	Yes
Frequency of administration	Annual	Annual

   2) Children younger than 18 years
   3) Adults and children with chronic cardiac or pulmonary disease, including asthma
   4) Adults and children who have chronic metabolic disease, renal disease, hemoglobinopathy, or immunodeficiency
   5) Adults and children who have an underlying condition that compromises respiratory function or that increases the risk of aspiration
   6) Residents of long-term care facilities
   7) Caregivers and household contacts of persons at high risk of influenza-related complications, as listed above
   8) Health care workers
  3. Contraindications
   a. Severe egg allergy
   b. LAIV only: age younger than 2 years or older than 50, immunosuppression, chronic medical problems, or pregnancy
 E. Measles, Mumps, and Rubella Vaccine
  1. Characteristics
   a. Live, attenuated vaccine
   b. Schedule: 2 doses separated by at least 4 weeks, anytime after first birthday
   c. Dose: 0.5 mL subcutaneously
   d. In the United States, the first dose is generally given at age 12 to 15 months and the second dose at age 4 to 6 years
  2. Indications
   a. One dose of measles, mumps, and rubella (MMR) vaccine is recommended for all adults born during or after 1957 unless they have a medical contraindication, history of measles based on health care provider diagnosis, or evidence of immunity
   b. Indications for second dose of MMR vaccine for adults born after 1957
    1) Recent exposure to measles or an outbreak situation
    2) Previous vaccination with a killed measles vaccine or with an unknown type of vaccine in 1963 to 1967
    3) Student in postsecondary institution
    4) Health care worker
    5) Upcoming international travel
   c. The above recommendations were made primarily to ensure measles immunity, but a mumps outbreak in Iowa (2005-2006) was a reminder that the other components of the vaccine are also important
  3. Contraindications
   a. Pregnancy
   b. Severe immunosuppression
  4. Side effects and precautions
   a. Fever
   b. Rash
   c. Parotid swelling
   d. Joint pain and swelling, primarily due to the rubella component; typically occurs only in adults who lack immunity to rubella
 F. Meningococcal Vaccine
  1. Characteristics
   a. Protects against meningococcal disease caused by *Neisseria meningitidis*
   b. Protects against 4 most common *Neisseria* serotypes: A, C, Y, and W135
   c. Two types of vaccine
    1) Quadrivalent meningococcal conjugate vaccine (MCV4): Menactra and Menveo
     a) Menactra is approved for persons aged 11 to 55 years; Menveo, for persons aged 2 to 55 years
     b) Given as a single intramuscular injection
     c) Longer-lasting protection compared with polysaccharide vaccine
     d) In 2009, the ACIP recommended revaccination with meningococcal conjugate vaccine every 5 years for persons at increased risk of meningococcal disease for prolonged periods

2) Meningococcal polysaccharide vaccine (MPSV4): Menomune
   a) Approved for use in children older than 2 years and in adults (no upper age limit)
   b) Given subcutaneously as a single dose
   c) Provides protection for 3 to 5 years
   d) Revaccination is recommended every 3 to 5 years if risk factor for meningococcal disease is still present
2. Indications for vaccination with meningococcal vaccine
   a. Anatomical or functional asplenia or terminal complement deficiency
   b. First-year college students living in dormitories
   c. Military recruits
   d. Laboratory workers or microbiologists who are routinely exposed to meningococci
   e. Travelers to countries in which meningococcal disease is hyperendemic or endemic
      1) Meningitis belt of sub-Saharan Africa
      2) Travelers to Mecca during the annual Hajj
3. Indications for revaccination with meningococcal vaccine
   a. Persons who previously received the polysaccharide vaccine need revaccination every 3 to 5 years if the risk factor for meningococcal disease is still present
      1) Includes college freshmen if their previous dose of meningococcal vaccine was the polysaccharide vaccine and was received more than 5 years ago
      2) Revaccination of college freshmen is *not* necessary if they previously received the conjugate vaccine (MCV4)
   b. Persons who received the conjugate vaccine should be revaccinated every 5 years *only* if they are in 1 of the following groups (which have the highest risk of meningococcal infection)
      1) Persons with persistent complement deficiencies or functional or anatomical asplenia
      2) Microbiologists who routinely work with *Neisseria meningitidis* in the laboratory
      3) Travelers to or residents of countries where meningococcal disease is hyperendemic or epidemic
4. Side effects and precautions
   a. Mild injection site pain and redness
   b. Brief fever in less than 5%
   c. Cases of Guillain-Barré syndrome reported after vaccination with MCV4; no causal link found
G. Pneumococcal Vaccine
   1. Characteristics
      a. Inactivated vaccine
      b. Polyvalent polysaccharide vaccine
      c. Contains 23 *Streptococcus pneumoniae* capsular antigens that represent at least 85% to 90% of the serotypes (including the most drug-resistant serotypes) that cause invasive pneumococcal disease in children and adults in the United States
      d. Schedule
         1) Single dose, with revaccination necessary in some instances (see below)
         2) If elective splenectomy is planned, vaccinate at least 2 weeks preoperatively for maximal benefit
   2. Indications for vaccination with pneumococcal vaccine
      a. All persons older than 65 years
      b. Indications for persons 2 to 64 years old
         1) Chronic pulmonary disease, diabetes mellitus, cardiovascular disease, or chronic liver or kidney disease
            a) All smokers who are 19 years or older (new recommendation in 2008)
            b) All asthmatic patients who are 19 years or older (new recommendation in 2008)
         2) Anatomical or functional asplenia
         3) Immunosuppressive conditions, including congenital immunodeficiency, human immunodeficiency virus infection, generalized malignancy, organ or bone marrow transplant, and immunosuppressive therapy
         4) Cochlear implants
         5) Cerebrospinal fluid leaks
         6) Residents of nursing homes and other long-term care facilities
         7) Alaskan natives and certain Native American populations
   3. Indications for 1-time revaccination after 5 years (these indications are different from

those for the first dose of pneumococcal vaccine)
      a. Chronic renal failure, asplenia, or immunosuppressive conditions
      b. Age older than 65 years if person was younger than 65 years at primary vaccination
   4. Side effects and precautions
      a. Local: redness and pain at injection site
      b. Systemic: fever, myalgias
H. Tetanus and Diphtheria Toxoids Vaccine
   1. Characteristics
      a. Schedule
         1) Primary series: 0, 1, and 6 months
         2) Booster every 10 years
   2. Indications
      a. Routine: booster every 10 years after primary series has been completed
      b. Wound management: tetanus and diphtheria (Td) booster recommended if wound is contaminated with soil and if latest Td was given more than 5 years earlier
   3. Side effects and precautions
      a. Pain and swelling at injection site
      b. Vaccine should be avoided in persons with a history of Guillain-Barré syndrome within 6 weeks after receipt of a vaccine containing tetanus toxoid or a history of Arthus reaction to tetanus toxoid vaccine administered within the previous 10 years
I. Tetanus, Diphtheria, and Acellular Pertussis Vaccine
   1. Characteristics
      a. Protects against pertussis, tetanus, and diphtheria
      b. Two tetanus, diphtheria, and acellular pertussis (Tdap) products are licensed in the United States; they are similar in composition
         1) Boostrix: licensed for use in persons 10 to 64 years old
         2) Adacel: licensed for use in persons 11 to 64 years old
   2. Indications
      a. Single dose of Tdap should replace the next scheduled booster of Td for all adults 19 to 64 years old
      b. Persons in contact with infants (who are at highest risk of serious complications of pertussis): health care workers, parents of newborns, grandparents, persons 65 years or older, and childcare providers
         1) Ideally, Tdap should be received at least 4 weeks before contact with infants
      c. For adults receiving a primary tetanus series, Tdap should be substituted for 1 of the Td doses
   3. Side effects and precautions
      a. Injection site redness, pain, and swelling
         1) Side effects may be increased in persons who recently received Td
         2) In general, a 2-year Td-Tdap interval is recommended unless the benefits of vaccination (eg, close contact with a neonate) outweigh the risk of side effects
      b. Vaccine should not be given to persons with a history of serious allergic reaction to any of the vaccine components or a history of encephalopathy not attributable to any other cause within 7 days after receipt of a pertussis-containing vaccine
      c. Contraindications to Td apply to this vaccine also
J. Varicella Vaccine
   1. Characteristics
      a. Live attenuated viral vaccine
      b. Schedule: 2 doses separated by 4 to 8 weeks
   2. Indications
      a. All adults without evidence of immunity to varicella
         1) Evidence of immunity
            a) Birth in the United States before 1966
            b) History of chicken pox or herpes zoster
            c) Evidence of previous vaccination with 2 doses of varicella vaccine separated by at least 4 weeks
            d) Positive serology
      b. Vaccination is especially important for persons who have close contact with others at high risk of severe disease: health care workers and family contacts of immunocompromised persons
   3. Contraindications
      a. Immunosuppression
      b. Pregnancy (women should be cautioned not to become pregnant within 4 weeks of vaccination)
      c. Allergy to gelatin, neomycin, or a previous dose of varicella vaccine
   4. Side effects and precautions
      a. Injection site pain and swelling in 33% of recipients
      b. Fever in less than 10%
      c. Rash in less than 5% (rash is usually mild and can occur up to 1 month after vaccination)

d. Vaccine strain virus can be transmitted to household contacts who are highly immunosuppressed (eg, bone marrow transplant recipients); close contact should be avoided for 4 weeks after vaccination
K. Zoster Vaccine
1. Characteristics
a. Licensed in 2006 for the prevention of herpes zoster in persons older than 60 years
b. Live attenuated vaccine
c. Contains the same vaccine strain as the varicella vaccine
d. Contains 14 times the viral antigen as the varicella vaccine
e. Is not interchangeable with the varicella vaccine
f. Schedule: single dose given as subcutaneous injection
2. Indication
a. Adults older than 60 years without prior history of shingles
3. Contraindications
a. Immunosuppression
b. Allergic reaction to neomycin, gelatin, or other vaccine component
c. Pregnancy
d. Active untreated tuberculosis
e. Persons in close contact with pregnant women who are not immune to varicella

Suggested Reading

National Center for Immunization and Respiratory Diseases. General recommendations on immunization: recommendations of the Advisory Committee on Immunization Practices (ACIP). MMWR Recomm Rep. 2011 Jan 28;60(2):1–64.

Pickering LK, Baker CJ, Freed GL, Gall SA, Grogg SE, Poland GA, et al. Immunization programs for infants, children, adolescents, and adults: clinical practice guidelines by the Infectious Diseases Society of America. Clin Infect Dis. 2009 Sep 15;49(6):817–40.

Mark P. Wilhelm, MD, FACP

Agents of Bioterrorism

I. Introduction
   A. Bioterrorism
      1. *Bioterrorism*: the intentional use of biological agents (living organisms or biological toxins) by persons or groups motivated by political, religious, or other ideological objectives to harm or kill civilians
      2. Goal of biological warfare: to kill or disable the largest possible number of enemy combatants as quickly as possible
      3. Goal of bioterrorism
         a. To generate pervasive fear among the civilian population, which can lead to panic, civil disorder, economic loss, and undermining of confidence in government
         b. Goal may be accomplished with relatively limited casualties attributable to the biological agent used
   B. Biological Agents as Inexpensive Weapons
      1. Biological agents suitable for use as bioweapons can in many cases be produced and developed in small facilities at relatively modest expense
      2. The human devastation that could be caused by certain biologic agents can rival that of a nuclear device at a small fraction of the cost
   C. History of Biological Agents
      1. Efforts to use biological agents for warfare were described in ancient times
      2. In modern times, governments of several countries have had extensive programs for developing and stockpiling biological agents for warfare
         a. The Imperial Japanese Army Unit 731 used prisoners as subjects in human experiments with *Bacillus anthracis*, *Yersinia pestis*, *Vibrio cholerae*, and other pathogens in Manchuria in the 1930s and 1940s
         b. Former Union of Soviet Socialist Republics
            1) Developed a vast biological weapons program and stockpiled agents, including variola virus and *B anthracis* in quantities of tens to hundreds of tons
            2) In 1979, the accidental release of weapons-grade anthrax spores from a secret production facility in Sverdlovsk resulted in at least 72 civilian deaths
         c. United States
            1) Maintained an extensive biological weapons research program, headquartered at Fort Detrick, Maryland, from 1942 until 1970

            2) Biological agents were never actually used for warfare
        d. Iraq
            1) In 1995, the Iraqi government disclosed that it had produced and stockpiled extensive quantities of anthrax spores, botulinum toxin, and aflatoxin
            2) These weapons were not used during the Persian Gulf War
            3) No stockpiled weapons or active production sites were discovered subsequent to the April 2003 invasion of Iraq
    3. Recent incidents of bioterrorism
        a. In 1984, the Rajneeshee cult contaminated salad bars in restaurants in Oregon with *Salmonella typhimurium* (in an attempt to influence the outcome of local elections), resulting in 751 cases of enteritis with 45 hospitalizations but no deaths
        b. In 1995, the Japanese cult Aum Shinrikyo attacked passengers in the Tokyo subway with sarin nerve gas after several unsuccessful attempts to aerosolize anthrax spores and botulinum toxin
        c. In the fall of 2001, an outbreak resulting in 22 cases of anthrax (11 inhalational and 11 cutaneous) occurred in Florida, the District of Columbia, New York, New Jersey, and Connecticut
            1) Traced to letters containing weapons-grade anthrax spores sent through the US Postal Service
            2) Inhalational anthrax caused 5 deaths
        d. Ricin
            1) In 2003, the US Department of Transportation received 2 letters containing small amounts of ricin
            2) In February 2004, a letter containing ricin was sent to a US senator
            3) There was no associated documented morbidity or mortality
    4. International agreements involving biological weapons
        a. The 1925 Geneva Protocol prohibited use but not research, production, or possession of biological warfare agents
        b. The Biological Weapons Convention (1972) prohibits the development, production, stockpiling, or retention of any biological agent "of types and in quantities that have no justification for prophylactic, protective, or other peaceful purposes"

II. Microorganisms as Weapons
    A. Advantages of Biologic Agents as Weapons
        1. Generally relatively easy to produce
        2. May be more cost-effective than ballistic or nuclear weapons
        3. Organisms and biotoxins are colorless, odorless, and invisible
        4. Potential for dissemination over a large geographic area
        5. Attacks are difficult to detect before presentation of initial clinical cases
        6. Potential to cause high morbidity and mortality
        7. Incite panic, creating additional "psychological casualties"
        8. Person-to-person transmission is possible
        9. Illness is often difficult to diagnose or treat
        10. Incubation period usually allows escape of the perpetrator
    B. Limitations of Biologic Agents as Weapons
        1. May adversely affect the health of the perpetrator as well as the intended victims
        2. Weather conditions affect aerosol dispersion
        3. Environmental conditions may kill organisms
        4. A contaminated area can be uninhabitable for a long time if the agent remains in the environment (eg, *B anthracis*)
        5. Agent may undergo secondary aerosolization
        6. Morbidity and mortality are unpredictable because they vary with agent delivery, environmental conditions, and the public health response
    C. Factors Affecting the Suitability of a Biological Agent for Offensive Use
        1. Availability
        2. Ability to be produced in adequate quantities
        3. Ability to deliver doses that can kill or incapacitate humans
        4. Potential for person-to-person spread
        5. Potential to be weaponized
        6. Ability to remain stable and virulent in storage, in the delivery vehicle, and in the environment
        7. Susceptibility of intended victims
        8. There is no generally available or effective treatment, prophylaxis, or vaccine
    D. Weaponization of Biological Agents
        1. Agent is purified and processed to maximize its effectiveness to cause disease (ie, creation of a weapons-grade agent)
            a. Optimal particle size of 1 to 5 μm to facilitate entry into the lower respiratory tract

b. Electrostatically neutral and nonclumping particles allow for optimal aerosolization
     2. Agent is placed in an effective delivery device
        a. Aerosol delivery: generally considered to be the most effective and most likely mode of delivery (eg, linear aerosol cloud delivered by an aerosol device aboard an aircraft)
        b. Bomblets loaded into missile warheads: explosive munitions are less effective since heat from the explosion could inactivate a large amount of agent
        c. Letter or package delivered by mail or package delivery systems
        d. Food or water contamination
III. Threat Agents
   A. Categories of Risk
      1. The Centers for Disease Control and Prevention (CDC) has categorized potential agents of bioterrorism into 3 categories based on risk for possible use in a bioterrorist attack (Box 45.1 and Table 45.1)
         a. Category A agents
            1) Considered to be the most important agents likely to be used in a bioterrorist attack
            2) Associated with high mortality
            3) Confer the greatest potential for substantial adverse public health impact
         b. Category B agents
            1) Associated with considerably lower mortality
            2) Generally considered to be incapacitating agents
         c. Category C agents
            1) Emerging pathogens
            2) Could be engineered for mass dissemination in the future
      2. Past research into the genetic engineering of microorganisms for use in biological warfare
         a. Underlines the possibility that a bioterrorist attack may involve novel or significantly modified organisms
         b. Modified organisms may have unexpected clinical manifestations and resistance profiles or be able to overcome vaccine-induced immunity
   B. *Bacillus anthracis* (Anthrax)
      1. Microbiology
         a. A gram-positive, aerobic, spore-forming bacillus
         b. Anthrax toxin is composed of 3 proteins: edema factor, lethal factor, and protective antigen

---

Box 45.1

CDC Categorization of Potential Agents of Bioterrorism

Category A: High-priority agents include those that pose a risk to national security because they a) can be easily disseminated or transmitted from person to person, b) result in high mortality rates and have the potential for a major public health impact, c) might cause public panic and social disruption, and d) require special action for public health preparedness
Bacillus anthracis (anthrax)
Clostridium botulinum toxin (botulism)
Yersinia pestis (plague)
Variola virus (smallpox)
Francisella tularensis (tularemia)
Viral hemorrhagic fever agents (filoviruses [eg, Ebola, Marburg] and arenaviruses [eg, Lassa, Machupo])

Category B: Second-highest priority agents include those that a) are moderately easy to disseminate, b) result in moderate morbidity rates and low mortality rates, and c) require specific enhancements of diagnostic capacity and disease surveillance
Brucella species (brucellosis)
Clostridium perfringens ε toxin
Food safety threats (eg, *Salmonella* species, *Escherichia coli* O157:H7, *Shigella* species)
Burkholderia mallei (glanders)
Burkholderia pseudomallei (melioidosis)
Chlamydophila psittaci (psittacosis)
Coxiella burnetii (Q fever)
Ricin toxin from *Ricinus communis* (castor bean)
Staphylococcal enterotoxin B
Rickettsia prowazekii (typhus fever)
Viral encephalitis agents (eg, Venezuelan equine encephalomyelitis, eastern equine encephalomyelitis, western equine encephalomyelitis)
Water safety threats (eg, *Vibrio cholerae*, *Cryptosporidium parvum*)

Category C: Third-highest priority agents include emerging pathogens that could be engineered for mass dissemination in the future because of a) availability, b) ease of production and dissemination, and c) potential for high morbidity and mortality rates and major public health impact
Emerging infectious disease agents such as Nipah virus and hantavirus

Abbreviation: CDC, Centers for Disease Control and Prevention.

Adapted from Centers for Disease Control and Prevention. Bioterrorism agents/disease [Internet]. [cited 2010 Aug 6]. Available from: http://www.bt.cdc.gov/agent/agentlist-category.asp.

---

         c. Toxin is responsible for the clinical manifestations of hemorrhage, edema, and necrosis
         d. An antiphagocytic capsule is also necessary for full virulence
      2. Epidemiology
         a. Naturally acquired disease occurs through direct contact with infected livestock, wild animals, or contaminated animal products
         b. The ultimate reservoir is the soil

Table 45.1
Clinical Features of Diseases Caused by CDC Category A Agents and Biotoxins

Disease	Etiologic Agent	Incubation	Clinical Presentation	Diagnosis	Person-to-Person Transmission	Treatment	Postexposure Prophylaxis
Inhalational anthrax	*Bacillus anthracis*	Usually 1-6 d but may be prolonged to ≥42 d	Widened mediastinum, fever, cough or dyspnea, shock	Gram stain and culture of blood, CSF, sputum; PCR; Wright stain of peripheral blood smear	No	Ciprofloxacin or doxycycline (plus 1 or 2 other agents with documented susceptibility, such as clindamycin or rifampin); Initial therapy should be intravenous; Duration 60 d	Ciprofloxacin or doxycycline; Amoxicillin can be used for susceptible strains; Duration 60 d; Anthrax vaccine adsorbed may be administered concomitantly
Cutaneous anthrax	*Bacillus anthracis*	1-12 d	Skin lesion (papule, eschar)	Culture of skin; PCR	No	Ciprofloxacin or doxycycline (penicillin or amoxicillin can be used with susceptible strains for naturally acquired disease); Duration 60 d for bioterrorist attack (7-10 d for naturally acquired disease with no systemic symptoms)	Same as for inhalational anthrax
Pneumonic plague	*Yersinia pestis*	1-6 d	Fulminant pneumonia, hemoptysis	Culture of blood, sputum; DFA; PCR	Yes	Streptomycin or gentamicin; Alternatives include doxycycline or ciprofloxacin; Duration 10 d	Doxycycline or ciprofloxacin for 7 d

Disease	Agent	Incubation	Clinical Features	Diagnosis	Person-to-person Transmission	Treatment	Prophylaxis
Smallpox	Variola virus	7-17 d (typically 12-14 d)	Synchronous vesicopustular rash	PCR of vesicular fluid, scab material, pharyngeal swab; Culture in biosafety level 4 laboratory	Yes	Possibly cidofovir	Vaccinia vaccine
Tularemia	*Francisella tularensis*	1-14 d (typically 3-5 d)	Fever, headache, cough; Pneumonitis likely with aerosol exposure	Culture of blood, sputum; PCR; Serology	No	Streptomycin or gentamicin for 10 d; Doxycycline or ciprofloxacin for 14 d	Doxycycline or ciprofloxacin for 14 d
Botulism	Toxin of *Clostridium botulinum*	2 h to 8 d (typically 1-3 d)	Alert patient with cranial nerve palsies and progressive descending paralysis	Clinical diagnosis; Mouse bioassay; Toxin immunoassay	No	Supportive care; Antitoxin	Antitoxin
Viral hemorrhagic fever	Filoviruses and arenaviruses (bunyaviruses and flaviviruses are not classified as category A agents)	2-21 d	Fever, shock syndrome, bleeding diathesis	Clinical diagnosis; ELISA; PCR; Culture in biosafety level 4 laboratory	Yes (with certain agents)	Supportive care; Ribavirin for arenaviruses and bunyaviruses	Ribavirin for certain arenaviruses and bunyaviruses in high-risk situations

Abbreviations: CDC, Centers for Disease Control and Prevention; CSF, cerebrospinal fluid; DFA, direct fluorescence assay; ELISA, enzyme-linked immunosorbent assay; PCR, polymerase chain reaction.

c. Spores can survive for decades in the environment
   d. Naturally occurring human disease in the United States
      1) From 1993 to 2000: 1 case of cutaneous anthrax
      2) From 1976 to 2001: no cases of inhalational anthrax reported
   e. No documented person-to-person transmission
3. Clinical manifestations
   a. Inhalational anthrax
      1) Spores are inhaled and transported by the lymphatics to hilar and mediastinal nodes
      2) Germination occurs after a variable period of spore dormancy
      3) Incubation period: generally 1 to 6 days but may be prolonged to 42 days or more
      4) Toxins cause hemorrhagic necrosis and edema of the mediastinal lymph nodes
      5) Hemorrhagic necrosis extends to the pleura, resulting in bloody effusions
      6) Hematogenous spread may lead to hemorrhagic meningitis in about 50% of cases
      7) Biphasic clinical pattern
         a) Initially 1 to 3 days of fever, cough, malaise, nausea, vomiting, and substernal pain
         b) Then sudden onset of fulminant illness with dyspnea, diaphoresis, cyanosis, and shock
   b. Cutaneous anthrax
      1) Usually occurs on exposed skin at the site of an abrasion or laceration
      2) Lesion begins as a painless, pruritic papule associated with localized edema
         a) Subsequently enlarges and ulcerates over 1 to 2 days, often with surrounding vesiculation
         b) An eschar forms over the ulcer, which then dries, loosens, and separates within 1 to 2 weeks
      3) Mild systemic symptoms with painful regional lymphadenopathy
      4) If untreated, may progress to septicemia and death
         a) Without treatment, case fatality rate is about 20%
         b) With treatment, death is rare
   c. Gastrointestinal anthrax
      1) Caused by ingestion of undercooked meat from infected animals
      2) Two clinical manifestations (both may lead to sepsis syndrome and death)
         a) Intestinal
            i) Ulcerative lesions occur most commonly in the terminal ileum or cecum
            ii) Symptoms include nausea, vomiting, fever, abdominal pain, bloody diarrhea, and ascites
         b) Oropharyngeal
            i) Edema and tissue necrosis with ulceration involving the oral cavity or esophagus
            ii) Symptoms include sore throat, fever, and dysphagia
      3) Gastrointestinal anthrax is thought to be a very unlikely manifestation of anthrax due to a bioterrorist attack
4. Diagnosis
   a. Chest radiography shows a widened mediastinum, often with pleural effusion with or without pulmonary infiltrates
   b. Computed tomographic scan of the chest shows hyperdense mediastinal nodes, edema, and effusions with or without infiltrates
   c. Organisms may be seen on a Gram-stained peripheral blood smear
   d. Blood cultures are usually positive with inhalational anthrax
   e. Organisms may be recovered from pleural fluid and cerebrospinal fluid
   f. For diagnosis of cutaneous anthrax: Gram stain and culture of vesicular fluid or skin (punch biopsy)
   g. Polymerase chain reaction (PCR) testing or immunostaining of blood, cerebrospinal fluid, pleural fluid, or skin
   h. Nasal swab culture
      1) An epidemiologic tool and not a means for clinical diagnosis of disease
      2) Predictive value of a positive nasal swab culture is unknown
5. Treatment
   a. Early antibiotic administration is essential
   b. Most naturally occurring *B anthracis* strains are susceptible to penicillin, doxycycline, ciprofloxacin, clindamycin, rifampin, imipenem, aminoglycosides, chloramphenicol, and vancomycin
   c. Inducible β-lactamases may confer clinical penicillin resistance in the presence of a large bacterial burden

d. Penicillin, doxycycline, and ciprofloxacin are approved by the US Food and Drug Administration for treatment of inhalational anthrax
e. An engineered strain resistant to tetracycline and penicillins has been reported
f. Combination therapy
   1) Use of 2 or 3 intravenous drugs is recommended for initial treatment of inhalational or gastrointestinal anthrax
   2) For example: ciprofloxacin or doxycycline in combination with 1 or 2 other drugs that have documented susceptibility, such as clindamycin and rifampin
g. Treatment duration is prolonged (≥60 days) because of possible recurrence of disease due to delayed spore germination
h. Treatment duration for cutaneous disease
   1) If exposure is unknown or suspected to be due to a bioterrorist attack: treatment should be for at least 60 days
   2) If exposure is known to have occurred through livestock exposure: treatment for 7 to 10 days may be adequate
6. Prevention
   a. Postexposure prophylaxis for 60 days with either ciprofloxacin or doxycycline (amoxicillin may be used, particularly in children, for susceptible strains)
   b. Anthrax vaccine adsorbed
      1) An inactivated cell-free product given in a 6-dose series
      2) Currently licensed only for preexposure administration, but may be given after exposure in addition to antibiotic prophylaxis
   c. Environmental decontamination of the exposed facility is required to prevent the possibility of delayed casualties due to aerosolization of spores persisting in the environment
C. Variola Virus (Smallpox)
   1. Microbiology
      a. A double-stranded DNA virus
      b. Member of family Poxviridae: genus *Orthopoxvirus*
   2. Epidemiology
      a. Last naturally occurring cases occurred in the United States in 1949 and worldwide in 1977
      b. Vaccination ceased in the United States in 1972 and worldwide about 1982
      c. Spreads from person to person by droplet nuclei or aerosol
      d. No known animal or insect reservoirs or vectors
      e. Transmission begins with onset of rash and wanes rapidly as scabs form
      f. Natural infection confers lifelong immunity
   3. Clinical manifestations
      a. Incubation period: 12 to 14 days (range, 7-17 days)
      b. Flulike symptoms (fever, back pain, headache, prostration) precede rash
      c. Maculopapular rash
         1) Develops after 2 to 3 days
         2) Begins on the oropharyngeal mucosa and face before involving the arms, legs, and trunk (centripetal spread)
         3) Lesions are most dense on the face and extremities
         4) Lesions often involve the palms and soles
      d. Synchronous lesions
         1) All lesions appear in the same stage of development
         2) An important clinical feature differentiating smallpox from varicella-zoster virus infection
      e. Lesions become vesiculopustular, and crusts form 8 to 9 days after onset of rash
      f. Pitted scars develop after scabs separate
      g. Variola major
         1) Overall case fatality rate: 30%
         2) Clinical forms
            a) Ordinary smallpox: the most frequent
            b) Modified smallpox: mild disease occurring in previously vaccinated persons
            c) Hemorrhagic smallpox
               i) Shorter incubation
               ii) More severe prodromal illness
               iii) Pregnant women are unusually susceptible
               iv) Uniformly fatal
            d) Malignant (flat) smallpox
               i) Confluent lesions remain soft, flat, and velvety
               ii) Lesions do not progress to pustules
               iii) Usually fatal
      h. Variola minor
         1) Case fatality rate: less than 1%
         2) Less severe illness with a sparse rash
         3) Also called alastrim

4. Diagnosis
      a. PCR testing
      b. Electron microscopy
      c. Culture of vesiculopustular fluid (in biosafety level 4 facility)
   5. Treatment: cidofovir
      a. Active in vitro
      b. Untested in humans
   6. Prevention: live vaccinia virus vaccine
      a. Efficacy about 95%
      b. Provides full immunity for 5 to 10 years, but immunity wanes thereafter (imprecisely defined)
      c. Rare but severe complications include eczema vaccinatum, progressive vaccinia, myopericarditis, and encephalitis
D. *Yersinia pestis* (Plague)
   1. Microbiology: gram-negative, bipolar staining ("safety pin"), aerobic coccobacillus
   2. Epidemiology
      a. Rodents are natural reservoirs of infection
      b. Disease is transmitted to humans by infected fleas
      c. Primary pneumonic plague results from inhalation of organisms
      d. Secondary pneumonic plague results from hematogenous spread to the lungs in patients with bubonic or septicemic plague
      e. Plague from a bioterrorist aerosol attack would most likely manifest as primary pneumonic plague
      f. If disease is untreated, mortality is high
      g. Human-to-human transmission occurs with pneumonic plague
   3. Clinical manifestations
      a. Incubation period: 1 to 6 days
      b. Three clinical forms: pneumonic, bubonic, and septicemic
         1) Pneumonic plague
            a) Fever, cough, dyspnea, and hemoptysis
            b) Chest radiograph usually shows lobar consolidation
            c) Fulminant course with rapid progression to respiratory failure and shock
         2) Bubonic plague
            a) Fever, malaise, tender lymph nodes (buboes)
            b) Results from bite of plague-infested flea
            c) May progress to septicemic form, with spread to central nervous system, lungs, or other organs
         3) Septicemic plague
            a) Bacteremia without lymphadenopathy
            b) Purpuric skin lesions and necrotic digits seen in advanced disease
   4. Diagnosis
      a. Gram stain and culture of blood, sputum, bubo aspirate
      b. PCR testing
      c. Direct fluorescence assay
   5. Treatment
      a. Gentamicin or streptomycin for 10 days
      b. Ciprofloxacin or doxycycline are therapeutic alternatives
   6. Prevention: doxycycline or ciprofloxacin for 7 days
E. *Francisella tularensis* (Tularemia)
   1. Microbiology: a small gram-negative aerobic coccobacillus
   2. Epidemiology
      a. Organism is hardy and may survive for weeks in water, soil, or decaying animal carcasses
      b. High infectivity: as few as 10 organisms may cause disease
      c. Various small mammals are natural reservoirs of infection
      d. Transmission to humans occurs through infected ticks, mosquitoes, or flies or through contact with infected animal tissues
      e. Transmission by inhalation is very uncommon, but it is the most likely mode in a bioterrorist attack (resulting in primary pneumonic or typhoidal tularemia)
      f. No person-to-person transmission
   3. Clinical manifestations
      a. Incubation period: usually 3 to 5 days (range, 1-14 days)
      b. Natural infection
         1) Typically has abrupt onset
         2) Nonspecific systemic symptoms (eg, fever, chills, headache, myalgias, nonproductive cough)
         3) Evidence of inflammation (regional lymphadenopathy with or without skin ulcer, conjunctivitis, and pharyngitis) where the organism entered the tissue
      c. Clinical forms of tularemia
         1) Ulceroglandular (most common naturally occurring disease manifestation)
         2) Glandular
         3) Oculoglandular

4) Oropharyngeal
5) Typhoidal
   a) Systemic infection
   b) No findings that suggest either a focal site of inoculation or an anatomical localization of infection
6) Pneumonic (primary or secondary)
   a) Clinically, pneumonic tularemia often resembles an acute systemic illness without prominent respiratory symptoms or signs
   b) Progression to frank pulmonary involvement may be subacute or fulminant
   c) May lead to respiratory failure, multisystem organ failure, and death
   d) Chest radiographs typically show subsegmental or lobar infiltrates, pleural effusion, and hilar adenopathy
    d. Any form of tularemia may be complicated by hematogenous spread (eg, to lungs or rarely to meninges)
    e. Tularemia probably would have a slower progression of illness and a considerably lower case fatality rate than inhalational plague or anthrax
  4. Diagnosis
    a. Culture of sputum and blood
    b. Serology
    c. PCR testing of primary lesion
  5. Treatment
    a. Parenteral streptomycin or gentamicin for 10 days
    b. Therapeutic alternatives include doxycycline or ciprofloxacin for 14 days
  6. Prevention: doxycycline or ciprofloxacin for 14 days
F. Botulinum Toxin (Botulism)
  1. Microbiology
    a. Polypeptide neurotoxins (7 antigenically distinct forms, designated *A* through *G*) produced by *Clostridium botulinum*, a spore-forming obligate anaerobe
    b. Botulinum toxin
      1) The most toxic substance known
      2) It is estimated that 1 g evenly dispersed and inhaled could kill 1 million people
      3) Toxin is colorless, odorless, and tasteless
  2. Epidemiology
    a. Natural habitat: soil
    b. Natural illness occurs after consumption of contaminated food (preformed toxin) or through a wound or bowel infected with *C botulinum*
    c. Aerosol dispersion and food contamination are the most likely modes of transmission in a bioterrorist attack
    d. No person-to-person transmission
    e. A major bioweapon threat
      1) Extreme potency and lethality
      2) Ease of production
      3) Documented historical evidence of large-scale production
      4) Need for prolonged intensive care of victims
  3. Clinical manifestations
    a. Botulism results from absorption of toxin from mucosal surfaces (eg, gut, lung) or wounds
    b. Toxin binds irreversibly to the neuromuscular junction and enzymatically blocks acetylcholine release, causing flaccid paralysis
    c. Three natural clinical forms of disease
      1) Foodborne botulism
      2) Wound botulism
      3) Intestinal botulism (infant, adult)
    d. Inhalational botulism is a man-made form of disease that manifests like foodborne disease
    e. Rapidity of onset and severity of disease depend on rate and quantity of toxin absorption
    f. Neurologic signs and symptoms
      1) Always begin in the bulbar musculature: difficulty seeing, speaking, and swallowing
      2) Symmetrical cranial neuropathies (eg, *d*ysarthria, *d*ysphonia, *d*ysphagia, and *d*iplopia and ptosis and sluggish pupils)
      3) Symmetrical descending weakness in a proximal-to-distal pattern, leading to respiratory failure
    g. Patients are alert and oriented with no fever or sensory findings
  4. Diagnosis
    a. Clinical features
    b. Detection of toxin (mouse bioassay, toxin immunoassay) in blood, gastric aspirate, feces, or food samples
    c. Isolation of *C botulinum* from the wound site in cases of wound botulism
  5. Treatment
    a. Supportive care, which may include intubation and mechanical ventilation
    b. Equine heptavalent botulism antitoxin

c. Human-derived botulism immune globulin for infants younger than 1 year
d. Paralysis can persist for weeks to months and may require prolonged assisted ventilation and other supportive care
6. Prevention: antitoxin
G. Viral Hemorrhagic Fever Agents
1. Microbiology
   a. The term *viral hemorrhagic fever* refers to clinical illness associated with fever and a bleeding diathesis caused by viruses belonging to 4 distinct families
      1) Filoviridae: Ebola virus, Marburg virus
      2) Arenaviridae: Junin virus, Machupo virus, and other New World arenaviruses and Lassa virus
      3) Bunyaviridae: agents of Rift Valley fever, Crimean-Congo hemorrhagic fever, hemorrhagic fever with renal syndrome, and hantavirus pulmonary syndrome
      4) Flaviviridae: agents of dengue, yellow fever, Omsk hemorrhagic fever, and Kyasanur forest disease
   b. Zoonotic RNA viruses with lipid envelope
2. Epidemiology
   a. Natural reservoir
      1) An arthropod or other animal host
      2) Reservoir of filoviruses is unknown
   b. Transmission to humans (depends on specific virus) through handling of animal carcasses, contact with sick animals or humans, and arthropod bites
   c. Potential for aerosol transmission with a bioterrorist attack
   d. Filoviruses and arenaviruses are transmissible from person to person with the potential for airborne transmission
3. Clinical manifestations
   a. Target organ: the vascular bed
      1) Dominant clinical features are attributable to microvascular damage and vascular permeability changes
      2) Initial symptoms include fever, dizziness, rash, myalgias, and prostration
      3) Signs of bleeding follow: from mild subconjunctival hemorrhage and petechiae to shock with generalized mucous membrane hemorrhage
   b. Pulmonary, hematopoietic, and neurologic dysfunction may occur
   c. Renal insufficiency is usually proportional to cardiovascular compromise (except with hemorrhagic fever with renal syndrome, in which it is an integral part of the disease)
   d. Patients usually improve or become moribund within 1 to 2 weeks
   e. Mortality: 1% to 90%, depending on virus
4. Diagnosis
   a. Epidemiologic and clinical features
   b. Serology
   c. Tissue immunohistochemistry
   d. PCR testing
   e. Virus isolation (requires biosafety level 4 facility)
5. Treatment
   a. No proven effective treatment for most viral hemorrhagic fevers
   b. Mainstay of therapy is supportive in the setting of intensive infection control precautions
   c. Ribavirin may be useful for bunyavirus and arenavirus infections
6. Prevention
   a. No known effective chemoprophylaxis or vaccines available for the filoviruses
   b. Ribavirin postexposure prophylaxis in high-risk situations with susceptible arenaviruses and bunyaviruses
   c. Vaccine available for yellow fever (preexposure)
H. Ricin Toxin
1. An important category B agent
   a. Ease of production
   b. Notorious history of use in warfare and espionage
   c. Recent bioterrorist attacks with ricin powder
2. Ricin
   a. A ribosome-inhibiting protein toxin
   b. Derived from *Ricinus communis* (castor bean)
3. Clinical manifestations of inhalational exposure
   a. Limited data from humans
   b. Lethal human aerosol exposures have not been described
   c. Onset of cough, shortness of breath, chest tightness, fever, and nausea approximately 4 to 8 hours after exposure
   d. Severity of signs and symptoms depends on inhaled dose
   e. Symptoms may last several hours and then resolve spontaneously
   f. Airway necrosis with capillary leak may occur, resulting in pulmonary edema

4. Clinical manifestations of ingestion of ricin
   a. Gastrointestinal tract symptoms, including nausea, vomiting, and abdominal pain
   b. High-dose exposure may result in necrosis of the gastrointestinal tract and other abdominal viscera
5. Parenteral exposure may cause myonecrosis followed by multiorgan failure and death
6. Diagnosis: there are currently no generally available tests for the diagnosis of ricin poisoning
7. Treatment: supportive

IV. General Clinical Principles
   A. Clinical Features Suggestive of a Biological Agent Attack
      1. Point-source exposure pattern with illness limited to 1 or more fairly localized or circumscribed geographical areas
      2. Apparent aerosol route of infection
      3. High attack rate among exposed persons
      4. Cluster of unusual, severe, or unexplained illnesses with high morbidity and mortality
      5. Highly unusual disease for geographic region
      6. Sentinel dead animals of multiple species
      7. Multiple cases of flulike illness when influenza would not typically be expected
      8. Absence of a competent natural vector where the outbreak occurred (for a biological agent that is vector-borne in nature)
      9. Clinical syndrome suggestive of a suspicious agent (eg, widened mediastinum, hemorrhagic fever syndrome, vesicopustular rash)
   B. Clinical Syndromes Suggestive of a Bioterrorism-Associated Illness
      1. Anthrax
         a. Systemic illness
         b. Widened mediastinum on chest radiography
      2. Smallpox
         a. Vesiculopustular rash involving palms and soles
         b. Facial involvement more than chest involvement
         c. All lesions in same phase of development
      3. Botulism
         a. Prominent neurologic symptoms in an alert patient
         b. Descending paralysis beginning with cranial nerve palsies
      4. Plague
         a. Fulminant pneumonia
         b. Hemoptysis
      5. Tularemia: increased incidence of atypical pneumonia
      6. Viral hemorrhagic fever: shock syndrome with hemorrhagic diathesis
   C. Clinical Management
      1. Maintain high degree of awareness: clinical presentation may be atypical because of an unusual method of dissemination (eg, aerosol) or possible alteration of organism resulting from genetic engineering
      2. Consider possibility of contagion, and institute appropriate isolation precautions (if indicated) promptly
      3. Consider use of rapid diagnostic technology (eg, PCR testing) in addition to routine testing (eg, Gram stain and culture)
      4. Notify county, state, and federal health authorities expeditiously
      5. Prompt initiation of antiinfective treatment (if available) and appropriate supportive care
      6. Obtain susceptibility data to determine appropriateness of therapy
      7. Assess extent of outbreak and potential for secondary transmission
   D. Perspectives From History
      1. Most attempts to deliberately use microorganisms or their toxins to effect large-scale disease and death have failed
      2. Natural pandemics probably pose significantly greater risks
      3. Most deliberate outbreaks, as with naturally occurring ones, can probably be curtailed through the vigorous application of public health measures
      4. It is difficult to obtain reliable real-time information on terrorist or state-sponsored clandestine biological weapons programs
      5. Current "threat assessments" are often no more than best guesses
      6. Assessments of the likely effect of a bioterrorist attack generally rely heavily on untested "theoretical data"
      7. Despite a history of extensive government-sponsored biological warfare programs with demonstrated capabilities, the large-scale use of biologic agents or toxins for warfare has not been successfully undertaken
      8. Owing to the effect of deterrence against the governmental use of biologic agents for warfare or terrorism, the principal ongoing threat is posed by rogue individuals or groups with no government affiliation
         a. Terrorists who hope to further ideologic or religious objectives
         b. Sociopathic persons
         c. Nihilistic groups waging war against society

Suggested Reading

Grey MR, Spaeth KR. The bioterrorism sourcebook. New York (NY): McGraw-Hill Medical Pub. Division; c2006.

Moran GJ, Talan DA, Abrahamian FM. Biological terrorism. Infect Dis Clin North Am. 2008 Mar;22(1):145–87.

Woods JB, Darling DG, Dembek ZF, Carr BK, Cieslak TJ, Lawler JV, et al. USAMRIID's medical management of biologic casualties handbook. 6th ed. Frederick (MD): U.S. Army Medical Research Institute of Infectious Diseases; 2005. [cited 2010 Aug 5]. Available from: http://www.usamriid.army.mil/education/bluebookpdf/USAMRIID%20BlueBook%206th%20Edition%20-%20Sep%202006.pdf.

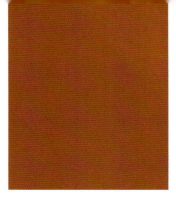

Special Hosts and Situations

Questions and Answers

Questions

Multiple Choice (choose the best answer)

1. Which of the following statements is *false* about cytomegalovirus (CMV) infection and disease after transplant?
   a. The most common clinical presentation is fever and myelosuppression.
   b. The most common organ-invasive disease involves the gastrointestinal tract (colitis and gastritis).
   c. Preemptive therapy is the preferred method for prevention of CMV disease in solid organ transplant recipients who have the following CMV-mismatch status: CMV-seropositive donor (D+) and CMV-seronegative recipient (R–).
   d. Antiviral prophylaxis with ganciclovir is not commonly used because of drug-induced neutropenia after allogeneic hematopoietic stem cell transplant.
   e. CMV disease after transplant has been associated with the occurrence of acute and chronic allograft rejection and a higher risk of opportunistic infections.

2. Which of the following statements is *false* about risk factors for cytomegalovirus (CMV) after transplant?
   a. Solid organ transplant recipients at highest risk are the CMV-seronegative recipients (R–) of organs from CMV-seropositive donors (D+).
   b. CMV D+/R– allogeneic hematopoietic stem cell transplant recipients are at higher risk of CMV disease compared with CMV-seropositive (R+) patients.
   c. Allograft rejection increases the risk of CMV disease after solid organ transplant.
   d. Graft-vs-host disease is a common risk factor for CMV disease after allogeneic hematopoietic stem cell transplant.
   e. Mycophenolate mofetil at dosages of more than 3 g daily has been associated with increased risk of tissue-invasive CMV disease.

3. Which of the following statements is *false* about the methods for the diagnosis of cytomegalovirus (CMV) disease after transplant?
   a. CMV polymerase chain reaction (PCR) assay is more sensitive than shell vial culture assay.
   b. CMV pp65 antigenemia assay, which detects CMV-infected leukocytes, is a clinically useful method for guiding antiviral treatment.
   c. The quantitative nature of viral PCR assays has helped in predicting CMV disease and in guiding the duration of antiviral treatment.
   d. CMV serology to detect IgM is a very reliable method for diagnosing acute CMV disease in transplant patients.
   e. In situ hybridization is a very useful method for demonstrating the tissue-invasive nature of CMV.

4. Which of the following statements is *false* about the epidemiology of infections after transplant?
   a. Dermatomal zoster occurs in approximately 10% of transplant recipients.
   b. Herpes simplex virus is the most common viral opportunistic pathogen during the first month after transplant.
   c. *Aspergillus fumigatus* is the most common fungal pathogen after transplant.
   d. Epstein-Barr virus infection is the cause of most lymphoma after transplant.
   e. *Coccidioides immitis* is an endemic fungus that can cause multisystemic disease after solid organ transplant.

5. Which of the following statements is *false* about the risk factors for infections after transplant?
   a. Fulminant hepatic failure may be complicated by disseminated fungal infection after liver transplant.
   b. Solid organ transplant recipients who are cytomegalovirus (CMV) seropositive (R+) have the highest risk of CMV disease after transplant.
   c. Allogeneic hematopoietic stem cell recipients who are CMV R+ have a higher risk of CMV disease compared with CMV-seronegative recipients (CMV R−).
   d. Invasive aspergillosis is observed more commonly after lung transplant than after liver transplant.
   e. Patients infected with *Strongyloides stercoralis* may present with disseminated bacterial and fungal superinfection after transplant.

6. A 48-year-old man is admitted to the hospital with an acute febrile illness with headache, confusion, and hypotension. A chest radiograph shows enlargement of the mediastinum with bilateral pleural effusions. Anthrax is suspected. Which of the following tests is *not* appropriate to establish the clinical diagnosis?
   a. Blood cultures with routine media
   b. Gram stain and culture of cerebrospinal fluid
   c. Culture of a nasopharyngeal swab
   d. Gram stain of blood
   e. Polymerase chain reaction (PCR) testing of blood and pleural effusion

7. Bioterrorist attacks would most likely occur by the aerosol route. Which of the following organisms could cause pneumonia in victims and pose a risk for secondary person-to-person transmission of infection?
   a. *Bacillus anthracis*
   b. *Francisella tularensis*
   c. *Coxiella burnetii*
   d. *Yersinia pestis*
   e. *Clostridium botulinum*

8. Early detection of a bioterrorist attack relies primarily on the astute clinical judgment of physicians treating initial disease cases. Which clinicoepidemiologic feature should *not* provoke a heightened suspicion of a possible bioterrorist attack?
   a. Illness occurring in otherwise healthy persons with epidemiologic features suggesting a point-source exposure pattern
   b. Occurrence of disease not usually seen in the geographic region
   c. Cluster of severe, unexplained illness with high morbidity and mortality
   d. Unusual clinical syndrome consistent with disease due to a suspect microorganism
   e. Cluster of cases of acute diarrheal illness

9. A 59-year-old man who has not received any medical care in the past 12 years presents for a general medical examination. No new medical problems are identified. Which of the following vaccinations would you recommend at this time?
   a. Tetanus, diphtheria, and acellular pertussis (Tdap)
   b. Tetanus and diphtheria (Td) and influenza
   c. Tdap and measles, mumps, and rubella (MMR)
   d. Tdap, varicella, and influenza
   e. Tdap and influenza

10. A 45-year-old teacher in a school for the developmentally disabled presents with questions about hepatitis B vaccination. She received 1 dose of hepatitis B vaccine 3 years ago, but she did not complete the series. What would be the most appropriate action at this point?
    a. Restart the vaccine series, and give 3 doses at 0, 1, and 6 months.
    b. Give a second dose now and the next dose in 5 months.
    c. Give a second dose now and the next dose in 1 month.
    d. Do nothing. The patient does not need the vaccination.
    e. Give the second dose now and the next dose in 2 months.

11. Which of the following patients should *not* be revaccinated with meningococcal conjugate vaccine?
    a. A healthy college freshman who received meningococcal conjugate vaccine 4 years ago at age 15
    b. An asplenic patient who received meningococcal conjugate vaccine 6 years ago
    c. An asplenic patient who received meningococcal polysaccharide vaccine 6 years ago
    d. A 45-year-old microbiologist who received meningococcal conjugate vaccine 8 years ago
    e. A healthy college freshman who received meningococcal polysaccharide vaccine 6 years ago, before a trip to sub-Saharan Africa

12. Which of the following are contraindications to the inactivated influenza vaccine?
    a. History of serious egg allergy
    b. History of multiple myeloma
    c. Pregnancy
    d. Age older than 65 years
    e. History of asthma

13. Which of the following statements about vaccines is *false*?
    a. Two parenteral live vaccines can be given at the same time.
    b. A live vaccine and an inactivated vaccine can be given at the same time.
    c. If a dose of a multidose vaccine series is missed, the entire series needs to be restarted.
    d. An inactivated vaccine can be given at the same time or at any time before or after another inactivated vaccine or live vaccine.
    e. Blood products can interfere with the immune response to live vaccines.

14. Which of the following is *not* included in the Institute for Healthcare Improvement Ventilator Bundle?
    a. Oral care
    b. Elevation of the head of the bed
    c. Sedation vacations and daily assessment of readiness to extubate
    d. Peptic ulcer prophylaxis
    e. Deep vein thrombosis (DVT) prophylaxis

15. What is the most common health care–associated infection (HAI)?
    a. Catheter-associated urinary tract infection (UTI)
    b. Ventilator-associated pneumonia
    c. Surgical site infection
    d. Bloodstream infection
    e. Aspiration pneumonia

16. During an elective cholecystectomy, the surgeon encounters dense adhesions and accidentally nicks the colon, with spillage of fecal material. How would this operation be classified?
    a. Type I/clean surgery
    b. Type II/clean-contaminated
    c. Type III/contaminated
    d. Type IV/dirty-infected
    e. Untypeable

17. An intensive care unit (ICU) patient requires intravenous access for rapid fluid administration. Which of the following options would be associated with the lowest risk of bloodstream infection?
    a. Triple-lumen catheter in a femoral site
    b. Triple-lumen catheter in the internal jugular vein
    c. Peripheral intravenous site
    d. Peripherally inserted central catheter (PICC) line
    e. Triple-lumen catheter in the subclavian position

18. Which of the following statements about respiratory syncytial virus (RSV) bronchiolitis is *false*?
    a. It is the most common cause of severe respiratory illness in infants.
    b. Children with underlying heart or lung conditions are at increased risk of severe disease.
    c. Patients present with wheezing due to inflammation of small airways.
    d. The disease is preventable by administering inactivated vaccine at 2, 4, and 6 months of age.
    e. Treatment is primarily supportive.

19. A 2-year-old boy had a cold last week and is now seen in the emergency department for a fever and a dry, barking cough. On physical examination he has intercostal retractions and inspiratory stridor. Of the following, which is the most appropriate therapy?
    a. Oral amoxicillin and oral albuterol
    b. Intramuscular ceftriaxone
    c. Intramuscular dexamethasone and nebulized racemic epinephrine
    d. Intravenous theophylline and nebulized albuterol
    e. Oral rimantidine

20. A full-term 1-week-old boy is seen for irritability, fever, and a generalized seizure. He has no skin rash. His mother was previously healthy, and the pregnancy was uncomplicated, although his mother noticed a burning sensation in the perineal area after delivery. Yesterday small red blisters developed in that area. Which of the following is true about this patient?
    a. Herpes simplex virus (HSV) infection in the infant is unlikely because he does not have a vesicular rash.
    b. Because his mother does not have a past history of genital herpes, bacterial meningitis is the most likely cause of this child's symptoms.
    c. Before the results are available for HSV serology on the infant, ampicillin and gentamicin are appropriate therapy.
    d. Prompt administration of acyclovir may be lifesaving for the infant.
    e. The infant should be observed carefully for evidence of a rash, and a Tzanck preparation should be performed if skin lesions develop.

21. A 2-year-old girl is seen for low-grade fever, abdominal cramps, and bloody diarrhea. Her family lives on a farm, where she has contact with pigs, goats, sheep, and cows. In addition, her 10-year-old brother has a pet snake. She attends day care 3 days a week. Which of the following is the most appropriate course of action?
    a. Order a stool culture and, while awaiting the results, treat her empirically with trimethoprim-sulfamethoxazole.

b. Do not order a stool culture, but treat her empirically with erythromycin.
c. Order a stool culture, and wait for the results before deciding whether to treat with antibiotics.
d. Do not order a stool culture, and treat with antibiotics only if the symptoms get worse.
e. Order a stool culture, and treat with antibiotics only if the culture grows *Escherichia coli* O157:H7.

22. A 45-year-old man presents with a 3-week history of progressive dyspnea, increasing fatigue, fever, and malaise. He has a history of intravenous drug abuse and has received a new diagnosis of AIDS, with a viral load of 300,000 copies/mL and a CD4 cell count of 5/μL. He began receiving antiretroviral therapy with zidovudine-lamivudine and indinavir. On examination, he appears ill. His temperature is 39.4°C, blood pressure 100/60 mm Hg, and pulse 120 beats per minute. Oxygen saturation on room air is 90%. Oral thrush is noted, and findings on lung examination are normal. Results for arterial blood gases on room air are the following: P_{O_2} 60 mm Hg, P_{CO_2} 22 mm Hg, and pH 7.58. Complete blood cell count results include the following: white blood cells 5.8 ×10⁹/L, hemoglobin 9.9 g/dL, and platelets 203×10⁹/L. Chest radiography shows bilateral symmetrical infiltrates. What is the most likely etiologic agent of his respiratory illness?
    a. *Streptococcus pneumoniae*
    b. *Histoplasma capsulatum*
    c. *Pneumocystis jiroveci*
    d. *Pneumocystis carinii*
    e. *Mycobacterium tuberculosis*

23. For the patient described in the preceding question, what initial therapy should be instituted?
    a. Levofloxacin 500 mg daily intravenously (IV)
    b. Rifampin-pyrazinamide-ethambutol-isoniazid
    c. Trimethoprim-sulfamethoxazole, with 5 mg/kg of the trimethoprim component every 8 hours
    d. Trimethoprim-sulfamethoxazole, with 5 mg/kg of the trimethoprim component every 8 hours and prednisone 40 mg daily
    e. Amphotericin B 0.7 mg/kg daily IV

24. A 30-year-old African American woman who is positive for human immunodeficiency virus (HIV) presents with waxing and waning headache, irritability, and malaise over the past 4 weeks. She was extensively treated with antiretrovirals in the past, but all previous antiretroviral regimens failed. She has a low-grade fever of 38.3°C with stable blood pressure and heart rate. She has no nuchal rigidity or neurologic deficits on examination. Computed tomographic scan of the head shows no abnormalities except for mild cerebral atrophy. Other results are CD4 cell count 75/μL and HIV type 1 RNA 100,000 copies/mL. What is the next most appropriate diagnostic test?
    a. Stereotactic brain biopsy
    b. Positron emission tomographic scan of the brain
    c. Magnetic resonance imaging of the brain
    d. Lumbar puncture and cerebrospinal fluid (CSF) studies
    e. *Toxoplasma* serology

25. A 36-year-old white homeless man with a known diagnosis of AIDS presents with cough, night sweats, hemoptysis, and weight loss of several months' duration. On examination his temperature is 38.7°C, blood pressure 135/80 mm Hg, heart rate is 72 beats per minute, and respiratory rate is 28 breaths per minute. Results of laboratory evaluations are shown.

Component	Value
Hemoglobin, g/dL	11.6
White blood cell count, ×10⁹/L	7.5
Platelet count, ×10⁹/L	140
Serum creatinine, mg/dL	1.0
CD4 cell count, cell/μL	180
Human immunodeficiency virus (HIV) type 1 RNA, copies/mL	150,000
Tuberculin skin test, mm	8

Chest radiographs show bilateral lower lobe consolidations. You are asked about the likelihood of tuberculosis in this patient. Which of the following statements is correct?
    a. The CD4 cell count is too high for tuberculosis to be likely.
    b. The HIV type 1 RNA value is too low for tuberculosis to be likely.
    c. A tuberculin skin test result of 8 mm is considered negative.
    d. The presence of abnormalities in the lower lung zones and the absence of cavities rules out tuberculosis.
    e. Sputum samples for acid-fast bacilli smear and culture are indicated.

26. A 28-year-old white man with no significant previous medical history presents with a lesion on his penis. He denies discharge or other symptoms. He admits to unprotected sex with a prostitute approximately 3 weeks ago. On examination, he is afebrile with normal vital signs. He has an indurated, clean-based ulcer on the shaft of his penis that is painless. He also has bilateral, enlarged inguinal lymph nodes. The rest of the examination findings are unremarkable. Which of the following statements about this infection is *false*?
    a. In general, the clinical manifestations of this infection are similar to those among persons not infected with human immunodeficiency virus (HIV).

b. In general, the serologic response to this infection seems to be the same in HIV-positive and HIV-negative persons.
c. There are no specific clinical manifestations of this infection that are unique to HIV infection.
d. Closer follow-up of HIV-infected patients with this infection is not indicated.
e. Penicillin-based regimens, whenever possible, are preferred for all stages of this infection in HIV-infected persons.

27. A 24-year-old man with a history of myasthenia gravis is referred to your clinic for pretravel recommendations for travel to the Republic of the Congo in central Africa for a 3-month stay. He is healthy now and has not received any immunosuppressants since his thymectomy 2 years ago. You advise him that a person traveling to the Republic of the Congo needs protection against several vaccine-preventable diseases; however, he is unable to receive 1 of the following vaccines. Which should he *not* receive?
    a. Hepatitis A vaccine
    b. Yellow fever vaccine
    c. Hepatitis B vaccine
    d. Injectable typhoid vaccine
    e. Conjugated meningococcal vaccine

28. An 86-year-old healthy African man immigrated to the United States at the age of 55 years and is now planning a trip to Tanzania for 1 month to visit his friends and family. His last trip back to Tanzania was 15 years ago. At that time, he was found to have immunity to hepatitis A from prior exposure, and he received yellow fever vaccine, injectable typhoid vaccine, and a poliovirus vaccine booster. Now you advise him to receive the typhoid vaccine. What should you tell him about the yellow fever vaccine?
    a. He should not receive the yellow fever vaccine because of his age.
    b. His yellow fever vaccination is still valid, and he does not need to receive additional vaccine.
    c. He should receive yellow fever vaccine, and his risk from the vaccine is minimal.
    d. Yellow fever vaccine is no longer indicated for travel to Tanzania.
    e. Yellow fever vaccine is contraindicated with concurrent typhoid vaccine.

29. A 26-year-old Sudanese female immigrant is planning to travel back to Sudan in 3 weeks and stay for 1 month. She is 11 weeks pregnant. She immigrated 5 years ago and traveled back to Sudan last year. At that time, her hepatitis A IgG serology was positive. She received the following vaccines: hepatitis B series, yellow fever, oral typhoid, meningococcal, inactivated poliovirus, and tetanus, diphtheria, and acellular pertussis. You tell the patient that it is best for her not to travel to Africa at this time; however, she has bought her ticket and is unwavering in her decision to go. Which of the following would you recommend to her for malaria prevention?
    a. Chloroquine
    b. Mefloquine
    c. Malarone (atovaquone-proguanil)
    d. Doxycycline
    e. Insect repellents only

30. A 13-year-old boy is planning a 2-month trip to Thailand, Cambodia, and Vietnam with his immigrant family. He is quite healthy except for a history of severe idiopathic urticaria, for which he is taking an antihistaminic agent on a regular basis. Which of the following vaccines is contraindicated for him for this trip?
    a. Hepatitis A vaccine
    b. Injectable typhoid vaccine
    c. Rabies vaccine
    d. Japanese encephalitis vaccine
    e. Hepatitis B vaccine

31. A 36-year-old healthy woman is planning to travel to Thailand for leisure for 1 week. You counsel her about vaccinations, insect precautions, and food and water precautions. She tells you that a friend took a new prescription medication daily for prevention of diarrhea on his trip, and the patient asks you about this new medication for prevention of traveler's diarrhea. Which of the following statements would be most accurate regarding this medication?
    a. It is effective in preventing diarrhea, but it is not needed for most people or for most trips.
    b. It is highly absorbed and can cause liver damage; therefore, its use is best avoided.
    c. It is extremely effective against preventing severe diarrhea.
    d. It is safe to use during pregnancy.
    e. It is most effective against traveler's diarrhea caused by *Campylobacter* species.

32. A 26-year-old woman, gravida 1 at 12 and 3/7 weeks' gestation, presents to the obstetrics clinic for routine prenatal care. Her new test results show the following: hemoglobin 13.2 g/dL, blood type O Rh-negative, negative for human immunodeficiency virus types 1 and 2 antibodies, negative polymerase chain reaction results for gonorrhea and *Chlamydia*, negative for IgG and IgM syphilis antibodies, and negative for immunity to hepatitis B virus. The urinalysis showed many gram-negative bacilli, few red blood cells, and few white blood cells. The patient denies having vaginal bleeding, dysuria, abdominal pain or cramping, nausea or vomiting, or fevers. What should be the next step in the care of this patient?
    a. Treatment of asymptomatic bacteriuria

b. Administration of Rh$_o$(D) immune globulin (RhoGAM)
   c. Addition of oral ferrous sulfate
   d. Dark-field examination of vaginal secretions
   e. Culture and sensitivity

33. A 23-year-old day care provider presents to the obstetrics clinic with concerns about exposure to cytomegalovirus (CMV). She is at 32 and 4/7 weeks' gestation with an accurate date of conception. Her pregnancy was complicated by 1 episode of bleeding in the first trimester but is otherwise unremarkable. CMV testing shows positive IgG and negative IgM titers in serial evaluation. What additional testing is needed?
   a. No further evaluation
   b. Amniocentesis and CMV polymerase chain reaction (PCR) testing of fluid
   c. Ultrasonography to evaluate for hydrops
   d. Antibody testing again in 2 to 4 weeks
   e. Avidity testing

34. A 17-year-old adolescent girl, gravida 1 at 36 and 5/7 weeks' gestation, has had ongoing evaluation in the high-risk obstetrics clinic for her positive human immunodeficiency virus (HIV) status. She started Combivir therapy at 9 weeks' gestation when the diagnosis of HIV was confirmed by Western blot. Viral loads and CD4 cell counts were followed in all 3 trimesters. Laboratory results at 36 weeks include viral load 1,200 copies/mL, CD4 cell count 600/µL, and positive *Chlamydia* polymerase chain reaction test. According to American Congress of Obstetricians and Gynecologists (ACOG) guidelines, which statement is true about cesarean delivery in HIV patients?
   a. This patient's viral load is an indication for cesarean delivery.
   b. This patient's CD4 cell count is an indication for cesarean delivery.
   c. This patient's *Chlamydia* superinfection is an indication for cesarean delivery.
   d. Cesarean delivery should always be performed for HIV patients.
   e. Cesarean delivery is contraindicated for HIV-infected women.

35. A 28-year-old woman, gravida 4, para 3, at 29 and 4/7 weeks' gestation, was transferred to your tertiary care center with a complicated hospital course characterized by fevers, epigastric pain, anorexia, and headaches for 1 week. She appeared ill and had an increased respiratory rate, decreased breath sounds, and right upper quadrant tenderness. The rest of the physical examination findings were normal. Her past medical history and family history were noncontributory. Laboratory results from the previous hospital are as follows:

Component	Finding
Aspartate aminotransferase, U/L	890
Alanine aminotransferase, U/mL	450
Lactate dehydrogenase, U/L	1,300
24-h urine protein, mg	329
Leukocytes, ×10^9/L	4.2
Platelets, ×10^9/L	130
Albumin, g/dL	2.6
Fibrinogen, mg/dL	450
Urinalysis	
Protein, mg/dL	20
Ketones, mg/dL	75
Virologic testing	
Hepatitis A IgM	Negative
Hepatitis B surface antigen	Negative
Hepatitis B core antibody	Negative
Hepatitis C antibody	Negative
Epstein-Barr virus IgM	Negative
Cytomegalovirus IgM antibody	Negative
Blood cultures	Negative
Urine drug screen	Negative
Imaging	
Chest radiography	Negative
Magnetic resonance cholangiopancreatography	Negative
Right upper quadrant ultrasonography	Negative
Amniocentesis for chorioamnionitis	Negative
Obstetric ultrasonography and fetal testing	
Fetal weight, g	1,142
Amniotic fluid index	18.5
Placenta	Posterior
Presentation	Breech

On the basis of these findings, what is the most likely diagnosis?
   a. Budd-Chiari syndrome
   b. Autoimmune hepatitis
   c. Acute human immunodeficiency virus (HIV) infection
   d. HELLP syndrome or acute fatty liver disease of pregnancy
   e. Viral hepatitis

36. A 45-year-old woman received a diagnosis of acute myelogenous leukemia 4 months ago and has been receiving chemotherapy through a surgically placed Hickman central venous catheter. She is admitted to the hospital with a temperature of 38.5°C and chills. Blood cultures from samples drawn through the catheter and peripherally are growing an organism. Which of the following conditions allows for retaining the central line with appropriate antimicrobial therapy?
   a. Evidence of tunnel infection
   b. Candidal line infection
   c. Coagulase-negative staphylococci bacteremia

d. *Pseudomonas aeruginosa* bacteremia
e. Mycobacterial line infection

37. A 50-year-old man with myelodysplastic syndrome and chronic leukopenia presents with cough of 1 week's duration with intermittent hemoptysis. Computed tomography of the chest shows right lower lobe central consolidation with early cavitation. The bronchial lavage preliminary results identify a few broad, nonseptate hyphae that appear fragmented with short branches at right angles. Which of the following statements is true?
    a. Invasive aspergillosis is the most likely fungal pathogen, and treatment should be started promptly with amphotericin B lipid complex.
    b. An agent of mucormycosis is likely, and treatment should be started with voriconazole.
    c. *Rhizopus* species or *Mucor* species is likely, and treatment should be started with amphotericin B lipid complex.
    d. *Candida albicans* is the most likely pathogen, and intravenous caspofungin therapy should be started.
    e. *Cryptococcus neoformans* is the most likely pathogen, and a spinal fluid examination should be performed promptly.

38. In splenectomized or functionally asplenic patients, which organism does *not* characteristically cause severe disease?
    a. *Capnocytophaga canimorsus*
    b. *Aspergillus fumigatus*
    c. *Streptococcus pneumoniae*
    d. *Haemophilus influenzae* type b
    e. *Neisseria meningitidis*

39. In which setting of an intravascular catheter–associated bloodstream infection should a surgically placed, tunneled catheter be retained with appropriate antimicrobial therapy?
    a. Infection with coagulase-negative staphylococci that involves a line-associated tunnel infection
    b. Infection with *Enterococcus faecalis* that is persistent 4 days after starting antimicrobial therapy that is active according to susceptibility testing
    c. Infection with *Pseudomonas aeruginosa* in a critically ill patient
    d. Infection with *Candida albicans* that clears after starting fluconazole therapy
    e. Infection with *Enterococcus faecalis* with mild exit site erythema and prompt resolution of bacteremia after starting antimicrobial therapy that is active according to susceptibility testing

40. Which of the following statements about the Retroviridae is *false*?
    a. The enzyme reverse transcriptase is unique to this group of viruses.
    b. They infect only humans.
    c. Human T-lymphotropic virus (HTLV)-1 and HTLV-2 belong to this group of viruses.
    d. Infection is usually followed by a latent period.
    e. They are RNA viruses.

41. A 26-year-old white man presents with a 1-week history of sore throat and malaise. On physical examination, he is afebrile; a maculopapular rash is noted on the trunk. There is bilateral cervical adenopathy. The liver edge is palpable. The rest of the examination findings are unremarkable. Laboratory results included the following: hemoglobin, 12 g/dL; white blood cell count, 8.4×10^9/L; platelet count, 180×10^9/L; and serum creatinine, 1.0 mg/dL. No atypical lymphocytes were noted. Liver function test values (aspartate aminotransferase, alanine aminotransferase, bilirubin, and alkaline phosphatase) were all normal. Results of monospot and cytomegalovirus antibody testing were negative. Which of the following statements regarding this condition is *false*?
    a. It occurs within days to weeks after exposure.
    b. The most common presentation is a mononucleosis-like syndrome.
    c. Results of human immunodeficiency virus antibody testing may be negative.
    d. Patients are not usually infectious during this period.
    e. The CD4 cell count may be reduced.

42. A 25-year-old white woman was referred to you to evaluate results of testing for human immunodeficiency virus (HIV). She is 18 weeks pregnant, and testing for HIV infection was performed as part of a routine prenatal evaluation. She had positive HIV antibodies on the screening enzyme-linked immunosorbent assay, but the confirmatory Western blot test results were indeterminate. She is married, is in a monogamous relationship, and denies other HIV risk factors. She had no complications with her previous 3 pregnancies. Which of the following is *not* a cause of false-positive HIV antibody test results?
    a. The presence of cross-reacting antibodies in certain patients, such as multiparous women
    b. Patients who have had multiple transfusions
    c. Participation in HIV vaccine studies
    d. Preseroconversion (window) period
    e. Technical or laboratory error

43. Which of the following descriptions of human immunodeficiency virus (HIV) type 2 is *false*?
    a. Primarily in West Africa
    b. Less efficient transmission
    c. Higher viral load
    d. Lower rate of decrease in CD4 cell count
    e. Slower clinical progression

44. A 35-year-old white man in whom you have diagnosed human immunodeficiency virus (HIV) infection recently came to your office with his HIV-uninfected wife and requested information about the risk of HIV transmission. They were interested in having children. Which of the following statements regarding HIV transmission is *false*?
    a. The proper use of condoms greatly reduces the risk of HIV transmission.
    b. Traumatic intercourse increases the risk of HIV transmission.
    c. Ulcerative genital infections increase the risk of HIV transmission.
    d. Kissing increases the risk of HIV transmission.
    e. Antiretroviral therapy decreases the rate of transmission from an HIV-infected pregnant mother to her fetus.

45. A nurse caring for a human immunodeficiency virus (HIV)-positive patient incurs a needlestick injury. Which statement does *not* provide information pertinent to the proper management of this situation?
    a. The average risk of HIV transmission from a needle stick is 0.3%.
    b. The HIV RNA value (viral load) influences the likelihood of transmission.
    c. Depth of injury influences the likelihood of transmission.
    d. The likelihood of transmission is influenced by whether blood was visible on the needle or device.
    e. If postexposure prophylaxis is initiated, it will need to be given for 12 weeks.

Answers

1. Answer c.
The American Society of Transplantation guidelines recommend the use of antiviral prophylaxis instead of preemptive therapy for the prevention of primary CMV disease in high-risk CMV D+/R− solid organ transplant recipients.

2. Answer b.
CMV R+ patients are at higher risk of CMV disease, especially if they receive tissue from CMV D− donors.

3. Answer d.
Serology results often lag behind and may remain negative for transplant patients who are severely immunosuppressed. All other statements are true.

4. Answer c.
Candida albicans is the most common fungal pathogen.

5. Answer b.
CMV-seropositive donor/R− patients have the highest risk of CMV disease.

6. Answer c.
Bacillus anthracis is often detected with Gram staining of body fluids, including blood, pleural effusion, and cerebrospinal fluid. It can also be recovered in cultures of these fluids with routine laboratory media. The presence of *B anthracis* DNA can be detected with PCR testing. Nasopharyngeal swab cultures may be useful in an epidemiologic investigation of an anthrax outbreak, but they would have no significant role in clinical diagnosis.

7. Answer d.
Bacillus anthracis, the agent of anthrax, typically causes necrotizing mediastinal infection rather than pneumonia and is not transmissible from person to person. *Francisella tularensis* (tularemia) and *C burnetii* (Q fever) are also not transmitted from person to person. *Clostridium botulinum* toxin does not cause pneumonia. *Yersinia pestis*, the agent of plague, can cause primary hemorrhagic pneumonia, however, which is readily transmitted from person to person.

8. Answer e.
Although cases of deliberate microbial contamination of food have been documented, clusters of foodborne enteric disease occur relatively frequently owing to inadvertent contamination at various stages of food production. Thus, although it is possible, the occurrence of an outbreak of diarrheal illness generally does not strongly suggest biological terrorism. All the other scenarios should raise considerable suspicion of a possible bioterrorist attack. Disease due to the deliberate release of microbial agents is thought to be more likely to occur through aerosol rather than foodborne transmission.

9. Answer e.
Tdap and influenza vaccines should be given. Since the patient is older than 50, he is presumed to be immune to varicella, measles, mumps, and rubella. Tdap vaccine is recommended to replace the next scheduled Td vaccine for adults younger than 65 years.

10. Answer b.
Staff and residents in centers for the developmentally disabled should be vaccinated against hepatitis B because of the increased risk of blood and body fluid exposure in these settings. It is not necessary to add doses or restart the series if doses are delayed; the series can be continued. The usual interval between the second and third doses is 5 months.

11. Answer a.
Revaccination after prior vaccination with meningococcal conjugate vaccine is recommended only for persons at highest risk of meningococcal disease. This includes persons with asplenia, complement deficiencies, or prolonged exposure risk such as microbiologists with laboratory exposure to *Neisseria meningitidis* or persons exposed by virtue of travel to or residence in areas where the disease is hyperendemic. Revaccination is not currently recommended for college freshmen who have received the conjugate vaccine. Revaccination is recommended 3 to 5 years after vaccination with meningococcal polysaccharide vaccine for all patients at risk, including college freshmen.

12. Answer a.
Among the choices listed, only a serious egg allergy is a contraindication to the inactivated influenza vaccine. All the other choices are conditions that increase the risk of complications from influenza; therefore, vaccine would be indicated.

13. Answer c.
It is not necessary to restart a multidose vaccine series if the interval between doses is longer than recommended. Previously administered doses count as valid doses, and the series can be continued with administration of the remaining doses. All the other statements are true.

14. Answer a.
The Ventilator Bundle does not include oral care. However, oral care with chlorhexidine or other products has been shown to decrease ventilator-associated pneumonia (VAP) rates, especially among cardiac surgery patients. Elevation of the head of the bed decreases VAP rates by decreasing the risk of aspiration. Daily sedation vacations and assessments of readiness to extubate decrease the duration of intubation and thereby reduce the risk of VAP. Peptic ulcer prophylaxis and DVT prophylaxis decrease the risk of complications that may prolong the need for mechanical ventilation.

15. Answer a.
Catheter-associated UTI is the most common HAI, accounting for 40% of all HAIs.

16. Answer c.
The elective cholecystectomy would have generally been classified as type II surgery (ie, clean-contaminated) since it involved entering a tract—in this case, the biliary tract. However, the accidental colon injury, with spillage of fecal material, would make this a type III surgery.

17. Answer c.
A peripheral intravenous site is associated with the lowest risk of catheter-related bloodstream infection. Large-volume infusions can be accomplished through large-bore peripheral catheters. The risk of infection increases with the number of lumens and increased frequency of use. Generally, subclavian lines are associated with a lower risk than internal jugular lines. Femoral sites carry a high risk of infection and should be avoided if possible. PICC lines generally carry a lower risk of infection than lines inserted directly into a central vein and are good options for long-term use. When used in the ICU, they are associated with higher infection rates than in general care or outpatient settings but are still safer than central lines.

18. Answer d.
RSV is the most common cause of severe respiratory illness in infants. During the first year of life, 1% to 2% of all infants are hospitalized with this condition. Children with congenital heart disease or chronic lung disease of prematurity are at highest risk of severe disease and are the target population for passive prophylaxis during the RSV season. Wheezing is the primary manifestation of infant bronchiolitis. No vaccine is available. However, palivizumab, a humanized monoclonal antibody administered intramuscularly, is given to selected high-risk children monthly during the winter to prevent RSV infection. Treatment is primarily supportive, although ribavirin is sometimes used, particularly for immunocompromised hosts.

19. Answer c.
This boy's presentation is typical for croup, which is usually caused by parainfluenza virus. The primary treatment consists of corticosteroids and nebulized epinephrine, both of which decrease inflammation of the subglottis, the region affected by the infection.

20. Answer d.
This presentation is typical for an infant with either disseminated or central nervous system HSV infection. Approximately 50% of infants with those forms of the disease will not have a rash at presentation. In addition, the mothers of most infants born with HSV infection do not have a history of genital herpes. Primary infection in the mother, rather than reactivation of a previous infection, is much more likely to result in transmission to the infant. HSV serology is an insensitive and poor test for diagnosis of HSV in the neonatal period. Ampicillin and gentamicin therapy is appropriate for neonatal bacterial meningitis or sepsis, but adding acyclovir to the regimen to cover HSV infection may be lifesaving. Tzanck smears are neither sensitive nor specific tests for HSV infection and should never be relied on. HSV polymerase chain reaction (PCR) testing should be performed on cerebrospinal fluid. An HSV PCR test (or direct fluorescence assay or viral culture) should be performed on skin lesions.

21. Answer c.
In children, bloody diarrhea should not be treated empirically with antibiotics unless there is strong epidemiologic evidence for infection with *Shigella* or *Campylobacter* (eg, a close contact had culture results that were positive for 1 of these organisms). Shiga toxin–producing *E coli* infections (especially with *E coli* O157:H7) are relatively more common in children than in adults. Treatment of *E coli* O157:H7 infection with antibiotics is associated with an increased risk of hemolytic uremic syndrome.

22. Answer c.
Pneumocystis jiroveci is the causative agent of pneumocystis pneumonia (PCP). PCP occurs primarily in patients with a new diagnosis of AIDS and in untreated immunocompromised patients. Despite a CD4 cell count of 5/μL, this patient was not receiving PCP primary prophylaxis. The subacute onset distinguishes PCP from bacterial pneumonia. Lung examination findings may be normal in PCP, or diffuse rales may be present. Histoplasmosis can be insidious in immunocompromised patients with exposure in areas where the disease is endemic. Serum *Histoplasma* antigen testing results are usually positive. Tuberculosis in this situation typically shows lower or middle lobe and miliary infiltrates. *Pneumocystis carinii* infects rats.

23. Answer d.
Trimethoprim-sulfamethoxazole is the treatment of choice for PCP, with dosing based on the trimethoprim component. Prednisone is indicated for this patient because the P_{O_2} of 60 mm Hg is low.

24. Answer d.
The patient's symptoms suggest a central nervous system process. In the absence of a focal mass on imaging studies, cryptococcal meningitis becomes prominent in the differential diagnosis and requires CSF analysis for confirmation. Common CSF findings include an elevated opening pressure, mild mononuclear pleocytosis, and elevated protein. The India ink preparation is positive in more than 70% of cases. The serum and CSF cryptococcal antigen tests have a sensitivity of 93% to 99%. CSF fungal cultures are the gold standard. Up to 75% of patients have positive blood cultures for *Cryptococcus neoformans*.

25. Answer e.
There are no CD4 cell count or HIV-1 RNA cutoff values for tuberculosis. When tuberculosis occurs later (CD4 cell

count <350/μL) in the course of HIV infection, it tends to have atypical features, such as extrapulmonary disease, disseminated disease, and an unusual chest radiographic appearance (lower lung zone lesions, intrathoracic adenopathy, diffuse infiltrations, and lower frequency of cavitation). HIV-positive patients who have skin reactions of more than 5 mm to 5 tuberculin units of purified protein derivative and who do not have active tuberculosis are considered to have latent tuberculous infection.

26. Answer d.
While clinical presentation, serologic response, and general management of syphilis are similar for HIV-positive and HIV-negative persons, closer follow-up of HIV-positive patients with syphilis is indicated to detect potential treatment failures or disease progression.

27. Answer b.
Yellow fever vaccine is a live viral vaccine and should not be given to persons with thymic dysfunction resulting from thymus disorders, thymoma, or thymectomy. Yellow fever vaccine is also contraindicated in congenital or acquired immunodeficiency states.

28. Answer c.
The risk of yellow fever vaccine–associated viscerotropic disease is for first-time recipients of the vaccine. The risk from yellow fever vaccine in those who have had the vaccine previously is negligible.

29. Answer b.
She is traveling to Sudan to visit friends and family for a long time. The risk of malaria and the risk of congenital malaria are high. She should not travel without malaria prophylaxis. Insect repellent alone is not adequate. Chloroquine is not appropriate for chloroquine-resistant areas such as Sudan. Malarone should be avoided in pregnant and lactating women because data on fetal and infant toxicity are limited. Doxycycline and primaquine are contraindicated in pregnant women. Mefloquine is the appropriate choice. Although animal studies suggest potential teratogenicity or embryotoxicity with mefloquine, clinical experience has not demonstrated such effects in humans.

30. Answer d.
The JE-VAX Japanese encephalitis vaccine can cause anaphylactic reaction (up to 10 days after the last dose) in persons with a history of allergic predisposition, such as urticaria. Therefore, this is a contraindication for this traveler. His best option is to use insect repellants regularly. The newer Japanese encephalitis vaccine, Ixiaro, is given to persons aged 17 years or older and does not carry the same anaphylactic risk.

31. Answer a.
This question refers to rifaximin, which is a nonabsorbable rifamycin that has been shown to be effective in preventing traveler's diarrhea when compared with placebo. It is effective in prevention and treatment of diarrhea caused by Escherichia coli but less so if diarrhea is caused by invasive organisms, such as Campylobacter, Shigella, and others. When used for primary prophylaxis for TD, it is best used in persons with immunocompromise or in those on a critical trip with a need to decrease any chance of change in itinerary. It is contraindicated for use in pregnancy.

32. Answer a.
Asymptomatic bacteriuria is a common finding in pregnancy and, if untreated, is associated with preterm labor and low infant birth weights. It occurs in 2% to 11% of all pregnancies, with a similar prevalence in nonpregnant women. However, pregnancy is associated with smooth muscle relaxation and ureteral dilatation. This leads to easier transport of bacteria from the bladder to the kidney and is associated with a much higher rate of pyelonephritis in pregnancy (up to 65%). If treated, less than 5% of asymptomatic bacteriuria cases progress to pyelonephritis. Treatment consists of a short course (usually 3 days) of antibiotics followed by another urinalysis 1 week after finishing the antibiotics for test of cure. If recurrent infection occurs or if pyelonephritis develops, suppressive therapy until 2 weeks after delivery can be considered. RhoGAM is not indicated at this time. It should be administered at 28 weeks for prophylaxis and, if abdominal trauma or vaginal bleeding occurs, for prevention of isoimmunization. The current hemoglobin level is within the reference range. The use of a prenatal vitamin is adequate for iron administration at this time. The hemoglobin level can be rechecked at 24 to 28 weeks, and if anemia is present, additional iron can be supplemented. The latest results were negative for IgG and IgM antibodies; the patient does not have syphilis. No further work-up with dark-field evaluation is needed at this time.

33. Answer d.
CMV is the most common cause of perinatal infections. In primary maternal infections, 40% to 50% of fetuses are affected by the virus. The transmission rate is lower when the infection occurs earlier in pregnancy; however, the fetal prognosis is worse if a primary infection occurs in the first trimester. A higher percentage of congenital transmission occurs if the infection occurs in the third trimester, but the sequelae are less severe. Of the infants who have congenital CMV, 90% have no symptoms. Symptoms include hepatosplenomegaly, jaundice, petechiae, and neurologic sequelae (microcephaly, chorioretinitis, mental retardation, hearing disorders, and seizures). Antibody testing is the standard of care. It should be repeated in 2 to 4 weeks with serial testing by the same laboratory so that accurate changes in concentrations can be identified. A positive IgG titer indicates that a prior infection has occurred. If the IgM titer is negative at the first test and remains negative at the second test, no current infection or reactivation is present and no further fetal testing is needed. A positive IgM titer with seroconversion of IgG suggests a primary CMV infection, and

invasive fetal testing of the amniotic fluid is indicated. PCR testing for viral DNA is the best test of the amniotic fluid. Positive results for IgM and IgG are suggestive of a recurrent CMV infection, and noninvasive monitoring of the fetus by ultrasonography is indicated. Classic congenital CMV infection findings on ultrasonography include cerebral ventriculomegaly, microcephaly, intracranial calcifications, hyperechoic bowel, hepatosplenomegaly, ascites, fetal growth restriction, and placental enlargement. However, normal ultrasonographic findings do not exclude a congenital infection, and postpartum evaluation of the infant is still suggested. Congenital CMV infection is not an indication for induction of labor.

34. Answer a.

HIV during pregnancy presents several important management issues. The biggest concern is maternal-fetal transmission. The majority of transmission is thought to occur intrapartum, so programs to prevent transmission have focused on identifying infected women as early as possible. Early identification includes universal opt-out testing, in which patients are told that testing is done on all patients unless they choose to decline. After an infection has been identified, standard treatment with highly active antiretroviral therapy is recommended. The goal is undetectable viral loads, with CD4 cell counts in the normal range. These values should be tested every trimester. If the viral load is greater than 1,000 copies/mL at 34 to 36 weeks of gestation, ACOG guidelines recommend cesarean delivery at 38 weeks to minimize transmission to the infant. The risk of transmission is less than 2% if viral loads are less than 1,000 copies/mL, so it is unlikely that cesarean delivery would offer any additional benefit for reducing transmission. Intravenous zidovudine therapy should be started 3 hours before surgery or delivery, and the infant should receive 6 weeks of postpartum prophylaxis. A concomitant *Chlamydia* infection is not an indication for cesarean delivery. The infection should be treated before delivery to prevent transmission, and a test of cure should be performed before delivery.

35. Answer e.

Although the patient had no history of herpetic lesions, further testing with enzyme immunoassay (EIA) and immunofluorescence assay (IFA) showed positive results for herpes simplex virus (HSV) IgM, suggestive of primary simplex herpes hepatitis. False-positive results for HSV IgM, with EIA and IFA, have been reported for pregnant females. However, on further testing, results were negative for autoimmune hepatitis, hepatotropic viruses, influenza, and HIV. Patients with HSV infection can present with fulminant hepatitis with high serum transaminase levels (thousands of units per liter). Pregnant women are at higher risk in the second and third trimesters. Both HSV type 1 and HSV type 2 can cause hepatitis. Diagnosis is confirmed by liver biopsy, which one tries to avoid in pregnancy. HSV hepatitis is associated with high mortality for both the fetus and the mother.

Treatment with acyclovir, compared with no therapy, has improved survival in a small series of patients. This patient began acyclovir therapy, with both clinical and laboratory improvement. She was discharged at 30 weeks' gestation with valacyclovir oral suppression therapy until delivery. She was induced at term. The baby was treated with acyclovir, but all testing was negative for HSV.

Neonatal herpes symptoms usually appear in the first 6 weeks of life. The estimated rate of neonatal herpes is 1 in 2,000 to 1 in 5,000 deliveries per year. The highest risk of infection is for babies born to mothers who have primary infection at the time of birth, with an infection rate of 30% to 50%. The risk of transmission for women with known genital herpes is less than 1%. Intrauterine infection is responsible for less than 5% of infections: 85% of infections occur during delivery, and less than 15% occur after delivery.

36. Answer c.

Indications for central line removal generally include evidence of tunnel infection and central line infections with fungi (including *Candida* species), *Mycobacteria* species, *Pseudomonas aeruginosa*, and other virulent or drug-resistant organisms. Failure to clear the bloodstream is another indication for line removal. Uncomplicated central line infections with coagulase-negative staphylococci often can be successfully managed with line retention.

37. Answer c.

Under the microscope, the agents of mucormycosis typically appear as broad, nonseptate or pauciseptate hyphae that commonly branch at right angles. The lack of septations makes the agents of mucormycosis fragile and subject to fragmentation with tissue processing. *Aspergillus* species typically have regular septations and branch more commonly at 45°. Although voriconazole is active against most *Aspergillus* species, it is inactive against the agents of mucormycosis. *Candida* species and *Cryptococcus* species are both yeasts and do not morphologically appear like the more filamentous molds.

38. Answer b.

In asplenic patients, *C canimorsus*, *S pneumoniae*, *H influenzae* type b, and *N meningitidis* all can cause severe, life-threatening disease. Disease manifestation and severity with *A fumigatus* is more dependent on the presence of functioning neutrophils.

39. Answer e.

Among the options listed, line removal is recommended in settings of tunnel infection, persistent bacteremia beyond 72 hours after starting active antimicrobial therapy according to in vitro testing, and infections with *P aeruginosa*, *Staphylococcus aureus*, *Candida* species, and mycobacteria. Long-term intravascular catheter–associated bloodstream infections with *Enterococcus* species may be treated with both systemic and intraluminal antimicrobial lock therapy if the patient has no complications or if bacteremia is persisting in a clinically stable patient.

40. Answer b.
The Retroviridae family is a large group of ubiquitous viruses that infect all classes of vertebrates.

41. Answer d.
Viral loads are typically very high (usually >100,000 copies/mL). Therefore, acute human immunodeficiency virus infection represents a period of high infectivity.

42. Answer d.
The preseroconversion period is a cause of false-negative HIV antibody test results.

43. Answer c.
Patients with HIV-2 tend to have lower viral loads than patients with HIV-1.

44. Answer d.
HIV is not transmitted by kissing.

45. Answer e.
Four weeks is the recommended duration for postexposure prophylaxis.

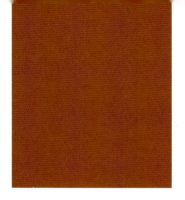

Index

Abacavir, 400, 401t, 410, 413
Abacavir hypersensitivity, 400–402
Abdominal disease, 143–44
Abelcet. *See* Amphotericin B lipid complex
Abscess
 brain, 336–38, 337t
 Candida infection and, 148f
 epidural, 338–39
 hepatic, 290, 290f
 intra-abdominal, 289
 liver, 290, 290f, 291b
 pancreatic infection and, 291
 pelvic, 483
 periapical, 245
 perinephric and intrarenal, 272
 skin, 342
Acalculous cholecystitis, 289
Acanthamoeba, 195f, 325
Acetaminophen, 23
Acid-fast bacilli (AFB), 42, 42f
Acinetobacter, 100, 264
Acinetobacter calcoaceticus-baumannii
 complex, 91
ACIP. *See* Advisory Committee on
 Immunization Practices
Actinomyces, 142–46
Activated protein C (APC), 278
Acute histoplasmosis, 159
Acute meningitis
 diagnosis of, 320–21, 321t
 epidemiology of, 319
 etiology of, 319–20, 320t, 325, 326b
 pathogens and, 321–25
 prevention and chemoprophylaxis for,
  326–27
 special situations regarding, 325–26
 treatment of, 321, 322t, 323t
Acute otitis media, 486
Acute Physiology and Chronic Health
 Evaluation (APACHE), 151, 278
Acute postpartum endometritis, 481–82,
 481b, 482b
Acute pyelonephritis, 271, 465–66, 466t
Acute rheumatic fever, 83–84
Acute uncomplicated cystitis, 270
Acyclovir, 21, 29t, 63t, 65, 69, 73, 334, 453
Adefovir dipivoxil, 297, 454
Adenovirus, 73–75
Advisory Committee on Immunization
 Practices (ACIP), 32, 517
Aeromonas species, 100
AFB. *See* Acid-fast bacilli
Albendazole
 for helminths, 206, 207, 209, 210, 213, 214
 for intestinal protozoa, 191, 193
Albumin, 7
Altitude sickness, 498
Amantadine, 22
AmBisome. *See* Amphotericin B liposomal
 complex
Amebic keratitis, 195
American trypanosomiasis (Chagas disease),
 200–201, 201f
Amikacin, 17, 18, 24, 27t, 132t, 137,
 141–42, 425
Aminoglycosides, 12, 25t, 137, 263, 468, 530

Aminopenicillins, 26t
Amoxicillin, 14, 145, 253, 303
Amoxicillin-clavulanate potassium
 (Augmentin), 14, 91, 141
ampC-mediated resistance, 29t
Amphotericin B, 12, 151, 167, 172, 176, 179,
 181, 184, 185, 204, 421
Amphotericin B deoxycholate, 23, 27t, 176
Amphotericin B lipid complex (Abelcet), 23
Amphotericin B liposomal complex
 (AmBisome), 23, 156, 203
Ampicillin, 14, 15, 91, 468, 487
Ampicillin sodium-sulbactam sodium
 (Unasyn), 14, 142, 309t, 310t, 311t,
 312t, 313t, 314t
Ancef. *See* Cefazolin sodium
Angiostrongylus cantonensis (rat lungworm),
 208–209, 325
Anidulafungin, 24
Animal bite prevention, 497
Anisakis species (herring worm), 208
Anthrax. *See* Bacillus anthracis
Antibacterials, 25–27t. *See also* specific drugs
 aminoglycosides, 17–18
 carbapenems, 17
 cephalosporins, 15–16
 clindamycin, 20
 daptomycin, 21
 fluoroquinolones, 18–19
 linezolid, 21
 macrolides and ketolides, 20
 metronidazole, 20–21
 monobactam, 16–17

Antibacterials (*continued*)
  penicillins, 14–15
  quinupristin-dalfopristin, 21
  tetracyclines and glycylcycline, 19
  trimethoprim-sulfamethoxazole, 20
  vancomycin, 18
Anti-CMV agents, 22, 28*t*
Antifungal agents, 23–24, 27–28*t*
Anti–hepatitis virus agents, 22
Anti–herpes simplex virus agents, 21
Anti-herpesvirus agents, 29*t*
Anti–influenza virus agents, 22, 28*t*
Antimicrobials, 25–29*t*
  activity patterns and, 12–13, 12*b*
  antibacterials, 14–21, 25–27*t*
  antifungal agents, 23–24, 27–28*t*
  antimycobacterial agents, 24
  antiviral agents, 21–22
  bacterial resistance issues and, 29–30*t*
  bioavailability, 4*b*
  for diarrhea, 283*t*
  for face, head, and neck infections, 254–55*t*
  for infectious arthritis due to bacteria, 356
  for liver abscesses, 291*b*
  for osteomyelitis, 354*t*
  in pregnancy, 465*t*
  for prosthetic joint infection, 358
  resistance to, 39–40
  stewardship, 40
  for transplant infections, 451*t*
Antimycobacterial agents, 24
Antiretroviral therapy (ART), 407
  agents for, 22
  benefits of, 409–10
  guidelines for, 409–10
  HIV-drug resistance testing for, 410–11, 411*b*
  pregnancy and, 414–15
  recommendations for, 409
  regimens for, 410
Antitubercular agents, 27*t*
Antiviral agents, 21–22
APACHE. *See* Acute Physiology and Chronic Health Evaluation
APC. *See* Activated protein C
Aphthous stomatitis, 251
APIC. *See* Association for Professionals in Infection Control and Epidemiology
Appendicitis, 291–92, 293*f*
Aqueous crystalline penicillin G sodium, 304*t*, 305*t*, 306*t*, 309*t*, 310*t*
Arboviruses, 324, 334
ART. *See* Antiretroviral therapy
Arthritis. *See* Gonococcal arthritis; Infectious arthritis, due to bacteria; Septic arthritis, in children
Arthropods, 190
Ascaris lumbricoides, 206
Aseptic meningitis, 76, 319
Aspergillosis, 50, 154, 155*t*, 156
Aspergillus flavus, 50
Aspergillus fumigatus, 50, 261
Aspergillus niger, 50
Aspergillus species, 153–56, 154*f*, 337–38, 455
Aspergillus terreus, 50, 156
Aspirin, 497

Association for Professionals in Infection Control and Epidemiology (APIC), 32
Asymptomatic bacteriuria, 271, 464–65, 466*t*
Atazanavir, 5, 401, 405*t*
Atovaquone, 123, 199, 419
Atypical pneumonia, 257–58, 258*t*
Augmentin. *See* Amoxicillin-clavulanate potassium
Azathioprine, 24
Azithromycin, 5, 20, 123, 137, 199, 366, 367, 424
Azole antifungals, 24
Aztreonam, 16, 25*t*

Babesia microti, 199, 200*f*
Babesiosis, 120–22, 122*f*
Bacillus anthracis (anthrax), 89, 527, 528–29*t*, 530–31, 535
Bacillus cereus, 89, 437
Bacillus species, 88
Bacillus subtilis, 89
Bacterial meningitis. *See* Acute meningitis
Bacterial vaginosis, 370, 371*f*, 372*b*, 466, 466*t*
Balamuthia mandrillaris, 195–96
Balantidium coli, 194–95, 194*f*
Bartonella bacilliformis, 99–100
Bartonella henselae, 99–100
Bartonella quintana, 99–100
Baylisascaris procyonis (raccoon roundworm), 210
Beef tapeworm. *See Taenia saginata*
Benznidazole, 201
BIG-IV. *See* Human Botulism Immune Globulin Intravenous
Biliary tract infection, 289–90
Bilirubin, 7
Biological agents, 525–27
Bioterrorism, 525, 526, 527*b*, 535
Bismuth subsalicylate (BSS), 514, 515
Bivalent vaccine (HPV2), 520
Black piedra, 46
Blastocystis hominis, 193
Blastomyces dermatitidis, 164
Blastomycosis, 48, 48*f*, 164–67, 166*f*, 167*t*
Bloodstream infections, 437–38
Bordetella parapertussis, 98
Bordetella pertussis, 98
Borrelia, 110–12, 111*f*
Borrelia burgdorferi, 324
Botulinum toxin (botulism), 528–29*t*, 533–34, 535
Botulism. *See also* Botulinum toxin; *Clostridium botulinum*
  diagnosis of, 106, 106*b*, 107*t*, 108, 108*t*
  epidemiology of, 106
  management of, 107*t*, 108–9
  prevention of, 109
  prognosis and outcome of, 109
  vaccine for, 109
  wound, 106*f*
Brain abscess, 336–38, 337*t*, 338*t*
Bronchiolitis, 486–87
Brucella abortus, 100
Brucella melitensis, 100
Brucella species, 96–97
Brucella suis, 100

BSS. *See* Bismuth subsalicylate
Bubonic plague, 94, 532
Buccal space infection, 247
Burkholderia, 95
Burkholderia mallei, 96
Burkholderia pseudomallei, 95–96, 100
Burkitt lymphoma, 72

Calculous cholecystitis, 289
California encephalitis virus group, 324, 334
Candida infection, 148, 148*f*, 425–26
  diagnosis of, 151
  by organ involvement, 148*t*
  of stomach, 151*f*
  syndromes, 149–50*t*
  treatment of, 151–52
Candida species, 147–48, 147*f*, 337, 455
Candida vaginitis, 149*t*, 370, 371*f*
Candidemia, 149*t*, 151
Canine space infection, 247
CAP. *See* Community-acquired pneumonia
Capillaria philippinensis, 207
Capnocytophaga canimorsus, 99, 100
Capreomycin, 24, 27*t*, 132*t*
Carbapenem, 17, 25*t*, 95, 141, 253, 263, 278, 340
Carboxypenicillins, 26*t*, 278
Carbunculosis, 342
Cardiotoxicity, 428–29
Carotid artery erosion, 250
Caspofungin, 7, 24, 151, 156, 182
Cat ascarids. *See Toxocara catis*
Catheter-associated urinary tract infection (CAUTI), 271, 458, 459, 459*b*
CAUTI. *See* Catheter-associated urinary tract infection
CDC. *See* Centers for Disease Control and Prevention
Ceclor. *See* Cefaclor
Cedax. *See* Ceftibuten
Cefaclor (Ceclor), 15
Cefadroxil (Duricef), 15
Cefamandole, 16
Cefazolin sodium (Ancef), 15, 286, 307*t*
Cefdinir (Omnicef), 15, 16
Cefditoren pivoxil (Spectracef), 15
Cefepime (Maxipime), 15, 16, 289, 314*t*
Cefixime (Suprax), 15, 16
Cefmetazole, 16
Cefoperazone, 16
Cefotan. *See* Cefotetan
Cefotaxime (Claforan), 15, 16, 112, 142
Cefotetan (Cefotan), 15, 16
Cefoxitin (Mefoxin), 15, 16, 24, 137
Cefpodoxime proxetil (Vantin), 4, 5, 15, 16
Cefprozil (Cefzil), 15
Ceftazidime (Fortaz), 15, 16
Ceftibuten (Cedax), 15, 16
Ceftizoxime, 146
Ceftobiprole, 15, 16
Ceftriaxone (Rocephin), 15, 16, 25*t*, 91, 112, 119, 141, 142, 146, 306*t*, 366
Ceftriaxone sodium, 304*t*, 305*t*, 312*t*, 313*t*
Cefuroxime (Zinacef), 15, 16
Cefuroxime axetil, 4, 5
Cefzil. *See* Cefprozil

Cellulitis, 342
  gangrenous, 349
  mucormycotic necrotizing angioinvasive, 349–50
  necrotizing, 343
  syndromes, 344–47t
  syndromes mimicking, 343t
Centers for Disease Control and Prevention (CDC), 31, 266, 295, 357, 527
Central nervous system (CNS)
  candidiasis, 150t
  diseases of
    Actinomyces and, 144–45
    cryptococcal, 178
    Nocardia and, 139–40
    presentation of, 145
    zygomycosis, 183
  infections of
    acute meningitis, 319–27
    chronic meningitis, 327–32
    CSF shunt, 340
    encephalitis, 332–35
    myelitis, 335
    postinfectious encephalitis, 335–36
    suppurative infection of, 336–40
  sepsis syndrome and, 276
  tuberculoma of, 128
Cephalexin (Keflex), 15, 341
Cephalosporins, 12, 15–16, 25t, 91, 95, 119, 253, 263, 278, 286, 483
Cerebrospinal fluid (CSF), 321t, 340
Cervarix, 505
Cervical adenitis, 252
Cestodes, 211–14
Chagas disease. *See* American trypanosomiasis
Chancroid, 366, 367f
Chemokine receptor CCR5 antagonist, 398, 407–8
Chemotherapy, 429–31, 429b, 430t
Chickenpox. *See* Varicella
Childhood immunizations, 485–86
Child-Pugh score, 7
Chlamydia trachomatis infection, 369, 369b
Chloramphenicol, 6, 112, 124, 530
Chloroquine, 199, 513
Cholangitis, ascending, 289
Cholecystitis, 289
Cholera vaccine, 509
Chromoblastomycosis, 47
Chronic bacterial parotitis, 251–52
Chronic meningitis
  diagnosis of, 328, 328t, 329b, 331b
  differential diagnosis for, 329, 331–32
  etiology of, 327, 327b
  evaluation of immunocompetent patient, 330f
  evaluation of immunocompromised patient, 330f
  treatment of, 328–29
Chronic mucocutaneous candidiasis, 149t
Chronic pelvic pain syndrome, 272
Chronic pulmonary histoplasmosis, 159
Cidofovir (HPMPC), 22, 28t, 75, 532
Cierny-Mader classification, for osteomyelitis, 351, 352b

Ciprofloxacin, 18, 19, 146, 286, 313t, 314t, 327, 366, 367
  for infection from bioterrorism agents, 530, 531, 532, 533
Cisplatin, 429
Claforan. *See* Cefotaxime
Clarithromycin, 7, 20, 137, 424
Clindamycin, 6, 12, 20, 25t, 123, 145, 199, 250, 253, 348, 420
  for infection from bioterrorism agents, 530, 531
Clindamycin-primaquine, 419
Clinical and Laboratory Standards Institute (CLSI), 10
Clofazimine, 24
Clonorchis sinensis, 216, 216f
Clostridium botulinum, 104–6
Clostridium difficile, 439, 463, 488
Clostridium tetani, 102, 104t
Clotrimazole, 426
CLSI. *See* Clinical and Laboratory Standards Institute
CMV. *See* Cytomegalovirus
CNS. *See* Central nervous system
Coagulase-negative *Staphylococcus* species, 81
Coccidioidal meningitis, 331
Coccidioides species, 168, 169f
Coccidioidomycosis, 48–49, 49f, 168–70, 170f
Cockcroft-Gault equation, 6
Codworm. *See Pseudoterranova decipiens*
Colistin, 264
Colorado tick fever, 335
Combivir, 479
Community-acquired pneumonia (CAP), 256–60, 257t, 258t, 259t
Computed tomography (CT)
  of appendicitis, 293f
  of diverticulitis, 293f
  of hepatic abscess, 290f
  of hydatid cyst, 290f
  of necrotic lesion, 291f
  of nocardiosis, 139f
Congenital rubella syndrome, 477b
Consensus Panel Report, 32
Contiguous-focus osteomyelitis, 351
Corticosteroids, 24, 209
Corynebacterium diphtheriae, 86
Corynebacterium jeikeium, 86, 437
Coxsackievirus, 78–79
Croup (laryngotracheobronchitis), 486
Cryptococcal CNS disease, 178
Cryptococcal meningitis, 329
Cryptococcal pneumonia, 178
Cryptococcosis
  clinical features and treatment of, 180t
  diagnosis of, 178, 178f, 179f, 421
  epidemiology of, 177, 421
  pathogenesis of, 177–78
  treatment of, 179–80, 421–22
Cryptococcus neoformans, 177–81, 178f, 455
Cryptosporidiosis, 425
Cryptosporidium, 191–92, 191f
CSF. *See* Cerebrospinal fluid
CT. *See* Computed tomography
Cutaneous anthrax, 530
Cutaneous infections, 440–41

Cutaneous leishmaniasis, 204
Cutaneous sporotrichosis, 176
Cutaneous zygomycosis, 183
Cyclophosphamide, 429
Cycloserine, 24, 27t, 133
Cyclospora cayetanensis, 192
Cyclosporine, 24
Cysticercosis, 212–13, 212f, 332
Cystitis. *See* Acute uncomplicated cystitis; Recurrent uncomplicated cystitis
Cytomegalovirus (CMV), 469t
  diagnosis of, 422, 451–52, 472, 473f
  direct and indirect effects of, 450
  epidemiology of, 422, 472
  fetus and newborn and, 490
  outcomes of, 472
  in pregnancy, 472, 473f
  prevention of, 452
  risk factors for, 450–51
  treatment of, 422, 452, 472

Dalfopristin-quinupristin, 25t
Dapsone, 24, 141, 456
Daptomycin, 5, 12, 21, 25t, 278
Darunavir, 405t
DEC. *See* Diethylcarbamazine citrate
Deep vein thrombosis (DVT), 496–97
DEET repellent, 496
Delavirdine, 402t, 408, 413
Dematiaceous fungal infection, 187, 188t
Dematiaceous molds, 51
Dentoalveolar disease, 246
Dermatophytes, 46–47
Dexamethasone, 321, 431
DHQP. *See* Division of Healthcare Quality Promotion
Diarrhea. *See* Infectious diarrhea
Diazepam, 24
Dicloxacillin, 14, 483
Didanosine, 400, 401, 401t, 413
Dientamoeba fragilis, 193
Diethylcarbamazine citrate (DEC), 210
Digoxin, 24
Diphenhydramine, 23
Diphyllobothrium latum (fish tapeworm), 211, 212f
Disseminated disease, 145
Disseminated histoplasmosis, 159
Disseminated sporotrichosis, 176
Diverticulitis, 292, 293f
Division of Healthcare Quality Promotion (DHQP), 31
Dog ascarids. *See Toxocara canis*
Donovanosis. *See* Granuloma inguinale
Doripenem, 17
Doxycycline, 19, 25, 115, 137, 145, 211, 294, 314t
  for treatment and prevention of malaria, 198, 199, 512, 513
  for treatment of bioterrorism agent infections, 530, 531, 532, 533
  for treatment of sexually transmitted diseases, 364–65b, 366, 367, 369b, 370b
  for treatment of tick-borne diseases, 119, 120, 124, 125
Dracunculus medinensis (guinea worm), 209

Duncan syndrome. *See* X-linked lymphoproliferative disease
Duricef. *See* Cefadroxil
DVT. *See* Deep vein thrombosis

Eastern equine encephalomyelitis virus, 324, 334
EBV. *See* Epstein-Barr virus
Echinocandins, 12, 24, 29t, 151, 152, 156
Echinococcosis, 213–14
Ecthyma gangrenosum, 349
Efavirenz, 8, 402t, 404, 404t, 408, 410, 414
Efavirenz-associated neuropsychiatric adverse events, 403–4
Eflornithine, 202
EHEC. *See* Enterohemorrhagic *E coli*
Ehrlichiosis, 120, 121f
   HGA, 119, 120
   HME, 119, 120
Eikenella corrodens, 100
Elimination
   of aminoglycosides, 17–18
   of anti-CMV agents, 22
   of anti–herpes simplex virus agents, 22
   of anti–influenza virus agents, 22
   of carbapenem, 17
   of cephalosporins, 16
   of clindamycin, 20
   of daptomycin, 21
   of echinocandins, 24
   of fluoroquinolones, 19
   half-life of, 9–10
   of infectious agents, 277–78
   of linezolid, 21
   of macrolides and ketolides, 20
   metabolism and, 6–9
   of metronidazole, 21
   of monobactam, 17
   of penicillins, 15
   of polyenes, 24
   of quinupristin-dalfopristin, 21
   renal, 6
   of tetracyclines and glycylcycline, 19
   of triazoles, 23
   of trimethoprim-sulfamethoxazole, 20
   of vancomycin, 18
ELISA. *See* Enzyme-linked immunosorbent assay
Employee and occupational health, 37–39
Emtricitabine, 400, 401t, 413, 414
Encephalitis
   Balamuthia mandrillaris and, 195
   diagnosis of, 333–34
   epidemiology and etiology of, 332–33
   noninfectious causes of, 333b
   nonviral infectious causes of, 332b
   pathogens for, 334–35
   postinfectious, 335–36, 336b
   postvaccinal, 336b
   signs and symptoms suggesting, 333t
   tick-borne, 509
   treatment of, 334
   viral causes of, 332b
Endobronchial tuberculosis, 127
Endometritis. *See* Acute postpartum endometritis

Endophthalmitis, 150t
Enfuvirtide, 406, 408
Entamoeba dispar, 194
Entamoeba histolytica, 193–94, 193f
Entecavir, 298
Enterobacteriaceae, 91–101
Enterobius vermicularis (pinworm), 207, 207f
Enterococci, 82t, 85
Enterohemorrhagic *E coli* (EHEC), 92
Enterovirus, 324
Enzyme-linked immunosorbent assay (ELISA), 118
Epidermophyton, 47
Epididymitis, 370, 370b
Epididymo-orchitis, 76
Epidural abscess, 338–39
Epstein-Barr virus (EBV), 70–73, 71f, 453
Ertapenem, 17
Erysipelas, 342
Erysipelothrix rhusiopathiae, 89
Erythema migrans, in Lyme disease, 118, 118f
Erythromycin, 7, 12, 20, 112, 146, 294, 366, 367
ESBL. *See* Extended-spectrum β-lactamase-producing gram-negative bacilli
Escherichia coli, 100, 488
Ethambutol, 24, 27t, 129, 132t, 423, 425
Ethionamide, 24, 132t
Etravirine, 402t, 404t, 408
Eumycotic mycetoma, 47–48
Extended-spectrum β-lactamase-producing (ESBL) gram-negative bacilli, 29t, 92
Extraintestinal nematodes, 208–10
   Angiostrongylus cantonensis, 208–209
   Baylisascaris procyonis, 210
   Dracunculus medinensis, 209
   Gnathostoma spinigerum, 209
   Toxocara canis and *Toxocara catis*, 209–10
   Trichinella spiralis, 209
Extraintestinal protozoa
   Babesia microti, 199, 200f
   free-living amebae, 195–96, 195f
   hemoflagellates, 199–204
   Plasmodium, 196, 197–98
   Toxoplasma gondii, 204–6
   Trichomonas vaginalis, 204
Extrapulmonary tuberculosis, 127–28, 131
Eyeworm. *See Loa loa*

Face, head, and neck infections, 246–49, 252–53
   anatomical relations, 247f
   antimicrobial regimens for, 254–55t
   general management of, 253, 255
   potential pathways of, 248f
   specimen acquisition and diagnosis of, 253
Facial tetany, 103f
Famciclovir, 4, 21, 29t, 63, 65, 69, 453
Fansidar. *See* Sulfadoxine-pyrimethamine
Fasciola hepatica, 216
Fasciolopsis buski. *See* Intestinal flukes
Fetus and newborn
   CMV and, 490
   congenital infections of, 490, 490t
   febrile evaluation for, 493–94
   GBS prevention for, 494

   HIV and, 491–92
   HSV-1 and HSV-2 in, 490–91
   human parvovirus 19 and, 491
   rubella and, 492
   syphilis and, 492
   toxoplasmosis and, 491
Fever of unknown origin (FUO), 237–43
   causes of, 237–38, 238b
   diagnosis of, 238–41
   drugs associated with, 241b
   early testing for, 237b
   historical clues for, 238b, 239t
   imaging and invasive testing for, 242–43t
   laboratory evaluation for, 239–40, 241t
   physical examination for, 239, 240t
   recurrent causes of, 240b
Fibrosing mediastinitis, 160
Fifth disease, 489
Filarial nematodes, 210–11
Fish tapeworm. *See Diphyllobothrium latum*
Flaccid paralysis, 335
Fluconazole, 23, 151, 170, 173, 179, 181, 182, 189, 196, 293, 371, 421, 426
Flucytosine, 28t, 152, 179, 196, 421
Fluoroquinolones, 12, 18–19, 24, 25t, 131, 137, 253, 286, 450, 515
Folliculitis, 341
Fortaz. *See* Ceftazidime
Fosamprenavir, 4, 405t, 410
Foscarnet, 22, 28t, 69
Francisella tularensis (tularemia), 97, 101, 532–33
   clinical features of, 528–29t
   clinical syndromes suggesting, 535
Free-living amebae, 195–96, 195f
Fungal infections
   dematiaceous, 187
   diagnostic tools for, 46
   Fusarium infection, 184–86, 185f
   Malassezia infection, 187
   opportunistic, 50–52, 51f
   Paecilomyces infection, 189
   Pseudallescheria boydii infection, 186–87, 186f
   risk factors for, 455
   Saccharomyces cerevisiae infection, 189
   subcutaneous, 47–48
   superficial and cutaneous mycoses and, 46–47
   systemic, 48–50, 48f, 49f, 50f
   transplant recipient infections and, 455–56
   Trichosporon infection, 189
   zygomycosis, 182–84, 183f, 184f
Fungal sinus infections, 439
FUO. *See* Fever of unknown origin
Furazolidone, 191
Furunculosis, 342
Fusarium infection, 184–86, 185f
Fusidic acid, 341
Fusion inhibitor, 398, 406–8

Ganciclovir, 22, 28t, 75, 334, 452
Gangrenous cellulitis, 349
Gardasil, 505
Gastrointestinal anthrax, 530
Gastrointestinal tract infections
   in children, 487–88

Clostridium difficile colitis, 439
  typhlitis, 439
Gastrointestinal zygomycosis, 183
Gatifloxacin, 132t
GBS. *See* Group B streptococci
Gemifloxacin, 18, 19
Generalized tetanus, 103
Genital ulcer disease, 360
Gentamicin, 17, 18, 308t, 532
Gentamicin sulfate, 305t, 306t, 307t, 309t, 311t, 314t
German measles. *See* Rubella
Giardia lamblia, 190–91, 191f
Glycopeptides, 278
Glycylcycline, 19
Gnathostoma spinigerum, 209
Gonococcal arthritis, 356–57
Gonorrhea, 368, 368f, 369f
Gram-negative aerobic bacteria, 90–100, 324
  epidemiologic associations and disease, 100–101
Gram-negative bacilli
  ampC-mediated resistance in, 29t
  Enterobacteriaceae, 91–101
  extended-spectrum β-lactamase-producing, 29t
  Vibrio, 91
Gram-negative cocci
  Acinetobacter calcoaceticus-baumannii, 91
  Moraxella catarrhalis, 91
  Neisseria meningitidis, 90–91, 90f
Gram-positive aerobic bacteria, 80–89
  Corynebacterium species, 86–89
  enterococci, 85
  staphylococci, 80–81
  streptococci, 81, 83–85
Gram-positive bacilli
  Bacillus species, 88–89
  Corynebacterium species, 86
  Listeria monocytogenes, 86–88
Granuloma inguinale (donovanosis), 366, 367, 368f
Granulomatous amebic encephalitis, 195
Group B streptococci (GBS)
  antibiotic prophylaxis indications for, 474b, 474t
  conditions associated with, 472
  fetus and newborn prevention of, 494
  prevention of, 473
  specimen collection of, 474b
Guinea worm. *See Dracunculus medinensis*

HAART. *See* Highly active antiretroviral therapy
HACE. *See* High-altitude cerebral edema
Haemophilus influenzae, 96, 323, 326–27
HAIs. *See* Health care–associated infections
Haloperidol, 24
Hand hygiene, 33–34
HAPE. *See* High-altitude pulmonary edema
HAV. *See* Hepatitis A virus
HBV. *See* Hepatitis B virus
HCAP. *See* Health care-associated pneumonia
HCV. *See* Hepatitis C virus
HDV. *See* Hepatitis D virus
Head infections. *See* Face, head, and neck infections

Health care–associated infections (HAIs), 31
  antimicrobial resistance and, 39–40
  antimicrobial stewardship and, 40
  of bloodstream, 461–62
  CAUTIs as, 458–59
  employee and occupational health and, 37–39
  environmental sources of, 36–37
  investigation of, 33
  medical waste management and, 37
  organizations influencing, 31–32
  patient care items and, 35–36
  SSIs as, 459–61
  standard precautions for, 34–35
  surveillance of, 32–33
  transmission-based precautions for, 35, 35t
  transmission modes of, 33–34, 33t
  VAP as, 260, 261, 462
  viral infections and outbreaks as, 464
Health care–associated pneumonia (HCAP), 260
Healthcare Infection Control Practices Advisory Committee (HICPAC), 31, 37, 266
Helminths, 190
  acute meningitis and, 325
  cestodes, 211–14
  nematodes, 206–11
  trematodes, 214–17
Hematogenous osteomyelitis, 352
Hematologic malignancy and infections
  approach to, 428
  chemotherapy for, 428–31, 430t
  syndromes and, 435–41
Hemoflagellates, 199–200
  American trypanosomiasis and, 200–201, 201f
  Human African trypanosomiasis and, 201–2
  leishmaniasis and, 202–3
Hemophagocytic lymphohistiocytosis, 72
Hepatic abscess, 290, 290f
Hepatic metabolism, 6–9, 8b
Hepatitis A virus (HAV), 295–96, 469t
  vaccine for, 296, 506, 519
Hepatitis B virus (HBV), 296–98, 297f, 454, 469t
  vaccine for, 506–507, 519–20
Hepatitis C virus (HCV), 298, 298f, 299, 470t
  treatment of, 454
Hepatitis D virus (HDV), 299, 470t
Hepatitis E virus (HEV), 299, 470t
Hepatitis G virus (HGV), 300
Hepatobiliary infections, 439–40
Hepatosplenic candidiasis, 150t, 293, 294f
Hepatotoxicity, 429
Herpes simplex virus type 1 (HSV-1), 62f, 334, 452, 470t
  acyclovir for, 63t
  characteristics of, 61–62
  diagnosis of, 62–63, 63f
  in fetus and newborn, 490–91
  in pregnancy, 473–75
Herpes simplex virus type 2 (HSV-2), 325, 366f, 452, 470t
  diagnosis of, 363
  epidemiology of, 363

  in fetus and newborn, 490–91
  in pregnancy, 473–75
  treatment of, 366, 367t
Herring worm. *See Anisakis* species
HEV. *See* Hepatitis E virus
HGA. *See* Human granulocytic anaplasmosis
HGV. *See* Hepatitis G virus
HICPAC. *See* Healthcare Infection Control Practices Advisory Committee
High-altitude cerebral edema (HACE), 498
High-altitude pulmonary edema (HAPE), 498
Highly active antiretroviral therapy (HAART), 409, 422, 424
Histoplasma capsulatum, 157
Histoplasma meningitis, 331–32
Histoplasmosis, 49–50, 49f, 50f
  acute, 158–59
  chronic pulmonary, 159
  diagnosis of, 160, 161t, 162, 162f
  disseminated, 159
  distribution map of, 158f
  epidemiology of, 157–58
  fibrosing mediastinitis and, 160
  ocular, 160
  risk factors for, 158
  treatment of, 159–60t, 159b
HIV. *See* Human immunodeficiency virus
HIV drug-resistance testing, 410–11, 411b
HME. *See* Human monocytic ehrlichiosis
Hodgkin disease, 73
Hookworms, 207
HPMPC. *See* Cidofovir
HPV. *See* Human papillomavirus
HPV2. *See* Bivalent vaccine
HPV4. *See* Quadrivalent vaccine
HSV-1. *See* Herpes simplex virus type 1
HSV-2. *See* Herpes simplex virus type 2
Human African trypanosomiasis (sleeping sickness), 201–2
Human Botulism Immune Globulin Intravenous (BIG-IV), 108
Human granulocytic anaplasmosis (HGA), 119, 120
Human herpesviruses 6 and 7, 453–54
Human immunodeficiency virus (HIV), 325
  acquiring risk for, 414t
  acute infection of, 396
  associated malignancies with, 426–27
  chronic infection of, 397
  classification of, 391–92
  diagnostic testing for, 397–98, 399f
  epidemiology of, 478
  evaluation algorithm for, 415f
  exposure to, 411–12
  in fetus and newborns, 491–92
  genetic organization of, 392f
  genome and gene product functions of, 393, 393f
  immune deficiency due to, 396
  immunopathogenesis of, 396
  life cycle of, 393–95, 394f, 395f
  mother-to-child transmission, 478b
    prevention of, 479b
  natural history of, 396, 397f
  origin of, 392
  postexposure management for, 412–13

Human immunodeficiency virus
    (HIV) (continued)
  postexposure prophylaxis and, 411–14,
      412t, 413t
  in pregnancy, 477–78
  structure of, 392
  TB in, 128
  testing recommendations for, 478b, 480b
  transmission of, 395–96
  treatment of, 398–416, 478–81
    antiretroviral drugs and, 398–408, 400b
    ART guidelines for, 409–10
    ART regimens for, 410
    postexposure prophylaxis, 411–14
    pregnancy and, 414–15
    TB, 129–31, 130t
Human monocytic ehrlichiosis (HME), 119, 120
Human papillomavirus (HPV), 371–72,
    373f, 374b
  vaccine for, 505–506, 520
Human parvovirus B19, 454, 471t
  diagnosis of, 77–78, 475, 476f
  epidemiology of, 475
  in fetus and newborn, 491
  infection of, 475
  pathology of, 77
  prevention of, 78
  rash of, 77f
Hyaline molds, 50–51
Hyaluronidase, 83
Hydatid cyst, 290f
Hydroxyurea, 400
Hyperlactatemia, 399–400

IDSA. See Infectious Diseases Society of
    America
IE. See Infective endocarditis
Imidazoles, 24, 173
Imipenem, 17, 24, 137, 141, 146, 530
Imipenem-cilastatin, 312t
Imiquimod, 372
Immune reconstitution inflammatory
    syndrome, 131
Immunologic deficiencies, 432t
Immunomodulating virus, 446
Impetigo, 341
Indinavir, 405t
Infected embryologic cysts, 252
Infectious arthritis due to bacteria, 355–37
Infectious diarrhea, acute
  antimicrobial therapy for, 283–84, 283t
  diagnosis of, 280–81, 281b
  etiology of, 280, 281t
  foods associated with, 282t
  pathogenesis of, 282t
  special situations for, 282–83
Infectious Diseases Society of America
    (IDSA), 32
Infective endocarditis (IE)
  cardiac conditions associated with, 318b
  case definitions of, 302
  in clinical practice, 301
  dental procedure and, 317t, 318b
  echocardiography, 302b
  epidemiology, 301, 316–17t
  etiology of, 302

  pathogenesis of, 301–2
  prophylaxis for, 303
  surgical intervention suggested for, 303b
  therapy for, 301, 303, 309t
    for culture-negative, 314–15t
    enterococcal, 310t, 311t, 312t
    by HACEK microorganisms, 313t
    of prosthetic valves, 306t
    by staphylococci, 307t, 308t
    by viridans streptococci, 304–5t
Influenza vaccine, 260, 504
  characteristics of, 520, 521t
  contraindications for, 521
  indications for, 520–21
Inhalational anthrax, 530
Insect bite prevention, 496
Integrase inhibitor, 398, 408
International travel
  altitude sickness and, 498
  animal bite prevention and, 497
  DVT and, 496–97
  general advice for, 496–98
  insect bite precautions for, 496
  jet lag and, 497–98
  motion sickness and, 497
  pretravel preventive strategies for, 495–96
  recommended vaccines for, 501–2t, 506–9
  required vaccines for, 503t, 509–11
  routine vaccines for, 498, 499–500t, 504–6
  sexual exposure during, 498
  vaccine-preventable diseases and, 498,
      504–9
Intestinal flukes (Fasciolopsis buski), 216–17
Intestinal nematodes, 206–8
  Ascaris lumbricoides, 206
  Capillaria philippinensis, 207
  clinical disease, 206
  diagnosis of, 206
  distribution of, 206
  herring worm and codworm, 208
  hookworms, 207
  pinworm, 207
  Strongyloides stercoralis, 207–8
  treatment for, 206
  Trichuris trichiura, 206–7, 206f
Intestinal protozoa
  Balantidium coli, 194–95, 194f
  Blastocystis hominis, 193
  Cryptosporidium, 191–92
  Cyclospora cayetanensis, 192
  Dientamoeba fragilis, 193
  Entamoeba histolytica, 193–94, 193f
  Giardia lamblia, 190–91, 191f
  Isospora belli, 192
  Microsporida, 192–93
Intestinal tapeworms, 211–12
Intra-abdominal abscesses, 289
Intra-abdominal infections, 285–94
  appendicitis, 291–92, 293f
  biliary tract infections, 289–90
  community-acquired treatment of, 288t
  diverticulitis, 292
  health care–acquired treatment of, 288t
  hepatic abscess, 290, 290f
  hepatosplenic candidiasis, 293, 294f
  intra-abdominal abscess, 289

  pancreatic infection, 291, 292f
  peliosis hepatis, 293–94, 294f
  peritoneal dialysis, infection related to, 286
  primary peritonitis, 285–86
  secondary peritonitis, 286–89
  tertiary peritonitis, 289
  typhlitis, 293
Intra-amniotic infection, 467–68, 468t
Intrauterine device (IUD), 144
Intravascular catheter infections, 441–42
Iodoquinol, 193, 194, 195
Isoniazid, 24, 27t, 129, 130, 132t, 423
Isospora belli, 192
Itraconazole, 23, 28t, 156, 167, 170, 173, 176,
    179, 181, 182, 185, 189
Itraconazole capsule, 4, 6
IUD. See Intrauterine device
Ivermectin, 206, 207, 208, 209, 210
Ixiaro, 508

Japanese encephalitis virus, 335, 507–8
Jet lag, 497–98
The Joint Commission (TJC), 21

Kanamycin, 27t, 132t
Kaposi sarcoma, 426–27
Keflex. See Cephalexin
Ketoconazole, 5, 173
Ketolides, 12, 20
Ketolides (telithromycin), 20
Klebsiella pneumoniae carbapenemase
    (KPC), 29t
KPC. See Klebsiella pneumoniae carbapenemase

Lady Windermere syndrome, 135
Lamivudine, 297, 400, 401t, 410, 413, 454
Larval infections, 212–14
Laryngotracheobronchitis. See Croup
LAT. See Latency-associated transcript
Latency-associated transcript (LAT), 61
Latent TB infection (LTBI)
  screening for, 424
  treatment of, 424
    in HIV-negative patients, 129–30
    in HIV-positive patients, 130
Lateral pharyngeal space infections, 248–49
Legionella infections, 98–99
Legionella micdadei, 98
Legionella pneumophila, 98
Leishmaniasis, 202–204, 203f
Lemierre syndrome, 250
Leptospira, 112–15, 113f
Leuconostoc species, 437
Levofloxacin, 18, 19, 132t
Linear pharmacokinetics, 7
Linezolid, 12, 21, 24, 26t, 141, 263, 312t
Lipid amphotericin B product, 28t
Lipopolysaccharide (LPS), 274–75
Listeria monocytogenes, 86, 88, 322–23
Listeriosis, 470t
Liver abscess, 290, 290f, 291b
Liver flukes, 216
Loa loa (eyeworm), 211
Lopinavir-ritonavir, 405t, 410, 413, 414
Lorabid. See Loracarbef
Loracarbef (Lorabid), 15

Lower lung field tuberculosis, 127
LPS. See Lipopolysaccharide
LTBI. See Latent TB infection
Ludwig angina, 249–50
Lumpy jaw, 143f
Lung fluke. See Paragonimus westermani
Lyme disease, 117–19
   erythema migrans in, 118, 118f
Lymphatic filariasis, 210–11, 210f
Lymphocutaneous disease, 140
Lymphocutaneous sporotrichosis, 176
Lymphocytic choriomeningitis virus, 325
Lymphogranuloma venereum, 366, 367f
Lymphoma
   Burkitt, 72
   nasal or nasal-type angiocentric, 73
   non-Hodgkin, 427
   primary CNS, 427
   T-cell, 73
Lymphomatoid granulomatosis, 72
Lymphoproliferative disorders
   Burkitt lymphoma, 72
   Duncan syndrome, 72
   hemophagocytic lymphohistiocytosis, 72
   Hodgkin disease, 73
   lymphomatoid granulomatosis, 72
   nasal or nasal-type angiocentric lymphoma, 73
   nasopharyngeal carcinoma, 72–73
   T-cell lymphoma, 73

Macrolide, 20, 26t, 91
Madura foot. See Mycetoma
Malaria
   diagnosis of, 198
   falciparum, 199
   geographic distribution of, 196
   life cycle of, 196, 197f
   patient education on, 513
   from *Plasmodium falciparum*, 196, 197f, 198
   from *Plasmodium vivax*, 198–99
   prevention of, 198–99, 511–12
   species causing, 196
   transmission of, 196
   treatment of, 199, 512t
Malarone, 198, 199, 513
Malassezia infection, 187
Mandibular molar infections, 248
Maraviroc, 408
Masticator space infection, 246
Mastitis, 483–84
MAT. See Microscopic agglutination test
Maxillofacial trauma, 253
Maxipime. See Cefepime
MDROs. See Multidrug resistant organisms
Measles, mumps, and rubella (MMR) vaccine, 504, 521
Mebendazole, 206
Medical waste management, 37
Mefloquine, 198, 199, 512, 513
Mefoxin. See Cefoxitin
Melarsoprol, 202
Meleney synergistic gangrene, 343
Menactra, 521
Meningitis, 140. See also Acute meningitis; Chronic meningitis
   aseptic, 76, 319
   benign recurrent aseptic, 325–26
   coccidioidal, 331
   cryptococcal, 329
   Histoplasma, 331–32
   neoplastic, 331
   recurrent community-acquired, 325
   recurrent nosocomial, 325
   sarcoid, 331
   tuberculous, 127–28, 329
   vaccine for, 509–10, 521–22
Meningococcal polysaccharide vaccine (MPSV4), 522
Menveo, 521
Men who have sex with men, STDs and, 372–74
Meperidine, 23
Meropenem, 17, 141–42
Metformin, 400
Methadone, 25
Methicillin-resistant *Staphylococcus aureus* (MRSA), 29t, 81, 263
Methotrexate, 429
Metronidazole, 12, 20–21, 26t, 109, 250, 289, 290
   for parasitic infections, 191, 193, 194, 195, 204
MIC. See Minimum inhibitory concentration
Micafungin, 24
Miconazole, 426
Microorganisms, disinfection and sterilization resistance of, 36f
Microscopic agglutination test (MAT), 115
Microsporida, 192–93, 192f
Microsporum, 47
Miliary tuberculosis, 127
Miltefosine, 204
Minimum inhibitory concentration (MIC), 10–11
Minocycline, 19, 141, 142, 145
MMR. See Measles, mumps, and rubella vaccine
Monobactam, 16–17
Moraxella catarrhalis, 91
Motion sickness, 497
Moxalactam, 16
Moxifloxacin, 18, 19, 132t
MPSV4. See Meningococcal polysaccharide vaccine
MRSA. See Methicillin-resistant *Staphylococcus aureus*
MTBC. See *Mycobacterium tuberculosis* complex
Mucocutaneous leishmaniasis, 204
Mucorales, 338
Mucormycotic necrotizing angioinvasive cellulitis, 349–50
Multidrug resistant organisms (MDROs), 263, 463
   nosocomial pneumonia caused by, 263, 263b
   treatment strategy for, 264f
Mumps virus, 75–77, 325
Mupirocin, 341
Musculoskeletal disease, 145
Mycetoma (Madura foot), 140
Mycobacteria, 126–37
   classification of, 41
   clinical manifestations of, 126–27
   epidemiology of, 126
   etiology of, 126
   extrapulmonary TB and, 127
   nontuberculous, 133–37
   TB diagnosis and, 127
   tests for LTBI and, 128–29
Mycobacterium avium complex, 135
Mycobacterium avium-intracellulare complex, 424–25
Mycobacterium kansasii, 135
Mycobacterium marinum, 136
Mycobacterium tuberculosis complex (MTBC), 41–43
Myelitis, 335
Myelosuppression, 428
Myopericarditis, 79

Naegleria fowleri, 196, 325
Nafcillin, 14, 307t, 308t
Nasal or nasal-type angiocentric lymphoma, 73
Nasopharyngeal carcinoma, 72–73
National Healthcare Safety Network (NHSN), 32
National Institute for Occupational Safety and Health (NIOSH), 39
Neck infections. See Face, head, and neck infections
Necrotizing cellulitis, 343
Necrotizing fasciitis, 343, 348
Neisseria meningitidis, 90–91, 90f, 322, 327
Nelfinavir, 406t
Nematodes
   extraintestinal, 208–10
   filarial, 210–11
   intestinal, 206–8
Neonatal tetanus, 103, 104f
Neoplastic meningitis, 331
Neuroborreliosis, 331–32
Neutropenia, 431
   infections during, 435
   management of, 435–36, 436b
   therapy response evaluation and, 437b
Neutrophil dysfunction, 431
Nevirapine, 8, 402t, 404t, 408, 410, 413
Nevirapine-associated rash, 403
Nevirapine-related hepatotoxicity, 402–3
Newborn. See Fetus and newborn
NHSN. See National Healthcare Safety Network
Nifurtimox, 201
NIOSH. See National Institute for Occupational Safety and Health
Nitazoxanide, 191, 192, 425
NNRTI. See Nonnucleoside reverse transcriptase inhibitor
Nocardia, 138–42, 337
   CT scan, 139f
   Gram stain of, 139f
Nocardia asteroides, 138
Nocardia brasiliensis, 138
Nocardia farcinica, 138
Nocardia nova, 138
Nocardia otitidiscaviarum, 138
Nocardia transvalensis, 138

Non-Hodgkin lymphoma, 427
Nonlinear pharmacokinetics, 7
Nonnucleoside reverse transcriptase inhibitor (NNRTI), 398, 402–4, 402t, 404t, 480
Nonodontogenic orofacial infections, 251–52
Nontuberculous mycobacteria (NTM), 133–37
   diagnosis of, 44–46, 134
   diseases caused by, 134t
   epidemiology of, 133–34
   Mycobacterium avium complex and, 135
   Mycobacterium kansasii and, 135
   Mycobacterium marinum and, 136
   noncultivatable, 45
   rapidly growing, 135–36
   Runyon classification and, 44–45
   susceptibility testing of, 46
   treatment of, 136–37, 136–37t
Norfloxacin, 286
Nosocomial pneumonia
   biologic markers and, 262
   diagnosis of, 261–62
   due to *Aspergillus fumigatus*, 261
   due to *Staphylococcus aureus*, 261
   due to viruses, 261
   epidemiology of, 260
   etiology of, 260
   intubation and mechanical ventilation for, 266
   MDROs causing, 263, 263b
   pathogens in, 261t
   prevention of, 266
   treatment of, 262–64, 263b, 264f, 265f
NRTI. See Nucleoside/nucleotide analogue reverse transcriptase inhibitor
NTM. See Nontuberculous mycobacteria
Nucleoside/nucleotide analogue reverse transcriptase inhibitor (NRTI), 398–402, 401t
Nystatin, 426

Occupational health. See Employee and occupational health
Occupational Safety and Health Administration (OSHA), 31
Odontogenic infections
   face, head, and neck infections from, 246–49
   primary sources of, 244–45
   prophylaxis of, 255
   spreading routes of, 245f
   syndromes and, 249–50
Omnicef. See Cefdinir
Onchocerca volvulus, 211
Ophthalmologic disease, 140
Opioids, 25
Opportunistic infections
   candidiasis, 425–26
   CMV and, 422
   cryptococcosis, 421–22
   cryptosporidiosis, 425
   fungal, 50–52, 51f
   HIV-associated malignancies and, 426–27
   immune status and, 417–18
   LTBI as, 424
   Mycobacterium avium-intracellulare complex and, 424–25
   occurrence of, 417
   pneumocystis pneumonia, 418–19, 419t
   progressive multifocal leukoencephalopathy, 426
   TB, 422–24
   toxoplasma encephalitis, 419–21
Opsonophagocytosis resistance, 83, 84f
Oral contraceptives, 24
Oral hairy leukoplakia, 72
Oral hypoglycemic agents, 24
Oral mucosal infections, 251
Orocervicofacial disease, 143
Oseltamivir, 22, 28t
OSHA. See Occupational Safety and Health Administration
Osteoarticular sporotrichosis, 175, 176
Osteomyelitis, 250
   in children, 489
   Cierny-Mader classification for, 351, 352b
   classification schemes of, 351
   as consequence of open fracture, 352
   contiguous-focus, 351
   diagnosis of, 352–53
   hematogenous, 352
   hyperbaric oxygen therapy for, 355
   microbiology of, 351, 352b
   pathogenesis of, 351
   therapy for, 353–55, 354t
   vertebral, 352
Ovarian vein thrombosis, 482–83, 483b
Oxacillin, 14, 307t, 308t
Oxazolidinones, 278

PAE. See Postantibiotic effect
Paecilomyces infection, 189
p-Aminosalicylic acid (PAS), 24, 27t, 132t
Pancreatic infection, 291, 292f
Panton-Valentine leukocidin, 80
Paracoccidioides brasiliensis, 171, 172f
Paracoccidioidomycosis, 50, 171–73
Paragonimus westermani (lung fluke), 215–16, 216f
Parasitic infections
   extraintestinal protozoa and, 195–206
   helminths and, 206–17
   intestinal protozoa and, 190–95
   transplant recipient infections and, 456–57
Paromomycin, 191, 193, 194, 195
Parotid space infection, 247–48
Parotitis, 76, 251–52
PAS. See p-Aminosalicylic acid
Pasteurella multocida, 101
Pasteurella species, 97–98
Pediatric diseases. See also Fetus and newborn
   acute otitis media, 486
   bronchiolitis, 486–87
   croup, 486
   gastrointestinal tract infections and, 487–88
   osteomyelitis, 489
   rash illnesses and, 488–89
   septic arthritis, 489
   STDs and, 487
   UTI, 487
Peliosis hepatis, 293–94, 294f
Pelvic abscess, 483

Pelvic inflammatory disease (PID), 369–70, 370b
   IUD role in, 144
Penicillin, 91, 112, 115, 145, 251, 253, 530, 531
Penicillin G, 14, 109, 250, 492
Penicillin G benzathine, 14
Penicillin G procaine, 14
Penicillins, 12, 14–15, 26t
Penicillin V, 14
Penicilliosis, 50, 50f
Pentamidine, 196, 202, 419, 456
Periapical abscess, 245
Perinephric and intrarenal abscesses, 272
Periodontal disease, 245–46
Peripherally inserted central catheter (PICC), 462
Peripheral neuropathy, 429
Peritoneal dialysis, infection related to, 286–87
Peritonitis
   antibiotic dosing for, 287b, 287t
   primary, 285–86, 286b
   secondary, 286–89
   tertiary, 289
Phaeohyphomycosis, 48, 188f
Pharmacodynamics, 3
   antimicrobial activity patterns and, 12–13, 12b
   concepts of, 10–13
   efficacy predictors of, 11f
   MIC and, 10–11
   PAE and, 11
   pharmacokinetic interrelationship with, 4f
   time course factors and, 11–12
Pharmacokinetics, 3
   absorption and, 3
   clearance and, 6
   concepts of, 3–10
   distribution and, 5–6
   dosing and, 3
   efficacy predictors of, 11f
   elimination half-life and, 9–10
   linear and nonlinear, 7
   metabolism and elimination and, 6–9
   oral route and, 3–5
   pharmacodynamic interrelationship with, 4f
   serum level interpretation and, 10
Phenytoin, 7, 24
PHN. See Postherpetic neuralgia
PI. See Protease inhibitors
PICC. See Peripherally inserted central catheter
PID. See Pelvic inflammatory disease
Pinworm. See *Enterobius vermicularis*
Piperacillin, 14, 15
Piperacillin sodium-tazobactam sodium (Zosyn), 14
Piperacillin-tazobactam, 15, 289
Plague. See *Yersinia pestis*
Plaque, 244–45
Plasmodium falciparum, 196, 197–98, 197f
Plasmodium vivax, 198–99
Pleurodynia, 79
Pneumococcal vaccine, 260, 504–505, 522
Pneumocystis, 52
Pneumocystis jiroveci, 456
Pneumocystis pneumonia, 418–19, 419t

Pneumonia
    atypical, 257–58, 258t
    CAP, 256–60
    cryptococcal, 178
    nosocomial, 260–66, 261t
    viral, 257
Pneumonic plague, 94, 528–29t, 532
Podofilox, 372
Polyenes, 24
Polyomavirus, 454
Pontiac fever, 99
Pork tapeworm. See Taenia solium
Posaconazole, 6, 23, 156, 181, 184, 189
Postantibiotic effect (PAE), 11
Postherpetic neuralgia (PHN), 67
Postinfectious encephalitis, 335–36, 336b
Postpartum wound infection, 483
Postsplenectomy sepsis (PSS), 431
Postvaccinal encephalitis, 336b
Praziquantel, 212, 215, 216, 217
Prednisone, 202
Pregnancy
    antimicrobials in, 465t
    ART and, 414–15
    bacterial vaginosis in, 466, 466t
    CMV in, 472, 473f
    drug use in, 465t
    GBS in, 472–73, 474b, 474t
    German measles in, 475, 476b
    HIV in, 477–78
    HSV-1 in, 473–75
    HSV-2 in, 473–75
    human parvovirus B19 in, 475, 476f
    infection in, 464, 472–81
        etiology, diagnosis, and management of, 469–71t
    syphilis in, 475–77
    toxoplasmosis in, 476, 476b
    vaccines in, 516b
    VZV in, 476
Premature membrane rupture. See Preterm labor
Preterm labor, 466–67, 467f
Pretracheal space infections, 249
Primaquine, 199, 512
Primary CNS lymphoma, 427
Primary peritonitis. See Peritonitis
Progressive multifocal leukoencephalopathy, 426
Propranolol, 24
Prostatitis, 271–72
Prosthetic joint infection, 357
    therapy for, 358–59, 358t
Protease inhibitor (PI), 24, 398, 404–6, 480
    characteristics of, 405–6t
    drugs cautiously used with, 407t
    drugs not used with, 407b
Protozoa. See Extraintestinal protozoa; Intestinal protozoa
Pseudallescheria boydii infection, 186–87, 186f
Pseudomonas, 264
Pseudomonas aeruginosa, 95
Pseudoterranova decipiens (codworm), 208, 208f
PSS. See Postsplenectomy sepsis
Puerperal infection and fever
    acute postpartum endometritis and, 481–82
    mastitis, 483–84
    pelvic abscess, 483
    postpartum wound infections, 483
    septic pelvic thrombophlebitis and ovarian vein thrombosis, 482–83
Pulmonary toxicity, 429
Pulmonary zygomycosis, 183
Pulpitis, 245
Pyrazinamide, 24, 27t, 129, 132t, 423
Pyridoxine, 129
Pyrimethamine, 206, 420

Quadrivalent vaccine (HPV4), 520
QuantiFERON-TB Gold test, 44, 129
Quinacrine, 191
Quinidine, 24, 199
Quinine, 123, 199
Quinolones, 12, 91, 95, 99, 263, 355, 358, 401
Quinupristin-dalfopristin (Synercid), 21, 312t

Rabies vaccine, 508–9
Raccoon roundworm. See Baylisascaris procyonis
Raltegravir, 408
Ramsay Hunt syndrome, 68
Rapid HIV testing, 398
Rat lungworm. See Angiostrongylus cantonensis
Recurrent uncomplicated cystitis, 270–71
Renal elimination, 6
Respiratory tract infections, 438–39
Retropharyngeal space infections, 249
Rhinocerebral zygomycosis, 182–83, 183f
Ribavirin, 400, 402, 454, 534
Ricin toxin, 534–35
Rifabutin, 7, 8, 132t, 423, 425
Rifampin, 6, 8, 24, 120, 129, 132t, 294, 308t, 314t, 327, 408, 423
    anthrax treatment, 528t, 530–31
    prosthetic joint infection treatment, 358–59, 358t
Rifamycins, 24, 27t, 130, 131, 423
Rifapentine, 130, 132t
Rifaximin, 514–15
Rimantadine, 22
Ritonavir, 406t, 410
Rituximab, 428, 453
Rocephin. See Ceftriaxone
Rocky Mountain spotted fever, 123–24, 123f, 335
Roseola infantum, 489
Rubella (German measles), 471t, 475, 489, 492
Rubeola, 471t
Runyon classification, of NTM, 44–45

Saccharomyces cerevisiae infection, 189
Salivary gland infections
    chronic bacterial parotitis, 251–52
    suppurative parotitis, 251
    tuberculous parotitis, 252
    viral parotitis, 252
Salmonella infections, 92–93, 93f, 488
Salmonella paratyphi, 92
Salmonella typhi, 92, 101
SAPHO syndrome. See Synovitis, acne, pustulosis, hyperostosis, and osteitis
Saquinavir, 406t, 410
Sarcoid meningitis, 331
Scarlet fever, 488
Scedosporium apiospermum, 338
Schistosoma, 214–15, 214f
Schistosomiasis, 214
Secondary peritonitis. See Peritonitis
Sepsis, 274
Sepsis syndrome
    cellular injury from, 275
    complications of, 276–77
    diagnosis of, 275–76
    epidemiology of, 274
    incidence of, 274
    pathogenesis of, 274–75
    prognosis and prevention and control of, 279
    treatment of, 277–79
Septic arthritis, in children, 489
Septic cavernous sinus thrombosis, 250
Septicemic plague, 94
Septic pelvic thrombophlebitis, 482–83
Serum level interpretation, 10
Sexually transmitted diseases (STDs), 360–74
    chancroid, 366, 367f
    in children, 487
    Chlamydia trachomatis infection, 369, 369b
    donovanosis, 366–67, 368f
    epididymitis, 370, 370b
    estimations regarding, 360
    genital ulcer diseases, 360
    gonorrhea, 368–69, 368f, 369f
    HPV and, 371–72
    HSV genital infection, 363, 366
    lymphogranuloma venereum, 366, 367f
    men who have sex with men and, 372–74
    PID, 369–70, 370b
    syphilis, 360–63, 361f, 362f, 363f, 364–65f, 364f
    urethritis, 367
    vaginal discharge syndromes, 370–71, 371t
SHEA. See Society of Healthcare Epidemiology of America
Shigella boydii, 94
Shigella dysenteriae, 94
Shigella flexneri, 94
Shigella sonnei, 94
Shingles vaccine, 505
SIRS. See Systemic inflammatory response syndrome
Skin abscess, 342
Skin and soft tissue infections
    animal and human bites and, 349
    cellulitis, 342
    erysipelas, 342
    folliculitis, 341
    furunculosis and carbunculosis, 342
    immunocompromised hosts and, 349–50
    impetigo, 341
    necrotizing, 342–43, 348
    situation influencing, 348–50
    skin abscess, 342
    water exposure influencing, 348–49
Sleeping sickness. See Human African trypanosomiasis
Smallpox. See Variola virus

Society of Healthcare Epidemiology of America (SHEA), 32
Soft tissue infection. *See* Skin and soft tissue infections
Spectracef. *See* Cefditoren pivoxil
Spinal tuberculosis arachnoiditis, 128
Spirillum minus, 98
Spirochetes, 324
Splenic rupture, 71
Sporothrix schenckii, 174–76
Sporotrichosis, 47, 47f
   cutaneous, 176
   diagnosis of, 175, 175f
   disseminated, 176
   epidemiology of, 174
   immunity for, 175
   lymphocutaneous, 176
   osteoarticular, 175, 176
   pulmonary, 176
   treatment of, 176
SSIs. *See* Surgical site infections
St Louis encephalitis virus, 324, 334
Staphylococci
   common species of, 80t
   features of, 80
   IE caused by, 307t, 308t
Staphylococcus aureus, 80, 257, 261, 437
Staphylococcus epidermidis, 437
Staphylococcus lugdunensis, 81
Staphylococcus species, 81, 324
Stavudine, 400, 401t, 413
STDs. *See* Sexually transmitted diseases
Stem cell transplant infection, 433f, 448f, 449–50
   in late-risk period, 434–35
   in postengraftment period, 434
   in preengraftment period, 433–34
   timing of, 433–34
Stenotrophomonas maltophilia, 95
Stibogluconate, 204
Streptobacillus moniliformis, 98
Streptococci, 81, 82t, 85
Streptococcus agalactiae, 84, 323
Streptococcus pneumoniae, 85, 256–57, 327
Streptococcus pyogenes, 81, 83f
Streptogramin, 278
Streptokinase, 83
Streptomycin, 17, 18, 27t, 132t, 425, 532
Streptomycin sulfate, 310t
Strongyloides stercoralis, 207–8, 208f, 456–57
Subcutaneous fungal infections
   chromoblastomycosis, 47
   eumycotic mycetoma, 47–48
   phaeohyphomycosis, 48
   sporotrichosis, 47, 47f
Subdural empyema, 339
Sublingual space infections, 248
Sulfadiazine, 196, 206
Sulfadoxine-pyrimethamine (Fansidar), 199
Sulfonamides, 137
Superantigen, 80, 81f
Suppurative intracranial venous sinus thrombosis, 339–40
Suppurative parotitis, 251
Suppurative thyroiditis, 252

Suprax. *See* Cefixime
Suramin, 202
Surgical site infections (SSIs), 459–61
   classification of, 460, 460f
   clinical importance of, 459
   microbiology of, 460
   risk stratification of, 460
   surgical prophylactic antibiotics and, 461
   treatment of, 460
   wound classification and, 459–60, 459b
Synercid. *See* Quinupristin-dalfopristin
Synergistic necrotizing cellulitis, 343
Synovitis, acne, pustulosis, hyperostosis, and osteitis (SAPHO syndrome), 353
Syphilis, 471t, 492
   chancres of, 361f
   clinical importance of, 475–76
   clinical manifestations of, 360–61
   condyloma lata in, 363f
   diagnosis of, 361–62
   epidemiology of, 360
   mucous patches of, 363f
   in pregnancy, 475–77
   rash of, 362f
   test interpretation of, 364f
   treatment of, 477
   treatment guidelines for, 364–65b
Systemic fungal infections
   blastomycosis, 48, 48f
   coccidioidomycosis, 48–49, 49f
   histoplasmosis, 49–50, 49f, 50f
   paracoccidioidomycosis, 50
   penicilliosis, 50, 50f
Systemic inflammatory response syndrome (SIRS), 274

Taenia saginata (beef tapeworm), 211
Taenia solium (pork tapeworm), 211
TB. *See* Tuberculosis
T-cell lymphoma, 73
Tdap. *See* Tetanus, diphtheria, and acellular pertussis vaccine
Telbivudine, 298
Telithromycin. *See* Ketolides
Tenofovir, 298, 398–99, 400, 401t
Teratogen Information System (TERIS) rating system, 464
TERIS. *See* Teratogen Information System rating system
Tertiary peritonitis, 289
Tetanus. *See also Clostridium tetani*
   clinical manifestations of, 103, 103b
   diagnosis of, 104, 104t
   epidemiology of, 102–103
   generalized, 103
   localized, 103
   management of, 104, 105t
   neonatal, 103, 104f
   prevention of, 104
   prognosis and outcome of, 104
   vaccine for, 104, 504, 523
Tetanus, diphtheria, and acellular pertussis vaccine (Tdap), 504, 523
Tetracycline, 19, 26t, 112, 145, 193, 195, 401, 531

Thalidomide, 429
Theophylline, 24
Thiabendazole, 207
Thoracic disease, 144
Thyroiditis, suppurative, 252
Ticarcillin, 14, 15, 253
Ticarcillin-clavulanate, 95
Ticarcillin disodium-clavulanate potassium (Timentin), 14
Ticks, 116–17
Tick-borne encephalitis virus vaccine, 509
Tick-borne infections, 116–25
   babesiosis, 120–23, 122f
   coinfections and, 125
   ehrlichiosis, 119–20, 121f
   Lyme disease, 117–19
   prevention of, 124–25
   Rocky Mountain spotted fever, 123–24, 123f
Tigecycline, 13, 19, 24, 27t
Timentin. *See* Ticarcillin disodium-clavulanate potassium
Tinea nigra, 47
Tinea versicolor, 47
Tinidazole, 191, 194, 204
Tipranavir, 406t, 408
TJC. *See* The Joint Commission
TMP-SMX. *See* Trimethoprim-sulfamethoxazole
Tobramycin, 17, 18, 24
Tolbutamide, 24
Toxocara canis (dog ascarid), 209–10
Toxocara catis (cat ascarid), 209–10
Toxoplasma encephalitis, 419–21
Toxoplasma gondii, 204–205, 205f, 338, 456
Toxoplasmosis, 205–206, 471t, 477
   in fetus and newborn, 491
   risk of, 477b
Transplant recipient infections
   allogeneic hematopoietic stem cell and, 456
   antimicrobials for, 451t
   bacterial, 450
   community-acquired, 446
   early diagnosis of, 444
   epidemiologic exposures and, 444–45, 444b
   fungal, 455–56
   from health care environment, 445–46
   heart and, 455
   immunomodulating viruses and, 446
   importance of, 443
   kidney and pancreas and, 455–56
   liver and, 455
   lung and, 455
   parasitic, 456–57
   pharmacologic immunosuppression and, 443
   prevention of, 457
   risk determinants for, 443
   screening tools before transplant and, 445b
   after solid organ transplant, 445b
   timing of, 446–50
      after allogeneic hematopoietic stem cell transplant, 448f, 449–50
      after solid organ transplant, 446–49, 447f
      temporal patterns, 446
   treatment of, 444
   vaccines and, 457

viral, 450–54
Transverse myelitis, 335
Traveler's diarrhea, 513–15
Trematodes
  intestinal fluke, 216–17
  life cycles of, 214
  liver fluke, 216
  lung fluke, 215–16
  Schistosoma, 214–15, 214f
Treponema pallidum, 324
Triazoles, 23, 28t
Trichinella spiralis, 209
Trichomonas vaginalis, 204, 204f
Trichomoniasis, 371, 372b, 372f
Trichophyton, 47
Trichosporon infection, 189
Trichuris trichiura (whipworm), 206–207, 206f
Triclabendazole, 216, 217
Trimethoprim-sulfamethoxazole (TMP-SMX), 20, 24, 27t, 91, 95, 141, 192, 286, 367, 418, 420, 448, 450, 456
Tropheryma whipplei, 89
Trypanosoma cruzi, 456
TST. *See* Tuberculin skin test
Tuberculin skin test (TST), 43–44, 423
  booster phenomenon of, 128
  false-negative results of, 129
  interpretation of, 43b, 128–29
Tuberculoma, 127, 128
Tuberculosis (TB), 126
  antitubercular drugs for, 132t
  clinical manifestations of, 423
  diagnosis of, 127, 423
  drug-resistant, 133t
  endobronchial, 127
  epidemiology of, 422–23
  extrapulmonary, 127–28
  in HIV-infected patients, 128
  in HIV-negative patients, 130, 130t
  in HIV-positive patients, 130–31
  immunodiagnostics for, 43–44
  laboratory diagnosis of, 41–44
  lower lung field, 127
  miliary, 127
  pericarditis, 128
  reactivation of, 126–27
  in special situations, 131, 133
  spinal arachnoiditis, 128
  susceptibility testing for, 44
  tests for latent infection of, 128–29
    nucleic acid amplification assay, 129
    TST, 128–29
    whole blood interferon-γ assay, 129
  treatment of, 423–24
Tuberculous meningitis, 127–28, 329
Tuberculous parotitis, 252
Tuberculous pericarditis, 128
Tularemia. *See Francisella tularensis*
Typhlitis, 293
Typhoid vaccine, 507

Unasyn. *See* Ampicillin sodium-sulbactam sodium
United Nations World Tourism Organization (UNWTO), 495
UNWTO. *See* United Nations World Tourism Organization
Ureidopenicillin, 26t
Urethritis, 367
Urinary tract candidiasis, 150t
Urinary tract infection (UTI)
  asymptomatic bacteriuria and, 271, 464–65, 466t
  in children, 487
  diagnosis of, 269–70
  epidemiology of, 268–69, 464
  hosts and, 268–69
  imaging of, 272–73
  management of, 270–73, 466t
  in men, 271
  natural history of, 269
  nosocomial, 458–59
  pathogenesis of, 267–68
  prevention of, 273
  relapsing of, 271
UTI. *See* Urinary tract infection

Vaccines
  antibody-containing product and, 519
  bivalent, 520
  for botulism, 109
  in childhood, 485–86
  cholera, 509
  commonly available, 517b
  for diphtheria, 523
  hepatitis A, 296, 506, 519
  hepatitis B, 506–507, 519–20
  HPV, 505–506, 520
  influenza, 260, 504, 520–21
  for international travel
    recommended, 501–502t, 506–509
    required, 503t, 509–11
    routine, 498, 499–500t, 504–506
  Japanese encephalitis, 335, 507–508
  meningococcal, 509–10, 521–22
  for men who have sex with men, 374
  MMR, 504, 521
  multidose series and, 516–17
  multiple administration of, 519
  pneumococcal, 260, 504–505, 522–23
  in pregnancy, 516b
  quadrivalent, 520
  rabies, 508–509
  recommended schedules, 517f, 518f
  safety of, 516
  shingles, 505
  Tdap, 504, 523
  for tetanus, 104, 504, 523
  tick-borne encephalitis virus, 509
  timing and spacing of, 516
  transplant recipient infections and, 457
  typhoid, 507
  varicella, 505, 523–24
  VZV, 65, 453
  yellow fever, 510–11
  zoster, 524
Vaccine Adverse Event Reporting System (VAERS), 505
VAERS. *See* Vaccine Adverse Event Reporting System

Vaginal discharge syndromes, 370–71, 371t
Vaginal trichomoniasis, 204
Vaginosis, bacterial, 370, 371f, 372b, 466, 466t
Valacyclovir, 4, 21, 29t, 63, 65, 69, 453
Valganciclovir, 4, 22, 28t, 452
Vancomycin, 13, 18, 27t, 81, 87f, 263, 286, 340, 450, 530
  for IE, 304t, 305t, 306t, 307t, 308t, 309t, 310t, 311t, 314t
  for hematology patients, 435–38
Vancomycin-intermediate *Staphylococcus aureus* (VISA), 30t
Vancomycin-resistant enterococci (VRE), 30t
Vancomycin-resistant *Staphylococcus aureus* (VRSA), 30t
Vantin. *See* Cefpodoxime proxetil
VAP. *See* Ventilator-associated pneumonia
Varicella (chickenpox), 63–66, 489
  vaccination for, 65, 505, 523–24
Varicella zoster immune globulin (VZIG), 64
Varicella-zoster virus (VZV), 425–53, 471t, 477
  vaccine for, 65, 453
  varicella and, 63–66
  zoster and, 66–70
Variola virus (smallpox), 528–29t, 531–32, 535
VariZIG, 66
Venezuelan equine encephalomyelitis virus, 324, 334
Ventilator-associated pneumonia (VAP), 260–61, 462
Vertebral osteomyelitis, 352
Vibrio cholerae, 91, 101
Vibrio parahaemolyticus, 91
Vibrio vulnificus, 91, 101
Viral hemorrhagic fever agents, 528–29t, 534, 535
Viral hepatitis, 295–300
Viral infections, 450–54, 464
Viral parotitis, 252
Viral pneumonia, 257
Viridans streptococci, 85, 304–305t, 305t, 437
VISA. *See* Vancomycin-intermediate *Staphylococcus aureus*
Visceral leishmaniasis, 202–204
Viscerotropic leishmaniasis, 204
Voriconazole, 6, 7, 23, 28t, 156, 181, 182, 184, 185, 189
VRE. *See* Vancomycin-resistant enterococci
VRSA. *See* Vancomycin-resistant *Staphylococcus aureus*
Vulvovaginal candidiasis, 370, 371f
VZIG. *See* Varicella zoster immune globulin
VZV. *See* Varicella-zoster virus

Waldvogel classification, 351
Warfarin, 24
Western equine encephalomyelitis virus, 324, 334
West Nile virus, 325, 334–35
Whipworm. *See Trichuris trichiura*
White piedra, 46

X-linked lymphoproliferative disease (Duncan syndrome), 72

Yeasts, 51–52
Yellow fever vaccine, 510–11
Yersinia enterocolitica, 94
Yersinia pestis (plague), 94, 101, 528–29t, 532, 535
Yersinia pseudotuberculosis, 94
Yersiniosis, 94–95

Zalcitabine, 413
Zanamivir, 22, 28t
Zidovudine, 400, 401t, 402, 410, 413, 414, 479t
Zinacef. *See* Cefuroxime
Zoster, 66–70
    Ramsay Hunt syndrome, 68

    vaccine for, 524
Zosyn. *See* Piperacillin sodium-tazobactam sodium
Zygomycosis, 51, 51f, 182–84, 183b, 183f, 184f